MODERN BLOOD BANKING AND TRANSFUSION PRACTICES

MODERN BLOOD BANKING AND TRANSFUSION PRACTICES

Editor-in-Chief   D. HARMENING PITTIGLIO, Ph.D., M.S. MT(ASCP)

Director of Educational Services
American Association of Blood Banks
Arlington, VA
Assistant Director/Assistant Professor
University of Maryland School of Medicine
Program in Medical Technology
Baltimore, MD

Guiding Editor   ANNA JURTSCHENKO BALDWIN, B.S., MT(ASCP)SBB

Formerly Clinical Education Coordinator
University of Maryland School of Medicine
Program in Medical Technology
Baltimore, MD

Guiding Editor   PAUL R. SOHMER, M.D.

Associate Director of Laboratories
Department of Pathology
St. Thomas Hospital
Nashville, TN

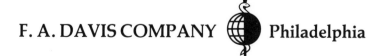

F. A. DAVIS COMPANY   Philadelphia

Library of Congress Cataloging in Publication Data

Main entry under title:

Modern blood banking and transfusion practices.

Includes bibliographies and index.
1. Blood—Transfusion.   2. Blood banks.   I. Pittiglio, D. Harmening (Denise Harmening) [DNLM: 1. Blood banks.   2. Blood transfusion.   3. Blood group-ing and crossmatching.   WH 460 M688]
RM171.M58   1983   615'.39   82-17989
ISBN 0-8036-6948-8

To all students, full-time, part-time, past, present, and future, who have touched and will continue to touch the lives of so many educators . . .

It is to you this book is dedicated in the hope of inspiring an unquenchable thirst for knowledge and love of mankind.

FOREWORD

Blood transfusion science is one of the newest branches of medical laboratory science. Blood groups were only discovered approximately 80 years ago and most of them have only been recognized in the last 30 years. Although transfusion therapy was used soon after the ABO blood groups were discovered, it was not until after World War II that blood transfusion science really started to become an important branch of medical science in its own right. Thus, compared with many branches of medicine, or even pathology, blood transfusion science is an infant, growing fast, changing continually, and presenting a great potential for research and future development.

To be able to grow, our young infant needs to be nurtured with a steady flow of new knowledge generated from research. This knowledge then has to be applied at the bench. To understand and best take advantage of the continual flow of new information being generated by blood transfusion scientists, and to apply it to everyday work in the blood bank, technologists (and pathologists) need to have a good understanding of basic immunology, genetics, biochemistry (particularly membrane chemistry), and the physiology and function of blood cells. To apply new concepts they need technical expertise and enough flexibility to reject old dogma when necessary and accept new ideas when they are supported by sufficient scientific data.

High standards are always expected and strived for by technologists who are working in blood banks or transfusion service. I very much believe that technologists should understand the principles behind the tests they are performing, rather than performing tasks like a machine does. Because of this, I do not think that "cook book" technical manuals have much value in *teaching* technologists; they do have a place as reference books in the laboratory. Over the years (too many to put in print) that I have been involved in teaching medical technologists, it has been very difficult to select *one* book to cover all that technologists in training need to know about blood transfusion science, without confusing them. Classic texts used regularly in teaching SBB students and pathology residents often contain too much information for the average medical technologist, especially those in training. They contain certain sections that can, and perhaps should, be read, but sometimes even these sections may serve to confuse learners rather than help and stimulate them. Some of them are written to be encyclopedic reference tomes, and others contain a great deal of clinical material or esoterica that are unnecessary for medical technologists who are not yet greatly experienced in blood transfusion practice.

Dr. Harmening Pittiglio has produced a single volume that covers everything a student of medical technology needs to know about blood transfusion science. She has been involved in teaching medical technologists for most of her career, and after seeing how she has arranged this book, I would guess that her teaching philosophies are close to those of my own. She has gathered together a group of experienced scientists and teachers who together with her cover all the important areas of blood transfusion science.

The chapters on the basic principles of cell preservation, genetics, and immunology provide a firm base for the learner to understand the practical and technical importance of the other chapters. The chapters on the blood groups and transfusion practice provide enough information for medical technologists, without overwhelming them with esoterica and clinical details.

Although this book was primarily designed for medical technologists, I believe it is admirably suited to pathology residents, hematology fellows, and others who want to review any aspect of modern blood transfusion science.

George Garratty, F.I.M.L.S., M.R.C. Path.

Scientific Director
American Red Cross Blood Services
Los Angeles, California

PREFACE

This book is designed to provide the medical technologist or blood bank specialist with a concise and thorough guide to transfusion practices and immunohematology. A problem-oriented approach to the subject matter has been incorporated to provide the practitioner with a working knowledge of modern, routine blood banking.

An introduction to the historical aspects of blood transfusion and preservation is presented as a prelude to current procedures utilized in donor phlebotomy, component preparation, and blood storage and preservation. In addition, new approaches to the above are discussed as an introduction to current research. Federal regulations have also been included in an attempt to clarify the issues of required quality control procedures for the routine blood bank laboratory.

Basic physiology as affected by blood loss will be examined as well as the pathophysiology of the red cells utilized in transfusion, both routine and massive. Consideration will be given to red cell metabolism, hemoglobin structure and function, and assessment of the need for transfusion therapy in a variety of clinical situations (e.g., trauma, chronic anemia, hemorrhagic disorders, and leukemia). A discussion of the adverse effects of blood transfusion will be incorporated in light of previously evaluated clinical disorders.

A thorough and current overview of blood group serology will be presented in the text in terms of basic immunology, inheritance and synthesis of blood group systems, and serologic activity of the associated antibodies. Certain clinical situations that are particularly relevant to blood banking will be discussed in detail, including hemolytic transfusion reactions, hemolytic diseases of the newborn, and autoimmune hemolytic anemia. In addition, a detailed discussion of compatibility testing and autoantibodies will be emphasized as it pertains to the clinical situations already described. Both federal and AABB regulations will be cited throughout the text as well as references at the conclusion of each chapter for further consideration. Finally, this text will also include chapters on human leukocyte antigens (HLA) and paternity testing, two areas that are often neglected in other texts.

This book is intended to bring about improved patient care by providing the reader with a basic understanding of the function of blood, the involvement of blood group antigens and antibodies, the principles of transfusion therapy, and the physiologic mechanisms of blood loss and replacement. It has been designed to generate an "unquenchable thirst for knowledge" in all medical technologists, blood bankers, and practitioners whose education, knowledge, and skills provide the public with excellent health care.

D. Harmening Pittiglio, Ph.D., M.S., MT(ASCP)

CONTRIBUTORS

ANNA JURTSCHENKO BALDWIN, B.S., MT(ASCP)SBB
Department of Pathology
Blood Bank
Greater Baltimore Medical Center
Baltimore, MD

MARGARET A. BROOKS
Supervisor
Baltimore Rh Typing Laboratory
Baltimore, MD

SANDRA ALM BUCK B.S., MT(ASCP)SBB
Johns Hopkins Hospital
Baltimore, MD

JOHN CASE, F.I.M.L.S.
Director of Regulatory Affairs
Gamma Biologicals, Inc.
Houston, TX

HELENA M. GLIDDEN, B.S., MT(ASCP)SBB
Arlington, VA

L. RUTH GUY, Ph.D.
Emeritus Professor
Department of Pathology
Southwestern Medical School
University of Texas Health Science Center
Dallas, TX

P. ANN HOPPE, B.A., MT(ASCP)SBB
Assistant to Director
Division of Blood and Blood Products
Office of Biologics
National Center for Drugs and Biologics
Bethesda, MD

ELLIOTT KAGAN, M.D.
Associate Professor of Pathology
Schools of Medicine and Dentistry
Georgetown University Medical Center
Washington, DC

BARBARA G. MCKEEVER, M.S., MT(ASCP)SBB
Deputy Associate Director
Service to Regional Centers
American Red Cross Blood Services
National Headquarters
Washington, DC

WILLIAM V. MILLER, M.D.
Chief Executive Officer
American Red Cross Blood Services
Missouri-Illinois Region
St. Louis, MO

DENISE HARMENING PITTIGLIO, Ph.D., M.S. MT(ASCP)
Director of Educational Services
American Association of Blood Banks
Arlington, VA
Assistant Director/Assistant Professor
University of Maryland
School of Medicine
Program in Medical Technology
Baltimore, MD

HERBERT F. POLESKY, M.D.
Director
The Minneapolis War Memorial Blood Bank
Minneapolis, MN

BRIAN E. RITCHEY, R.N.
Pheresis Specialist
City of Hope National Medical Center
Duarte, CA

PAUL R. SOHMER, M.D.
Associate Director of Laboratories
Department of Pathology
St. Thomas Hospital
Nashville, TN

EDWIN A. STEANE, Ph.D.
Associate Professor of Clinical Pathology
Southwestern Medical School
University of Texas Health Science Center
Dallas, TX

SUSAN M. STEANE, M.S., MT(ASCP)SBB
Clinical Coordinator
Blood Bank Technology Program
Department of Medical Technology
University of Texas Health Science Center
Dallas, TX

MARY ANN TOURAULT, M.A., MT(ASCP)SBB
Consumer Safety Officer
Division of Compliance
Office of Biologics
National Center for Drugs and Biologics
Bethesda, MD

FRANCES K. WIDMANN, M.D.
Associate Professor of Pathology
Duke University School of Medicine
Durham, NC
Assistant Chief, Laboratory Service
Veterans Administration Medical Center
Durham, NC

PATRICIA A. WRIGHT, MT(ASCP)SBB
Technical Education Coordinator
American Red Cross Blood Services
Chesapeake Region
Baltimore, MD

CONTENTS

CHAPTER 1

BLOOD PRESERVATION: HISTORICAL PERSPECTIVES AND CURRENT TRENDS

DENISE HARMENING PITTIGLIO, PH.D., MT(ASCP)

HISTORICAL ASPECTS

Man has always been fascinated by blood. Ancient Egyptians bathed in it. Aristocrats drank it. Authors and playwrights used it as themes. And modern man transfuses it. The road to an efficient, safe, and uncomplicated transfusion technique has been at best rough. But great progress is being made.

In 1492 blood was taken from three young men and was given to the stricken Pope Innocent VII in the hope of curing him. All four died. For the first time, a blood transfusion was duly recorded in history. The path to the successful transfusions so familiar today is marred by many reported failures. But man's physical, spiritual, and emotional fascination with blood is primordial. Why did success elude experimenters for so long?

Clotting was the principal obstacle. Attempts to find a nontoxic anticoagulant began in 1869 when Braxton Hicks recommended sodium phosphate. This was perhaps the first example of blood preservation research. Karl Landsteiner went further. He discovered the ABO blood groups and explained the serious reactions that occur in humans as a result of incompatible transfusions.

Next came appropriate devices designed for performing the transfusions. Lindemann was the first to succeed. He carried out vein-to-vein transfusion of blood by using multiple syringes and a special cannula for puncturing the vein through the skin. But this time-consuming, complicated procedure required many skilled assistants. It was not until Unger designed his syringe-valve apparatus that transfusions from donor to patient by an unassisted physician became practical.

An unprecedented accomplishment in blood transfusion was achieved in 1914 when Hustin reported the use of sodium citrate and glucose as a diluent and anticoagulant solution for transfusions. Later, in 1915 Lewisohn determined the minimum amount of citrate needed for anticoagulation and demonstrated its nontoxicity in small amounts. Transfusions became more practical and safer for the patient.

The development of preservative solutions to enhance the metabolism of the red cell followed. Glucose was tried as early as 1914, but its function in red cell metabolism was not understood until the 1930s. Therefore, the common practice of using glucose in the preservative solution was delayed.

World War II stimulated blood preservation research because the demand for blood and plasma increased. Efforts in several countries resulted in the landmark publication of the July 1947 issue of the *Journal of Clinical Investigation*, which devoted nearly a dozen papers to blood preservation. Hospitals responded immediately, and in 1947 blood banks were established in many major cities of the United States. Transfusion became commonplace. The daily occurrence of transfusions led to the discovery of numerous blood group systems. And antibody identification surged to the forefront as sophisticated techniques were developed. The interested student can review historical events during World War II in Kendrick's *Blood Program in World War II, Historical Note.*[1]

Frequent transfusions and the massive use of blood soon resulted in new problems, such as circulatory overload. Component therapy has solved these. Before, a single unit of whole blood could serve only one patient. With component therapy, however, one unit may be used for multiple transfusions. Today, the physician can select the specific component for his patient's particular needs without risking the inherent hazards of whole blood transfusions. He can transfuse only the required fraction in concentrated form, without overloading the circulation. Appropriate blood component therapy now provides more effective treatment and more complete use of blood products. Extensive use of blood during this period, coupled with component separation, led to increased comprehension of erythrocyte metabolism and a new awareness of the problems associated with red cell storage.

RED BLOOD CELL METABOLISM

The goal of blood preservation is to provide viable and functional blood components for patients needing blood transfusion. Research in this area has focused on maintaining red cell viability during storage and lengthening red cell post-transfusion survival. These are paramount considerations in blood preservation research.

Viability is a measure of in vivo red cell survival following transfusion. Seventy percent survival of transfused red cells after 24 hours is the lower limit for a successful transfusion. This arbitrary figure was first introduced by Rous and associates[2] in 1947. As storage time increases, red cell viability decreases. As a result, blood has always been assigned a limited, predetermined storage or shelf-life.

The loss of red cell viability has been correlated with the "lesion of storage," which is associated with various biochemical changes. These changes include a decrease in pH, a buildup of lactic acid, a decrease in glucose consumption, a decrease in ATP (adenosine triphosphate) levels, and a loss of red cell function, expressed as a shift to the left of the hemoglobin-oxygen dissociation curve or an increase in hemoglobin-oxygen affinity.

Viability is usually associated with both red cell ATP levels and membrane integrity. If viability can be maintained, the storage time of blood can be increased and the 70-percent post-transfusion survival of red cells ensured. Survival time of transfused red cells has been shown to correlate with ATP levels.[3] When ATP levels fall below approximately 1.5 μmole per g hemoglobin, viability is markedly impaired. In fact, Dern and coworkers[3] have established 1.5 μmoles per g hemoglobin as the minimum acceptable ATP level for 70-percent post-transfusion survival of red cells stored in acid-citrate-dextrose (ACD) and citrate-phosphate-dextrose (CPD) preservatives (Fig. 1-1). Therefore, any preservative that does not maintain ATP levels above approximately 1.5 μmole per g hemoglobin is unlikely to maintain adequate viability of stored red cells. Adequate ATP levels are necessary for maintenance of (1) red cell membrane integrity and deformability; (2) red cell volume, by sustaining the Na^+/K^+ ATPase pumps; (3) hemoglobin function; (4) adequate amounts of red cell reduced pyridine nucleotides; and (5) red cell plasma-lipid exchange.

Red cells generate energy almost exclusively through the breakdown of glucose, since the metabolism of the anucleated erythrocyte is more limited than that of other body cells. The adult red cell possesses little ability to metabolize fatty acids and amino acids. Additionally, mature erythrocytes contain no mitochondrial apparatus for oxidative metabolism. The red cell's metabolic pathways are mainly anaerobic, as one expects, since the function of the red cell is to deliver oxygen, not to consume it. Red cell cellular energetics may be divided into the *anaerobic glycolytic pathway* and three ancillary pathways that serve to maintain the function

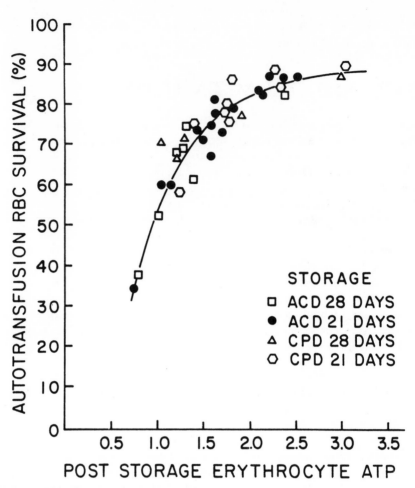

FIGURE 1-1. ATP levels and post-transfusion RBC survival.

of hemoglobin[4] (Fig. 1-2). All of these processes are essential if the erythrocyte is to transport oxygen and maintain those physical characteristics required for its survival in circulation.

Ninety percent of the ATP needed by red blood cells is generated in glycolysis, the erythrocyte's main metabolic pathway. Approximately 10 percent of the red cell's ATP is provided by the *pentose phosphate pathway*, which couples oxidative metabolism with pyridine nucleotide and glutathione reduction. The activity of this pathway increases following increased oxidation of glutathione or retardation of the glycolytic pathway.[5]

When the pentose phosphate pathway is functionally deficient, the amount of reduced glutathione becomes insufficient to neutralize intracellular oxidants. This results in globin denaturation and precipitation as aggregates (Heinz bodies) within the cell.[4] If this process results in sufficient membrane damage, cell destruction occurs.

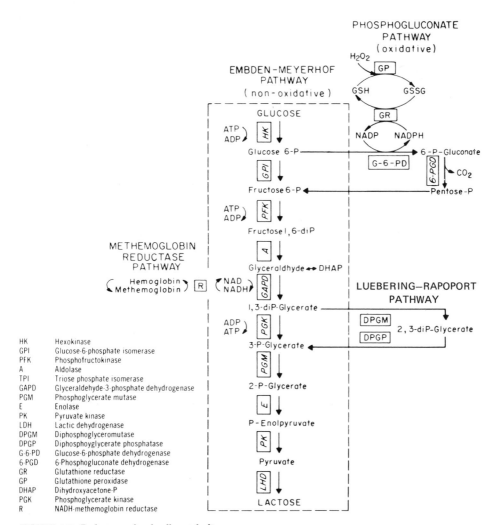

FIGURE 1-2. Pathways of red cell metabolism.

Such oxidative destruction of the red cells usually occurs as a result of an increased oxidant load with a latent decrease in pathway capacity. It is clear, therefore, that some activity in this pathway is essential for normal red cell survival.

The *methemoglobin reductase pathway* is another important component of red cell metabolism. Two methemoglobin reductase systems are important in maintaining hemoglobin in a reduced functional state. Both pathways are dependent on the regeneration of reduced pyridine nucleotides and are referred to as NADH methemoglobin reductase and NADPH methemoglobin reductase. Of the two pathways, there is a physiologic preference for the NADH methemoglobin reductase activity. This pathway is necessary to maintain the heme iron of hemoglobin in the ferrous (Fe^{++}) functional state.

In the absence of the enzyme methemoglobin reductase and the reducing action of the pyridine nucleotide (NAD), methemoglobin, which results from the conversion of the ferrous iron of heme to the ferric form, accumulates. Methemoglobin represents a nonfunctional form of hemoglobin and a loss of oxygen transport capabilities, since the metheme portion cannot combine with oxygen. Normal efficiency of the methemoglobin reductase pathway is exemplified by the fact that usually no greater than 1 percent of methemoglobin exists in the erythrocytes of normal, healthy individuals. A defect in the methemoglobin reductase pathway is, therefore, significant to red cell post-transfusion survival and function.

Another pathway that is crucial to red cell function is the *Luebering-Rapoport shunt*.[4] This pathway permits the accumulation of another important red cell organic phosphate, 2,3-diphosphoglycerate (2,3-DPG). A large amount of this compound is found in the red cell in a one-to-one molar relationship with hemoglobin, representing approximately 5 mM.[4] The apparent reason for this extraordinary amount of 2,3-DPG lies in its profound effect on the affinity of hemoglobin for oxygen.[6]

HEMOGLOBIN STRUCTURE AND FUNCTION

Hemoglobin makes up approximately 95 percent of the dry weight of a red cell or approximately 33 percent of its weight by volume.[4] Owing to its multichain structure, hemoglobin, which has a molecular weight of 68,000, is capable of considerable allosteric change as it loads and unloads oxygen. When the individual heme groups unload oxygen, the beta chains are pulled apart, permitting the entrance of 2,3-DPG and the establishment of salt bridges between the individual chains. This is known as the tense (T) form of the hemoglobin molecule and results in a progressively lower affinity of the hemoglobin molecule for oxygen.[7,8]

Recent work indicates that 2,3-DPG actually exerts an effect on intracellular pH, which may be of extreme importance in oxygen delivery. With oxygen uptake, salt bridges are broken, and the beta chains are pulled together, expelling DPG and causing the affinity of the hemoglobin molecule for oxygen to increase. This is known as the relaxed (R) form of the hemoglobin molecule.[7]

These allosteric changes that occur as the hemoglobin loads and unloads oxygen are known as the "respiratory movement."[4] This respiratory movement between the relaxed and tense state of the hemoglobin molecule can be illustrated by the hemoglobin-oxygen dissociation curve (Fig. 1-3).

Hemoglobin affinity for oxygen is also expressed by P_{50} values. This designates the partial pressure of oxygen at which hemoglobin is 50 percent saturated with oxygen under standard in vitro conditions of temperature and pH.[4] The P_{50} of normal blood is from 26 to 30 mm Hg.[4] A decrease in hemoglobin affinity for oxygen results in a "shift to the right" of the hemoglobin-oxygen dissociation curve and an increase in P_{50} (Fig. 1-4).[6] An increase in hemoglobin affinity for oxygen results in a "shift to the left" of the hemoglobin-oxygen dissociation curve and a decrease in P_{50} (Fig. 1-5).[6]

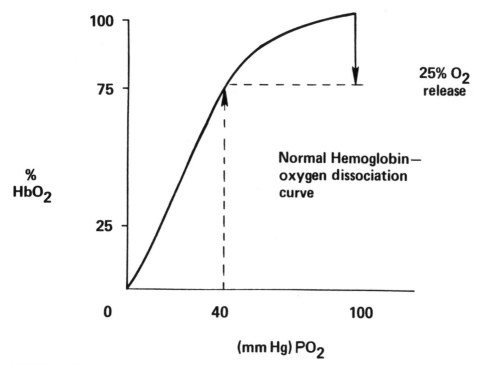

FIGURE 1-3. Hemoglobin-oxygen dissociation curve.

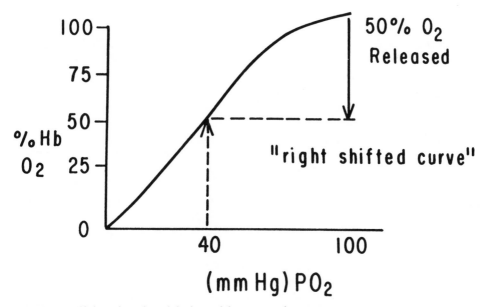

FIGURE 1-4. "Shift to the right" of the hemoglobin-oxygen dissociation curve.

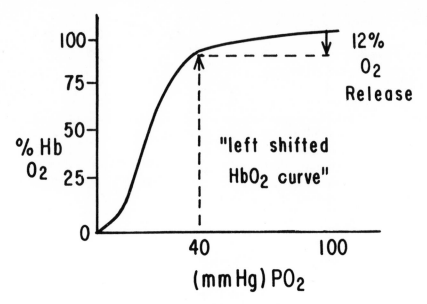

FIGURE 1-5. "Shift to the left" of the hemoglobin-oxygen dissociation curve.

The normal position of the oxygen dissociation curve depends on three different ligands normally found within the red cell: H^+ ions, CO_2, and organic phosphates.[4] Of these three, 2,3-DPG plays the most important role physiologically. The dependence of normal hemoglobin function on 2,3-DPG levels in the red cell has been well documented.[9,10]

In 1954 Valtis and Kennedy[11] found that hemoglobin oxygen affinity increases during blood storage. The relationship of oxygen affinity to 2,3-DPG remained unclear until the work of Chanutin and Curnish[10] and Benesch and Benesch.[9] These investigators defined a linear inverse relationship between 2,3-DPG concentrations and hemoglobin oxygen affinity.[10] As 2,3-DPG levels decrease, hemoglobin oxygen affinity increases. Akerblom[12] and Bunn[13] confirmed these findings as they demonstrated that the increase in oxygen hemoglobin affinity correlates well with a decrease in 2,3-DPG concentrations during storage. A change of 0.43 μmol per ml RBC of 2,3-DPG produces a change of 1 mm Hg in the P_{50}.[14] High concentrations of 2,3-DPG stabilize the hemoglobin molecule in the deoxygenated form, thereby decreasing hemoglobin affinity for oxygen and shifting the O_2 curve to the right.[15]

Since low 2,3-DPG levels profoundly influence the oxygen dissociation curve of hemoglobin, DPG-depleted cells may have an impaired capacity to deliver oxygen to the tissues. The rate of restoration of 2,3-DPG is influenced by the acid-base status of the recipient, phosphorus metabolism, and the degree of anemia.[6]

Blood storage, however, is associated with low 2,3-DPG levels and a shift to the left of the hemoglobin-oxygen dissociation curve.[16,17] A loss of red cell function, oxygen delivery to tissues, is also associated with this.[16,17] Therefore, an effective blood preservative must be capable of maintaining both viability reflected in ATP levels and hemoglobin function reflected in 2,3-DPG levels.

MODERN BLOOD BANKING AND TRANSFUSION PRACTICES

APPROVED PRESERVATIVE SOLUTIONS

In acid-citrate-dextrose (ACD) preservative, most of the 2,3-DPG is lost early in the first week of storage. Therefore, a substitute preservative, citrate-phosphate-dextrose (CPD), came into widespread use in the United States because it was superior for preserving this organic phosphate. This effect is presumably due to a higher pH (Table 1-1). Even in CPD, red cells become low in 2,3-DPG by the second week. Subsequent studies led to the addition of various chemicals along with the currently approved anticoagulant CPD in pursuit of a means to stimulate glycolysis.[18-20]

One of the chemicals, adenine, was approved for addition to CPD by the Food and Drug Administration in August 1978. The incorporation of adenine (CPDA-1) into blood storage seems to increase ADP levels, thereby driving glycolysis toward the synthesis of ATP. CPDA-1 contains 0.25 mM of adenine plus 25 percent more glucose than is required in CPD. Adenine-supplemented blood can be stored on the shelf for 35 days. The majority of blood now collected in the United States is drawn into CPDA-1 preservative solution. CPDA-2, containing 0.5 mM of adenine plus 75 percent more glucose than CPD or 1.4 times more glucose than CPDA-1, is currently under investigation for future use and is now before the FDA for approval. However, blood stored in CPDA-1 also becomes depleted of 2,3-DPG by the second week of storage.

The reported pathophysiologic effects of the transfusion of red blood cells with low 2,3-DPG levels and increased affinity for oxygen include either an increase in cardiac output or a decrease in mixed venous PO_2 tension or a combination of these. The physiologic importance of these effects is *not* easily demonstrated. This is a complex mechanism and there are numerous variables involved that are beyond the scope of this text.

TABLE 1-1. Comparison of the composition of acid-citrate-dextrose (ACD) and citrate-phosphate-dextrose (CPD) preservatives

	ACD	CPD	CPDA-1	CPDA-2
Tri-sodium citrate	22.0 g	26.30 g	26.30 g	26.30 g
Citric acid	8.0 g	3.27 g	3.27 g	3.27 g
Dextrose	24.5 g	25.50 g	31.90 g	34.70 g
Monobasic sodium phosphate	–	2.22 g	2.22 g	2.22 g
Adenine	–	–	0.27 g	0.54 g
Water	1000 ml	1000 ml	1000 ml	1000 ml
Volume/100 ml blood	15 ml	14 ml	14 ml	14 ml
Approximate volume of preservative solution/bag	67.5 ml	63.0 ml	63.0 ml	63.0 ml
Initial pH of solution*	5.0	5.6	5.6	5.6
pH of blood on initial day drawn into storage bag*	7.0	7.2	7.4	7.3
pH of blood at day 28*	6.7	6.8	6.8	6.8
pH of blood at day 35*	–	–	6.8	6.8

*Indicates measurement at room temperature.

Stored red cells do regain the ability to synthesize 2,3-DPG after transfusion, but levels necessary for optimal hemoglobin oxygen delivery are not reached immediately. It requires approximately 24 hours to restore normal levels of DPG after transfusion.[9,10,21,22] The 2,3-DPG concentrations after transfusion have been reported to reach normal levels as early as 6 hours.[23] Most of these studies have been performed on normal, healthy individuals. There is, however, evidence to suggest that in the transfused subject, whose capacity is limited by an underlying physiologic disturbance, even a brief period of altered oxygen hemoglobin affinity is of great significance.[24]

It is quite clear now that 2,3-DPG levels in transfused blood are important in certain clinical conditions. Recent animal studies demonstrate significantly increased mortality associated with transfusing blood that is low in 2,3-DPG levels in persistent anemia, hypotension, hypoxia, and cardiac and hemorrhagic shock. Human studies demonstrate that myocardial function improves following transfusion of blood with high 2,3-DPG levels during cardiovascular surgery.[25]

Several investigators suggest that the patient in shock who is transfused with 2,3-DPG-depleted erythrocytes may have already strained his compensatory mechanisms to their limits.[6] Perhaps for this type of patient the poor oxygen delivery capacity of 2,3-DPG-depleted cells makes a significant difference in recovery and survival.

It is apparent that factors other than ATP levels may limit the viability of transfused red cells. One of these factors is the plastic material utilized for the storage container. The plastic must be sufficiently permeable to carbon dioxide in order to maintain higher pH levels during storage. As a result, glass storage containers are a matter of history in the United States. Currently all blood is stored in polyvinyl chloride (PVC) plastic bags. Another problem, associated with PVC bags, is the plasticizer that is used in the manufacture of the bags. It has been found to leach into the blood itself. The effect of this leaching is being investigated. The accumulation of excessive amounts of acid from glucose utilization even at low storage temperatures is also a major problem in liquid preservation of red cells.[26] Research, therefore, has been focused on the development of an improved plastic blood bag as well as better preservative solutions.

PLATELET METABOLISM AND PRESERVATION

Not only are preservative solutions of profound importance in the maintenance of red cell function and viability, but they also have a direct influence on platelet function and viability. This is an important issue to examine because of the expanding use of component therapy for transfusion practices and because of the large number (2.2 million in 1979) of platelet concentrates (PC) transfused annually.[28] Existing controversies regarding platelet storage have resulted in attempts to interpret discrepancies regarding the effect of storage on the hemostatic function of transfused PCs. In the 1950s, platelet transfusions were given as freshly drawn whole blood or platelet-rich plasma. These platelets disappeared within 4 to 5 days after injection into the blood stream of patients with thrombocytopenia secondary to marrow failure.[28] An alternative method is to prepare PCs. A unit of blood is drawn into a plastic bag containing an anticoagulant and centrifuged at 22°C to prepare platelet-rich plasma (PRP). The PRP is centrifuged a second time and the excess plasma expelled to prepare PC.

Current regulations permit platelets to be stored for 3 to 5 days, depending upon the type of plastic bag used by the collection facility (for further information, refer to Chapter 10). Storage conditions, by necessity, do cause alterations in the metabolism and function of platelets. Initial pH, temperature of storage, total platelet count, volume of plasma, duration of storage, agitation during storage, and hydrogen ion accumulation are some of the controversial factors known to influence platelet metabolism and function.

A number of other inter-related variables can also affect platelet viability and function during storage, namely, the anticoagulant used for blood collection, the method used to prepare platelet concentrates, and the composition, surface area, and thickness of the walls of the storage container.

A major advance in the development of platelet storage occurred in 1969, when Murphy and Gardner[29] demonstrated with survival studies that the optimal storage temperature for platelets was 22°C rather than 4°C. Platelets stored at 4°C are associated with an irreversible disk-to-sphere transformation. When stored for several hours at 4°C, platelets do not return to their disk shape upon rewarming and are irreversibly sphered.[30] This loss of shape in platelets stored at 4°C is probably a result of microtubule disassembly, which may also be a major contributor to decreased survival of platelets stored at 4°C. The major objections to platelets stored at 4°C are their shortened life span after reinfusion,[31] and their marked decrease in survival after only 18 hours of storage.[32]

In light of these developments, PCs are now prepared and stored at 22°C. However, even storage at 22°C for platelets has several disadvantages. One major difficulty is the regulation of pH. Virtually all units of PC demonstrate a decrease in pH from their initial value of 7.0.[33] This decrease is primarily due to the production of lactic acid by platelet glycolysis and to a lesser extent to accumulation of CO_2 from oxidative phosphorylation.[34] As pH falls from 6.8 to 6.0, the platelets progressively change shape from disks to spheres. In this pH range, the changes of shape are reversible if the platelets are resuspended in plasma with physiologic pH. However, if the pH falls below 6.0, a further irreversible change occurs that renders the platelets nonviable after infusion in vivo.[34]

The present goal of platelet preservation is to prevent the deleterious changes associated with decreases in pH. Apparently, oxygen supply to the platelets within the plastic bag is also intimately related to pH maintenance. If the supply is sufficient, glucose will be metabolized oxidatively, resulting in CO_2 production, which diffuses out of the walls of the plastic PC container. If the supply of oxygen is insufficient, glucose will be metabolized anaerobically, resulting in the production of lactic acid, which must remain within the container and thus lowers the pH. The oxygen tension within the container is governed by several factors: the concentration of platelets, which consume oxygen; the permeability of the wall of the plastic PC bag; the surface area of the container available for gas exchange; and the type of agitation used, since this facilitates gas exchange. Federal regulations require that some form of gentle agitation be used.[35] This has also led to the controversial question regarding the type of agitator to be used. Both platform and elliptical rotators are currently in use. It appears that future recommendations will advocate the use of the platform rotator in light of the new plastics being used for platelet storage.

The only variable that the blood bank can modulate is the concentration of platelets. PCs with a platelet count greater than 1.6×10^6 per μl commonly show evidence of inadequate oxygenation and a decline in pH over a 72-hour period.[34,36,37] For this reason many blood banks now favor a PC plasma volume of 50 ml. Volumes are determined by maintenance of pH of not less than 6.0 by federal regulations. Although this may result in a large volume for clinical use, especially for pediatric patients, it does minimize platelet concentration. Studies by Murphy and Gardner[34] indicate that oxygenation can be maintained by using a container with increased oxygen permeability. In conclusion, all research is aimed at increasing the storage time of platelets while also maintaining platelet viability and function.

CURRENT TRENDS IN BLOOD PRESERVATION RESEARCH

Research in blood preservation has developed in five directions: (1) chemical incorporation, (2) rejuvenation studies, (3) red cell freezing, (4) blood substitutes, and (5) the use of solid buffers.

CHEMICAL INCORPORATION

Numerous chemical additives, after incorporation into stored blood, have been assessed for their ability to maintain the essential organic phosphates. Purine nucleosides were the first group to be investigated, with adenosine the first substance investigated. These investigations led to a more practical method for maintaining ATP levels: the addition of adenine to the preservative media.

Alternative sugars in addition to glucose, such as mannose and fructose, have also been investigated.[23] All three sugars share equal ability to sustain ATP levels during storage.

Dihydroxyacetone (DHA) is a chemical used to maintain the other important organic phosphate in the red cell, 2,3-DPG. DHA enters directly into the glycolytic pathway as a three-carbon sugar. Red cells are able to metabolize DHA at a rate approximately equal to that at which glucose is metabolized. DHA has also been shown experimentally to be essentially nontoxic. When added to the presently approved anticoagulants, DHA markedly enhances 2,3-DPG maintenance during red cell storage.[23]

Selected chemicals incorporated into the preservative medium can alter red cell metabolism, modifying the levels of various intermediates within the cell without directly being metabolized by the red cell. These modifiers include ascorbic acid, ascorbate-6-phosphate, and pyruvate.[23] Each of these chemicals, in combination with other additives, aids in maintaining 2,3-DPG levels. Modifiers alone in the preservative medium produce only slight improvement. When used, however, in combination with other chemicals to improve 2,3-DPG levels, these mixtures very rapidly deplete red cell ATP.

In 1974, Hogman and associates[20] proposed a new approach to red blood cell preservation using an artificial storage medium after removal of blood plasma. In the Hogman system (referred to as SAG) after collection of whole blood into CPD the accompanying plasma and platelets are removed and the remaining red blood cell concentrate is resuspended in approximately 75 to 100 ml of saline containing adenine and glucose. Resuspension and storage of red blood cells in the SAG system offer a number of advantages: (1) the lower viscosity of the red cell suspension yields flow properties superior to those of conventional red cell concentrates; (2) although the red blood cells are supplied with sufficient adenine and glucose, by removal of the majority of platelets from the red blood cell preparation, platelet exposure to adenine and added glucose is avoided; and (3) by removal of the majority of platelets and white blood cells from the red blood cell preparation, the formation of microaggregates is strongly diminished. Results obtained from a now extensive clinical experience in Sweden indicate that the SAG approach is effective. Increased hemolysis of red blood cells during storage in SAG has been eliminated by the addition of mannitol to the saline-adenine-glucose diluent. Clinical trials with this improved SAG formulation (ADSOL) were reported by Heaton and coworkers[38] to demonstrate excellent post-transfusion red cell viability for a minimum of 35 days without significant hemolysis in vitro. FDA approval of ADSOL is expected in the future.

Despite all the research generated to date, the search for the best chemical preservative that has the ability to simultaneously maintain red cell survival and function continues.

REJUVENATION STUDIES

Solutions containing phosphate, inosine, glucose, pyruvate, and adenine (PIGPA), incubated with outdated erythrocytes, can regenerate both ATP and DPG levels. Valeri and coworkers[6,15,21] have been the forerunners in these rejuvenation studies on outdated blood. Subsequent investigations have led to the removal of glucose from the original mixture, and the resulting solution is designated PIPA. This solution is anticipated to be federally approved in the near future. Generally, outdated blood can be rejuvenated by incubation for 1 hour at 37°C with these solutions. The red cells are washed before transfusion to remove the rejuvenation mixture and deleterious amounts of extracellular potassium. FRES, another rejuvenation solution, is presently approved and available on the market. The practicality and efficiency of these solutions in routine blood banking are debatable. The procedures are time-consuming and require extensive manipulation.

RED CELL FREEZING

Red blood cells stored by conventional methods have a shelf-life of 21 to 35 days, depending upon the preservative solution employed in the collection bag. This storage period is usually quite satisfactory for the routine storage of bank blood. There are, however, occasions when a much longer shelf-life is desirable and even necessary. Development of the technology for freezing red blood cells without subsequently hemolyzing them upon thawing has fulfilled this need and has also shown other advantages beyond long-term storage.

The procedure for freezing a unit of packed red cells is simple. Basically, it involves the addition of a cryoprotective agent to the red cells, which are less than 6 days old. Glycerol is used most commonly and is added to the red cells slowly with vigorous shaking, thereby enabling the glycerol to permeate the red cells. The cells are then rapidly frozen and stored in a freezer. The usual storage temperature is below $-65°C$, although storage (and freezing) temperature depends upon the concentration of glycerol used.

Transfusion of frozen cells *must* be preceded by a deglycerolization process, otherwise the thawed cells would hemolyze in vivo. Removal of glycerol is achieved by systematically replacing the cryoprotectant with decreasing concentrations of saline. The usual protocol involves washing with 12-percent saline, followed by 1.6-percent saline, with a final wash in normal saline. A cell washer system, such as those manufactured by IBM or Haemonetics, Inc., is utilized in the deglycerolizing process.

The final cell product, resuspended in the saline used for the last wash sequence, is used in transfusion. Excessive hemolysis is monitored by noting the hemoglobin concentration of the wash supernatant. Osmolality of the unit should also be monitored to ensure adequate deglycerolization. Because the unit of blood is entered to incorporate the glycerol (prior to freezing) or the saline solutions (for deglycerolization), the outdating period of thawed red cells is 24 hours.

Frozen red cells provide a method for long-term storage of blood. Currently, the FDA licenses frozen red cells for a period of 3 years from the date of freezing, that is, frozen red cells may be stored up to 3 years prior to thawing and transfusion. Once thawed, these cells demonstrate function and viability near that of fresh blood. Experience has shown that storage periods longer than 3 years do not adversely affect viability and function. Very rare blood types, such as Bombay or Tj(a−), have been transfused after greater than 3 years' storage. These products are no longer licensed blood products, but to the patient with a very rare blood type, they may be lifesaving. Hemolysis during the washing procedure must be closely examined prior to issuing these rare cells.

Experience has also shown that frozen-thawed red cells have several other advantages. The final red cell product has very low quantities of residual leukocytes and platelets, often 1 to 5 percent of the original quantity. The washing procedure also removes significant amounts of plasma proteins. In accordance with these observations, deglycerolized red cells are often the product of choice for patients with histories of severe febrile or allergic transfusion reactions. Finally, it was felt at one time that frozen-thawed red cells carried a reduced risk of transmitting post-transfusion hepatitis, owing to the freezing and washing processes. This conjecture has not been verified and evidence to the contrary has been presented. Consequently, there is no evidence at this time that this blood product carries less of a hepatitis risk than other red cell products.[39,40]

The major disadvantages of this system are twofold. Preparation of these red cells, both for freezing and thawing, is a time-consuming process. In addition, the cost of the equipment, materials, and the time of the technologist greatly inflates the cost of the product to the potential recipient. These disadvantages, however, should be weighed against the potential benefits to the patient.

BLOOD SUBSTITUTES

Another area of blood research deals with the development of "blood substitutes" such as stroma-free hemoglobin solution (SFHS) and the perfluorochemicals (PFCs). PFCs are currently being used clinically in Japan and are undergoing clinical trials in the United States. It is expected that SFHS will also undergo clinical trials in the near future. Consequently, it is only a matter of time before they come into use in the United States. A common feature of these products is their ability to carry oxygen.

SFHS has been considered for use as a medium to carry oxygen for many years. These solutions are prepared by hemolyzing outdated red blood cells and removing all of the contaminating stroma, which is quite toxic to the kidney. These solutions have several shortcomings. One is their short intravascular persistence. SFHS, although *not* toxic to the kidney, is very quickly eliminated in the urine. Messmer[41] found intravascular half-life of SFHS to be 100 minutes. Another factor that poses problems is the high oxygen affinity of native SFHS. Work has shown a shift to the left of the hemoglobin-oxygen dissociation curve and P_{50} values in the range of 12 to 17 mm Hg.[41,42]

Attempts to correct these deficiencies have been made. SFHS polymerized with dextran remained in the circulation a much longer time, but it had an even greater affinity for oxygen than the unmodified SFHS.[43] Attempts to decrease the oxygen affinity have met with better results. SFHS linked to pyridoxal-5'-phosphate (PLP) has an improved oxygen release capacity. Messmer[42] tested the SFH-PLP in animal studies and found no associated side effects. SFH-PLP has shown P_{50} values of 24 to 34 mm Hg, a significant improvement over the raw solution. The circulation half-life of SFH-PLP (2 to 6 hours) is also an improvement, but still limits its application as a blood-replacing fluid on a routine basis.

Intramolecular linkage with ATP shows some promise for improving both oxygen delivery and total retention time.[44] Perhaps future SFHS products having both phosphates and high molecular weight compounds attached to the hemoglobin molecule may prove to be the "ideal" product.

Finally, modern SFHS preparations have shown a long shelf-life and are very stable. They may be stored as liquids or in the lyophilized form for up to 18 months.

In addition, they do not appear to be antigenic, so that patient immunization is not likely to be a problem, as it is with blood products. This would also eliminate the blood bank testing procedures normally performed prior to blood transfusion.

Perfluorochemicals have experienced a tremendous amount of research and testing, as well as publicity. Also known as perfluorocarbons or PFCs, these are hydrocarbon structures in which all the hydrogen atoms have been replaced with fluorine. They carry oxygen and CO_2 by dissolving them. Most PFCs can dissolve as much as 60 percent oxygen by volume compared with whole blood, which can dissolve only about 20 percent.[45] These chemicals are injected as emulsions with albumin, fats, or other chemicals; otherwise, they may cause pulmonary embolism, asphyxia, and death.[46] Geyer[43] exchanged the blood of rats with PFCs to a hematocrit of 1 percent without any sign of complication. Reperfusion of the rats was also accomplished successfully.

Fluosol-DA, produced in Japan, is the most widely studied PFC thus far. This compound contains both perfluorodecalin and perfluorotripropylamine, as well as hydroxy ethyl starch (to maintain blood volume) and electrolytes (to maintain osmotic pressure). It has been used successfully in both Japan and the United States, while undergoing clinical trials. It is also used in the United States under very limited circumstances when the patient absolutely refuses blood transfusion, even in a life-threatening emergency.

One problem associated with PFCs is that some of these chemicals are retained in the tissues for very long periods of time. Accumulations of these chemicals have been shown in liver, spleen, and other organs. The long-term effects of these deposits need to be evaluated. PFCs are also excreted unmetabolized in the urine and from the lungs and skin.

Another problem that has been observed involves the atmosphere under which Fluosol transfusions are carried out. Fluosol has required a simultaneous administration of 100 percent O_2 both during and after the transfusion. However, recent modifications by Japanese researchers have eliminated the need for O_2 administration, and such transfusions are now carried out under normal atmospheric conditions.

Another problem with PFCs that needs to be solved is that of storage requirements. Fluosol-DA must be maintained under deep-freeze storage temperatures. This aspect also puts constraints on its applicability as a blood substitute, but certain compounds now under investigation have been freeze-dried successfully. Their capabilities as oxygen-carriers are unknown.

Research needs to focus on the production of a perfluorocarbon that is very stable, does not have a prolonged tissue retention time, does not require O_2 administration for effectiveness, and has practical storage requirements.

USE OF SOLID BUFFERS

Research of an entirely new concept in blood preservation—solid buffers—shows promise for better viability reflected in ATP levels, and for functional ability reflected in 2,3-DPG levels. Ion-exchange resins as a preservative system may solve the problem of maintaining levels of both organic phosphates in stored red cells. An investigation during a 28-day storage period showed that the resin system yields high 2,3-DPG levels without an incorporation of any chemicals other than CPD preservative.

Several types of ion-exchange resins were investigated, but Amberlite IR-45 anion-exchange resin seems to be most promising for future blood banking. These resin beads are approximately 400 microns large and completely filterable at the time of transfusion. The resins are biologically and chemically inert. They are easily sterilized because they possess great thermal stability. IR-45 resin is pretreated and charged with dibasic phosphate to replace the hydroxyl functional group present on the commercially available bead. This replacement allows mobile phosphate ions to be slowly released to the blood in the free monomeric form. The phosphate ion, a normal constituent of blood, buffers best throughout the pH range of stored blood. This phosphate resin system, therefore, is tantamount to inserting a strong buffer into the closed blood storage bag, preventing a marked change in pH. The introduction of sufficiently strong buffers into a closed system, preventing pH change of stored blood, has been a research goal for many years. Regulation of pH significantly extends the shelf-life of blood because deleterious amounts of lactic acid are made as the red cell metabolizes glucose. Ordinarily, hydrogen ion concentration, or pH, changes during storage. The pH has a great and complex influence on red cell metabolism and function. Thus, the answer to the blood preservation problems may lie in pH maintenance.

The resin system described slowly releases phosphate to the blood when needed. Its function is twofold: (1) as a buffer, it combines with H^+ to form H_2PO_4, thereby maintaining a narrower pH range; (2) as a source of inorganic phosphate, it maintains ATP levels and yields high 2,3-DPG levels by accelerating its synthesis due to increases in the substrates needed for its production.

The resin system is associated with the following advantages: (1) an increase in initial pH promotes greater glucose use, (2) inorganic phosphate is provided to maintain ATP and DPG simultaneously, (3) CO_2 can be bound by the resin molecule and a narrow pH range is maintained to enhance enzyme activity, (4) the resin is inert, filterable, and uses no additional chemicals other than CPD, and (5) bacteria are absorbed, apparently irreversibly.

These research areas described are all working toward the common goal of providing not only functional and viable red blood cells, but also providing a practical blood preservation system.

REFERENCES

1. KENDRICK, DB: *Blood Program in World War II, Historical Note.* Washington, D.C., 1964.
2. ROUS, P and TURNER, JR: *The preservation of living red blood corpuscles in vitro. II. The transfusion of kept cells.* J Exp Med 23:234, 1947.
3. DERN, RJ, BREWER, GJ and WIORKOWSKI, JJ: *Studies on the preservation of human blood. II. The relationship of erythrocyte adenosine triphosphate levels and other in vivo measures to red cell storageability.* J Lab Clin Med 69:968, 1967.
4. BREWER, GJ: *General red cell metabolism.* In Surgenor, D (ED): *The Red Blood Cell,* ed 2. Academic Press, New York, 1975.

5. RAPOPORT, S: *Control mechanisms of red cell glycolysis.* In Greenwalt, TJ and Jamieson, GA (EDS): *The Human Red Cell in Vitro.* Grune & Stratton, New York, 1974, p 153.

6. VALERI, CR: *Oxygen transport function of preserved red cells.* In Valeri, CR (ED): *Blood Banking and the Use of Frozen Blood Products.* CRC Press, Cleveland, 1976, Ch 7, p 141.

7. MONOD, J, WYMAN, J and CHANGEUX, JP: *On the nature of allosteric transitions. A plausible model.* J Mol Biol 12:88, 1965.

8. DUHM, J, DEUTIKLE, B and GERLACH, E: *Complete restoration of oxygen transport function and 2,3-diphosphoglycerate concentration in stored blood.* Transfusion 11:147, 1971.

9. BENESCH, R and BENESCH, RE: *The effect of organic phosphates from the human erythrocyte on the allosteric properties of hemoglobin.* Biochem Biophys Res Commun 26:162, 1967.

10. CHANUTIN, A and CURNISH, RR: *Effect of organic and inorganic phosphates on the oxygen equilibrium of human erythrocytes.* Arch Biochem Biophys 121:96, 1967.

11. VALTIS, DJ and KENNEDY, AC: *Defective gas-transport function of stored red blood cells.* Lancet 1:119, 1954.

12. AKERBLOM, O and KREUGER, R: *Studies on citrate-phosphate-dextrose (CPD) blood supplemented with adenine.* Vox Sang 29:90, 1975.

13. BUNN, HF, et al.: *Hemoglobin function in stored blood.* J Clin Invest 48:311, 1969.

14. OSKI, FA, et al.: *The effects of deoxygenation of adult and fetal hemoglobin on the synthesis of red cell 2,3-diphosphoglycerate and its in vivo consequences.* J Clin Invest 49:400, 1970.

15. VALERI, CR: *Simplification of the methods for adding and removing glycerol during freeze-preservation of human red blood cells with the high or low glycerol methods: Biochemical modification prior to freezing.* Transfusion 15:195, 1975.

16. VALERI, CR: *Oxygen transport function of preserved red cells.* Clin Haematol 3:649, 1974.

17. VALERI, CR: *Metabolic regeneration of depleted erythrocytes and their frozen storage.* In Greenwalt, TJ and Jamieson, GA (EDS): *The Human Red Cell in Vitro.* Grune & Stratton, New York, 1974, pp 281–321.

18. DAWSON, RB and KOCHOLATY, WF: *Hemoglobin function in stored blood. VI. The effect of phosphate on erythrocyte ATP and 2,3-DPG.* Am J Clin Pathol 56:656, 1971.

19. DAWSON, RB and KOCHOLATY, WF: *Hemoglobin function in stored blood. XII. Effects of varying phosphate concentrations on red cell ATP and 2,3-DPG with adenine and inosine.* Haematologia 7:295, 1973.

20. HOGMAN, CF, et al.: *Experience with new preservatives: Summary of the experiences in Sweden.* In Greenwalt, TJ and Jamieson, GA (EDS): *The Human Red Cell in Vitro.* Grune & Stratton, New York, 1974, p 217.

21. VALERI, CR and HIRSCH, NM: *Restoration in vivo of erythrocyte adenosine triphosphate, 2,3-diphosphoglycerate, potassium ion and sodium ion concentrations following the transfusion of acid-citrate-dextrose stored human red blood cells.* J Lab Clin Med 73:722, 1969.

22. BEUTLER E and WOOD, LA: *The in vivo regeneration of red cell-diphosphoglyceric acid (DPG) after transfusion of stored blood.* J Lab Clin Med 74:300, 1969.

23. BEUTLER, E: *Experimental blood preservatives for liquid storage.* In Greenwalt, TJ and Jamieson, GA (EDS): *The Human Red Cell in Vitro.* Grune & Stratton, New York, 1974, p 189.

24. VALERI, CR and COLLINS, FB: *Physiological effects of 2,3-DPG depleted red cells with high affinity for oxygen.* J Appl Physiol 31:823, 1971.

25. DENNIS, RC, et al.: *Improved myocardial performance following high 2,3-diphosphoglycerate red cell transfusions.* Surgery 77:741, 1975.

26. BEUTLER, E and WOOD, LA: *Preservation of red cell 2,3-DPG and viability in bicarbonate containing medium: The effect of blood bag permeability.* J Lab Clin Med 80:723, 1972.

27. American Blood Commission: *1979 Annual Report,* 1980.

28. STEFANINI, M and DAMESHAK, W: N Engl J Med 248:797, 1953.

29. MURPHY, S and GARDNER, F: *Platelet preservation effect of storage temperature on maintenance of platelet viability—deleterious effect of refrigerated storage.* N Engl J Med 280:1094, 1969.

30. KATTLOVE, HE and ALEXANDER, B: *The effect of cold on platelets. I. Cold-induced platelet aggregation.* Blood 38:39, 1971.

31. BECKER, GA, et al.: *Studies of platelet concentrates stored at 22°C and 4°C.* Transfusion 13:61, 1973.

32. Murphy, S: *Harvesting of platelets for transfusion and problems of storage.* In Greenwalt, TJ and Jamieson, GA (EDS): *Blood Platelets in Transfusion Therapy.* Alan R. Liss, New York, 1978, p 102.

33. Murphy, S, Sayar, SN and Gardner, FH: *Storage of platelet concentrates at 22°C.* Blood 35:15, 1970.

34. Murphy, S and Gardner, FH: *Platelet storage at 22°C: Role of gas transport across plastic containers in maintenance of viability.* Blood 46:209, 1975.

35. Federal Register (1975): *Federal Register 40.* January 29, 4300, Washington, DC.

36. Slichter, SJ and Harker, LA: *Preparation and storage of platelet concentrates. I. Factors influencing the harvest of viable platelets from whole blood.* Br J Haematol 34:395, 1976.

37. Slichter, SJ and Harker, LA: *Preparation and storage of platelet concentrates. II. Storage variables influencing platelet viability and function.* Br J Haematol 34:403, 1976.

38. Heaton, A, et al: *Improved storage of high hematocrit red cell concentrates using mannitol, adenine, saline, glucose solutions* (abstr). Transfusion 21:600, 1981.

39. Meryman, HT, et al.: *The effects of red cell freezing and deglycerolizing or of saline washing on post-transfusion hepatitis* (abstr). Transfusion 19:656, 1979.

40. Alter, HJ, et al.: *Transmission of hepatitis B virus infection by transfusion of frozen-deglycerolized red blood cells.* N Engl J Med 298:637, 1978.

41. Messmer, K, et al: *Oxygen supply by stroma free hemoglobin solution.* In Greenwalt, TJ and Jamieson, GA (EDS): *Blood Substitutes and Plasma Expanders.* Alan R. Liss, New York, 1978, pp 175–190.

42. Messmer, K and Jesch, F: *Oxygen affinity of stroma free hemoglobin solution and its effect on tissue oxygenation.* Bibl Anat 15:375, 1977.

43. Geyer, RP: *Substitutes for Blood—Experimental and Practical Considerations.* In *A Seminar of Blood Components: E Unum Pluribus.* 30th Annual Meeting of the American Association of Blood Banks, Atlanta, Georgia, November 1977, pp 75–88.

44. Greenburg, AG: *Hemoglobin solutions—new life for old blood.* Diagnostic Medicine 6:19, 1981.

45. Maugh, TH: *Blood substitute passes its first test.* Science 205: 205, 1979.

46. Rice, CL and Moss, GS: *Blood and blood substitutes: Current practice.* Adv Surg 13:93, 1979.

BIBLIOGRAPHY

American Association of Blood Banks: *Standards for Blood Banks and Transfusion Services,* ed 10. Washington, DC, 1980.

Antonini, E and Brunori, M: *Hemoglobin.* Ann Rev Biochem 39:977, 1970.

Arturson, G and Westman M: *Survival of rats subjected to acute anemia at different levels of erythrocyte 2,3-diphosphoglycerate.* Scand J Clin Lab Invest 35:745, 1975.

Bakker, JC, et al.: *The influence of the position of the oxygen dissociation curve on oxygen-dependent functions of the isolated perfused rat liver. I. Studies at different levels of hypoxic hypoxia.* Pfluegers Arch 362:21, 1976.

Baranowski, J: *Your hematocrit is zero, and you're doing fine.* Diagnostic Medicine 3:60, 1980.

Barrett, LA and Dawson, RB: *Avian erythrocyte development: Microtubules and the formation of the disk shape.* Dev Biol 36:72, 1974.

Bartlett, GR: *Effects of adenine on stored human red cells.* Adv Exp Med Biol 28:479, 1972.

Bartlett, GR and Barnet HN: *Changes in the phosphate compound of the human red blood cell during blood bank storage.* J Clin Invest 39:56, 1960.

Bauer, C, et al.: *Effect of 2,3-diphosphoglycerate and H^+ on the reaction of O_2 and hemoglobin.* Am J Physiol 224:838, 1973.

Behnke, O: *Some possible practical implications of the lability of blood platelet microtubules.* Vox Sang 13:502, 1967.

Benesch, R, Benesch, RE and Enoki, Y: *The interaction of hemoglobin and its subunits with 2,3-diphosphoglycerate.* Proc Natl Acad Sci USA 61:1102,1968.

BENESCH, R, BENESCH, RE and YU, CI: *Reciprocal binding of oxygen and diphosphoglycerate by human hemoglobin.* Proc Natl Acad Sci USA 59:526, 1968.

BENESCH, RE, BENESCH, R and YU, CI: *The oxygenation of hemoglobin in the presence of diphosphoglycerate. Effect of temperature, pH, ionic strength, and hemoglobin concentration.* Biochemistry 8:2567, 1969.

BENSINGER, TA, METRO, J and BEUTLER, E: *In vitro metabolism of packed erythrocytes stored in CPD adenine.* Transfusion 15:135, 1975.

BENSINGER, TA and ZUCK, TF: *Additional studies concerning the metabolism of packed erythrocytes in CPD-adenine.* Transfusion 16:353, 1976.

BEUTLER, E: *Red Cell Metabolism.* Grune & Stratton, New York, 1971.

BEUTLER, E and DURON, O: *Effect of pH on preservation of red cell ATP.* Transfusion 5:17, 1965.

BEUTLER, E and DURON, O: *The preservation of red cell ATP: The effect of phosphate.* Transfusion 6:124, 1966.

BEUTLER, E and WOOD, LA: *The viability of human blood stored in phosphate and adenine media.* Transfusion 7:401, 1967.

BEUTLER, E and WOOD, LA: *Preservation of red cell 2,3-DPG in modified ACD solution and in experimental artificial storage media.* Vox Sang 20:403, 1971.

BIRNDORF, NI and LOPAS, H: *Effects of red cell stroma free hemoglobin solution on renal function in monkeys.* J Appl Physiol 29:573-577, 1970.

BUNN, HF and JANDL, JH: *Control of hemoglobin function within the red cell.* N Engl J Med 282:1414, 1970.

BUNN, HF, RANSIL, BJ and CNAO, A: *The interaction between erythrocyte organic phosphates, magnesium ion and hemoglobin.* J Biol Chem 246:5273, 1971.

CHANUTIN, A: *The effect of the addition of adenine and nucleosides at the beginning of storage on the concentrations of phosphates of human erythrocytes during storage in acid-citrate-dextrose and citrate-phosphate-dextrose.* Transfusion 7:120, 1967.

COLLINS, JA: *Problems associated with massive transfusion of stored blood.* Surgery 75:274, 1974.

COLLINS, JA: *Massive blood transfusions.* Clin Hematol 5:201, 1976.

CROWLEY, JP, et al.: *The purification of red cells for transfusion by freeze-preservation and washing. V. Red cell recovery and residual leukocytes after freeze-preservation with high concentrations of glycerol and washing in various systems.* Transfusion 17:1, 1977.

DAWSON, RB, ELLIS, TJ and HERSHEY, RT: *Blood preservation. XVI. Packed red cell storage in CPD-adenine.* Transfusion 16:79, 1976.

DAWSON, RB, et al.: *Blood preservation. XXVI. CPD-adenine packed cells: Benefits of increasing the glucose.* Transfusion 18:339, 1978.

DAWSON, RB, et al.: *The hemoglobin function of blood stored at 4°C.* In Brewer, GJ (ED): *Red Cell Metabolism and Function.* Plenum Press, New York, 1970, p 305.

DENNIS, RC, et al.: *Transfusion of 2,3-DPG enriched red blood cells to improve cardiac function.* Ann Thorac Surg 26:17, 1978.

DERN, RJ: *The prediction of post storage red cell viability from ATP levels in erythrocyte metabolism and function.* In BREWER, GJ (ed): *Red Cell Metabolism and Function.* Plenum Press, New York, 1970, p. 269.

DUHM, J: *Effects of 2,3-diphosphoglycerate and other organic phosphate compounds on oxygen affinity and intracellular pH of human erythrocytes.* Pfluegers Arch 326:341, 1971.

FILIP DJ, ECKSTEIN, JD and SIBLEY, CA: *The effect of platelet concentrate storage temperature on adenine nucleotide metabolism.* Blood 45:749, 1975.

Food and Drug Administration: *Title 21, Code of Federal Regulations.* United States Government, 1980.

GABRIO, BW, et al: *Erythrocyte preservation. IV. In vitro reversibility of the storage lesion.* J Biol Chem 215:357, 1955.

GEYER, RP: *Substitute for blood and its components.* In Jamieson, GA and Greenwalt, TJ (EDS): *Blood Substitutes and Plasma Expanders.* Alan R. Liss, New York, 1978, pp. 1-21.

GONZALEZ, ER: *The saga of "artificial blood."* JAMA 243:719, 1980.

GREENBERG, J, SCHOOLEY, M and PESKIN, GW: *Improved retention of stroma free hemoglobin solution by chemical modification.* J Trauma 17:501, 1977.

HARMENING, DM, DAWSON, RB and MASTERS, JM: *The use of ion-exchange resins as a blood preservation system.* Transfusion 19:675, 1979.

HARRISON, RL: *Blood banking in the year 2000.* Medical Laboratory Observer 2:54, 1979.

HOLME, S, VAIDJA, K AND MURPHY, S: *Platelet storage at 22°C: Effect of type of agitation on morphology, viability and function in vitro.* Blood 52:425, 1978.

HOLMSEN, H and DAY, HJ: *Adenine nucleotides and platelet function.* Semin Hematol 4:28, 1971.

HOLSINGER, JW, SALHANY, JM and ELIOT, RS: *Physiologic observations on the effect of impaired blood oxygen release on the myocardium.* Adv Cardiol 9:81, 1973.

KATTLOVE, HE: *The effect of cold on platelets. III. Adenine nucleotide metabolism after brief storage at cold temperature.* Blood 42:557, 1973.

KOTELBA-WITKOWSKA, BK, HOLMSEN, H and MURER, EH: *Storage of human platelets: Effects on metabolically active ATP and on the release reaction.* Br J Haematol 22:4, 1972.

KOTELBA-WITKOWSKA, B, HARMENING-PITTIGLIO, DM and SCHIFFER, CA: *Storage of platelet concentrates using ion exchange resin charged with dibasic phosphate.* Blood 58:537, 1981.

KREUGER, A, AKERBLOM, O and HOGMAN, C: *A clinical evaluation of citrate-phosphate-dextrose-adenine blood.* Vox Sang 29:81, 1975.

KUNICKI, TJ, et al.: *A study of variables affecting the quality of platelets stored at "room temperature."* Transfusion 15:414, 1975.

LACELLE, PL: *Alteration of deformability of the erythrocyte in stored blood.* Transfusion 9:238, 1969.

MARTIN, GJ: *Ion Exchange and Adsorption Agents in Medicine.* Little, Brown & Co, Boston, 1954, p 89.

MESSETER, L, et al.: *CPD-adenine as a blood preservative—studies in vitro and in vivo.* Transfusion 17:210, 1977.

MUIRHEAD, H, et al.: *Structure and function of haemoglobin.* J Mol Biol 28:117, 1967.

MURPHY, S and GARDNER, FH: *Platelet storage at 22°C: Metabolic, morphologic, and functional studies.* J Clin Invest 50:370, 1971.

OHNISHI, Y and KITAZAWA, M: *Application of perfluorochemicals in human beings.* Acta Pathol Jpn 30:489, 1980.

ORENGO, A, LICHNGER, B and HARPER, JR: *Extended storage of human platelets at 22°C: Changes in glycogen and adenine nucleotide metabolism.* Transfusion 20:153, 1980.

OVERGAARD-HANSEN, K: *Rejuvenation of adenosine triphosphate in human erythrocytes by purine nucleosides.* Acta Pharmacol 14:67, 1957.

PERUTZ, MF: *Stereochemistry of cooperative effects of haemoglobin.* Nature 228:726, 1970.

PERUTZ, MF: *Hemoglobin structure and respiratory transport.* Sci Am 239:92, 1978.

RAPOPORT, S: *Regulation of metabolism in red cells.* Proceedings of the 11th Congress of the International Society of Blood Transfusion. Sydney, 1966. Bibl Haemat 29:133. S Karger, New York, 1968.

RICE, CL, et al.: *Benefits from improved oxygen delivery of blood in shock therapy.* J Surg Res 19:193, 1975.

ROBERTS, SC: *Cryopreserved red blood cells: Blood component.* In *A Seminar on Blood Components: E Unum Pluribus.* 30th Annual Meeting of the American Association of Blood Banks, Atlanta, Georgia, 1977.

ROSENTHAL, TB: *The effect of temperature on the pH of blood and plasma in vitro.* J Biol Chem 173:25, 1978.

SALZMAN, E, et al: *Platelet volume: Effect of temperature and agents affecting platelet aggregation.* Am J Physiol 217:1330, 1969.

SCOTT, EP and SLICHTER, SJ: *Viability and function of platelet concentrates stored in CPD-adenine (CPDA-1).* Transfusion 1980. Vol. 20 p. 489.

SHIELDS, CE: *Effect of plasma removal on blood stored in ACD with adenine.* Transfusion 11:134, 1971.

SHIVELY, JA, GOTT, CL and DEJONGH, DS: *The effect of storage on adhesion and aggregation of platelets.* Vox Sang 18:204, 1970.

SIMON, ER: *Workshop on Adenine and Red Cell Preservation.* Transcript of Proceedings, Bureau of Biologics, Food and Drug Administration, Department of Health, Education and Welfare, Washington, DC, October 1–2, 1976.

SLICHTER, SJ: *Preservation of platelet viability and function during storage of concentrates.* In Greenwalt, TJ and Jamieson, GA (EDS): *Blood Platelets in Transfusion Therapy.* Alan R. Liss, New York, 1978, p 83.

SLICHTER, SJ: *Controversies in platelet transfusion therapy.* Annu Rev Med 31:509, 1980.

SOHMER, PR and DAWSON, RB *The significance of 2,3-DPG in red blood cell transfusion.* CRC Crit Rev Clin Lab Sci, CRC Reviews, CRC Press, Boca Raton, Florida, November 1979.

SPECTOR, JI, et al.: *Physiologic effects of normal or low oxygen-affinity red cells in hypoxic baboons.* Am J Physiol 232: H-79, 1977.

VALERI, CR: *Blood Banking and the Use of Frozen Blood Products.* Chemical Rubber Company Press, Cleveland, 1976.

VALERI, CR, SZYMANSKI, IO and RUNCK, AH: *Therapeutic effectiveness of homologous erythrocyte transfusions following frozen storage at $-80°C$ for up to seven years.* Transfusion 10:102, 1970.

VALERI, CR, et al.: *Viability and function of red blood cell concentrates at 4°C for 35 days in CPD-A1, CPD-A2, and CPD-A3 anticoagulant solutions.* Abstract presented at the 33rd Annual Meeting of the American Association of Blood Banks, 1980.

ZUCK, TF, et al.: *The in vivo survival of red cells stored in modified CPD with adenine: Report of a multi-institutional cooperative effort.* Transfusion 17:374, 1977.

CHAPTER 2

BASIC GENETICS

EDWIN A. STEANE, PH.D.

I. MENDELIAN GENETICS
   A. Mitosis and Meiosis
   B. The Principle of Independent Segregation
   C. The Principle of Independent Assortment
   D. Population Genetics: The Hardy-Weinberg Equilibrium

II. BIOCHEMICAL GENETICS
   A. Deoxyribonucleic Acid (DNA)
   B. Ribonucleic Acid (RNA)
   C. Translation of Messenger RNA: Production of Proteins
   D. DNA Transcription and Replication

III. CONCLUSION

This chapter is divided into two major sections: Mendelian Genetics and Biochemical Genetics. In the first section, the "rules of inheritance" and the mathematics of dealing with population gene frequencies are discussed; in the second, the mechanisms by which genes produce their observed effects are covered. It must be stated at the outset that these topics are explored in a somewhat superficial manner, since each topic deserves a book to itself, not half a chapter. An outline of the essential concepts necessary to an understanding of modern genetics, together with a sufficient framework to support these concepts, is provided. Suggested books that will permit the interested reader to discover more fully the world of genetics are appended; however, the number of available books on genetics is seemingly endless, and any of them should enrich your knowledge.

As always, new science requires the assimilation of new language. Definitions of important terms in genetics are given the first time they are used in the text. A clear understanding of these terms is essential to progress in organizing your accumulation of knowledege of genetics.

MENDELIAN GENETICS

From the mid 1800s to the early 1900s revolutionary changes occurred in our knowledge of biology. These led inevitably to modern medical practice and provided the basis for a second revolution, beginning in the 1950s, which produced the new subscience we know today as molecular biology. Particularly important to the early revolution was the work of Darwin and of Mendel, together with the hypothesis that the basic unit of life was the cell, and the concept that since the sperm was largely composed of the same material as the cell nucleus, the nucleus was concerned with the material of inheritance. When Mendel's ideas were rediscovered independently by de Vries, Correns, and Tschermak in 1900, and Thomas Hunt Morgan began his work with fruit flies, all these notions came together to produce a genetic theory that we can conveniently call mendelian or classic genetics.

We must begin with the *gene*. As we have discovered more about how genes act, the gene has become more difficult to define, but for this section we shall describe a gene as a *unit of inheritance*. It had long been observed that characteristics were passed on from generation to generation; geneticists call them *traits*. Mendel proposed that these traits were the outward expression, the *phenotype*, of genes and enunciated two general principles governing their passage from generation to generation: the *principle of independent segregation* and the *principle of independent assortment*.

MITOSIS AND MEIOSIS

There is no need for us to take a strictly chronologic approach to genetics. As always, what was extremely puzzling to early investigators seems obvious by hindsight. Since we have the benefit of hindsight, it is appropriate to leave Mendel for a few moments to return to the nucleus and the cell theory.

As microscopy became more advanced and the cell theory was confirmed, it became obvious that as a cell produced two daughter cells by division, the nucleus of the cell also divided, and certain physical events were happening within the nucleus. Moreover, the production of new individuals by the combination of ovum and sperm required an explanation as to how the correct amount of nuclear material arrived at its final destination. Investigations led to an understanding that the nucleus is composed of long, thin strands of material called *chromosomes*, and that as a cell divides, this material is duplicated by the dividing cell and equally divided between the two daughter cells. This process is known as *mitosis*. In mitosis, not only is each chromosome duplicated, but one of each pair passes to each daughter cell, that is, each new cell has exactly the same complement of chromosomes as the cell from which it was derived. This is diagrammed in Figure 2-1. We speak of mitosis as the process that maintains the parental chromosome number—obviously an important concept if offspring are to resemble their parents.

But how do we explain the production of new individuals? If we were to combine an ovum and a sperm, would not the resulting individual have twice as many chromosomes as the preceding generation? This unsatisfactory state of affairs leads us to a new concept: cells such as ova and sperm are *haploid*, that is, they have only *one* copy of each chromosome. This necessarily means that other body cells are *diploid*—they have *two* copies of each chromosome. Now we have the necessary pieces to construct a reasonable explanation for the production of new individuals.

By a process known as *meiosis*, sex cells are produced that are haploid. When the ovum and sperm unite to form a *zygote*, the diploid state is produced, in which two copies of each chromosome are present, one copy being derived from each parent. Meiosis is diagrammed in Figure 2-2. Meiosis reduces the parental chromosome number. In the diagram, the male has two copies of chromosome A, designated as A_M, and the female also has two copies of A, designated as A_F. But remember, one of each of the two copies in the male must have come from each of his parents, and one of each in the female must have come from each of her parents; therefore, the labels are to identify the chromosomes, not to indicate that there is an A "male" chromosome and an A "female" chromosome.

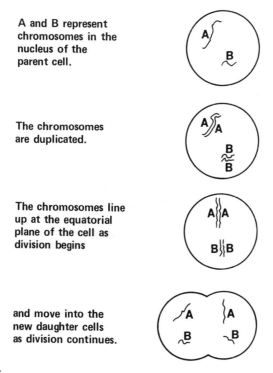

A and B represent chromosomes in the nucleus of the parent cell.

The chromosomes are duplicated.

The chromosomes line up at the equatorial plane of the cell as division begins

and move into the new daughter cells as division continues.

FIGURE 2-1. Mitosis.

Diploid cells, in which
there are two copies of
chromosome A_M (one from
father - f; one from
mother - m) and
chromosome A_F.

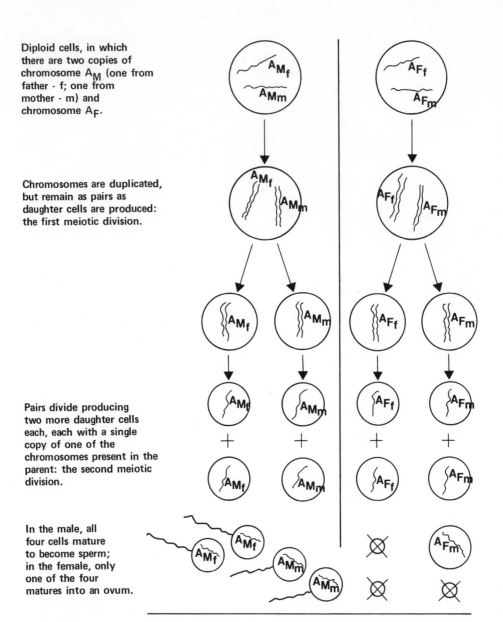

Chromosomes are duplicated,
but remain as pairs as
daughter cells are produced:
the first meiotic division.

Pairs divide producing
two more daughter cells
each, each with a single
copy of one of the
chromosomes present in the
parent: the second meiotic
division.

In the male, all
four cells mature
to become sperm;
in the female, only
one of the four
matures into an ovum.

At fertilization, copies of
chromosome A_M derived
from the father and
chromosome A_F derived from
the mother are present
in the zygote.

FIGURE 2-2. Meiosis.

How then is sex determined, and how many chromosomes are there? Sex is determined by a special pair of sex chromosomes, called X and Y. Since a female has two X chromosomes and must pass on one copy of each of her chromosomes to her offspring, each male must have one X chromosome derived from his mother; it is the Y chromosome, derived from the father, that determines "maleness." Chromosome number varies from species to species, but the pair of sex chromosomes is a common feature of higher animals. In humans, there are 46 chromosomes in the diploid nucleus; 1 pair of sex chromosomes and 22 pairs of *autosomes*. Techniques have been devised to categorize and examine the chromosomes. Such a display, a *karyotype*, is shown in Figure 2-3. In the human female, therefore, there are 23 *pairs* of chromosomes, one of which is the X pair; in the human male, there are 22 pairs of chromosomes and an XY combination. Now let us return to Mendel.

THE PRINCIPLE OF INDEPENDENT SEGREGATION

Mendel was able to achieve his conceptual breakthrough because he kept meticulous records of offspring in his experiments on crossing different types of plants. Much of the knowledge that Mendel used to begin his experiments was common to the horticulturists of the day; it is the observer who seeks the order beneath the results who makes the important discoveries.

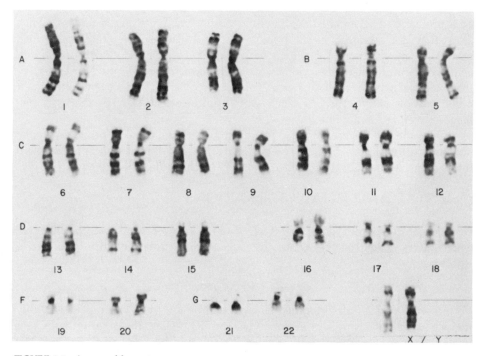

FIGURE 2-3. A normal karyotype.

Mendel cultivated sweet pea plants until they "bred true," that is, the offspring were identical to the parents in the trait observed. In this fashion, he bred plants that only produced red flowers, and plants that only produced white flowers. Then he crossed the red plants with the white and produced plants that had red flowers. But when he crossed these new generation plants with each other, he bred plants that produced red flowers and white flowers: the important observation was that the ratio was three red to one white. When he crossed the initial offspring with their true breeding forebears, he obtained two different results: If he crossed the new plants with the red plants, all the offspring plants produced red flowers; if he crossed the new plants with the white plants, one half of the offspring plants produced red flowers and the other half white.

We can reason more simply than did Mendel, since we know that each plant has two copies of each autosome. If the unit of inheritance (the gene) that produces "redness" is denoted as R, then we recognize that the genotype of the true breeding plants is RR; in the zygote, both autosomes carry the R gene, from which our term *homozygote* is derived. Similarly, in the white true breeding plants we can designate the gene that produces "no redness" as r; these plants are also homozygous, but rr. RR plants would produce sex cells carrying chromosomes bearing the R gene; rr plants sex cells carrying chromosomes bearing the r gene. When these sex cells are combined, a zygote that possesses both the R and r genes is produced: an Rr *heterozygote*. Why do these plants produce red flowers? Here we must introduce the concept of *dominance*, that is, when a plant has both R and r genes, only R is expressed. R is said to be dominant to r. When R is absent, that is, the plant genotype is rr, no red is produced. This is called the *recessive* state. Genes are either *dominant*, which means they are expressed in the homozygote and heterozygote; *recessive*, which means they are expressed only in the homozygous recessive individual; or *codominant*, which means there is no dominance of one gene over the other, and both are fully expressed whenever they appear. For instance, were R and r to be codominant in our example above, then Rr plants would produce pink flowers, that is, something between red and white.

Once these ideas are understood, the rest of classic genetics becomes simple, even the mathematics. The next few paragraphs summarize the concepts presented to this point. Make sure that you totally grasp all these ideas before going on.

PARENTAL AND FILIAL GENERATIONS

If we denote one homozygous parent as RR (all red flowers) and the other as rr (all white flowers), then the first cross, the *parental* or P cross, between these two is denoted as

$$P - RR \times rr$$

We recognize that all offspring of this cross will be Rr, since one parent can only produce sex cells carrying chromosomes bearing the R gene, the other only sex cells carrying chromosomes bearing the r gene. We call this the F (for *filial*, meaning son or daughter) generation.

If we now make a cross between these Rr heterozygotes, we can express this as

$$F_1 - Rr \times Rr \quad (F_1 \text{ indicates the first filial generation})$$

Offspring of this generation will produce red flowers versus white flowers in a ratio of three to one, since the R (red) gene is dominant.

Since each individual in the F_1 generation is able to produce sex cells carrying chromosomes bearing the R or r gene, these can recombine in all possible combinations. To diagram the possibilities, a simply constructed "magic square" is useful:

♂ ♀	R	r	parents haploid genotype
R	RR	Rr	offspring
r	Rr	rr	diploid genotype

Note that of the offspring (the F_2, or second filial generation), three fourths will have an R gene and produce red flowers, but that of these, one third will be homozygous RR and two thirds heterozygous Rr. Their *genotype* is their actual genetic makeup; their *phenotype* is the observed expression of their genotype.

If R and r were codominant, and if the Rr genotype plant produced pink flowers, the plants of the F_2 generation would produce red, pink, and white flowers in a ratio of one:two:one.

From this beginning we can construct Mendel's first law, which says that traits segregate independently. What this means is that the chance of any gene on a particular chromosome ending up in any particular individual is a random event. This is best demonstrated using genetic events with which we also wish to become familiar: the inheritance of the blood groups. Since most blood group genes have codominant expression, they provide an ideal set of markers to study mendelian principles. Figure 2-4 demonstrates independent segregation of the MN blood groups in two families, using different lettering to facilitate the following of a particular gene from generation to generation.

THE PRINCIPLE OF INDEPENDENT ASSORTMENT

Mendel continued his experiments by enumerating offspring ratio when two traits were observed simultaneously. For this he chose seed production by the plants. He noticed that there were seeds that were round and smooth and seeds that were wrinkled; also that some seeds were green, others yellow. Once again, he cultivated true breeding plants that only produced seeds of a particular type, for example, round and yellow or wrinkled and green. Then he proceeded to do parental and filial crosses as described earlier. Once again, he was confronted with a dominant-recessive inheritance, in that round was dominant to wrinkled and yellow dominant to

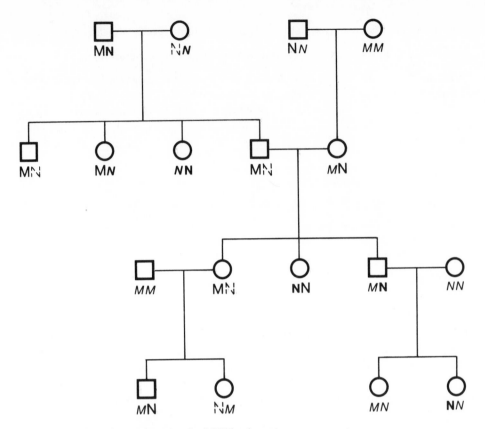

FIGURE 2-4. Independent segregation: the MN blood groups.

green. Here, inheritance becomes a little more complicated, but provided one makes use of simple diagrams and "magic squares," not at all difficult. We shall begin by knowing what Mendel actually discovered: that the chromosome carrying the round-wrinkled trait is not the same chromosome as that carrying the yellow-green trait. Figure 2-5 diagrams the results of experiments such as those Mendel performed.

Other factors require further explanation. For instance, what if the two traits being observed are *linked*, that is, they are on the same chromosome? One does not then observe independent assortment. Genes sometimes "travel together," as in the MNSs blood group gene complex. Occasional aberrant results seen in some experiments are explained by the phenomenon of *crossing over*. Crossing over is diagrammed in Figure 2-6.

Crossing over is a normal event in meiosis. It appears to be a natural means of further "shuffling" the genetic material; natural selection processes thus have greater variations among which to choose. The degree of crossing over between two particular genes can be calculated by observing the number of unexpected *recombinants*, that is, gene pairs not expected from the parental genotypes. If the recombinants occur with a frequency of more than 50 percent, this situation cannot be distinguished from ordinary independent assortment, but this does not mean the genes are not on the same chromosome. Genes that are linked, but that cannot be demonstrated to be linked by simple pedigree analysis, are said to be *syntenic*.

We know from many experiments that the degree of crossing over exhibited by two linked genes is determined by their distance from each other on the chromosome. Closely linked genes seldom show crossovers (once again, the MNSs complex is an example), but as the distance increases, the frequency of crossovers increases. By determining crossover frequency, one can map chromosomes and determine the relative position and distance of one *locus* (the region of a chromosome occupied by a gene) from another.

Crossovers, although rare, can occur *within* genes, as we now know from our studies of abnormal hemoglobins and other proteins.

Alleles are differing forms of the same gene that can occupy a given locus. The existence of allelic forms is referred to as *polymorphism*. For example, the *A*, *B*, and *O* genes are allelic; the ABO blood group system is a polymorphism.

Other accidents that can influence the results of experiments such as those conducted by Mendel are mutation, deletion, inversion, translocation, and nondisjunction. *Mutation* is a spontaneous change in a gene, which can be brought about by radiation or chemical damage. *Deletion* is the accidental loss of a portion of a chromosome. *Inversion* is the breaking of a chromosome during division, with reattachment occurring "upside down." *Translocation* is the transfer of a portion of one chromosome to the end of another. *Nondisjunction* is the failure of two chromosomes to separate during meiosis, resulting in one cell with both unseparated chromosomes, the other with none. All of these accidents can have lethal consequences, or they can be compatible with life but result in severely impaired performance. Down's syndrome results from a nondisjunction event in which the final zygote has three copies of chromosome 21. Most are familiar with the distressing consequences of this genetic accident. Medical genetics is the study of these (and other) causes of genetic disease. Refer to the Bibliography at the end of this chapter for further reading on the subject.

POPULATION GENETICS:
THE HARDY-WEINBERG EQUILIBRIUM

In a randomly mating, relatively large population, gene frequencies tend to remain constant unless subjected to some selective pressure; they reach an equilibrium. This equilibrium is given by the Hardy-Weinberg formula:

$$p^2 + 2pq + q^2 = 1$$

where p is the frequency of one gene, q the frequency of its allele, and $p + q = 1$. This formula and its application are so basic in blood banking that some time spent understanding its derivation is worthwhile.

Let us invent a randomly mating population with a gene *A* of frequency 50 percent (or 0.5) and its allele *a*, also of frequency 50 percent, and state that there are no selective pressures operating on *A* or *a*. The chance of any given sex cell bearing

[Text continues on page 34]

R = round; r = wrinkled;   = yellow; y = green.

Plant type 1: **seeds round and yellow. Since all plants breed true, we know they are homozygous for their trait observed.**

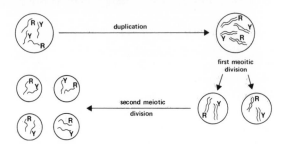

All sex cells produced carry an R — bearing chromosome and a Y — bearing chromosome.

Plant type 2: **seeds wrinkled and green. Similarly to above, all sex cells produced carry an r — bearing chromosome and a y — bearing chromosome.**

The cross between these two plant types can be diagrammed as follows:

P   RRyy x rryy

and the offspring would all be $RrYy$.
The first filial generation cross would be

F₁   RrYy x RrYy

and the offspring produced can be deduced from a "magic square" once the sex cells that can be produced have been determined. In this case the situation is

Diploid precursor

Duplication

First meiotic division

Second meiotic division

The chromosomes randomly (independently) assort, the only requirement being that an $R-$ bearing or $r-$ bearing and a $Y-$ bearing or $y-$ bearing chromosome be present in each cell.

♂ \ ♀	RY	Ry	rY	ry	parents haploid genotype
RY	RRYY	RRYy	RrYY	RrYy	
Ry	RRYy	RRyy	RrYy	Rryy	offspring
rY	RrYY	RrYy	rrYY	rrYy	diploid genotype
ry	RrYy	Rryy	rrYy	rryy	

The F_2 generation would be composed of

> 9 of every 16 plants producing round and yellow seeds
> (genotypes *RRYY, RRYy. RrYY,* and *RrYy*)
> 3 of every 16 plants producing round and green seeds
> (genotypes *RRyy* and *Rryy*)
> 3 of every 16 plants producing wrinkled and yellow seeds
> (genotypes *rrYY* and *rrYy*)
> 1 of every 16 plants producing wrinkled and green seeds
> (genotype *rryy*)

It was exactly this 9:3:3:1 ratio that Mendel obtained from which he formulated his Principle of Independent Assortment.

FIGURE 2-5. Mendel's second law: the principle of independent assortment.

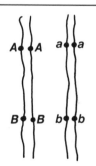

During meiosis, when the duplicated chromosomes are paired,

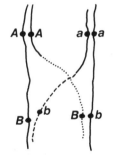

portions can "cross over," and exchange with the complementary (homologous) chromosome.

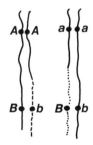

When the chromosomes separate, the alignment of the genes on the chromosomes is not as it was originally (a recombinant).

FIGURE 2-6. Crossing over.

the A gene in this population would be 0.5; similarly for a, 0.5. The genotypes of the population are therefore given by

	0.5 A	0.5 a
0.5 A	0.25 AA	0.25 Aa
0.5 a	0.25 Aa	0.25 aa

that is, 0.25 AA, 0.50 Aa, and 0.25 aa.

Now let us determine the frequency with which a person of genotype AA would mate with another person of genotype AA, and so on. This is given by

	0.25 AA	0.50 Aa	0.25 aa
0.25 AA	0.0625 AA/AA	0.1250 AA/Aa	0.0625 AA/aa
0.50 Aa	0.1250 AA/Aa	0.2500 Aa/Aa	0.1250 Aa/aa
0.25 aa	0.0625 AA/aa	0.1250 Aa/aa	0.0625 aa/aa

From this, possible mating combinations and their frequencies are as follows:

Mating	Frequency
$AA \times AA$	0.0625
$AA \times Aa$	0.2500
$AA \times aa$	0.1250
$Aa \times Aa$	0.2500
$Aa \times aa$	0.2500
$aa \times aa$	0.0625
	1.0000

The first and last matings can only produce homozygote AA and aa offspring, respectively, and the mating $AA \times aa$ can only produce Aa heterozygotes. We can diagram the other possibilities as follows:

AA x Aa

	A	A
A	AA	AA
a	Aa	Aa

Aa x Aa

	A	a
A	AA	Aa
a	Aa	aa

Aa x aa

	A	a
a	Aa	aa
a	Aa	aa

Thus, we can prepare a table of the proportion of offspring of given genotypes from each of our possible matings:

	Proportion of offspring of genotype		
Mating	AA	Aa	aa
AA × AA	all	none	none
AA × Aa	½	½	none
AA × aa	none	all	none
Aa × Aa	¼	½	¼
Aa × aa	none	½	½
aa × aa	none	none	all

If we now combine the frequency of the mating with proportion of offspring from each mating, we can construct the following table of the frequency of the genotypes in the next generation:

	Frequency of offspring of genotype		
Mating	AA	Aa	aa
AA × AA	0.0625	0.0000	0.0000
AA × Aa	0.1250	0.1250	0.0000
AA × aa	0.0000	0.1250	0.0000
Aa × Aa	0.0625	0.1250	0.0625
Aa × aa	0.0000	0.1250	0.1250
aa × aa	0.0000	0.0000	0.0625
	0.2500	0.5000	0.2500

We see that the proportion of each genotype remains constant, that is, the population is in equilibrium.

We obtain the frequency of any combination event as the product of the frequencies of the individual occurrences, that is, if the frequency of A is 0.5, then the frequency of an AA homozygote is 0.5 × 0.5 = 0.25. In each of the "magic squares," the simple way to do the calculations is to write the frequencies as shown at the beginning of this section, then enter the product of the individual frequencies at the head of each column into the proper box.

If A and a are present in equal proportions, one might expect a stable population. But what if they are decidedly unequal in frequency? Let us use the Kell blood group system as an example to see what happens if we go through the same process as before. In whites, the approximate gene frequency of K is 0.05 and of k 0.95 (remember, the gene frequencies must sum to 1). What would be the proportion of homozygous KK and kk and heterozygous Kk in our randomly mating population? We can diagram and calculate as before:

	0.05 K	0.95 k
0.05 K	0.0025 KK	0.0475 Kk
0.95 k	0.0475 Kk	0.9025 kk

Roughly 90 percent of the population will be Kell negative, 10 percent Kell positive. Now we must determine mating frequencies as before:

	0.0025 KK	0.0950 Kk	0.9025 kk
0.0025 KK	0.00000625 KK/KK	0.00023750 KK/Kk	0.00225625 KK/kk
0.0950 Kk	0.00023750 KK/Kk	0.00902500 Kk/Kk	0.08573750 Kk/kk
0.9025 kk	0.00225625 KK/kk	0.08573750 Kk/kk	0.81450625 kk/kk

The numbers get more difficult to deal with, but the mathematics is no more complicated. Note that although the mating $kk \times kk$ occurs only once in the square, it occurs with a frequency of better than 80 percent because k is so common. On the other hand, the mating $KK \times KK$ also occurs once in the square, but notice the frequency: about 1.6 times in every 100,000 matings. In this way, K, rare to begin with, remains rare. Let us list our six matings and their frequencies as before.

Mating	Frequency
$KK \times KK$	0.00000625
$KK \times Kk$	0.00047500
$KK \times kk$	0.00451250
$Kk \times Kk$	0.00902500
$Kk \times kk$	0.17147500
$kk \times kk$	0.81450625
	1.00000000

Although these frequencies are very different from those for A and a given earlier, remember that the *proportion* of offspring of a given genotype produced by a mating is *precisely* the same as before. This means that all of the offspring of a $KK \times KK$ mating will be KK; one-half of the offspring of a $KK \times Kk$ mating will be KK, one-half Kk, none kk; and so on.

We can then construct our final table:

| Mating | Frequency of offspring of genotype | | |
	KK	Kk	kk
$KK \times KK$	0.00000625	0.00000000	0.00000000
$KK \times Kk$	0.00023750	0.00023750	0.00000000
$KK \times kk$	0.00000000	0.00451250	0.00000000
$Kk \times Kk$	0.00225625	0.00451250	0.00225625
$Kk \times kk$	0.00000000	0.08573750	0.08573750
$kk \times kk$	0.00000000	0.00000000	0.81450625
	0.00250000	0.09500000	0.90250000

Once again the frequencies of KK and kk homozygotes and the Kk heterozygote have not changed.

How can we obtain the gene frequencies from the genotype frequencies? One simple way is to count them. Let us say we examine 10,000 persons at random. Of these, 25 will be KK, 950 Kk, and 9,025 kk. We now have a pool of 20,000 genes (each person has two), and in the pool 1,000 will be K (25 + 25 + 950) and 19,000 will be k (950 + 9,025 + 9,025). The gene frequency of K is 1,000/20,000 or 0.05; that of k is 19,000/20,000 or 0.95. Everything checks out.

All of this leads up to a much simpler approach: use of the Hardy-Weinberg formula, $p^2 + 2pq + q^2 = 1$. Let us draw a square and label it as follows:

	p	q
p	pp	pq
q	pq	qq

This is all we have been doing in our examples with Aa and Kk. Once we know the frequency of any gene in a two-allele combination, we can calculate the frequency of all genotypes, which remain stable.

For example, the frequency of the blood group gene S is about 0.30. This is all we need to know to calculate that the frequency of s is 0.70, and that the distribution of the genotypes is $0.30 \times 0.30 = 0.09$ SS, $2 \times 0.30 \times 0.70 = 0.42$ Ss, and $0.70 \times 0.70 = 0.49$ ss.

If, on the other hand, we only know the genotype frequency, we must work just a little harder. For example, let us say we test a population with anti-Jk[a] and discover that about 75 percent of those tested are positive. The situation is as follows:

$$
\left. \begin{array}{l} Jk(a+b-) \\ Jk(a+b+) \end{array} \right\} = 0.75
$$
$$
Jk(a-b+) = 0.25
$$

that is, both Jk^aJk^a homozygotes and Jk^aJk^b heterozygotes are included in our Jk^a positive group. We could solve the equation

$$
p^2 + 2pq = 0.75, \quad \text{where } p + q = 1
$$

but there is a much easier way. Since $p^2 + 2pq + q^2 = 1$, and $p^2 + 2pq = 0.75$, then $q^2 = 0.25$. If we take the square root of 0.25 we obtain q:

$$
q = q^2 = \sqrt{0.25} = 0.5
$$

Frequencies in the Kidd system are very close to those of A and a with which we began. In truth, Jk(a+) individuals are about 76.4 percent of the population, so $q^2 = 0.236$, $q = 0.4858$, and the actual genotype frequencies would be

$$
\begin{array}{llr}
Jk(a+b-) = p^2 = 0.5142^2 & = 0.2644 \\
Jk(a+b+) = 2pq = 2(0.5142)(0.4858) & = 0.4996 \\
Jk(a-b+) = q^2 = 0.4858^2 & \underline{= 0.2360} \\
& 1.0000
\end{array}
$$

Handling the mathematics involved with a two-allele system is not particularly difficult. With three or more alleles the equations are considerably more complex, and beyond the scope of this chapter. If you wish to read a lucid account of the mathematics of a system of three or more alleles, then I recommend that of Race and Sanger for the ABO blood group system in their classic book, *Blood Groups in Man*. After studying this section of their book you will appreciate why it needed a mathematician, Bernstein, to firmly establish the mendelian inheritance of the ABO blood group markers some 24 years after they were discovered.

INHERITANCE PATTERNS

Essentially, genes can be autosomal dominant (or codominant) or recessive, or X-linked dominant (or codominant) or recessive (the Y chromosome has few identifiable genes). It is useful to be able to recognize the characteristic pattern of inheritance that these different types of genes produce.

Before we proceed it will be necessary to learn a few more conventions regarding pedigree analysis. Figure 2-4 is a typical pedigree. Males are denoted by squares; females by circles. A line joining a male and female indicates a mating, and offspring are indicated by a vertical line drawn from the line joining the pair. Other conventions are diagrammed in Figure 2-7. The *propositus* (from the Latin *proponere*, to set forth) is usually designated by an arrow and indicates the family member who first draws attention to the pedigree. Sometimes the propositus is called the *proband* or *in-*

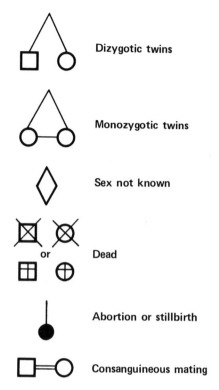

	Dizygotic twins
	Monozygotic twins
	Sex not known
or	Dead
	Abortion or stillbirth
	Consanguineous mating

FIGURE 2-7. Pedigree charting conventions.

dex case. Generations are given Roman numerals and individuals in each generation Arabic numbers from left to right. This makes referring to any given individual simple (II-3, V-8, etc.).

Autosomal dominant genes produce an effect whenever they are present; in this sense these genes have no definite pattern to their inheritance. The trait appears in parent and offspring; persons not showing the trait do not transmit it to their offspring.

Autosomal recessive genes, on the other hand, are only expressed in the homozygous state. In general, therefore, they only appear in the propositus or siblings of the propositus. Figure 2-8A is a typical example, demonstrating that the trait is usually not seen in the parents; one fourth of siblings of the propositus are, on average, affected. The parents of affected children may be consanguineous (blood relations, e.g., cousins). In dominant and recessive autosomal traits there is no sex preference for the appearance of the trait. This is not true of the X-linked traits, however, in which sex preference is the pattern that raises suspicions that one is dealing with X-linked inheritance.

Figure 2-8B is an example of X-linked dominant inheritance. Characteristically, males possessing the trait have no sons with the trait, whereas all their daughters express it. Females with the trait, on the other hand, can be heterozygous or homozygous. Transmission in females, then, is identical to that with an autosomal domi-

A. Autosomal recessive

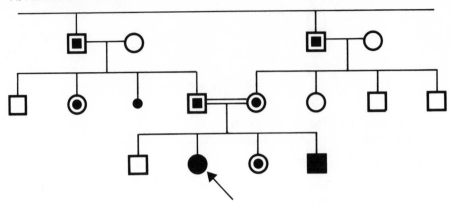

B. X—linked dominant

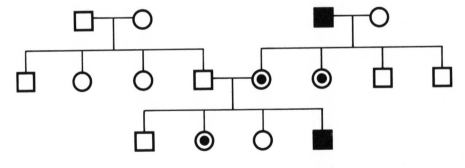

C. X—linked recessive

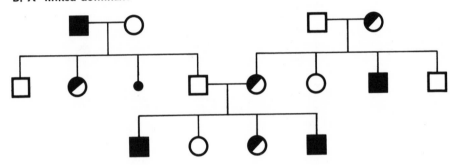

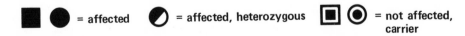

■ ● = affected   ◐ = affected, heterozygous   ▣ ◉ = not affected, carrier

FIGURE 2-8. Inheritance patterns.

MODERN BLOOD BANKING AND TRANSFUSION PRACTICES

nant trait. It is also a clue to note that in X-linked dominant traits, females bearing the trait are twice as common as males (females have two X chromosomes; males only one). For example, examine the frequency of Xgª-positive females as opposed to Xgª-positive males.

Figure 2-8C diagrams an example of X-linked recessive inheritance. Characteristically, the trait is never passed from father to son, but the trait is passed through all his daughters to half *their* sons; the trait "skips a generation." Since the trait is only expressed in the homozygous (XX) or hemizygous (XY) state, trait-bearing males are more common than trait-bearing females.

LINKAGE AND POSITION EFFECTS

Since this chapter is written for persons interested in blood banking, linkage and position effects are significant. Many blood group genes appear to be inherited as *linkage groups*. *MNSs* and *KkKpᵃKpᵇJsᵃJsᵇ* are examples. Linkage is confirmed or ruled out by pedigree analysis. Usually, inspection of the results of testing will demonstrate close linkage or independent assortment; however, where crossing over occurs, leading to recombinants, the problem becomes more difficult. If the recombinants are few, one can demonstrate that the genes are usually transmitted as a linkage group. If recombinants are more frequent, one must resort to mathematical analysis, often of many families, to confirm linkage. This is beyond the scope of this chapter, but covered in several of the books listed in the Bibliography.

Sometimes a gene on an homologous chromosome can have an effect on the expression of a given gene. In addition, it is possible for a gene within a linkage group to have an effect on the expression of another gene within the linkage group. We refer to these as *position effects*. To make discussion simple, we use the terms *cis* and *trans*. Cis position effects are those caused by a gene on the same chromosome; trans position effects are those caused by genes on the homologous chromosome. As an example, we often say that presence of the Rh antigen C (and by implication the Rh gene *C*) has an effect on the Rh antigen D (the *D* gene). This is seen both in the cis and trans positions, that is, when *C* is part of the same linkage group as *D* (*CDe*) or on the opposite chromosome (*Cde/cDe*).

BIOCHEMICAL GENETICS

In this section we discuss what is known about how genes work. Early work had shown that chromosomes were made of nucleic acids and associated proteins (called histones), and we knew that four nucleic acids were specifically required, those formed from the pyrimidine analogs thymine and cytosine, and those from the purine analogs adenine and guanine. Further, we knew that in any preparation of nuclear material the amount of thymine was always equal to that of cytosine, and the amount of adenine equal to that of guanine. We also were aware of another important fact: the ratio of thymine plus adenine to cytosine plus guanine was constant for any given species. It was apparent that in some manner these facts combined to pass critical information from one generation of cells to the next.

Today, the basic picture is so clear that one wonders why it took so long to establish the method by which four nucleic acids provide the entire information necessary to construct a new individual. A description of the exciting chase to unravel the secret of DNA can be found in J. D. Watson's 1968 book, *The Double Helix.* The story can be easily followed, but to do so a knowledge of biochemistry is necessary.

DEOXYRIBONUCLEIC ACID (DNA)

Chromosomes are constructed of DNA. DNA is made from the four nitrogenous bases referred to above, namely, thymine, cytosine, adenine, and guanine. The basic structure of these compounds and their "parents" is given in Figure 2-9. To each base is added a molecule of deoxyribose and a molecule of phosphoric acid. We call the compound formed from the joining of the base and the sugar deoxyribose a

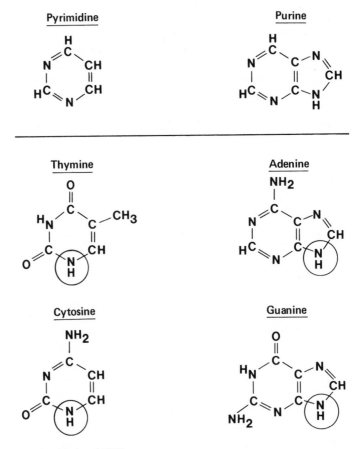

FIGURE 2-9. Building blocks of DNA.

nucleoside. When the phosphate group is attached to a nucleoside, we call the compound a *nucleotide*. The formula for deoxyribose is as follows:

$$\text{⑤CH}_2\text{OH} \quad \text{O} \quad \text{OH}$$

The linkage structure is shown with carbons numbered ④ C, ① , H, H H, H, ③ C—C ②, OH H.

Phosphoric acid (H_3PO_4) can attach in two places to deoxyribose, through the hydroxyl group at carbon 3 or the hydroxyl group at carbon 5. The importance of these dual sites of attachment will become apparent later. Phosphoric acid attaches (esterifies), with the elimination of a molecule of water, as follows:

$$-\text{C}-\text{OH} \; + \; \text{HO}-\overset{\text{OH}}{\underset{\text{OH}}{\text{P}}}=\text{O} \; \longrightarrow \; \text{C}-\text{O}-\overset{\text{OH}}{\underset{\text{OH}}{\text{P}}}=\text{O} \; + \; H_2O$$

The linkage of the deoxyribose to the base is through the hydroxyl group at carbon 1. This is an N-glycosidic linkage, again with the loss of a water molecule, as follows:

$$\text{sugar} ——\text{OH} \; + \; \text{H}\,\text{N} —— \text{base}$$

$$\downarrow$$

$$\text{sugar} — \text{N} — \text{base} + H_2O$$

The NH group involved in each case is circled in Figure 2-9. The four nucleosides formed are called deoxythymidine, deoxycytidine, deoxyadenosine, and deoxyguanosine. When the phosphate group is added and the nucleotides are formed, the position of esterification is indicated by giving the carbon number; for ease of nomenclature in such complex compounds, the number sometimes has a prime (') sign attached. Primed numbers indicate that the carbon atom referred to is in the sugar molecule, nonprimed numbers indicate that the carbon atom is in the base. I have not included the numbering system for the bases, since it is not important to this discussion and can be found in most biochemistry textbooks. Natural nucleotides are esterified at carbon 5, so the nucleotides that correspond to the nucleosides above are deoxythymidine 5'-phosphate, deoxycytidine 5'-phosphate, deoxyadenosine 5'-phosphate, and deoxyguanosine 5'-phosphate, respectively.

The key to understanding DNA came when it was realized that the bases form natural pairs: thymine with adenine and cytosine with guanine. These natural pairs are illustrated in Figure 2-10. Paired nucleosides, each nucleoside linked to its

Thymine—adenine

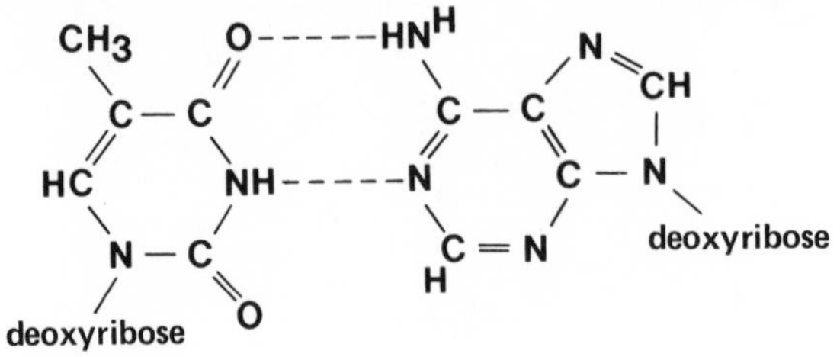

Cytosine—guanine

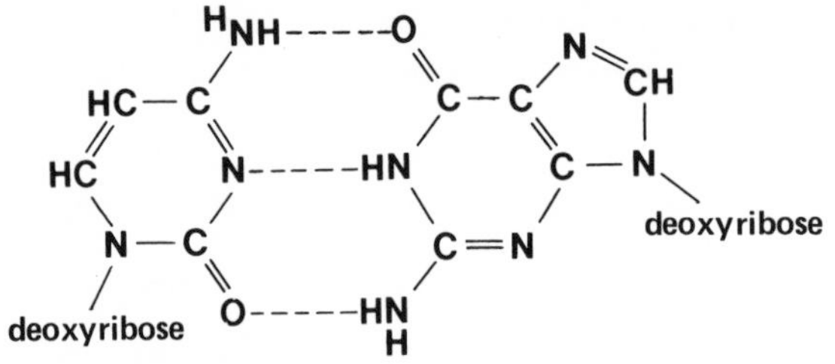

Dotted lines represent interatomic hydrogen bonds, which hold the base pairs together.

FIGURE 2-10. Base pairing in DNA.

neighbor through a phosphate bridge, form the double-stranded molecule of DNA; the "twist" or helix of the molecule is also a natural outcome of its composition. A side-view sketch is seen in Figure 2-11. Obviously, DNA can be of any length, and inspection of the chromosomes in the karyotype presented in Figure 2-3 points out these varying lengths.

INFORMATION STORAGE AND PROCESSING

Given a molecule such as that described above, how can we explain the ability of the molecule to transmit information from cell to cell? Once again, it is unnecessary for us to struggle as did the early chemists; we can go right to the heart of the matter. Essentially, the genetic material has but two capabilities: self-replication and the production of proteins. The manner in which DNA is replicated and proteins are produced is discussed later. Given that the information contained in DNA is processed into proteins, and knowing that proteins are, like DNA, linear molecules composed of amino acids rather than nucleic acids, the problem is discovering the information available in a four-base "code" that permits the specification of some 20 amino acids. For deciphering the code, Nirenberg received the Nobel prize.

It is readily apparent that one base cannot specify one amino acid; if this were so, we could only code for four different amino acids. If we use two bases as our code, we obtain 16 (4 × 4) possibilities (TT, TA, TC, TG, AT, AA, AC, AG, and so

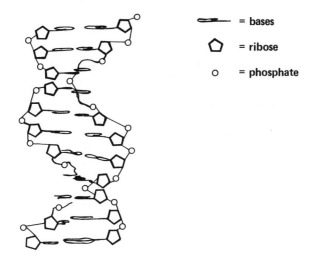

Note: It is not intended that the molecules and their spacings be to scale in this sketch. Rather, an idea of the position of the various components that make up DNA and the essentially planar (flat) nature of the base pairs is intended.

FIGURE 2-11. A sketch of the DNA molecule.

on). This is still not enough to code for 20 amino acids. But a three-base code provides 64 (4 × 4 × 4) possibilities, which are too many. However, the code *is* three bases; there is "redundancy" in the code, that is, several triplets of bases code for the same amino acid. The DNA triplets GAA, GAT, GAC, and GAG, for example, all code for leucine. When the information in DNA is processed, each set of three bases specifies an amino acid (the next two sections deal with how this is accomplished). Figure 2-12 gives the complete genetic code.

RIBONUCLEIC ACIDS (RNAs)

DNA, as we have seen, is composed of four nitrogenous bases, each with an associated deoxyribose and phosphate group, linked through a phosphate "backbone" into a long strand, and paired with another strand through base bonding. This second strand is complementary to the first in that the "opposite" base appears, as follows:

first strand ———— TATAGGGCTCAGA ————
second strand ———— ATATCCCGAGTCT ————

We must now discuss some similar molecules, the ribonucleic acids, which consist of a base, ribose (rather than deoxyribose), and phosphate. The bases are the same as in DNA, except that uracil replaces thymine. The nucleoside is called uridine, and

2nd position

		A	G	T	C		
DNA		A	G	T	C		
mRNA		U	C	A	G		

1st position							3rd position
DNA	**mRNA**					**mRNA**	**DNA**
A	U	Phe	Ser	Tyr	Cys	U	A
		Phe	Ser	Tyr	Cys	C	G
		Leu	Ser	Stop	Stop	A	T
		Leu	Ser	Stop	Trp	G	C
G	C	Leu	Pro	His	Arg	U	A
		Leu	Pro	His	Arg	C	G
		Leu	Pro	Gln	Arg	A	T
		Leu	Pro	Gln	Arg	G	C
T	A	Ile	Thr	Asn	Ser	U	A
		Ile	Thr	Asn	Ser	C	G
		Ile	Thr	Lys	Arg	A	T
		Met	Thr	Lys	Arg	G	C
C	G	Val	Ala	Asp	Gly	U	A
		Val	Ala	Asp	Gly	C	G
		Val	Ala	Glu	Gly	A	T
		Val	Ala	Glu	Gly	G	C

Amino acid abbreviations:

Phe = phenylalanine
Ser = serine
Tyr = tyrosine
Cys = cysteine
Leu = leucine
Trp = tryptophan
Pro = proline
His = histidine
Arg = arginine
Gln = glutamine

Ile = isoleucine
Thr = threonine
Asn = asparagine
Lys = lysine
Met = methionine
Val = valine
Ala = alanine
Asp = aspartic acid
Gly = glycine
Glu = glutamic acid

FIGURE 2-12. DNA/RNA genetic code.

the nucleotide is uridine 5'-phosphate. Structures for ribose and uracil are given in Figure 2-13. Compare these to the structures of deoxyribose and thymine given earlier.

There are three species of ribonucleic acid, each with defined functions: *messenger* RNA (mRNA), *ribosomal* RNA (rRNA), and *transfer* RNA (tRNA). Essentially, messenger RNA is the molecule from which the protein is made, ribosomal RNA is the major constituent of ribosomes (the structures on which the protein is made), and transfer RNA is the molecule that brings the proper amino acid into place as

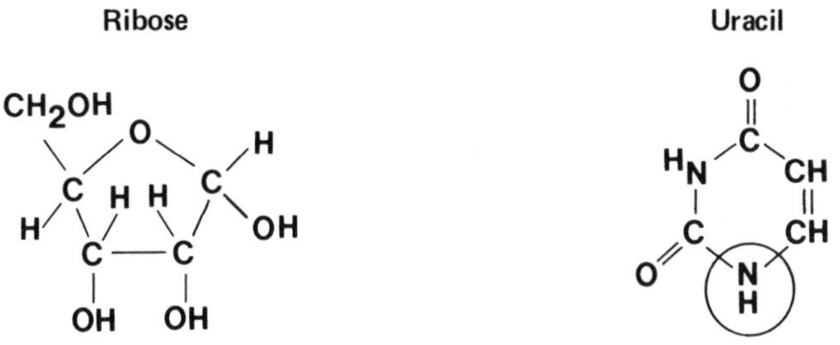

Ribose

Uracil

FIGURE 2-13. Structures of ribose and uracil.

the protein is constructed. All are derived from the information encoded in the DNA. Exactly how mRNA, rRNA, and tRNA are made from DNA is beyond the scope of this chapter. We call the process of production of RNA *transcription*; it requires an enzyme, RNA polymerase. Messenger RNA is then *translated* into protein according to the genetic code. Note that RNAs are complementary to the DNA strand from which they are transcribed. In Figure 2-12, both the DNA code and the complementary RNA code are shown. There is a tRNA specific for each mRNA triplet, which we call a *codon*, and also specific for the proper amino acid. The tRNA has an *anticodon* that recognizes the mRNA codon and positions the amino acid; thus, an anticodon is complementary to its codon.

TRANSLATION OF MESSENGER RNA: PRODUCTION OF PROTEINS

Protein production is usually discussed in three phases: *initiation, elongation,* and *termination*. Initiation refers to the process by which all the complex macromolecules are brought together to begin the production of a protein. Elongation is the mechanism through which specified amino acids are linked through peptide bonds to form the protein—the polypeptide chain. Termination is the signal for and release of the finished polypeptide.

You will have noted the added complexity introduced by all this into our concept of the gene. DNA also specifies rRNA and tRNA, as well as the essential protein-specifying "gene material," mRNA. As knowledge accumulated, genes were redefined using a concept known as "one gene, one polypeptide chain," and other names such as cistron and operon began to appear to describe those portions of the DNA that were not involved in making proteins, but were nevertheless vital to their production. It is doubtful that this definition is suitable today, given the recent work, particularly on immunoglobulins, from which we now know that messages can be varied by processes as yet incompletely understood, and genes themselves may be varied in given cells.

INITIATION

Proteins are formed by linkage of the amino group of one amino acid to the carboxyl (acid) group of the next:

$$NH_2 \quad C\!-\!\!\fbox{OHH}\!-\!N \quad C-OH$$

All protein synthesis, however, begins with an amino acid called N-formyl methionine. In this amino acid, the amino group is "blocked" by the N-formyl group, and thus cannot participate in peptide linkage. In this way, the linkages of further amino acids can only proceed in one direction. The carboxyl group of N-formyl methionine is attached to the amino group of the next amino acid, and the carboxyl group of this amino acid to the amino group of the next to be added, and so on.

Proteins are formed on ribosomes, which are complex structures made up of proteins and rRNA. Each ribosome is composed of two subunits, one large and one smaller. We call the large one the 60S subunit and the smaller one the 40S subunit, referring to the speed with which they sediment in the ultracentrifuge. Protein synthesis is started by the binding of the tRNA bearing N-formyl methionine to the 40S subunit. This step requires two proteins, called initiation factor 2 and initiation factor 3 (IF2 and IF3), and a supply of energy. Most biochemical energy is provided by nucleotide polyphosphates, adenine triphosphate (ATP) being the most commonly used. In protein synthesis the energy source is usually guanosine triphosphate (GTP), but some ATP is also consumed.

Once this step has occurred, the mRNA binds to the complex. Another initiation factor (IF4) and ATP are required. It appears that at initiation, the matching of the message with the triplet of bases in the tRNA occurs in exactly the opposite fashion to the majority of synthesis. As we shall see below, the reading of the triplet codons provides the attachment site for each of the amino acids. In initiation, the N-formyl methionine-tRNA/40S ribosome complex attaches the AUG codon of the message. When this is complete, the 60S subunit is complexed, and the process of translation is ready to proceed.

ELONGATION

On the 60S subunit are two "sites," called the A and P sites. In these two sites the joining of amino acids takes place. A diagram (Fig. 2-14) is helpful in following what is relatively simple in essence, but seems difficult when written down.

When the 60S subunit is complexed, the tRNA and its attached N-formyl methionine lie in the P site. Another protein is required, elongation factor 1 (EF-1) plus GTP. Three bases in the mRNA (i.e., the next codon) now attract and direct the next tRNA with its attached amino acid into the A site. The tRNA is a rigid, somewhat cloverleaf-shaped molecule, as represented below:

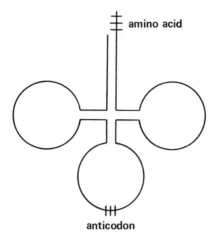

The shape of the molecule is due to internal bonding between complementary base pairs, similar to the bonding in DNA. At the top the amino acid is attached, and at the base is a three-base anticodon, which base pairs with the codon in mRNA. Each amino acid has a specific tRNA with the appropriate anticodon. An enzyme, peptidyl transferase, then catalyzes the peptide bond formation between the two amino acids.

Another enzyme, aminoacyl synthetase, "loads" the amino acid onto its tRNA. ATP provides the energy for this linking. Exactly how the tRNA recognizes its amino acid is not yet known.

A further elongation factor (EF-2) and considerable energy is required for the next step, called translocation. Both the mRNA and the linked amino acids are moved. The most recently attached amino acid moves from the A to the P site, and the N-formyl methionine leaves the ribosome. Now the next codon of mRNA is opposite the A site, and the next tRNA and its attached amino acid are brought into the A site. Repeating this process over and over again, the polypeptide grows until the termination signal in mRNA is reached.

TERMINATION

There are three codons that signal the completion of the protein (see Fig. 2-12). As one might expect by this time, termination requires a protein, called releasing factor (RF), and energy, supplied by GTP. Unlike the two preceding steps, in this case the codon recognizes and binds RF in the A site, not a tRNA. When this happens, a perturbation of the peptidyl transferase enzyme occurs, which now catalyzes the hydrolysis of the bond between the final amino acid, in the P site, and its tRNA. When this occurs the protein floats free from the ribosome, RF is released, the ribosome subunits separate, and the process is complete.

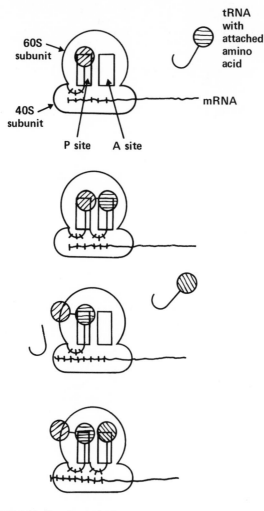

60S subunit	Complex of 40S subunit, first amino acid and its tRNA, and mRNA associate with 60S subunit. Next mRNA codon is opposite A site, attracting next tRNA and amino acid. First amino acid is bound to P site.
tRNA with attached amino acid	
mRNA	
40S subunit	
P site A site	

tRNA of next amino acid pairs with mRNA codon. Amino acid is bound in A site. Peptide bond formed between amino acids.

Complex is translocated. First amino acid leaves ribosome, and its tRNA floats free. Second amino acid is bound in P site. Next amino acid and its tRNA attracted to A site.

Third amino acid bound in A site. Peptide bond formed between second and third amino acids. Third and fourth steps now repeat until polypeptide is complete.

FIGURE 2-14. Protein synthesis.

We have only a few more points. First, apparently a single message can be simultaneously translated on more than one ribosome. As the AUG initiator codon leaves the first ribosome, it can eventually complex with another 40S subunit and begin another copy of the protein. This conservation of message is obviously useful if large quantities of a protein are required in a hurry.

Second, when mRNA dissociates from the ribosomes, it is rapidly degraded by enzymes. In other words, mRNA is only present when the protein is being made. This provides a control mechanism so that cells make just the proteins they require.

Third, the polypeptide chain may undergo some alteration before the cell transports it to its final destination. Although all proteins begin with the same amino acid, we do not find this amino acid when we analyze proteins. We know, from sequence analysis of the bases in mRNA, that the final protein is often "scissored" at both ends. After this, the protein folds into its characteristic shape through natural interactions between the amino acids and the intracellular environment. This alteration of proteins should not be too surprising, since clotting of blood requires the alteration of the inactive protein prothrombin to the active enzyme thrombin. Similar creation of active enzymes occurs in the complement cascade.

DNA TRANSCRIPTION AND REPLICATION

Transcription of DNA to form RNA occurs only in one direction. One can examine two complementary DNA strands, such as

TATGCCTTA— strand 1
ATACGGAAT— strand 2 (complementary)

If we transcribe the first strand from left to right, we would produce the following RNA:

AUACGGAAU

and (referring to Fig. 2-12) this codes for the following three amino acids:

isoleucine-arginine-asparagine

Transcribing the first strand right to left would produce

UAAGGCAUA

and code for

termination-glycine-isoleucine

Similarly, for strand 2 we would get

UAUGCCUUA
tyrosine-alanine-leucine

and

AUUCCGUAU
isoleucine-proline-tyrosine

Obviously, this is unsatisfactory. Each possibility produces a different protein. How then do we control the production of a protein? On each strand of DNA there are encoded signals: "starter" regions. When RNA polymerase initiates transcription, it binds to such a region and then travels in *one direction only*. If you remember, we remarked that we would return to the importance of the 3′ and 5′ linkage positions in the deoxyribose molecule. Remember, DNA is joined as follows:

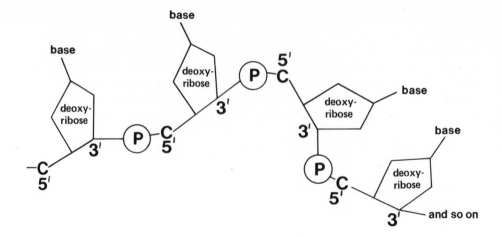

Transcription proceeds only in a 5′ → 3′ direction.

DNA produces copies of itself—replicates—in similar fashion. In this case the enzyme is DNA polymerase. This enzyme also repairs and corrects errors in transcription, but that is beyond the scope of this introductory chapter. You can find this well described in several of the books listed in the Bibliography. From these descriptions, the basis for meiosis, mitosis, and gene action should now be clear.

MUTATION

A change in a base in DNA can lead to a change in the amino acid incorporated into the polypeptide. It may not *necessarily* do so, because of the redundancy of the genetic code. We call such a change a *point mutation*. These changes can be brought about by radiation (particularly ultraviolet light) or chemical damage. Mutations of this type should be identifiable when we analyze the amino acids of the original protein and its mutant offspring. We know several: for example, the simple substitution of valine for glutamic acid in the β-chain of sickle hemoglobin. Importantly, when we examine the genetic code for these two amino acids, their codons should differ by but a single base. They do (refer to Fig 2-12): either GAA to GUA or GAG to GUG provides the change seen.

Alternatively, a message can be read incorrectly, perhaps because a base is missing, or an extra base is accidentally inserted. This causes a completely different result. Past the point at which the change occurs, an entirely new polypeptide region will result, since the triplet reading pattern is moved one base. We call this a *frame-shift mutation*.

Changes in proteins caused by mutation can result in ineffective proteins and genetic disease. This is the subject of many books, and we have made rapid advances in our understanding as we discovered the underlying molecular biology. Alternatively, a protein may function better than its predecessor, providing the advantage by which natural selection operates and preserves the favorable mutation.

CONCLUSION

This necessarily brief chapter is intended as an introduction to the subject of genetics. From it, one should derive enough information to understand blood group genetics and the mathematics of blood group systems, and also an understanding of the basic mechanisms by which glycosyltransferases and other protein gene products are produced. You might also desire to know more about subjects such as chromosomal aberrations, disorders of the sex chromosomes, multifactorial inheritance, studies with twins and chimeras, genetic counseling, prenatal genetic diagnosis, controls of gene action, mechanisms by which genetic diversity (particularly of immunoglobulins) is produced, and inborn errors of metabolism. The Bibliography is designed as a starting point.

BIBLIOGRAPHY

CASKEY, CT: *Peptide chain termination*. Trends in Biochemical Sciences 5:234, 1980.

CLARK, B: *The elongation step of protein biosynthesis*. Trends in Biochemical Sciences 5:207, 1980.

EDWARDS, JA: *Human Genetics*. Chapman & Hall, London, 1978.

GIBLETT, ER: *Genetic Markers in Human Blood*. Blackwell Scientific, Oxford, 1969.

HUNT, T: *The initiation of protein synthesis*. Trends in Biochemical Sciences 5:178, 1980.

McKUSICK, VA and CLAIBORNE, R: *Medical Genetics*. HP Publishing, New York, 1973.

MOURANT, AE, KOPEĆ, AC and DOMANIEWSKA-SOBCZAK, K: *The Distribution of the Human Blood Groups and Other Polymorphisms*, ed 2. Oxford University Press, Oxford, 1976.

MOURANT, AE, KOPEĆ, AC and DOMANIEWSKA-SOBCZAK, K: *Blood Groups and Diseases*. Oxford University Press, Oxford, 1978.

RACE, RR and SANGER, R: *Blood Groups in Man*, ed 6. Blackwell Scientific, Oxford, 1975.

SRB, AM, OWEN, RD and EDGAR, RS (eds): *Facets of Genetics*. WH Freeman, San Francisco, 1970.

STANBURY, JB, WYNGAARDEN, JB and FREDRICKSON, DS: *The Metabolic Basis of Inherited Disease*, ed 4. McGraw-Hill, New York, 1978.

STEVENSON, AC and DAVISON, BCC: *Genetic Counselling*, ed 2. JB Lippincott, Philadelphia, 1976.

THOMPSON, JS and THOMPSON, MW: *Genetics in Medicine*, ed 3. WB Saunders, Philadelphia, 1980.

VALENTINE, GH: *The Chromosome Disorders*, ed 3. JB Lippincott, Philadelphia, 1975.

WATSON, JD: *Double Helix: Being a Personal Account of the Discovery of the Structure of DNA*. Atheneum, New York, 1968.

WATSON, JD: *Molecular Biology of the Gene*, ed 3. WA Benjamin, Menlo Park, California, 1976.

WIDMANN, FK (ed): *Blood group immunogenetics*. In *Technical Manual of the American Association of Blood Banks*, ed 8. American Association of Blood Banks, Washington, DC, 1981, ch 8, pp. 99–104.

WOODS, RA: *Biochemical Genetics*. Chapman & Hall, London, 1973.

CHAPTER **3**

FUNDAMENTALS OF BLOOD GROUP IMMUNOLOGY

ELLIOTT KAGAN, M.D.

The immune system has evolved as a highly specialized adaptive function of vertebrates and is concerned with the recognition and elimination of substances considered "foreign" to the organism. It consists of a cellular component (primarily lymphocytes, plasma cells, and macrophages) and a humoral component (essentially comprising the antibody proteins and the complement system). Certain immunologic reactions also involve the participation of other mediator cells, including neutrophils, eosinophils, basophils, mast cells, and platelets. Since the field of blood group serology is mainly associated with the humoral arm of the immune system, only a brief overview will be given of the cellular immune system. More detailed descriptions are provided in other texts.[1-3]

CELLULAR IMMUNE APPARATUS

The lymphoid cells of the body are aggregated in specialized lymphoid organs such as the thymus, tonsils, lymph nodes, and spleen. They are also found as localized lymphoid collections in the bone marrow and beneath the mucosa of the respiratory and gastrointestinal tracts. There is a free communication between various lymphoid structures and the blood. All lymphoid cells are derived from common ancestral hemopoietic stem cells, which originate from the fetal yolk sac, the fetal liver, and from the bone marrow. Thereafter, the progeny of these stem cells may follow at least two independent pathways of development (Fig. 3-1). Some lymphocytes traffic through the thymus or are influenced by thymic hormones. These cells are thus referred to as *thymic-dependent* or *T lymphocytes.* Other lymphocytes are not processed by the thymus and, since they are bone marrow-derived, are designated *B lymphocytes.* By a process of morphologic and functional differentiation,

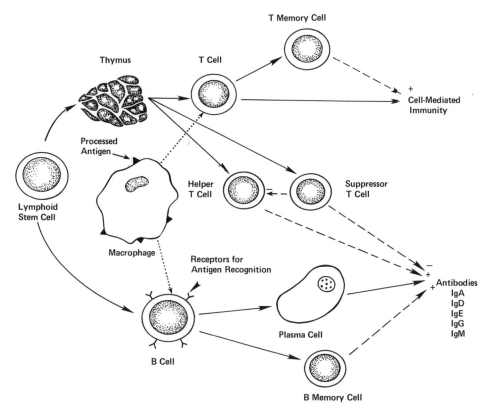

FIGURE 3-1. Schematic representation of the cellular immune apparatus. The events relating to cell-mediated immunity are beyond the scope of this text but are important in transplant rejection and in the body's defenses against cancer and against infection by certain bacteria, viruses, fungi, and parasites. The macrophage is involved in the processing and presentation of antigens to T and B cells. + = Enhancement of immune function; − = suppression of immune function.

B lymphocytes mature into plasma cells that secrete antibodies. There are several distinct subsets of T lymphocytes, some of which discretely regulate the amount of antibody produced by the B lymphocyte series. There are thus *helper T cells* (which augment B cell antibody production) and *suppressor T cells* (which inhibit antibody production). From this, it is apparent that the function of the immune apparatus is finely "tuned" by a number of regulatory influences that involve the collaboration of T cells and B cells. A variety of lymphocyte marker techniques can be used to identify both T and B lymphocytes in the blood and other organs. Table 3-1 lists the more commonly used techniques for identification of T and B cells. For instance, T cells (through a quirk of nature) have the ability to bind sheep erythrocytes, whereas B cells possess easily detectable amounts of antibodies on their cell surfaces. By identifying these characteristics, it can be shown that circulating lymphocytes in the peripheral blood comprise approximately 60 to 75 percent T cells and 15 to 30 percent B cells.[4]

TABLE 3-1. Techniques Most Commonly Used for Identification of T Cells and B Cells

	T Cells	B Cells	Comments
Rosette methods			Cytocentrifuge preparations are of value in evaluating lymphomas.
Spontaneous sheep red cell E rosette	+	−	Most useful T-cell marker.
EAC (IgM) (Compl. rec.)	(+)	+	Probably some T cells. Convoluted T-cell lymphomas are observed with complement receptors.
EA (IgG) (Fc receptor)	−	+	Limited usefulness.
Surface Ig*	−	+	By immunofluorescence. Monocytes may mark because of Fc receptors.
Cytoplasmic Ig	−	+	Immunoperoxidase more useful than immuno-fluorescence in lymphomas because it can be used on paraffin sections.
Antisera			
HTLA	+	−	Antigen source: thymus, brain; specificity is a problem.
HBLA	−	+	Antigen source: CLL cells, B lymphoblastoid cell lines; specificity is a problem.
Cytochemistry			
α-Naphthyl butyrase (NSE)	(+)	−	Focal staining reported in T cells. Specificity for T cells is not proved.
Acid phosphatase	(+)	−	Reported in convoluted T cell and T-cell ALL.
Tartrate-resistant acid phosphatase	−	(+)	Hairy cell leukemia.
Muramidase (lysozyme)	−	−	Immunoperoxidase method on paraffin sections or imprints.

*T cells have a small amount of surface Ig not detected by immunofluorescent methods.
Ig = Immunoglobulin; HTLA = human T-lymphocyte antibody; HBLA = human B-lymphocyte antibody; NSE = nonspecific esterase. Parentheses indicate that the finding lacks specificity, is controversial, or is seen only with certain types of lymphoma-leukemia. (Modified from Lukes, RJ, et al.: *A morphologic and immunologic surface marker study of 299 cases of non-Hodgkin's lymphomas and related leukemias.* Am J Pathol 90:463, 1978.)

IMMUNE RESPONSE

"Foreign" substances that are capable of stimulating the immune system are called *antigens*. When the immune apparatus is exposed to an antigenic stimulus, a series of orchestrated immunologic events occur. These are collectively designated the *immune* response. In order to be rendered antigenic, a substance must first be "processed" by mononuclear phagocytic cells (macrophages) residing within the liver, spleen, lymph nodes, and other reticuloendothelial organs. After macrophage processing, the antigen is "recognized" by a small number of genetically preprogrammed T and B cells, which are then transformed into mitotically active *immunoblasts*. The process of antigen recognition is governed by specific surface receptors for the antigen on the preprogrammed T and B cells. An important end product of the immune response to a given antigen is the production of specific antibody against that antigen by plasma cells. (Remember, however, that the immune response may not always be characterized by detectable circulating antibodies, as in cell-mediated immune responses such as graft rejection. As a result, the term *immunogen* has been suggested to replace the term antigen.) Since only a small proportion of the body's immune repertoire is involved in an immune response to a specific antigen at any time, each individual is capable of reacting to a large number of different antigens. Once the immune system has been "primed" after its first encounter with an antigen, the individual becomes *sensitized* to that antigen. This process of sensitization is associated with the development of specific *immunologic memory* for the antigen, which is mediated by both T and B "memory cells" (see Fig. 3-1). This has important clinical implications, since subsequent encounters with that antigen will evoke an accentuated immune response in a previously sensitized individual. Thus, an Rh-negative mother who becomes sensitized to her Rh-positive fetus (as evidenced by detectable anti-Rh antibodies in her serum) is likely to produce an enhanced antibody response in a subsequent Rh-positive pregnancy, or if she is transfused with Rh-positive blood.

Antibodies belong to a group of proteins that are mainly (but not exclusively) located within the gamma globulin fraction of serum. For this reason, antibodies are also designated *immunoglobulins.* When antibodies are produced in response to heterologous antigens (*xenoantigens*) of another species (as in the production of antisera for the Coombs' antiglobulin test—see Chapter 4), they are classed as *xenoantibodies* or *heteroantibodies.* When directed against antigens belonging to genetically different individuals of the same species (*alloantigens*), they are termed *alloantibodies* or *isoantibodies.* These are the immunoglobulins that cause transfusion-related problems. Antibodies that react against an individual's own antigenic determinants are referred to as *autoantibodies.*

PRIMARY AND SECONDARY IMMUNE RESPONSES

When an individual is first exposed to a foreign antigenic stimulus, there is an initial period of latency, during which no antibody response is detectable in the subject's serum. The duration of this latent period may extend from a few days to several months and is influenced by a number of factors, including the dose, solubility, and immunogenicity of the antigen. The earliest immune response is known as *the primary response* and is characterized by the detection in the subject's serum of increasing quantities of specific antibodies (Fig. 3-2). The antibody concentration soon reaches a plateau and then gradually declines to baseline (unstimulated) levels. The immunoglobulins constituting the primary immune response are predominantly of the IgM class, but are soon replaced by IgG antibodies.

After a subsequent exposure to the same antigen, there is a much shorter latent period, followed by a vigorous *secondary antibody response*, which peaks earlier and declines very slowly (see Fig. 3-2). The exuberant secondary response is the result of the generation of antigen-specific memory cells (which are both T and B cells) during the primary response to antigen. These memory cells amplify the sec-

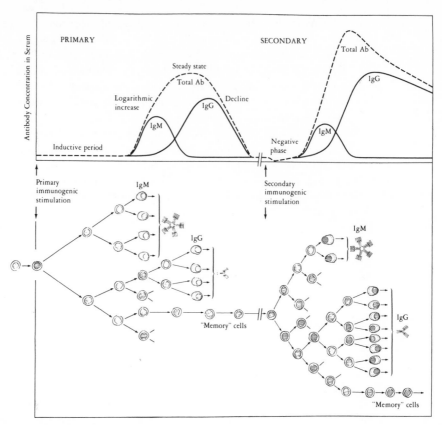

FIGURE 3-2. Schematic representation of primary and secondary (anamnestic) antibody responses. Note the greater antibody production and enhanced cellular activity seen during anamnestic response. (From Bellanti,[1] with permission.)

ondary response. The antibodies constituting the secondary response are almost exclusively of the IgG variety, with variable amounts of IgA and an evanescent IgM component. These immunoglobulins have a higher avidity for antigen and are produced at significantly lower doses of antigen than antibodies produced during the primary response. The importance of these phenomena in blood banking practice is seen in Rh-negative individuals who receive Rh-positive red cells. Unimmunized subjects may require a dose of at least 200 to 300 ml of Rh-positive erythrocytes before they are able to manifest a primary anti-Rh response. Previously sensitized individuals may, however, mount a brisk secondary anti-Rh response after the administration of as little as 0.1 ml of Rh-positive red cells.[3]

CHARACTERISTICS OF ANTIGENS

Not all substances are antigenic. Antigens are generally structurally complex molecules whose molecular weights usually exceed 10,000 daltons.[1] There is, however, considerable structural diversity among antigens. Red cell antigens, for instance, may be proteins, such as the Rh, M, and N blood group substances, or glycolipids, such as the ABH, Lewis, Ii, and P blood group substances. The HLA antigens, on the other hand, are glycoproteins, whereas the hepatitis B surface antigen (HB$_s$Ag) is a lipoprotein.[3,5] Paradoxically, antibodies may also under certain circumstances become antigenic. This explains why rabbits produce antibodies against human immunoglobulins after they have been immunized with purified human serum immunoglobulin fractions. These "anti-antibodies" are used as reagents in the Coombs' antiglobulin test.

A number of characteristics influence antigenicity. These include the molecular size and charge, solubility, the three-dimensional conformation or shape, and biologic and chemical properties of the antigen. The portion of the antigenic molecule that is directly involved in the interaction with antibody is designated the *antigenic determinant* or *epitope*.

TISSUE DISTRIBUTION OF ANTIGENS

Some blood group substances are widely distributed throughout the tissues. The ABH antigens are found on virtually all cells, and the serologically defined HLA antigens are found on all nucleated cells and occasionally on red cells.[3] Other blood group antigens, however, have a more restricted tissue distribution. Kell blood group substances, with one exception, are found only on red cells.[6] The immune associated (Ia) antigens, which are important in lymphocyte typing, are restricted to spermatozoa, B cells, monocytes, and macrophages.[3] It should be noted that a few blood group substances are detectable not only on red cells, but also in some body fluids. Saliva is a source of ABH, I, Lewis (Le^{a}Le^b), and Sd^a antigens, whereas milk contains I blood group substances.[3] These body fluids can be used to neutralize the agglutinating effect of specific serum antibodies in vitro.

Certain antigens (especially those of the Rh system) are integral structural components of the red cell membrane. When these antigens are genetically absent (as in some Rh-null individuals), the erythrocyte membrane is defective and this results in the development of a hemolytic anemia. When, however, antigens do not form part of the essential membrane structure of red cells (as occurs with ABH antigens), their absence (as reflected in individuals of the "Bombay" phenotype) does not predispose to early red cell destruction.[8]

CHARACTERISTICS OF IMMUNOGLOBULINS

There are five classes of immunoglobulins (Ig) in human body fluids. These classes have been designated IgA, IgD, IgE, IgG, and IgM. Individual immunoglobulin classes differ with respect to molecular size, carbohydrate content (all are glycoproteins), biologic activity, and plasma half-life, as illustrated in Table 3-2. Although IgA is the main immunoglobulin component of external secretions such as saliva, the predominant immunoglobulin in serum is IgG. Thus, approximately 80 percent of the

TABLE 3-2. Characteristics of Serum Immunoglobulins

Characteristic	IgA	IgD	IgE	IgG	IgM
Heavy chain type	Alpha	Delta	Epsilon	Gamma	Mu
Sedimentation coefficient(s)	7–15*	7	8	6.7	19
Molecular weight (daltons)	160,000–500,000*	180,000	196,000	150,000	900,000
Biologic half-life (days)	5.8	2.8	2.3	21	5.1
Carbohydrate (%)	7.5–9	10–13	11–12	2.2–3.5	7–14
Placental transfer	No	No	No	Yes	No
Complement fixation (classic pathway)	−	−	−	+	+++
Agglutination in saline	+	−	−	±	++++
Heavy chain allotypes	A_m	No	No	G_m	No
Percentage of total immunoglobulin	13	1	0.002	80	6

*May occur in monomeric or polymeric forms.

total serum immunoglobulin is IgG, 13 percent is IgA, 6 percent is IgM, and 1 percent is IgD, while IgE is normally present in only trace amounts.[2] The serum levels of IgA, IgG, and IgM are influenced by a number of factors, notably age and race. The concentrations of these immunoglobulins are lowest soon after birth and increase progressively with advancing age, generally peaking during adolescence. Several studies have shown that adult blacks have significantly higher serum immunoglobulin levels than whites in similar geographic locations.[5]

IMMUNOGLOBULIN STRUCTURE

All immunoglobulins share a common chemical structural configuration (Fig. 3-3). Each basic antibody unit is composed of four polypeptide chains: two identical light chains (with molecular weights of approximately 22,500 daltons) and two identical heavy chains (ranging in molecular weight from approximately 50,000 to 75,000 daltons).[1] The four chains are held together by covalent disulfide bonds. Thus, the two heavy chains are interconnected by disulfide linkages in an area of the molecule termed the *hinge region.* Similar forces tether each light chain to a heavy chain. The chemical structure of the heavy chain is responsible for the diversity of immunoglobulin classes, and the five types of heavy chain are designated alpha (in IgA), delta (in IgD), epsilon (in IgE), gamma (in IgG), and mu (in IgM). There are, on the other hand, only two types of light chains (designated kappa or lambda) that are common to all classes of immunoglobulins. In most instances, approximately two thirds of antibodies of any particular specificity contain kappa light chains and only one third contains lambda light chains.[2] Such antibodies are termed *polyclonal immunoglobulins,* since they are derived from multiple ancestral clones of antibody producing cells. In certain select situations, however, all antibodies of a given specificity may contain exclusively kappa or exclusively lambda light chains, but not both light chain varieties. These immunoglobulins of a more restricted nature are termed *monoclonal antibodies,* since they are derived entirely from a single ancestral antibody-forming

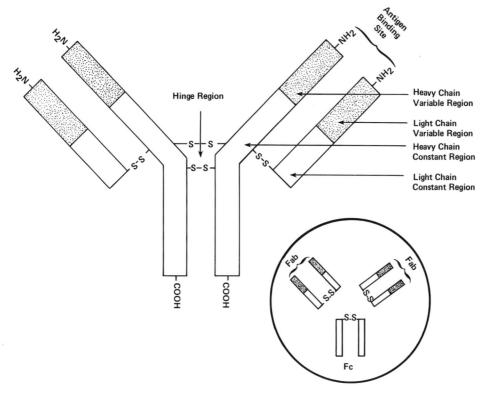

FIGURE 3-3. Schematic representation of basic immunoglobulin structure. The inset shows formation of Fab and Fc fragments after enzymatic cleavage of the IgG molecule by papain.

parent cell. The most notable examples of monoclonal antibodies that are likely to be encountered by blood bankers are to be found in patients with chronic cold hemagglutinin disease, a type of autoimmune hemolytic anemia associated with IgM antibodies directed against red cells (see Chapter 19). Rare examples of IgA or IgG monoclonal red cell agglutinins have been described in other clinical states.[3]

Analysis of the amino acid sequences of immunoglobulins has shown that a portion of the carboxyl ($-$COOH) terminal region of the heavy chain has a relatively constant amino acid sequence within any given antibody class. Analogous *constant regions* are present on the $-$COOH terminal portions of the immunoglobulin light chains. These constant regions of the molecule consequently play no role in the determination of antibody specificity for a given antigen. Each immunoglobulin molecule is, however, uniquely equipped to recognize its specific homologous antigen by virtue of the structural arrangement and characteristic amino acid sequences of the amino ($-$NH$_2$) terminal regions of the light and heavy chains. These $-$NH$_2$ terminal portions of the molecule are known as the *variable regions* of the light and heavy chains, since they account for the variations in antibody specificity against different antigens in nature. Embedded within the variable regions of adjacent light and heavy chains is the *antigen-combining site* of the molecule, which is also referred to as the antibody's *idiotype*. There is, thus, a reciprocal relationship between the idiotype and its corresponding antigenic epitope, a situation analogous to the "fit" of a lock and key.

Each light and heavy chain contains certain regions that are folded into compact globular loops designated *domains* (Fig. 3-4). The domains are stabilized by intrachain covalent disulfide bonds. There is one domain (designated V_L) in the variable region and one domain (designated C_L) in the constant region of each light chain. There is, similarly, one variable domain (designated V_H) on each heavy chain. The number of domains on the constant regions of each heavy chain is determined by the immunoglobulin class. Thus, there are four constant domains (numbered C_H1 to C_H4) on the heavy chains of IgA, IgD, and IgG and five constant domains (numbered C_H1 to C_H5) on the heavy chains of IgE and IgM.[1] It is believed that the antigen-binding idiotypic region of the antibody molecule is located within three-dimensional pockets created by the V_L and V_H domains.[9] Some of the biologic properties that are peculiar to IgG and IgM immunoglobulins appear to relate to certain constant domains on their heavy chains, since complement fixation is associated with the C_H2 domain. On the other hand, the cytophilic attachment of IgL on the macrophage cell membrane involves the C_H3 domain.

By treating the intact immunoglobulin with papain, it is possible to cleave the antibody molecule into three component parts (see Fig. 3-3): two identical antigen-

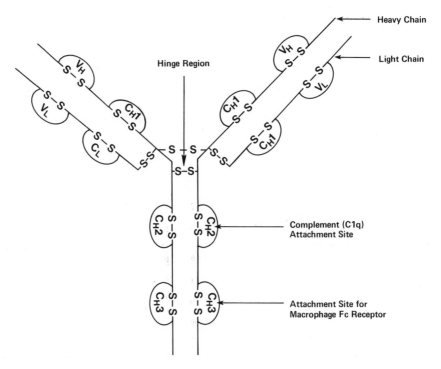

FIGURE 3-4. Schematic illustration of the domain structure within the IgG molecule.

MODERN BLOOD BANKING AND TRANSFUSION PRACTICES

binding fragments (Fab) and one crystalline fragment (Fc). The Fc fragment has diverse biologic functions, including complement activation, placental transfer, and macrophage attachment.

MONOMERIC AND POLYMERIC EXPRESSION OF IMMUNOGLOBULINS

Immunoglobulins D, E, and G are present in monomeric form in serum. Antibodies of the IgM variety, however, exist as pentamers comprising five identical monomeric subunits of IgM linked by covalent disulfide bridges and arranged in a circular fashion, as illustrated in Figure 3-5. Approximately 90 percent of serum IgA immunoglobulins are monomeric; the remainder occurs as dimers or trimers.[3] All polymerized expressions of immunoglobulins contain an additional chain, designated the J chain, which is a glycopolypeptide of approximately 15,000 daltons.[9] Since the polymerized molecules have significantly larger molecular weights than the monomeric varieties, their sedimentation coefficients are greater (see Table 3-2).

The pentameric configuration of IgM can be dissociated via the cleavage of covalent bonds interconnecting monomeric subunits and the J chain. This is usually accomplished by gentle reduction with sulfhydryl compounds such as 2-mercaptoethanol or dithiothreitol. These agents are commonly used in immunohematology to distinguish

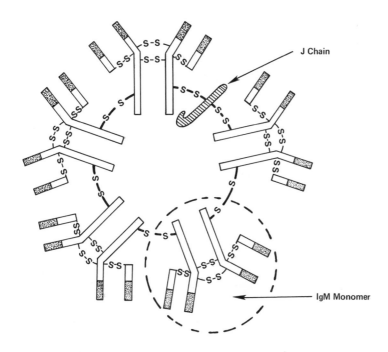

FIGURE 3-5. Schematic representation of the pentameric configuration of IgM immunoglobulin.

TABLE 3-3. Biologic Properties of IgG Isotypes

Characteristic	IgG_1	IgG_2	IgG_3	IgG_4
% Total serum IgG	65–70	23–28	4–7	3–4
Complement fixation (classic pathway)	Yes	Yes	Yes	No
Binding to macrophage Fc receptors	Yes	No	Yes	No
Placental transfer	Yes	Yes	Yes	Yes
Biologic half-life (days)	21	21	7–8	21

between IgM and IgG hemagglutinins, since only IgM agglutinating activity will be abolished by the use of such compounds.

IMMUNOGLOBULIN SUBCLASSES

The use of antisera obtained from animals immunized with different preparations of purified monoclonal human IgG has shown that IgG antibodies vary in their antigenic make-up. These studies have demonstrated that IgG immunoglobulins in serum are heterogeneous and are composed of four different *subclasses:* IgG_1, IgG_2, IgG_3, and IgG_4. The various subclasses reflect subtle differences in chemical structure within the constant regions of the gamma heavy chains.[3] These differences chiefly relate to the number of disulfide bonds bridging the two heavy chains in the hinge region of the molecule, and they account for variations in electrophoretic mobility and in biologic properties of the IgG subclasses. The distribution of IgG subclasses in normal serum and their major biologic characteristics are summarized in Table 3-3.

In most instances, IgG antibodies of a single specificity tend to show a "spread" of all four subclasses. In some situations, however, the antibodies tend to be predominantly or exclusively of one IgG subclass. Thus, anti-Rh antibodies are predominantly of the IgG_1 and IgG_3 subclasses, while anti-K (Kell) and anti-Fy^a (Duffy) antibodies are generally exclusively of the IgG_1 subclass. Anti-Jk^a (Kidd) immunoglobulins, however, are mainly of the IgG_3 variety. Patients with idiopathic thrombocytopenic purpura have an IgG immunoglobulin in their serum that is directed against platelets and that has been shown to be restricted to the IgG_3 subclass. Curiously, when hemophiliacs develop antibodies against the factor VIII coagulant protein, which they lack, the immunoglobulin has been shown to be of the IgG_4 subclass.

The reason for the biologic differences in subclass expression is an enigma, but these variations in immunologic responsiveness may possibly have underlying clinical significance. It is of interest that in one study of mothers whose infants developed Rh hemolytic disease of the newborn, those with IgG_3 antibodies had more severely affected infants than those whose antibodies were exclusively of the IgG_1 variety.[3] Subclasses have also been defined with respect to IgA (IgA_1 and IgA_2), and there is some evidence that IgD and IgM subclasses may also exist.

IMMUNOGLOBULIN ALLOTYPES

There are inherited variations of immunoglobulin structure between different individuals in the same way that there are inherited blood group differences. These genetic variations are termed immunoglobulin allotypes and are located on the C_L domains of kappa light chains (K_m markers), on the constant domains of IgA (A_m markers), and on the constant domains of IgG (G_m markers). Three K_m, two IgA, and seventeen IgG allotypic determinants have been defined. These genetic markers are inherited in an autosomal codominant fashion and exhibit isotype restriction, since they are not present on IgA_1 or IgG_4 subclasses of immunoglobulins.[9]

Typing for allotypic determinants is becoming a widely used resource in the field of immunohematology. G_m typing is employed in paternity exclusion testing and in studies of population genetics. Recently, an association has been shown between some G_m phenotypes and certain autoimmune diseases. The inheritance of specific G_m phenotypes may also determine, to some extent, the ability of an individual to mount an antibody response of a given immunoglobulin subclass. The genes that determine allotype expression may thus subserve an additional biologic role as "immune response regulators," in a manner analogous to genes residing within the HLA system.

Antibodies against G_m and A_m allotypic determinants are usually the consequence of maternal alloimmunization after multiple pregnancies or alloimmunization in patients who have received multiple transfusions of blood, plasma, or gamma globulin. Antibodies against A_m allotypes have been implicated in some transfusion reactions.

INDUCTION OF IMMUNOLOGIC UNRESPONSIVENESS

It has been shown in a variety of experimental situations that the immune system can be rendered selectively unresponsive or "tolerant" to a specific antigen. There are various ways of inducing *specific immunologic unresponsiveness*, including exposure to antigen during earliest fetal life. This occurs in the occasional human *chimera* who receives an unsolicited cross-transfusion of ABO-incompatible blood-forming cells from a dizygotic (nonidentical) twin sibling in utero. Such an individual will be a lifelong ABO phenotypic hybrid. The chimera will be permanently unable to mount an antibody response against red cells of the same ABO type as those of the twin sibling.

Of far greater importance in the field of blood banking is the prevention of a primary immune response in Rh-negative subjects who have been exposed to Rh-positive red cells. This exposure is most likely to occur in Rh-negative mothers who have recently delivered Rh-positive infants, or in Rh-negative individuals who have inadvertently received a transfusion of Rh-positive cells. Paradoxically, the immune response to the Rh antigen can be effectively suppressed in these people by the passive administration of IgG Rh immune globulin within 48 to 72 hours of antigenic exposure. The mechansim of suppression of Rh alloimmunization is not understood, but appears to relate to the clearance or elimination of Rh antigen prior to immunologic sensitization.

It is of interest that approximately 30 percent of Rh-negative subjects are unable to produce anti-Rh antibodies in spite of repeated transfusions of incompatible Rh-positive cells.[3] It is not known why there is such a large proportion of "immunologic nonresponders" in the Rh-negative population, but it is tempting to speculate that their immunologic unresponsiveness may be governed by as-yet-undefined "immune response genes."

FACTORS INFLUENCING ANTIGEN-ANTIBODY REACTIONS

Since the center of attention in blood group serology is red cell antigen-antibody reactions, this section will deal exclusively with factors influencing the agglutination of erythrocytes by antibodies. Serologic reactivity is determined by a number of variables that may influence the binding of antigen to its corresponding antibody. The degree of "fit" between antigen and antibody is known as the *binding* or *equilibrium constant*.

The visible clumping or agglutination of a red cell suspension by specific antibody occurs in two stages:

Stage 1. Antigenic determinants on the red cell membrane combine with the antibody idiotype on the variable regions of the immunoglobulin heavy and light chains. Antigen and antibody are held together by noncovalent forces. Visible agglutination does not yet occur.

Stage 2. A firmer union is established between antigen and antibody by the creation of a cohesive infrastructure or lattice (Fig. 3-6). The lattice is composed of multiple antigen-antibody bridges interconnecting adjacent red cells. Thus, a stable network of agglutinated cells is formed.

AGGLUTINATION REACTIONS

Agglutination reactions are routinely graded as a 1+ through 4+ during regular blood bank testing. The reader should refer to Color Plate 2 for examples of the various agglutination reactions.

The degree of positive agglutination reactions is reported differently by different individuals. The American Association of Blood Banks (AABB) recommends the following:

4+ = One solid aggregate of red cells
3+ = Several large aggregates
2+ = Medium-sized aggregates, clear background
1+ = Small aggregates; turbid, reddish background
+w = Tiny aggregates; turbid, reddish background; or microscopic aggregates only
Note: Complete or partial hemolysis = positive reaction

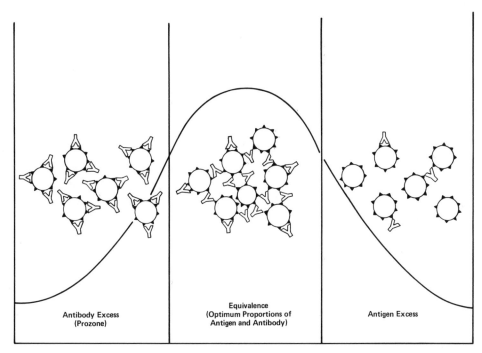

Equivalence
(Optimum Proportions of
Antigen and Antibody)

Antigen Excess

FIGURE 3-6. Schematic representation of the effects of varying concentrations of antigen and antibody on lattice formation.

The student should be aware of pseudoagglutination, which is a false appearance of clumping but not true agglutination. It is usually due to rouleau formation of red cells—a formation in which the cells under the microscope resemble a stack of coins that has been pushed over (see Color Plates 2I and 2J). Rouleau formation is due to high concentrations of globulins in a patient's serum or fibrinogen in plasma. Patients with multiple myeloma and those with high globulin content or abnormal globulins in their sera, as well as those who have received dextran as a plasma expander, frequently show pseudoagglutination in blood grouping tests. Adding a few drops of saline to the reaction and then mixing will usually break up rouleaux. This procedure is known as saline replacement. Saline is added *after, not before,* the reaction. If it is added before a reaction has had sufficient time to occur, it dilutes the antibody before the antibody can react, possibly producing a false-negative reaction. If added after the reaction, the antibody has already reacted and dilution will not affect true agglutination. Evaluation of rouleaux should include both a microscopic examination of the stacked cells as well as the saline replacement technique.

COMPLETE AND INCOMPLETE ANTIBODIES

Most IgM antibodies are capable of agglutinating red cells suspended in 0.85-percent saline medium and are termed complete antibodies. Most IgG antibodies, on the other hand, will not agglutinate erythrocytes in saline medium and are designated incomplete antibodies. These are unfortunate terms, since both antibody varieties are composed of complete immunoglobulin molecules. Their usage is, however, time-honored in blood banking. Examples of complete antibodies include agglutinins against ABH, Ii, MN, Lewis (Le^a, Le^b), Lutheran (Lu^a), and P blood-group determinants. Antibodies directed against Ss, Kell (Kk, Js^a, Js^b), Rh (CDEce), Lu^b, Duffy (Fy^a, Fy^b) and Kidd (Jk^a, Jk^b) antigens are of the incomplete variety.

EFFECT OF SURFACE CHARGE

Red cells normally repel one another because they have a surplus electronegative surface charge. This is due to a high sialic acid content of their cell membranes. When suspended in an ionic medium such as saline, the cations in solution arrange themselves around the erythrocytes in a diffuse double-layered *ionic cloud* (Fig. 3-7). The inner layer of cations is firmly bound to the erythrocytes and moves in tandem with the cells. The cations in the outer layer move freely in the medium. The difference in charge density between the inner and outer layers of the ionic cloud creates an electrostatic potential termed the *zeta potential*. This potential is measured at the boundary zone between the two cloud layers and the value of the zeta potential

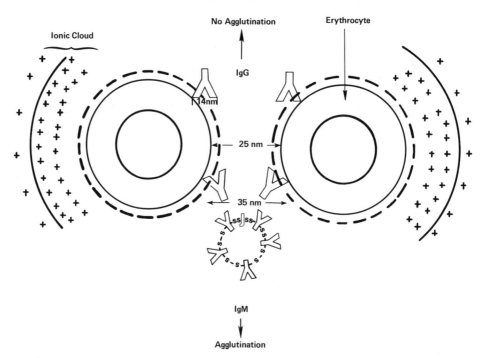

FIGURE 3-7. Schematic representation of the "ionic cloud" concept and its relevance to hemagglutination induced by IgG and IgM antibodies. Compare the size of the "incomplete" IgG antibody with the "complete" IgM molecule. The size of the IgG molecule is not large enough to span the distance between two adjacent red cells.

correlates directly with the distance between two erythrocytes. Under normal circumstances, the forces of mutual repulsion keep the red cells approximately 25 nm apart. Since IgM molecules can span a distance of 35 nm, because of their circular pentameric arrangement, they can effectively overcome the repulsive forces separating the erythrocytes and produce agglutination in saline medium. Because the maximum span of IgG molecules is only on the order of 14 nm, however, lattice formation is unstable and agglutination impossible. This explains the apparent inability of IgG incomplete antibodies to agglutinate red cells in the saline medium.[5] There are several methods whereby incomplete antibodies can be "transformed" into effective hemagglutinins.

PRETREATMENT OF RED CELLS WITH ENZYMES

When red cells are exposed to the action of certain proteolytic enzymes such as papain, bromelin, ficin or trypsin, cell-to-cell contact is enhanced by reduction of the zeta potential. This allows exposure of antigenic sites at defined points on the red cell membrane. The cells are then agglutinable by IgG antibodies, owing to the formation of multiple bridges between clusters on adjacent cells.

USE OF HIGH PROTEIN MEDIA

Various colloidal diluents, such as polymerized albumin, can enhance the agglutinating potential of IgG antibodies. They appear to act by increasing the *dielectric constant* (a measure of electrical conductivity) of the medium. This results in a lowered zeta potential. Other polymers such as polyvinylpyrrolidone (PVP), polybrene, and protamine also act by reducing the red cell electrostatic repulsion.

USE OF ANTIGLOBULIN REAGENTS

The addition of a xenoantibody (anti-human antibody) against human IgG gamma chains will cross-link adjacent IgG-coated erythrocytes to form a stable lattice. Thus, red cells sensitized by incomplete antibodies agglutinate, since the critical 25-nm distance between adjacent red cells has been spanned by the anti-human antibody. This forms the basis for the antiglobulin reaction (see Chapter 4).

CHEMICAL REDUCTION OF THE IgG MOLECULE

It has been recently demonstrated[10] that incomplete IgG antibody can be converted into an effective saline agglutinin by chemical reduction of the immunoglobulin molecule. Cleavage of the interchain disulfide bonds in the "hinge" region of the molecule results in greater flexibility of the immunoglobulin and, consequently, a wider "stretch" capacity. Once again, the net effect is to bridge the gap between adjacent red cells.

EFFECT OF pH

The equilibrium constant is influenced by pH. The binding of the majority of antibodies to red cells is optimal at a slightly acid pH of 6.5 to 7.5.

EFFECT OF TEMPERATURE

Agglutinating antibodies differ with respect to their thermal reactivities. *Cold agglutinins* are optimally reactive in the cold (4°C) and may produce no detectable effect above 20 to 30°C. They can, however, exhibit a wide thermal amplitude over the range of 4 to 37°C. Cold agglutinins are generally of the IgM variety. *Warm agglutinins*, on the other hand, react best at 37°C and are predominantly of the IgG class. Occasionally these antibodies belong to the IgA or IgM classes.

EFFECT OF IONIC STRENGTH

The equilibrium constant for most antibodies can be enhanced in media of low ionic strength. This has the effect of shortening the incubation period needed to demonstrate agglutination and appears to be related to the presence of fewer charged ions within the ionic cloud. Low ionic strength salt solution (LISS) containing 0.2 percent sodium chloride in 7 percent glucose is used for this purpose instead of 0.85 percent saline.

EFFECT OF RED CELL ANTIGEN DOSAGE

The number of antigen-determinant sites per red cell can influence the amount of agglutination. This is particularly well illustrated by the various subgroups of blood group A individuals. Maximal reactivity is obtained in A_1 adults (who have approximately 850,000 antigen sites per cell). Lesser degrees of reactivity are noted in A_2 adults and A_1 newborn children (both of whom have approximately 250,000 antigen sites per cell). Only about 35,000 determinants per cell are found in A_3 individuals, who exhibit even weaker agglutination reactions.[3] Red cells obtained from homozygous individuals (who possess a double dose of antigen) often give stronger reactions than those obtained from heterozygous subjects (who possess a single dose of antigen).

DETERMINATION OF OPTIMAL AMOUNTS OF ANTIGEN AND ANTIBODY

Each monomeric immunoglobulin molecule has two antigen combining sites. Under conditions of relative antibody excess, it is therefore to be expected that there will be a relative surplus of antigen-combining sites which are not bound to antigen (see Fig. 3-6). This produces an incomplete lattice and agglutination does not occur. This effect of excessive antibody concentration is known as the *prozone phenomenon*. It can result in an erroneously false-negative interpretation of an agglutination reaction by an inexperienced serologist. The prozone effect can be overcome simply by performing serial dilutions of the antibody until optimal amounts of antigen and antibody are present in the test system. This corresponds to the *equivalence zone,* where lattice formation is most stable. When, however, there are suboptimal amounts of antibody with respect to antigen, lattice formation again becomes unstable and the agglutination reaction disappears (see Fig. 3-6).

ROLE OF COMPLEMENT

The complement system is composed of at least 20 distinct serum proteins. Some of these proteins have specific enzymatic activity and some of these are inhibitors and regulators. These proteins differ in their size distributions and electrophoretic properties. The complement components discovered originally are numbered sequentially (in their order of discovery) C1 through C9. Some components are designated by letters (factor B and factor D) or trivial names (properdin). A number of complement regulatory proteins have also been defined (B1H, C1 esterase inhibitor, C3b inactivator, and C4 binding protein). The various components are normally present in an inactive state except factor D. Under appropriate circumstances, the inactive precursor molecules are sequentially activated to enzymatically active components. Divalent cations (Ca^{++} and Mg^{++}) are required for some of these processes. The complement proteins or complexes that have enzymatic activity are indicated by a bar symbol placed over the appropriate number or letter (e.g., $\overline{C4,2}$ or factor $\overline{D}$).

During the generation of a complement reaction, several smaller molecular weight fragments are produced as a consequence of the cleavage of parent complement proteins (e.g., C3b, C4b, and C5b). Some of these fragments (C3a, C5a) have strong biologic activity and can cause severe tissue damage or systemic anaphylaxis. These products are not, however, of immediate importance in the area of immunohematology and will not be considered further. The most important biologic role of complement in blood group serology is the production of *cell membrane lysis* of antibody-coated targets. Red cells may be used as target cells when evaluating the hemolytic potency of certain agglutinating antibodies, whereas lymphocytes are used as targets in HLA serotyping. The lytic potential of complement can be abolished by heating serum at 56°C for 30 minutes. Activation of the complement cascade may be accomplished through two independent pathways of activation and a common cytolytic pathway (Fig. 3-8). These have been designated, respectively, the *classic* and the *alternative* pathways of activation.

CLASSIC COMPLEMENT PATHWAY

This sequence may be activated by the interaction of antigen with its corresponding antibody (see Fig. 3-8). Only certain immunoglobulin classes (IgM and IgG) and subclasses (IgG_1, IgG_2, and IgG_3) can produce this effect (see Tables 3-2 and 3-3). After IgM, the IgG_3 subclass is the most efficient in complement activation.[9]

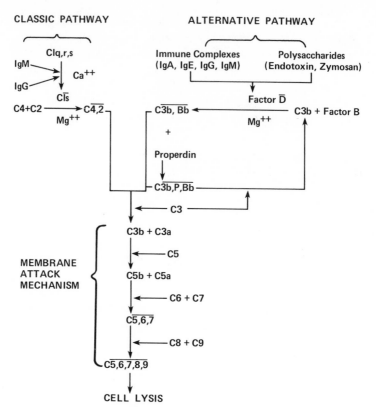

FIGURE 3-8. Schematic diagram illustrating the sequential activation of the complement system via the classic and alternative pathways. For simplicity, the role of complement regulator proteins ($\overline{\text{C1s}}$ inhibitor, C3b inactivator, and $\beta_1 H$) has been omitted.

The classic complement pathway activation sequence is initiated by the binding of C1 to the Fc fragment of IgG or IgM. The earliest reaction involves the sequential activation of the three C1 subunits (C1q,r,s). The generation of C1s activates C4 and C2, forming a bimolecular complex. This activated complex is a potent cleaving enzyme whose natural substrate is native, inactive C3. Important by-products of the classic pathway of complement activation include C4b, C3a, and C3b. Since human erythrocytes have surface receptors for C4b and C3b, some of these cleavage products attach to the red cell surface. Later, these fragments, C4b and C3b, are further degraded to C4d and C3d, respectively, through the action of C3b inactivator in the presence of trypsin.

ALTERNATIVE COMPLEMENT PATHWAY

This pathway can be activated immunologically by aggregates of IgA, IgE, and IgG molecules. Naturally occurring polysaccharides and lipopolysaccharides can also initiate this mechanism of complement activation in a nonimmunologic fashion. The main participants in this reaction sequence include factor D (analogous to C1), factor B (analogous to C2), and the C3b cleavage product of C3 (analogous to C4). When the complex comprising C3b and factor B (analogous to C4, 2) is acted upon by factor $\bar{\text{D}}$ (analogous to $\overline{\text{C1s}}$), the bimolecular complex $\overline{\text{C3b,Bb}}$ (analogous to $\overline{\text{C4,2}}$) is formed by a cleavage product of factor B (Bb). The $\overline{\text{C3b,Bb}}$ complex is stabilized by the presence of properdin ($\overline{\text{C3b,P,Bb}}$) and constitutes an esterase enzyme that cleaves native C3 into additional C3b fragments. These C3b molecules then attach to the red cell membrane via the erythrocyte C3b surface receptors. It is therefore evident that C3b acts as a "positive feedback" mechanism for driving the alternative pathway and that this activation sequence by-passes the $\overline{\text{C1,4,2}}$ activation sequence of the classic pathway. Although there is no firm evidence that red cell antibodies activate the alternative pathway, this cascade can be spontaneously activated by nonimmunologic means. This occurs in patients with paroxysmal nocturnal hemoglobinuria, an uncommon condition characterized by exquisite sensitivity of the patients' erythrocytes to the lytic action of complement in the absence of red cell antibodies.

MEMBRANE ATTACK MECHANISM

The terminal components of the complement sequence constitute the membrane attack system (see Fig. 3-8). This mechanism is initiated by cleavage of C5 via either the classic pathway (through $\overline{\text{C4b,2a,3b}}$) or the alternative pathway (through $\overline{\text{C3b,P,Bb,C3b}}$). Generation of C5b on the cell membrane is rapidly followed by sequential membrane attachment of $\overline{\text{C6,7,8,9}}$. When this occurs, a "leaky" transmembrane channel forms, which eventually results in osmotic lysis of the erythrocyte.

BINDING OF COMPLEMENT BY RED CELL ANTIBODIES

The effective activation of the classic pathway via C1q necessitates the binding of one C1 molecule to two adjacent immunoglobulin Fc regions. This is easily accomplished by a single pentameric IgM molecule, which can provide two Fc regions side-by-side. Monomeric IgG molecules, however, bind C1q far less efficiently, since they are distributed randomly on the red cell surface and are less likely to align themselves in a side-by-side "doublet" arrangement. As many as 800 IgG anti-A molecules may need to attach to one adult A_1 red cell in order to bind a single C1 molecule.[9] Since Rh antigens are sparsely distributed over the red cell surface, IgG anti-Rh antisera are not favorably sited to activate complement. This may explain the poor hemolytic potential of most anti-Rh agglutinins. Occasional IgG antibodies are, however, extremely efficient hemolysins. The most notable of such examples are encountered in patients with paroxysmal cold hemoglobinuria, who have antibodies directed against P blood group system determinants.

ROLE OF EFFECTOR CELLS IN ANTIBODY-MEDIATED RED CELL DESTRUCTION

Complement-mediated lysis is not the only mechanism that eliminates antibody-coated erythrocytes in vivo. Cells of the *mononuclear phagocyte system,* including monocytes, macrophages, and the cells lining the hepatic and splenic sinusoids, also play an important role in the clearance of antibody-coated red cells. These mononuclear phagocytes are equipped with two biologically important types of surface receptors: complement and immunoglobulin Fc (Fig. 3-9).

The biologic functions of complement and immunoglobulin Fc receptors have clinical relevance. Transfused erythrocytes coated with C3b alone, without antibody, are sequestrated only transiently in the reticuloendothelial organs, but thereafter survive normally. Since monocytes and macrophages lack IgM receptors, transfused IgM-coated erythrocytes are not eliminated via Fc receptor-mediated phagocytosis. Erythrocytes, coated with IgG (especially with associated C3b), however, will be rapidly cleared from the circulation via this mechanism.

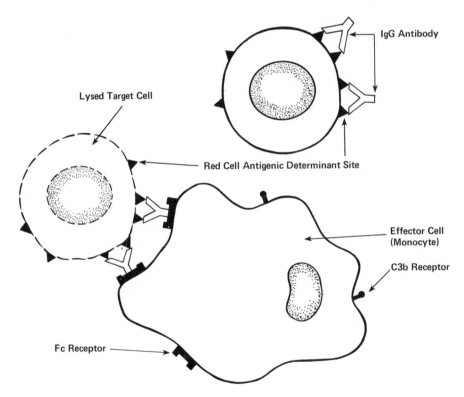

FIGURE 3-9. Schematic diagram represents the mechanism of antibody-dependent cellular cytotoxicity and illustrates the role of effector cell Fc surface receptors in this process.

COMPLEMENT RECEPTORS

Monocytes and macrophages have membrane receptors for the C3b cleavage product of complement activation. Consequently, when red cells are coated with C3b (generated from either the classic or alternative pathways), they will attach to the surface membranes of these phagocytes. Although the erythrocytes are attached, they are not internalized by the phagocytic cells. Thus, the surface receptor for C3b does not promote the phagocytosis of erythrocytes.

Membrane-bound C3b is usually rapidly degraded to C3d by C3b inactivator. Since the mononuclear phagocytes lack receptors for C3d, red cells coated with C3d detach from the surfaces of the phagocytic cells.

IMMUNOGLOBULIN Fc RECEPTORS

Macrophages and monocytes are also provided with receptors for the attachment of IgG immunoglobulin. These receptors can bind to the C_H3 domain in the Fc portion of the IgG molecule. Only the IgG_1 and IgG_3 subclasses are capable of cytophilic attachment to the immunoglobulin Fc receptors. Red cells coated with IgG_1 or IgG_3 will thus adhere to monocytes and macrophages. Unlike the C3b receptors, the immunoglobulin Fc receptors promote the phagocytosis of attached IgG-coated erythrocytes. When red cells are coated with both IgG and C3b, there is an accelerated phagocytic response, since the C3b and IgG receptors on the mononuclear cells act in concert.

ANTIBODY-DEPENDENT CELLULAR CYTOTOXICITY

When monocytes are incubated with IgG-coated erythrocytes in vitro, lysis of the red cells occurs (see Fig. 3-9). This phenomenon is not complement-mediated since it occurs in the absence of complement. The mechanism of hemolysis does not involve phagocytosis of the erythrocytes by the monocytes. Because there is a specific requirement for both antibody and cytotoxic effector cells in the test system, the phenomenon is known as antibody-dependent cellular cytotoxicity. Certain lymphocytes, known as *killer* or *K cells*, may be substituted for monocytes in the assay. IgM antibodies cannot replace IgG immunoglobulins because the process requires attachment of antibody-coated red cells via IgG Fc receptors on effector cells.

CLINICAL SIGNIFICANCE OF RED CELL ANTIBODIES

Not all serum hemagglutinins are a consequence of prior immunization with red cells. Alloantibodies in the serum of an individual that are not provoked by previous red cell sensitization are termed *"naturally occurring"* agglutinins. This time-honored term is not entirely appropriate, as it suggests that other antibodies should be regarded as "unnatural" or, perhaps, even "supernatural." The best known examples of such naturally occurring antibodies are the anti-A and anti-B isoagglutinins. Since these antibodies only begin to appear in the serum approximately 6 months after birth (at a time of established bacterial colonization of the large bowel), it appears that they are induced by heterologous bacterial antigens. Other less frequent examples of naturally occurring hemagglutinins include those directed against determinants within the Lewis (Le^a, Le^b), MNS, P(P$_1$), Rh (E), and Wr (Wr^a) blood group systems. Most of these antibodies are of the IgM variety, are present in low serum concentration, react optimally at 4°C, and do not generally react above 37°C. For this reason, most of them do not generally give rise to transfusion reactions.

On the other hand, *"immune" antibodies* are evoked by previous alloimmunization. The immunizing event is related to transfusion, pregnancy, or the administration of certain vaccines (which contain A and B blood group determinants). Immune antibodies are most frequently of the IgG class and react optimally at 37°C. They may or may not fix complement. These antibodies obviously have more serious clinical implications than do naturally occurring hemagglutinins.

Autoantibodies may be of either the cold or warm agglutinin variety. Cold autoagglutinins are generally IgM immunoglobulins, whereas warm autoagglutinins are mainly IgG or occasionally IgA antibodies. Many warm autoantibodies do not show antigen specificity within a single blood group system. Such antibodies may agglutinate all normal red cells as well as the subject's own cells and are termed *panagglutinins*. They create severe problems in crossmatching blood for transfusion purposes.

PLACENTAL TRANSFER OF IMMUNOGLOBULINS

Not all antibodies can cross the placenta. This property is restricted to IgG antibodies of the IgG$_1$, IgG$_2$, IgG$_3$, and IgG$_4$ subclasses. Placental transfer is effected via the Fc portion of the IgG molecule. The ability of a hemagglutinin to cross the placenta has obvious clinical significance, for it may result in fetal red cell destruction and hemolytic disease of the newborn. Transplacental antibodies are usually directed against Rh or A and B determinants. Hemolytic disease of the newborn caused by feto-maternal ABO incompatibility is usually associated with group O mothers. The disease is not associated with group A or B mothers whose corresponding isoagglutinins are of the IgM variety.

LABORATORY DETECTION OF CLINICALLY SIGNIFICANT ANTIBODIES

It should be evident from the foregoing description that in most instances in which serum hemagglutinins are identified by the serologist, it ought to be possible to predict the survival of transfused erythrocytes. Thus, individuals with serum antibodies to Rh, Kell, Kidd, or Duffy determinants are likely to rapidly eliminate transfused red cells containing those particular antigens.

It is not always possible to forecast whether maternal alloantibodies will cause fetal erythrocyte destruction. There are also situations confronting the hemotherapist in which compatible red cells for transfusion are unavailable. This may happen because the recipient has an autoreactive serum panagglutinin, an alloantibody against a high frequency antigen, or multiple alloantibodies. Such situations require a laboratory tool to predict the real clinical significance of these antibodies. Schanfield and associates[7] have recently developed a laboratory assay that holds promise for the evaluation of clinically relevant antibodies. The procedure is an in vitro mononuclear phagocyte assay that employs blood monocytes or peritoneal macrophages as phagocytic cells. The principle is based on the ability of the phagocytes to bind and phagocytose IgG-coated erythrocytes. The number of phagocyte-associated erythrocytes is expressed as an index. These investigators have noted a correlation between the assay score and the survival of transfused erythrocytes when certain serum antibodies are evaluated. The technique remains, however, a research tool at present.

REFERENCES

1. BELLANTI, JA: *Immunology II.* WB Saunders, Philadelphia, 1978.
2. BENACERRAF, B and UNANUE, EA: *Textbook of Immunology.* Williams & Wilkins, Baltimore, 1979.
3. MOLLISON, PL: *Blood Transfusion in Clinical Medicine.* Blackwell Scientific Publications, London, 1979.
4. KAGAN, E, ET AL.: *Immunological studies of patients with asbestosis. II. Studies of circulating lymphoid cell numbers and humoral immunity.* Clin Exp Immunol 28:268, 1977.
5. HENRY, JB: *Clinical Diagnosis and Management by Laboratory Methods.* WB Saunders, Philadelphia, 1979.
6. PIERCE, SR: *A review of erythrocyte antigens shared with leukocytes.* In *A Seminar on Antigens or Blood Cells and Body Fluids.* American Association of Blood Banks, 1980.
7. SCHANFIELD, MS, SCHOEPPNER, SL and STEVENS, JO: *New approaches to detecting clinically significant antibodies in the laboratory.* In Sandler, SG, Nusbacher, J and Schanfield, MS (EDS): *Immunobiology of the Erythrocyte.* Alan R Liss, Inc., New York, 1980.
8. SCHMIDT, PJ: *The hemolytic anemia of the Rh_{null} blood group.* In *Cellular Antigens and Disease.* American Association of Blood Banks, 1977.
9. FUDENBERG, HH, ET AL.: *Basic and Clinical Immunology.* Lange Medical Publications, Los Altos, California, 1980.
10. GRAHAM, HA, ET AL.: *Rh typing with saline agglutinating, chemically-reduced IgG anti-D.* Transfusion 19:657, 1979.

BIBLIOGRAPHY

ALEXANDER, JW and GOOD, R: *Fundamentals of Clinical Immunology.* WB Saunders, Philadelphia, 1977.
BIGLEY, NJ: *Immunologic Fundamentals.* Year Book Medical Publishers, Chicago, 1980.
ROITT, IM: *Essential Immunology*, ed 4. CV Mosby (Blackwell Scientific Publications), St Louis, 1980.

CHAPTER 4

THE ANTIGLOBULIN TEST

L. RUTH GUY, PH.D.

The antiglobulin test is one of the most useful and most universally applied tests employed in blood banks and immunohematology laboratories. However, the original publication by Moreschi[1] describing the procedure in 1908 attracted little attention. His experimental model consisted of sensitizing rabbits and goats. Coombs[2,3] independently rediscovered the principle of the test in 1945, when he prepared antihuman serum in rabbits. In this experiment, human serum was injected into rabbits, and the rabbit antibody produced against the human globulin was collected and purified. This rabbit antihuman globulin (AHG) was used to demonstrate incomplete human antibodies that were adsorbed to red blood cells but did not produce visual agglutination, unless Coombs' serum was used (see Color Plate 1).

This antihuman serum was useful in detecting nonagglutinating Rh antibodies in serum, and those coating the red blood cells of infants with hemolytic disease of the newborn. The antiglobulin test is frequently referred to as the Coombs' test in honor of R.R.A. Coombs, who rediscovered it. The versatility of the procedure soon became apparent and it gained widespread use, despite the lack of well-defined standards for preparation of the antiserum and information regarding its required reactivity. Other useful applications of the antiglobulin test include detection of autoimmune hemolytic anemia, investigation of transfusion reactions, and detection of red cell sensitization reactions caused by certain drugs (see Chapter 20).

The development of the current high-quality AHG reagents has been due in large part to the efforts of the manufacturers rather than the regulatory bodies. Actually, the Federal Regulations remain as published in 1948.

The antiglobulin test is routinely applied in two ways: direct and indirect. The *direct antiglobulin test* (DAT) is used to detect "in vivo" coating of red blood cells with antibody globulin (IgG) and/or complement. Therefore, the patient's red cells, when received in the laboratory, are already coated with antibody. No incubation with serum (a source of antibody) is necessary since the red cells are taken *directly* from the patient sample, washed with normal saline, and mixed with antihuman globulin (AHG).

Several applications of the direct Coombs' test include detection of hemolytic disease of the newborn, detection of autoimmune hemolytic anemia, investigation of transfusion reactions, and detection of red cell sensitization reactions caused by drugs (e.g., penicillin, cephalothin, and alpha-methyldopa) (see Direct Antiglobulin Test, Applications, below).

In *indirect antiglobulin tests* (IAT) serum serves as a source of antibody and red blood cells serve as a source of antigen. The IAT is performed by combining serum and red cells in vitro to permit attachment of the antibody to the corresponding red cell antigen (if present) prior to testing with AHG.

During the IAT, serum is incubated with a red cell suspension for the manufacturer's specified amount of time. The red blood cells are then washed free of uncombined globulin using physiologic saline. Next, antihuman globulin serum is added to the washed cells.

Several applications of the IAT include compatibility testing, antibody screening, antibody identification, testing for the weak Rh variant antigen D^u, and red cell phenotyping (see Indirect Antiglobulin Test, Applications, below). Regardless of the application of the antihuman globulin test, the presence of antibody globulin and/or complement on the red cells is demonstrated by the presence of agglutination after the addition of the AHG reagent.

In terms of Coombs' testing, whether direct or indirect, washing is a vital and mandatory step in the procedure. Inadequate washing of red cells will result in neutralization of the antihuman globulin reagent by trace amounts of residual globulin left in the patient's serum surrounding the red blood cells. This yields a false-negative reaction.

One drop of a 1:4000 dilution of human serum is capable of neutralizing one drop of antihuman globulin reagent.

PRODUCTION OF ANTIGLOBULIN SERUM

The antiglobulin serum is prepared by injecting human whole serum or plasma, purified IgG globulin, or complement components into a suitable animal. In the United States, rabbits and goats are most frequently used. Sheep have been used successfully, also. Although horses produce large amounts of antibody, their serum is not satisfactory because of its tendency to show unusual prozones.[4]

The commercially prepared antisera are satisfactory for most purposes. However, some workers prefer to make their own. The injections can be made intramuscularly or intravenously. Deep intramuscular injections result in a better antibody response than those given by the intravenous route unless the IgG has been heat aggregated. The injection of Freund's adjuvant with the antigen has been more satisfactory than alum-precipitated antigen for booster injections. For a detailed protocol of injections, the reader should refer to the publications of Ironside;[5] Boorman, Dodd, and Lincoln;[6] Müller-Eberhard and coworkers;[7,8] and Mollison.[9] In any case, the worker must be prepared to spend time in absorbing out the unwanted antispecies antibodies and in standardizing the reagent.

BROAD-SPECTRUM ANTIGLOBULIN SERUM

The polyspecific antiglobulin serum is the basic reagent most generally employed for routine crossmatching, antibody screening tests, preliminary investigation of hemolytic anemia, and antigen or antibody identification. It contains anti-IgG, anti-IgM, and anticomplement. If the test is positive with this reagent, the use of a monospecific reagent may or may not be indicated depending on the information desired. The anticomplement component is usually anti-C3d, or anti-C3d plus anti-C4.

MONOSPECIFIC ANTIGLOBULIN SERUM

Anti-IgG will detect almost all clinically significant coating antibodies encountered in compatibility testing and is helpful in studies of immune hemolytic anemias. Standards do not require anticomplement activity for crossmatching. Anti-IgG is particularly useful in determining whether or not a crossmatch is incompatible as a result of clinically significant alloantibodies or complement fixed onto cells by cold agglutinins.

Anti-IgM is not a practical reagent since most IgM antibodies are easily detected by simple agglutination technique.

Anticomplement was originally called anti-non-gamma. Anticomplement serum may contain both anti-C3d and anti-C4. Once C3 and C4 have been activated and have attached themselves to the cell membrane, they cannot be removed by washing. C3d is the final inactivated portion of C3 that remains on the cell membrane. C3, C3b, and C3c are very labile and are less likely to be detected by routine procedures.

Anti-C3d serum is somewhat more useful than C3d plus anti-C4, since excessive amounts of C4 may become attached to the membrane following activation by relatively low-titered, clinically insignificant cold agglutinins. Both anticomplement sera are useful in studying immune hemolytic anemias. Anti-IgA and anti-IgM are not readily available for use in the routine testing procedures, but special procedures described by Petz and Garratty[10] can be employed. They use a passive agglutination technique for detecting anti-IgA and anti-IgM. To perform this technique, normal red blood cells are coated in vitro with IgA or IgM, as the case may be. If the corresponding antibody is present in the serum to be tested, the coated cells are agglutinated. There is no commercial serum prepared for detecting IgA or IgM on red blood cells. However, anti-IgA and anti-IgM are available for use in immunoelectrophoresis or immunodiffusion procedures. Because these methods are relatively insensitive, they are not helpful in detecting IgA or IgM coating on red blood cells. Since the commercial antisera (prepared in animals) contain antispecies (e.g., antihuman) antibodies as well as specific anti-IgA or anti-IgM, it is necessary to absorb the serum with human red blood cells until the serum will no longer agglutinate red blood cells coated with IgG antibody.[10] Tests involving anti-IgA and anti-IgM are applicable for studies in sophisticated immunohematology laboratories but are neither required nor needed for routine purposes.

DIRECT ANTIGLOBULIN TEST (DAT)

The direct antiglobulin test is used to detect antibodies and/or complement that have coated red blood cells in vivo.[11] If one is interested in IgG coating only, the red blood cells may be harvested from either clotted or anticoagulated blood. For studies of red blood cells from patients with suspected immune hemolytic anemia, the blood sample should be collected in EDTA anticoagulant to stop in vitro activation of complement.

PROCEDURE

The technique is simple. A 2 to 4 percent suspension of red blood cells is prepared in saline.

1. Add 2 drops of 2 to 4 percent suspension of red blood cells to a 10 by 75 mm or 12 by 75 mm test tube.
2. Wash the cells by filling the tube with saline and centrifuging for 1 minute in a fixed speed centrifuge.

3. Remove the saline from the cell button either by suction or rapid decant and discard the supernatant.
4. Agitate cells to resuspend in residual saline. Repeat steps 2 and 3, three times.
5. Decant or suction final supernatant saline and drain or blot to remove excess saline.
6. Resuspend cells and add 2 drops antiglobulin serum according to manufacturer's directions. Centrifuge 15 to 20 seconds in a fixed-speed, table top centrifuge.
7. Gently resuspend the cell button by rocking the tube back and forth, letting the residual saline do most of the work.
8. Observe how the cells go into suspension. Look for agglutination using a visual aid. Grade and record the reaction using the directions for standard reading of agglutination tests.[11,12]

APPLICATIONS

The direct antiglobulin test is used to detect

1. Alloantibodies adsorbed onto red blood cells in
   a. Hemolytic disease of the newborn (see Chapter 18).
   b. Hemolytic transfusion reactions, particularly delayed reactions (see Chapter 16). Broad-spectrum antiglobulin serum and anti-IgG are well suited for these purposes.
2. Autoimmune antibodies in autoimmune hemolytic anemias (see Chapter 19).
   a. Cold autoantibodies.
   b. Warm autoantibodies.
3. Drug-induced antibodies (see Chapter 20).

The broad-spectrum or polyspecific reagent is used in the screening test for the detection and characterization of autoimmune antibodies directed against antigens on the patient's red blood cells and drug-induced antibodies. If the direct antiglobulin test is positive with this reagent, it is desirable to test the cells using both anti-IgG and anti-C3d. If the anti-IgG test is positive, eluates can be prepared from the cells and used in identification procedures (see Chapter 19). Anti-C3d and anti-C4 will not be eluted from the red blood cells.

Fluorescent antibody techniques make use of antihuman globulin serum to which a fluorescein dye has been conjugated. Few of these techniques are applicable to immunohematology at this time.

INDIRECT ANTIGLOBULIN TEST (IAT)

The indirect antiglobulin test is used to detect antibodies in serum samples that will react with red blood cells carrying the corresponding antigen(s).

PROCEDURE

1. Place 2 drops of the serum to be tested in a test tube (10 by 75 mm or 12 by 75 mm).
2. Add 2 drops of the 2 to 4 percent suspension red blood cells to be used in the test.
3. Incubate 15 to 30 minutes at 37°C, depending on the manufacturer's directions.
4. Centrifuge 15 to 20 seconds in a fixed-speed, table top centrifuge.
5. Gently dislodge the cell button and examine for agglutination.
6. Wash the cells 3 to 4 times with saline as described in the procedure for the direct antiglobulin test.
7. Drain or blot the excess saline after the last wash. Resuspend the cells by shaking the tube.
8. Add 1 to 2 drops of antiglobulin serum, according to manufacturer's directions.
9. Centrifuge and observe for agglutination as described above.

APPLICATIONS

The indirect antiglobulin test is used to

1. Detect unknown antigens on red blood cells using antiserum known to contain antibody directed against a specific antigen (e.g., anti-K, anti-Jk^a, anti-Fy^a). It is used in the test for the anti-Rh$_0$(D) variant. Cells negative for the Rh(D) antigen by routine tests are incubated with anti-Rh(D) and the indirect antiglobulin test applied in order to detect the weaker variant, D^u.
2. Detect unknown antibodies in serum using reagent red blood cells known to possess most of the common red blood cell antigens.
3. Identify antibodies using a panel of selected group O cells known to possess these common antigens in different combinations.
4. Titrate antibodies in which the relative strength of a known antibody is determined by testing various dilutions of the serum with cells known to possess the corresponding antigen.
5. Determine the serologic compatibility of donor's blood with recipient's serum. In compatibility testing the antigenic profile of the doner's cells is unknown. The test is used to determine whether or not the recipient has antibodies directed against some antigen on the donor's red blood cells.

CONTROLS

Group O red blood cells coated with IgG antibodies (Coombs' control or check cells) are used as the control to verify negative antiglobulin tests.[11] If there is no agglutination following the addition of the antiglobulin serum, the test may be negative

TABLE 4-1. Sources of Error in Antiglobulin Tests

False-Positive Results
1. Overcentrifugation
2. Contaminated or polyagglutinable *test cells*
3. Poorly prepared antiglobulin reagent with traces of antispecies or other antibodies
4. Dirty glassware
5. Already-coated test cells (prior to testing by the IAT)
6. In vitro coating of test cells by complement in patients with strong cold-autoagglutinins
7. Over-reading

False-Negative Results
1. Antiglobulin serum not added
2. Patient serum not added (in IAT)
3. Inadequate washing
4. Neutralization of the reagent
5. Delay in reading tubes
6. Undercentrifugation or overcentrifugation
7. Heavy cell suspension
8. Use of old serum (will not detect complement-dependent antibodies)
9. Under-reading
10. Failure to provide optimal temperatures and conditions during indirect testing
11. Omission of microscopic examination of all macroscopic negative results

because antibodies did not coat the test cells, antiglobulin serum was not added, or the antiglobulin had been neutralized. Agglutination of known coated cells after the original test reading confirms that the test is negative because no antibodies coated the cells in the original mixture. Omission or neutralization of the antiglobulin serum should be suspected if the Coombs' control cells do *not* agglutinate. No control is required for the positive test.

The antiglobulin test, either direct or indirect, will detect the presence of IgG or complement on red blood cells, but does not identify the specificity of the antibody activity. The specificity of the antigen or antibody in question is determined by the cells and serum used in the test.

SOURCES OF ERROR

There are many potential causes for either false-positive or false-negative results; the technologist should be aware of these as they may be difficult to identify. These sources of error are listed in Table 4-1.

REFERENCES

1.   Moreschi, C: *Neue Tatsachen die Blutkorperchen Agglutinationen.* Zentralbl Bakteriol 46:49, 1908. Cited by Mollison, PL: *Blood Transfusion in Clinical Medicine.* Blackwell Scientific Publications, Oxford, 1979.

2. Coombs, RRA, Mourant, AE and Race, RR: *A new test for the detection of weak and "incomplete" Rh agglutinins*. Br J Exp Pathol 26:255, 1945.

3. Coombs, RRA, Mourant, AE and Race, RR: *In vivo isosensitization of red cells in babies with hemolytic disease*. Lancet i: 264, 1946.

4. Medical Research Council: *Production of antibody against purified VG globulin in rabbits, goats, sheep and horses (report of a committee)*. Immunology 10:271, 1966.

5. Ironside, PN Jr: *Production of anti-human globulin in goats*. Immunology 15:503, 1968.

6. Boorman, KE, Dodd, BE and Lincoln, PJ: *Blood Group Serology*, ed 5. Churchill Livingstone, London, 1977, pp 466–473.

7. Müller-Eberhard, HJ and Nilsson, U: *Relation of a B-glycoprotein of human serum to the complement system*. J Exp Med 111:217, 1960.

8. Müller-Eberhard, HJ and Biro, CE: *Isolation and description of the fourth component of human complement*. J Exp Med 118:447, 1963.

9. Mollison, PL: *Blood Transfusion in Clinical Medicine*, ed 6. Blackwell Scientific Publications, Oxford, 1979, ch 11, pp 434–455.

10. Petz, LD and Garratty, G: *Acquired Immune Hemolytic Anemias*. Churchill Livingstone, London, 1980, pp 139–184.

11. American Association of Blood Banks: *Technical Manual of the American Association of Blood Banks*. Washington, DC, 1981, ch 7, pp 89–98.

12. American Association of Blood Banks: *Standards for Blood Banks and Transfusion Services*, ed 10, Washington, DC, 1981.

CHAPTER **5**

THE ABO BLOOD GROUP SYSTEM

DENISE HARMENING PITTIGLIO, PH.D., MT(ASCP)

HISTORICAL PERSPECTIVE

Karl Landsteiner truly opened the doors of blood banking with his discovery of the first human blood group system, ABO. This marked the beginning of the concept of individual uniqueness defined by the red cell antigens present on the red cell membrane. The ABO system still remains the most important of all blood groups in transfusion practice. Transfusion of an incorrect ABO type can result in death to the patient.

In 1901 Landsteiner drew blood from himself and five associates, separated the cells and the serum, and then mixed each cell sample with each serum. He was inadvertently the first individual to perform the forward and reverse grouping. *Forward grouping* is defined as using known sources of reagent antisera (antibodies) to detect antigens on an individual's red cells (Table 5-1). *Reverse grouping* is defined as using known reagent cells and testing the serum of the patient (Table 5-2).

Groups A, B, and O were the first blood groups described by Landsteiner. He found that serum from group B individuals agglutinated group A red blood cells and, therefore, that an antibody to A antigens was present in group B serum. Conversely, serum from group A individuals agglutinated group B red cells and, therefore, an antibody to B antigens was present in group A serum. Serum from group O individuals agglutinated both A and B cells, indicating the presence of antibodies to both A and B in group O serum (see Table 5-1).

In 1902 Landsteiner's associates, Sturle and von Descatello, discovered the fourth ABO blood group, AB.

Blood Group	Reaction with Anti-A	Reaction with Anti-B
AB	+	+

The frequency of these blood groups in the white population is as follows: Group O, 45 percent; Group A, 41 percent; Group B, 10 percent; and Group AB, 4 percent. Therefore, O and A are the most common blood group types. The rarest blood group is AB. However, frequencies of ABO groups differ in a few selected populations and ethnic groups (Table 5-3).[1] For example, group B is found twice as

TABLE 5-1. ABO Forward Grouping

Patient's Red Cells	Reaction with Anti-A	Reaction with Anti-B	Interpretation of Blood Group
#1	visual agglutination (+)	negative	A
#2	negative	visual agglutination (+)	B
#3	negative	negative	O

TABLE 5-2. ABO Reverse Grouping

Patient's Serum	Reaction with Reagent A_1 cells	Reaction with Reagent B cells	Interpretation of Blood Group
#1	negative	+	A
#2	+	negative	B
#3	+	+	O
#4	negative	negative	AB

TABLE 5-3. ABO Phenotype Frequencies[11-13]

Phenotype	White	Black	Mexican	Oriental
A_1	34%	19%	22%	27%
A_2	10%	8%	6%	Rare
B	9%	19%	13%	25%
A_1B	3%	3%	4%	5%
A_2B	1%	1%	Rare	Rare
O	44%	49%	56%	43%

frequently in blacks and Orientals as in whites. Subgroup A_2 is rarely found in Orientals.

Landsteiner concluded from the reactions he observed that the ABO blood group system has "naturally occurring" antibodies in the serum of individuals directed against the missing antigen they lack. This term "naturally occurring" is really a misnomer, since substantial evidence suggests that anti-A and anti-B are stimulated by substances that are ubiquitous in nature. Bacteria have been shown to be chemically similar to human ABO antigens and may serve as a source of stimulation of antibody formation. Springer and coworkers[2] have demonstrated that Leghorn chickens kept in a germ-free environment from birth lacked ABO antibodies in comparison to control chickens raised under normal conditions who had ABO antibodies. Various seeds from pollinating plants are also chemically similar to human ABO antigens, so much so that they can be used as a source of antisera (e.g., the reagent anti-A_1 lectin; see section on ABO Subgroups).

Whether the source of stimulation to ABO antigens the individual lacks is pollen particles, bacteria, or other substances present in nature, the fact remains that there is a general processing of that particular antigen. This results in a consistent immune response reflected in antibody production. These antibodies are always present in normal, healthy individuals. ABO antibodies are a result of cross-reactivity and are initiated at birth upon exposure to foreign substances ubiquitous in nature. Titers are generally too low for detection until the individual is 3 to 6 months of age. As a result, it is logical to perform only forward grouping on cord blood from newborn infants. The antibody production peaks at 5 to 10 years of age and then declines progressively with advanced age. Patients greater than 65 years of age usually have low titers, so that antibodies may be undetectable in the reverse grouping. The ABO blood group system is unique in that all normal, healthy individuals consistently have antibodies present in their serum to antigens they lack on their red cells. The other defined blood group systems do not have "naturally occurring" antibodies persistently present in their serum to antigens they lack. Most other blood systems require the introduction of foreign red cells by transfusion or pregnancy. Some blood groups, however, can occasionally have antibodies present that are not related to the introduction of foreign red cells. These antibodies are usually the IgM type and are not consistently present in everyone's serum. Performance of a reverse grouping is, therefore, unique to the ABO blood group system.

Testing of ABO is relatively easy; therefore, the regular occurrence of anti-A and/or anti-B in persons lacking the corresponding antigens serves as a confirmation of results of the forward grouping. Complete absence of anti-A and anti-B is very rare in healthy individuals (except AB subjects), occurring at less than 0.01 percent in a random population.[3]

The consistently present ABO antibodies, however, create a treacherous situation as far as blood transfusion is concerned. If group B (or A) red cells are given to a patient whose serum contains anti-B (or anti-A), the donor's red cells will be destroyed almost immediately, being lysed at a rate of approximately 1 ml of red cells per minute. This produces a very severe, if not fatal, transfusion reaction in the patient. Therefore, both forward and reverse grouping must be performed on all patients' samples, noting the correct reciprocal relationship of antigens and antibodies in a given blood group type (Table 5-4).

ABO ANTIBODIES

There is a wide variation in the titers of ABO isoagglutinins in a random population. Generally, anti-A from a group O individual has a higher titer than that of group B, and anti-A from a group B individual usually has a higher titer than anti-B from group A. ABO antibodies are generally IgM. Characteristically, IgM antibodies are cold reacting antibodies that do not cross the placenta and that can bind complement. (For a review of other characteristic properties of IgM antibodies, see Chapter 3.)

In a given serum from a group A and/or B individual, anti-B and/or anti-A may be IgM entirely, a mixture of IgM and IgG, a mixture of IgM and IgA, or a mixture of all three immunoglobulins.[4] However, the majority of anti-A from a group B individual and anti-B from a group A individual contains IgM antibody predominantly, with minor amounts of IgG or IgA present, if detectable at all. The "immune" form of anti-A or anti-B can be produced by individuals exposed to foreign red cell stimulation, either by transfusion or pregnancy.

Serum from group O individuals contains not only anti-A and anti-B, but also anti-A,B. Anti-A,B antibody activity, originally thought to be just a mixture of anti-A and anti-B, cannot be separated into a pure specificity when absorbed with either A or B cells. Activity toward both A and B cells still remains with anti-A,B, even

TABLE 5-4. Summary of Forward and Reverse Grouping

Patient	Patient Cells Tested with		Interpretation: Forward Group	Patient Serum Tested with		Interpretation: Reverse Group
	Anti-A	Anti-B		A_1 Cells	B Cells	
1	negative	negative	O	+	+	O
2	+	negative	A	negative	+	A
3	negative	+	B	+	negative	B
4	+	+	AB	negative	negative	AB

after repeated absorptions with A or B cells.[5,6] Anti-A,B, therefore, possesses serologic activity not found in mixtures of anti-A plus anti-B. Anti-A,B from group O individuals is a higher titer of anti-A and anti-B than found in group A and B individuals. This makes A,B antiserum a convenient reagent to use to detect weak ABO antigens; therefore, this serum from group O individuals is routinely utilized in the forward grouping.

Anti-A,B from group O individuals has been reported to be a mixture of IgG and IgM, or IgG, IgM, and IgA. Anti-A,B will cross the placenta more frequently than anti-A or anti-B, confirming the presence of IgG. The "immune" form of anti-A,B can be produced by O individuals exposed to A or B red cells either by transfusion or pregnancy. These anti-A,B "immune" antibodies are predominantly IgG. IgG anti-A and anti-B antibodies develop far more commonly in group O individuals than in A or B individuals. Knowledge of the amount of IgG anti-A or anti-B or anti-A,B in a woman's serum sometimes allows prediction or diagnosis of hemolytic disease of the newborn caused by ABO incompatibility (see Chapter 18).

INHERITANCE OF THE ABO BLOOD GROUPS

The theory for the inheritance of the ABO blood groups was first described by Bernstein in 1924. He demonstrated that each individual inherits one ABO gene from each parent and that these two genes determine which ABO antigens are present on the red cell membrane. One position or locus on each chromosome number nine is occupied by either an A, B, or O gene. The O gene is considered an amorph since no detectable antigen is produced in response to the inheritance of this gene. The designations A or B refer to phenotypes, whereas AA, BO, and OO denote genotypes. In the case of an O individual, both phenotype and genotype are the same since that individual would have to be homozygous for the O gene. Table 5-5 lists possible ABO genotypes from various matings. The inheritance of ABO antigens, therefore, follows simple mendelian genetics. ABO, like most other blood group systems, is codominant in expression. (For a review of genetics, refer to Chapter 2.)

FORMATION OF A, B, AND O ANTIGENS

The ABO genes do not actually code for the production of ABO antigens, but rather produce specific glycosyl-transferases that add sugars to a basic precursor sub-

TABLE 5-5. ABO Groups of the Offspring from the Various Possible ABO Matings

Mating Phenotypes	Mating Genotypes	Offspring Possible Phenotypes (and Genotypes)
A × A	AA × AA	A (AA)
	AA × AO	A (AA or AO)
	AO × AO	A (AA or AO) or O (OO)
B × B	BB × BB	B (BB)
	BB × BO	B (BB or BO)
	BO × BO	B (BB or BO) or O (OO)
AB × AB	AB × AB	AB (AB) or A (AA) or B (BB)
O × O	OO × OO	O (OO)
A × B	AA × BB	AB (AB)
	AO × BB	AB (AB) or B (BO)
	AA × BO	AB (AB) or A (AO)
	AO × BO	AB (AB) or A (AO) or B (BO) or O (OO)
A × O	AA × OO	A (AO)
	AO × OO	A (AO) or O (OO)
A × AB	AA × AB	AB (AB) or A (AA)
	AO × AB	AB (AB) or A (AA or AO) or B (BO)
B × O	BB × OO	B (BO)
	BO × OO	B (BO) or O (OO)
B × AB	BB × AB	AB (AB) or B (BB)
	BO × AB	AB (AB) or B (BB or BO) or A (AO)
AB × O	AB × OO	A (AO) or B (BO)

stance. Also, ABO genes genetically interact with several other separate, independent blood group systems, resulting in addition of sugar residues to a common precursor substance. The action of the H gene is intimately related to the formation of the ABO antigens. The inheritance of the H gene is independent of the inheritance of the ABO genes, but A, B, and H antigens are all formed from the same basic precursor material, which is itself a genetic product. The basic material has a glycoprotein or glycolipid backbone to which sugars are attached in response to specific enzyme transferases elicited by an inherited gene. The ABH glycolipid antigens are built upon a common carbohydrate residue, which represents a paragloboside (see Color Plate 3).

INTERACTION OF Hh AND ABO GENES

Inheritance of the H gene elicits an enzyme, L-fucosyltransferase, which transfers the sugar L-fucose to the terminal galactose of the precursor chain. The H gene is very common in the random population, with greater than 99.99 percent inheriting the H gene. The allele of H, h, is quite rare, with the genotype, hh, being extremely rare.

This hh genotype is called the "Bombay phenotype" and *lacks* normal expression of the ABO genes. Even though Bombay (hh) individuals may inherit ABO genes, normal expression reflected in the formation of A, B, or H antigens does not occur.

The H substance must be formed first by the inheritance of at least one H gene in order for the other sugars to be attached in response to an inherited ABO gene. Therefore, the Bombay phenotype is devoid of all antigens of the ABO system. Remember, however, for all practical purposes all individuals possess the H gene, in which H substance is formed first, and then other sugars attach onto this, dependent on the ABO genes inherited. The sugars which occupy the terminal positions of this precursor chain and confer blood group specificity are called the immunodominant sugars. Therefore, L-fucose is the sugar responsible for H specificity (see Color Plate 4).

The A gene codes for the production of N-acetylgalactosaminyltransferase, which transfers an N-acetylgalactosamine (GalNAc) sugar to the H structure. This sugar is responsible for A specificity (see Color Plate 5). The A-specific immunodominant sugar is linked to a type-2 chain glycolipid precursor. Only type-2 paragloboside chains are found in the erythrocyte membrane being synthesized by the red cell precursors. Type-2 chain refers to an alpha-1→4 linkage between the D-galactose and the N-acetyl*glucosamine* of the precursor substance, where the number one carbon of the D-galactose is linked to the number four carbon of the N-acetylglucosamine (see Color Plate 6).

The A gene tends to elicit higher concentrations of glycosyltransferase than the B gene. This leads to the conversion of practically all the H antigen on the red cell to A antigen sites. As many as 810,000 to 1,170,000 antigen sites exist on an A adult red cell in response to inherited A genes.

The B gene codes for the production of D-galactosyltransferase, which transfers a D-galactose (Gal) sugar to the H substance. This sugar is responsible for B specificity (see Color Plate 7). Anywhere from 600,000 to 830,000 B antigen sites exist on a B adult red cell in response to the conversion of the H antigen by the glycosyltransferase elicited by the B gene.

When A and B genes are both inherited, the B enzyme seems to compete more efficiently for the H structure and the A enzyme is not as successful. Therefore, the average number of A antigens on an AB adult cell is approximately 600,000 sites, compared with an average of 720,000 B antigen sites.

The O gene is an amorph that does not elicit a transferase and, therefore, adds no additional sugar to the H structure. As a result, the O blood group has the highest concentration of H antigen.

FORMATION OF A, B, AND H SOLUBLE ANTIGENS

All the ABH antigens develop as early as 37 days of fetal life but do not increase very much in strength during the gestational period. Typically, ABH reactivity of the newborn erythrocyte is not as strong as that of the adult cell. The red cells of the newborn have been estimated to carry anywhere from 25 to 50 percent of the number of antigenic sites found on the adult red cell. In addition to age, the phenotypic expression of ABH antigens may vary with race, genetic interaction, and disease states. The genetic interaction of the ABO blood group system with the Lewis, Ii, and P blood groups is reflected in the synthesis of all these antigens by the sequential addition of sugar residues to a common *precursor substance* previously described for ABO.

In addition to red cells, ABH antigens can be found on white blood cells and platelets, as well as all other tissue cells. In fact, ABH soluble antigens can be synthesized and secreted by tissue cells. Therefore, ABH blood group specific substances can be found in all the body secretions dependent on the ABO genes inherited, as well as the inheritance of another set of genes that regulates their formation.

INTERACTION OF Sese AND ABO GENES

The Se gene and its allele, se, are inherited independently of the ABO and the H gene. Approximately 78 percent of the random United States population has inherited the Se gene, possessing the genotype SeSe or Sese. This genotype is given the name "secretor." These individuals secrete *glycoproteins* containing A, B, or H antigenic specificity corresponding to their inherited ABO blood group. The remaining 20 percent possess the genotype sese and are called "nonsecretors," since their saliva as well as other secretions lack the A, B, or H glycoprotein substances or antigens. The exact mechanism of how the Se gene functions to regulate tissue secretory cells is not known. However, the H-specific transferase (L-fucosyltransferase) is found *only* in the secretions of secretors, indicating that the secretor gene controls the expression of the H gene in the secretory cells. The Se gene does *not*, however, affect the formation of A, B, or H antigens on the red cell. The Se gene does *not* control the presence of A, B, or H transferases in hematopoietic tissue. In fact, A or B transferase enzymes, *unlike* A or B glycoprotein substances or antigens, are found in the secretions of A_1 or B individuals regardless of their secretor status. However, it is the presence of the H gene-specified L-fucosyltransferase (which is dependent on the inheritance of the Se gene) that determines whether ABH soluble substances will be secreted, since H substance must be synthesized prior to the formation of A or B substances (see Color Plate 8).

DISTINCTION OF A, B, AND H ANTIGENS AND A, B, AND H SOLUBLE SUBSTANCES

The formation of A, B, and H substances is the same as described for the formation of A, B, and H antigens on the red cells, except for a few minor distinctions:

1. The secreted substances are glycoproteins; the red cell antigens are glycolipids.

2. The first sugar in the common carbohydrate residue of the precursor substance is N-acetylgalactosamine for the glycoprotein secretions, and glucose for the red cell antigens (review Color Plates 3, 4, 5, 7, and 8).

3. In the biosynthesis of the glycoprotein secretions, both type-1 and type-2 linkages occur in the precursor structures. In the case of the red cell ABH glycolipid

antigens, only type-2 precursor chains are involved. Note that type-1 chain refers to an alpha $1 \rightarrow 3$ linkage in which the number one carbon of the galactose is attached to the number three carbon of N-acetylglucosamine sugar of the precursor substance, as opposed to an alpha $1 \rightarrow 4$ linkage previously described for a type-2 chain.

4. Since the H structure or substance is the precursor or acceptor substrate for sugars transferred by the A or B gene-specified enzymes, the Sese system regulates the H-gene activity in secretions, but *not* in the red cell.

Tests for ABH secretion may help establish the true ABO group of an individual whose red cell antigens are poorly developed. The demonstration of the A, B, and H substances in saliva is evidence for the inheritance of an A gene, B gene, H gene, and Se gene. The term "secretor" refers only to secretion of A, B, or H antigens in body fluids. The glycoprotein soluble substances or antigens normally found in the saliva of secretors are listed in Table 5-6. The procedure for determination of secretor status can be found at the end of this chapter.

ABO SUBGROUPS

A SUBGROUPS

In 1911 von Dungern described two different A antigens based on reactions with anti-A and anti-A_1 antisera. Serum from group B individuals contains a mixture of two antibodies, anti-A and anti-A_1, which can be separated by absorption techniques using appropriate red cells. The A red cells that react with anti-A only and *not* with anti-A_1 are classified as A_2 subgroup. When anti-A is purposely absorbed from the serum of a group B individual using A_2 red cells, the serum left after the cells and attached anti-A are removed by centrifugation is referred to as "absorbed serum" (anti-A_1). Group A red cells that react with both anti-A and anti-A_1 are classified as A_1.

Another source of anti-A_1 besides absorbed serum is anti-A_1 lectin. Lectins are seed extracts that agglutinate human cells with some degree of specificity. The seeds of the plant Dolichos biflorus serve as the source of the anti-A_1 lectin. This reagent agglutinates A_1 or A_1B cells but does not agglutinate A_2 or A_2B cells.

TABLE 5-6. ABH Substances in the Saliva of Secretors (SeSe or Sese)*

	Substances in Saliva		
ABO Group	A	B	H
A	high concentration	none	some
B	none	high concentration	some
O	none	none	high concentration
AB	high concentration	high concentration	some

*Nonsecretors (sese) have no ABH substances in saliva.

Classification into A_1 and A_2 phenotypes accounts for 99 percent of all group A individuals. The cells of approximately 80 percent of the group A population are A_1, while the remaining 20 percent are A_2 or weaker subgroups. The difference between A_1 and A_2 is both quantitative and qualitative, and the production of both types of antigens is still a result of an inherited gene at the ABO locus (Table 5-7). Inheritance of an A_1 gene converts almost all the H precursor structure to A_1 antigens on the red cells, since this gene elicits high concentrations of the enzyme N-acetylgalactosaminyltransferase. Remember, this enzyme transfers the immunodominant sugar N-acetylgalactosamine to the H antigen conferring A specificity to these red cells. A_1 is a very potent gene that creates from 810,000 to 1,170,000 A_1 antigen sites on the adult A_1 red cell. Inheritance of an A_2 gene results in the production of only 240,000 to 290,000 A_2 antigen sites on the adult A_2 red cell. These quantitative differences have been reflected not only in the number of antigen sites but also in the concentration of N-acetylgalactosaminyltransferase. Studies on the transferases from A_1 and A_2 individuals have demonstrated greater activity in the sera of A_1 individuals than in A_2 individuals by their ability to convert group O cells to A cells.[7,8] Qualitative differences also exist since 1 to 8 percent of A_2 individuals produce anti-A_1 in their serum and 22 to 35 percent of A_2B individuals produce anti-A_1. In fact, some investigators have demonstrated that anti-A_1 can be found in the sera of all A_2B individuals if sensitive techniques are utilized. Therefore, some subtle qualitative differences between A_1 and A_2 antigens must exist, even though the same immunodominant sugar is attached by the same transferase in each case. There must be some change in the antigenic structure, since the A_2 and A_2B individuals cannot recognize the A_1 antigen as being part of their own red cell make-up and are immunologically stimulated to produce a specific A_1 antibody that does not cross-react with A_2 red cells.

Moreno and coworkers[9] have suggested that the A_1 specificity is conferred by the linkage of the immunodominant sugar to two different types of precursor chains, type 1 and type 2. According to this theory, the same immunodominant sugar is only attached to type-2 precursor chains in A_2 antigens. Other workers, however,

TABLE 5-7. Additional ABO Genotypes, Phenotypes, and Frequencies[11]

| Genotype | Phenotype | U.S. Frequencies | |
		Whites	Blacks
A_1A_1 A_1A_2 A_1O	A_1	33%	19%
A_2A_2 A_2O	A_2	7%	5%
A_1B A_2B	A_1B A_2B	2% 1%	2% 2%

have not been able to confirm these findings and contradict this theory by showing that only type-2 precursor chains are synthesized by red cells (see Color Plate 6) and that the A-active structures isolated from group A_1 and A_2 red cells are identical. However, perhaps in the formation of the A_2 antigen, the sugar N-acetylgalactosamine is attached in an alternative position to the galactose sugar of the precursor structure.

More recently, a new theory of ABO subgroups has been proposed by the identification of four different forms of H antigens, two of which are unbranched and two of which are branched chains. In order to avoid confusion of the issue of subgroups, this theory is presented later in this chapter under the heading ABO Subgroup Formation: A New Theory.

Whatever the case, the distinction of A_1 and A_2 does exist, and the groups A and AB are divided into A_1 and A_2 and A_1B and A_2B. It is generally presented, however, that A_1 has two antigens, A and A_1, while A_2 has only one, A antigen (see Color Plate 9). However, to simplify the concept, one can think of A_1 as having only A_1 antigen sites and A_2 as having only A antigen sites. Anti-A serum (from group B donors) contains two antibodies, anti-A plus anti-A_1; therefore, this antibody mixture will react with both A_1 and A_2 red cells. Pure anti-A_1 antibody will only react with A_1 antigen sites (see Color Plate 9). Regardless of which conceptual presentation is utilized, the fact remains that group A red cells can be subdivided by the results of tests with anti-A (from B donor sera), anti-A,B (from O donor sera), and anti-A_1 (absorbed serum or lectin).

Similar classifications can be made among group AB red cells. To include these subgroups in the genetic pathways of the biosynthesis of ABH antigens, we must again start with the basic precursor substance (Fig. 5-1). From this diagram one can see that the H gene appears to be necessary for the formation of the A,B and H antigens. H antigen is found in greatest concentration on the red cells of group O individuals. Group A_1 individuals will not possess a great deal of H antigen. In the presence of the A_1 gene, almost all of the H antigen is converted to the A_1 antigen by placing that large N-acetylgalactosamine sugar on the H substance. Since so many A_1 antigens exist, the H antigen may be so hidden that A_1 and A_1B red cells may not react with anti-H antisera. In the presence of an A_2 gene, only some of the H antigen is converted to A antigens and the remaining H antigen is expressed on the cell. Therefore, weak subgroups of the A antigen will often have large amounts of H antigen exposed and a lower number of A antigens formed. The same is usually true in subgroups of B (see Table 5-9). The H antigen in A_1 and A_1B red cells is so well hidden by the addition of that large immunodominant sugar that anti-H is occasionally found in their serum. This anti-H is a "naturally occurring" IgM cold agglutinin that reacts best below room temperature. As can be expected this antibody is formed in response to a natural substance and reacts most strongly with cells of group O individuals. It is an insignificant antibody in terms of transfusion purposes, as it has no reactivity at 37°C body temperature. However, high-titered anti-H may react at room temperature and may be a problem in compatibility testing (see Chapter 11). It can be detectable during antibody screening procedures, since the reagent cells used are all group O red cells (see Chapter 12). However, since 80 percent of the A and

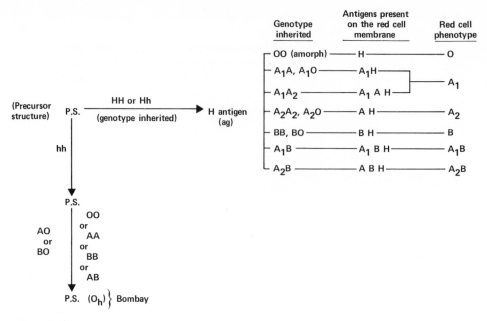

FIGURE 5-1. Summary of the genetic pathway for the biosynthesis of ABH antigens.

AB donors are A_1 and A_1B, these would probably be selected for the appropriate patient and would be compatible with anti-H in the patient's serum.

Anti-H lectin from the extract of Ulex europaeus closely parallels the reactions of human anti-H. Both agglutinate cells of group O and A_2 and react very weakly or not at all with A_1 and A_1B. Group B cells give reactions of variable strength (see Fig. 5-2). Apparently the difference in the accessibility of the fucose sugar that determines H specificity contributes to the reactivity of anti-H among the various red cell ABO groups (for review refer to Color Plates 4 through 7).

Reactivity with anti-H may be utilized to classify the weaker subgroups of A along with the reactions using anti-A, anti-A,B, and anti-A_1 previously mentioned. Also, the presence or absence of anti-A_1 in the serum as well as the ability of individuals to secrete A substance in saliva and the presence of A transferase in their serum can all be utilized to subdivide A individuals into A_1, A intermediate, A_2, A_3, and so on. Similar classifications can be made among AB red cells (Table 5-8). Most group A infants appear to be A_2 at birth, since ABO antigens are not fully developed on the red cells at this time. However, no difficulty is usually encountered in group-

$$O > A_2 > B > A_2B > A_1 > A_1B$$

greatest	least
amount of	amount of
H	H

FIGURE 5-2. Reactivity of anti-H antisera or anti-H lectin with ABO blood groups.

ing cord red cells, since most reagents contain potent anti-A and anti-A,B. Most cord A_2 cells will eventually group as A_1 individuals after a given amount of time for development, usually a few months.

B SUBGROUPS

Subgroups of B are infrequent. They are usually recognized by variations in the strength of the reaction using anti-B and anti-A,B (Table 5-9). An anti-B lectin, Bandeiraea simplicifolia (modified BS-1 lectin), has been prepared for differentiating group B variants. The most important finding of this new lectin, however, is its ability to differentiate true B antigens from "acquired B-like" antigens on red blood cells. Modified BS-1 lectin does not agglutinate "acquired B" antigens, only true B antigens. (A discussion of "acquired B" antigens can be found in the section ABH Antigens in Disease, later in this chapter). This lectin is not widely available yet and, therefore, is not routinely utilized, as is the anti-A_1 lectin, in the laboratory.

Since 99 percent of the subgroups encountered in the laboratory are A_2, subgroups are mainly of academic interest. Occasionally they may present practical problems if, for example, an A_x donor is mistyped as group O. This is potentially dangerous since the group O patient possesses anti-A,B, which will agglutinate and lyse A_x red cells. Occasional problems also arise when A_2 or A_2B individuals demonstrate anti-A_1 in their serum. Since anti-A_1 is a "naturally occurring" IgM cold antibody, it is unlikely to cause a transfusion reaction, but will be detected in the compatibility testing as well as in reverse grouping.

THE BOMBAY PHENOTYPES (O_h)

The H gene appears to be necessary for the formation of A and B antigens (see Fig. 5-1). It is very common; 99.99 percent of all individuals possess the H gene. The allele, h, is very rare and does *not* produce the L-fucose transferase *necessary* for formation of the H structure. The genotype hh is extremely rare and is known as the Bombay phenotype or O_h.

Bombay cells cannot be converted to group A or B by the specific transferases. This supports the concept that the H structure serves as the acceptor molecule or precursor substance for the product of the A or B gene-specified transferases. Bombay individuals lack all normal expression of the A, B, or O genes they inherited (see Fig. 5-1). The Bombay phenotype was first reported by Bhende in 1952 in Bombay, India. More than 30 Bombay phenotypes have now been reported in various parts of the world. These red cells are devoid of normal ABH antigens. The Bombay red cells fail to react with anti-A, anti-B, anti-A,B, and anti-H. Bombay serum contains anti-A, anti-B, anti-A,B, and anti-H. Unlike the anti-H found occasionally in the serum of A_1 and A_1B individuals, the Bombay anti-H is active over a wide thermal range. It is an IgM antibody that can bind complement and cause red cell lysis. Since the H antigen is common to all ABO blood groups, Bombay blood is incompatible with all ABO donors. Only blood from another Bombay individual can be transfused to a

TABLE 5-8 Characteristics of A Subgroups

	Forward Grouping							
	Reaction of Red Cells with					Presence of Anti-A$_1$ in Serum	Saliva of Secretors	Presence of A transferase in Serum
Classification or Phenotype	Anti-A	Anti-B	Anti-A,B	Anti-A$_1$ Lectin	Anti-H Lectin			
A$_1$	++++	neg	++++	++++	wk or neg	neg	A & H	pos
A$_2$	++	neg	+++	neg	+++	1–8% pos	A & H	pos
A$_{int}$	+++	neg	++++	++	+++	neg	A & H	pos
A$_3$	mf	neg	mf	neg	+++	neg	A & H	pos
A$_m$	wk or neg	neg	wk or neg	neg	+++++	usu pos	A & H	pos
A$_x$	wk or neg	neg	+	neg	+++++	usu neg	H	neg
A$_{end}$	mf	neg	mf	neg	+++++	uncertain	H	neg
A$_{el}$*	neg	neg	neg	neg	+++++	usu pos	H	neg
A$_{finn}$	mf	neg	mf	neg	+++++	usu pos	H	neg

*A specificity found only in eluate.
mf = mixed field; neg = negative; pos = positive; wk = weak; usu = usually

TABLE 5-9. Characteristics of B Subgroups

	Forward Grouping						
	Reaction of Red Cells with				Presence of Anti-B in Serum	Saliva of Secretors	Presence of B Transferase in Serum
Classification or Phenotype	Anti-A	Anti-B	Anti-A,B	Anti-H Lectin			
B$_3$	neg	mf	mf	++++	neg	B & H	pos
B$_x$	neg	wk	wk/+	+++++	pos	H	neg
B$_m$*	neg	neg	neg	+++++	neg	B & H	pos
B$_{el}$*	neg	neg	neg	++++	occasional	H	neg

*B specificity found only in eluate.
mf = mixed field; neg = negative; pos = positive; wk = weak

MODERN BLOOD BANKING AND TRANSFUSION PRACTICES

Bombay recipient. In routine forward grouping, using anti-A, anti-B, and anti-A,B, the Bombay would phenotype as an O blood group. However, giving normal group O (with the highest concentration of H antigen) would cause immediate cell lysis by the potent anti-H of the Bombay individual.

INHERITANCE

The genotype hh usually occurs in the children of consanguineous marriages. When family studies demonstrate which ABO genes are inherited in the Bombay pheno-type, then the genes are written as superscripts ($O_h{}^A$, $O_h{}^B$, $O_h{}^{AB}$).

The serum of Bombay individuals who are genetically A or B contains the specific A or B transferases, demonstrated by the ability of the Bombay serum to convert group O cells to A or B. O_h (hh) individuals are all nonsecretors of ABH substances, since both the H gene and the Se gene must be inherited for the ABH antigens to be found in secretions.

CLASSIFICATION

The Bombay phenotype has now been classified into four different categories that are dependent upon the inheritance of the alleles of H (hh) or modifying genes (zz) that are responsible for the variable expression of H and, in turn, A and B antigens (Fig. 5-3).

The deficiency of H characterizing the Bombay phenotype can be divided into four groups (Table 5-10):

Group 1. These Bombay individuals, previously described, inherit hh, result-ing in lack of H antigen in both the saliva and red cells, regardless of the ABO genes inherited. A wide thermal range anti-H is present in their sera. This group is desig-nated as O_h, $O_h{}^A$, $O_h{}^B$, and $O_h{}^{AB}$.

Group 2. These Bombay individuals inherit the modifying genes (zz), result-ing in a lack of H antigen on the red cells only. The saliva of secretors contains the H glycoprotein substance and the sera of these individuals contain a weak anti-H or

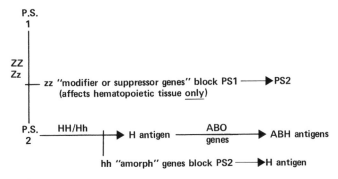

FIGURE 5-3. A possible pathway for the genetic control of the formation of the various groups of Bombay phenotypes.

TABLE 5-10. Bombay Phenotypes

Designation	Suggested Mode of Inheritance	Anti-A	Anti-B	Anti-AB	Antibody Present in Serum	Saliva of Secretor
Group 1: O_h, O_h^A, O_h^B, O_h^{AB}	hh	neg	neg	neg	anti-A,B anti-H	neg
Group 2: O_{HM}, O_{HM}^A, O_{HM}^B, O_{HM}^{AB}	zz	neg	neg	neg	anti-A,B wk anti-H or IH	H
Group 3: A_h	hh	wk/neg	neg	+	anti-B anti-H	neg
B_h		neg	wk/neg	+	anti-A anti-H	neg
Group 4: A_{HM}		neg	neg	++	anti-B wk anti-H or IH	A & H
B_{HM}	zz	neg	+	+	anti-A wk anti-H or IH	B & H

neg = negative; wk = weak

IH. This group is designated O_{Hm}, $O_{Hm}{}^A$, $O_{Hm}{}^B$, and $O_{Hm}{}^{AB}$. (Note: The "I" refers to the I blood group system.)

Group 3. These Bombay individuals probably inherit the hh, resulting in lack of H antigen in both the saliva and red cells; however, weakly reacting A or B antigens are detectable on the red cells dependent upon the inheritance of the A or B gene. The saliva of secretors contains no ABH substances and the sera of these individuals contain a wide thermal range anti-H. This group is designated A_h and B_h.

Group 4. These Bombay individuals probably inherit the modifying genes (zz), resulting in a lack of H antigen on the red cells only. However, weakly reacting A or B antigens are detectable on the red cells dependent on the inheritance of the A or B gene. The saliva of these subjects contains ABH glycoprotein substances and their sera contain a weak reacting anti-H or IH. This group is designated A_{Hm} and B_{Hm}.

ABH ANTIGENS IN DISEASE

Associations between ABH antigens and practically any disorder known to man can be found throughout medical literature. Even more profound are the associations of blood group specificity and such things as a more pronounced "hangover" in A blood groups, criminality in group B blood groups, and good teeth in group O individuals. There are also several papers correlating blood groups with personality traits. It is no surprise that many scientists refer to these associations as a part of blood group mythology. However, more relevant associations between blood groups and disease are important to the blood banker in terms of blood group serology.

Various disease states seem to alter red cell antigens and result in progressively weaker reactions or additional acquired "pseudo-antigens" during forward grouping. Leukemia, for example, has been shown to depress antigen strength. Often the cells will appear to be a mixed field agglutination (tiny agglutinates in a sea of unagglutinated cells). These weakened A or B antigens have been referred to as Ag or Bg, respectively, and demonstrate the type of serologic reactions seen below:

	Forward Grouping			Reverse Grouping	
Patient	Reaction of Patient Cells with			Reaction of Patient Serum with	
Phenotype	Anti-A	Anti-B	Anti-A,B	A_1 cells	B cells
Ag	+ mf	neg	+ + mf	neg	+ + +
Bg	neg	± / +	+	+ + + +	neg

mf = mixed field

The weakening of the antigen tends to follow the course of the disease. The antigen strength will increase again as the patient enters into remission. The isoagglutinins (anti-A, anti-B, or anti-A,B) may also be weak or absent in those leukemias demonstrating hypogammaglobulinemia, such as chronic lymphocytic leukemia (CLL). Various lymphomas, such as the malignant (non-Hodgkin's) variety, may yield weak isoagglutinins owing to moderate decreases in the gamma globulin fraction. Also, immunodeficiency diseases, such as congenital agammaglobulinemia, will also yield weak or absent isoagglutinins. If this problem is suspected, a simple serum protein electrophoresis will confirm or deny this condition. Hodgkin's disease has also been reported to weaken or depress ABH red cell antigens, resulting in variable reactions during forward grouping similar to those found during leukemia.

The very young and elderly will also have weak expression of the ABO isoagglutinins. In the elderly the production of immunoglobulin is depressed. In the infant population the production of ABO isoagglutinins is not detectable until 3 to 6 months of age. Also, A antigen production is not fully complete at birth and newborn cells will appear as the subgroup A_2. Discrepancies in the reverse grouping are thus observed even in the absence of a disease state.

Individuals with intestinal obstruction, carcinoma of the colon or rectum, or other disorders of the lower intestinal tract will have increased permeability of the intestinal wall, which allows passage of the bacterial polysaccharides from Escherichia coli serotype O_{86} into the patient's circulation. This results in the "acquired B" phenomenon in group A individuals. The patient's group A red cells absorb the B-like polysaccharide, which reacts with anti-B. This reaction is always weaker than the reaction of the true A antigen with anti-A. The "acquired B" phenomenon has also been associated with septicemic infections from Proteus vulgaris. An "acquired A" phenomenon has been associated with septicemic infections from Proteus mirabilis.

A lack of detectable ABO antigens can occur in patients with carcinoma of the stomach or pancreas. The patient's red cell antigens have not been changed, but their serum contains excessive amounts of blood group specific soluble substances (BGSS), which neutralize the antisera utilized in the forward grouping. The individual's red cells can be grouped correctly when they are washed three times with saline to remove any residual patient serum.

All these disease states previously mentioned result in discrepancies between the forward and reverse grouping, indicating that the patient's red cell group is not what it seems. All ABO discrepancies must be resolved before blood is to be released for that patient. Saliva studies may help in some cases to confirm the patient's true ABO group.

ABO DISCREPANCIES

ABO discrepancies are usually technical in nature and can be simply resolved by correctly repeating the testing and carefully checking reagents with meticulous reading and recording of results. Some of the more common causes of technical errors leading to ABO discrepancies in the forward and reverse grouping are listed in

TABLE 5-11. Common Sources of Technical Errors Resulting in ABO Discrepancies

1. Inadequate identification of blood specimens, test tubes, or slides
2. Cell suspension either too heavy or too light
3. Clerical errors
4. A mix-up in samples
5. Missed observation of hemolysis
6. Failure to add reagents
7. Failure to follow manufacturer's instructions
8. Uncalibrated centrifuge
9. Contaminated reagents
10. Warming during centrifugation

Table 5-11. Occasionally, however, the discrepancy may be due to a real problem with the patient's ABO group. Before trying to resolve the discrepancy it helps to acquire essential information regarding the patient's age, diagnosis, transfusion history, medications, immunoglobulin levels (if determined), and history of pregnancy.

ABO discrepancies may be arbitrarily divided into four major categories, which will each be considered separately.

GROUP I DISCREPANCIES

These discrepancies are between forward and reverse grouping owing to weak reacting or missing antibodies. Discrepancies in group I are more common than those in the other groups listed. When a reaction in the reverse grouping is weak or missing, weak or missing antibodies should be suspected since, normally, forward and reverse grouping reactions are very strong (4+). The reason for the missing or weak isoagglutinins is that the patient has depressed antibody production or cannot produce the ABO antibodies. Some of the more common populations with discrepancies in this group are

1. Newborns
2. Elderly patients
3. Patients with leukemias (which give hypogammaglobulinemia, e.g., CLL)
4. Patients with lymphomas (which give hypogammaglobulinemia, e.g., malignant lymphomas)
5. Patients using immunosuppressive drugs (which yield hypogammaglobulinemia)
6. Patients with congenital agammaglobulinemia
7. Patients with immunodeficiency diseases
8. Patients with bone marrow transplantations (patients develop hypogammaglobulinemia from therapy and start producing another different red cell population from the transplanted bone marrow)

An example of a typical ABO discrepancy caused by group I is given below:

	Forward Grouping			Reverse Grouping	
	Reaction of Patient Cells with			Reaction of Patient Serum with	
	Anti-A	Anti-B	Anti-A,B	A_1 Cells	B Cells
Patient	neg	neg	neg	neg	neg

Probable group: O patient associated with any of the causes (a) through (h) resulting in lack of detectable isoagglutinins.

One of the rare causes of a weak or missing ABO isoagglutinin is chimerism. Chimerism is defined as the presence of two cell populations in a single individual. Detecting a separate cell population may be easy or difficult depending upon what percentage of cells of the minor population is present. Reactions from chimerism will typically be mixed field agglutination. More commonly, artificial chimeras occur, yielding mixed cell populations that are due to (1) blood transfusions (e.g., group O cells given to an A or B patient); (2) transplanted bone marrows; (3) exchange transfusions; and (4) fetal-maternal bleeding. True chimerism is rarely found and occurs in twins in which two cell populations will exist throughout the life of the individual. In utero exchange of blood occurs because of vascular anastomosis. As a result, two cell populations emerge that are both recognized as self, and the individuals do not make anti-A or anti-B. Therefore, no detectable isoagglutinins are present in the reverse grouping. If the patient or donor has no history of a twin, then the chimera may be due to dispermy (two sperm fertilizing one egg) and indicates mosaicism.

GROUP II DISCREPANCIES

These discrepancies are between forward and reverse grouping owing to weak reacting or missing antigens. This group is probably the least frequently encountered. Some of the causes of discrepancies in this group include the following:

1. Subgroups of A and/or subgroups of B (see the section on ABO subgroups) may be present.

2. Leukemias may yield weakened A or B antigens referred to as Ag or Bg.

3. Hodgkin's disease has been reported in some cases to mimic the depression of antigens found in leukemia.

4. Excess amounts of blood group specific soluble substances (BGSS) present in the plasma in association with certain diseases, such as carcinoma of the stomach and pancreas, will neutralize the reagent anti-A or anti-B, leaving no unbound antibody to react with the patient cells. This yields a false-negative or weak reaction in the forward grouping. Washing the patient cells free of the BGSS with saline should alleviate the problem, resulting in a correlating forward and reverse grouping.

5. "Acquired B" phenomenon results from intestinal obstruction, carcinoma of the colon or rectum, and other disorders associated with the lower intestinal tract. This results from increased permeability of the intestinal wall and subsequent adsorption of the bacterial polysaccharide (E. coli O_{86}) onto the red cells yielding B specificity. The "acquired B" antigen has also been reported with septicemic infections from Proteus vulgaris. An "acquired A" antigen has been reported in association with an infection caused by Proteus mirabilis. The reaction of the appropriate antiserum with these acquired antigens demonstrates a weak reaction, often yielding a "mixed field" appearance. Below is the type of discrepancy in the forward and reverse grouping one may recognize owing to an "acquired B" antigen:

	Forward Grouping			Reverse Grouping	
	Reaction of Patient Cells with			Reaction of Patient Serum with	
	Anti-A	Anti-B	Anti-A,B	A_1 Cells	B Cells
Patient	+ + + +	+	+ + + +	neg	+ + + +

Recently it has been reported that acidifying the anti-B typing reagent to pH 6.0 would differentiate between "true" and "acquired" B antigens, since the acidified anti-B antisera will only agglutinate "true" B antigens.

6. Antibodies to low-incidence antigens may be present in the reagent anti-A or anti-B. It is impossible for manufacturers to screen reagent antisera against all known red cell antigens. It has been reported (although rarely) that this additional antibody in the reagent antisera has reacted with the corresponding low-incidence antigen present on the patient's red cell. This gives an unexpected reaction of the patient cells with anti-A, anti-B, or both, mimicking the presence of a weak antigen (see reactions below):

	Forward Grouping			Reverse Grouping	
	Reaction of Patient Cells with			Reaction of Patient Serum with	
	Anti-A	Anti-B	Anti-A,B	A_1 Cells	B Cells
Patient	+ + + +	+	+ + + +	neg	+ + + +

GROUP III DISCREPANCIES

These discrepancies are between forward and reverse grouping owing to protein or plasma abnormalities and have the following causes:

1. Elevated levels of globulin from certain disease states, such as multiple myeloma, Waldenström's macroglobulinemia, and other plasma cell dyscrasias, as

well as certain moderately-advanced cases of Hodgkin's lymphomas, result in rouleau formation. Also, increased levels of fibrinogen can enhance rouleau formation. Rouleaux of red cells result from a stacking of erythrocytes that adhere in a coin-like fashion, giving the appearance of agglutination. Washing the patient's red cells with saline or adding a drop or two of saline to the test tube will free the cells in the case of rouleau formation. In the case of true agglutination, red cell clumping will still remain after the addition of saline.

2. Plasma expanders, such as dextran and polyvinylpyrrolidone (PVP), will also cause rouleau formation as previously described. Washing the red cells with saline will also alleviate this problem. The type of discrepancy in the forward and reverse grouping caused by rouleau formation is shown below:

| | Forward Grouping | | | Reverse Grouping | |
| | Reaction of Patient Cells with | | | Reaction of Patient Serum with | |
	Anti-A	Anti-B	Anti-A,B	A_1 Cells	B Cells
Patient	$++++$	$++$	$++++$	$++$	$++++$

3. Wharton's jelly is a viscous mucopolysaccharide material present on cord bloods that causes spontaneous rouleauxing, resembling agglutination. Washing the cord cells six to eight times should alleviate this problem. Even though it is rather illogical to perform reverse groupings on cord samples, a small minority of hospitals still routinely carry out this procedure. Therefore, the student should be aware that washing the cord cells with saline will result in an accurate forward grouping. However, the reverse grouping may still be *non*correlating, since the antibodies detected are usually of maternal origin.

GROUP IV DISCREPANCIES

These discrepancies are between forward and reverse grouping owing to miscellaneous problems and have the following causes:

1. Polyagglutination (spontaneous red cell agglutination by most normal human serum) can occur owing to exposure of a hidden erythrocyte antigen (T antigen) in patients with bacterial or viral infections. Bacterial contamination in vitro or in vivo produces an enzyme that alters and exposes this hidden antigen on red blood cells, leading to "T activation." All normal human serum contains anti-T, which reacts with this now-exposed hidden antigen T. The strength of the reaction depends upon how much anti-T antibody is in the serum. An example of the type of discrepancy in the forward and reverse grouping caused by T activation is shown below:

	Forward Grouping			Reverse Grouping	
	Reaction of Patient Cells with			Reaction of Patient Serum with	
	Anti-A	Anti-B	Anti-A,B	A_1 Cells	B Cells
Patient	++	+	++++	++++	++++

"Tn activation," although rarely encountered, is another type of polyagglutinability. This condition is permanent, *not* transient, and is *not* associated with bacterial or viral infections. "Acquired A antigen" phenomenon has been reported in Tn activation (see Chapter 21).

2. Patients with potent cold autoantibodies will yield a positive direct Coombs test (see Chapter 19), and this can cause spontaneous agglutination of the patient's cells. If the antibody in the serum reacts with all adult cells, for example, anti-I (see I Blood Group System in Chapter 8), then the reagent A and B cells utilized in the reverse grouping will also agglutinate. The type of discrepancy in the forward and reverse grouping caused by cold autoantibodies is shown below:

	Forward Grouping			Reverse Grouping	
	Reaction of Patient Cells with			Reaction of Patient Serum with	
	Anti-A	Anti-B	Anti-A,B	A_1 Cells	B Cells
Patient	++	++++	++++	++++	+++

Patients with warm autoimmune hemolytic anemia or those on drugs such as alpha methyldopa may have red cells coated with sufficient antibody to promote spontaneous agglutination that will react more weakly at room temperature than at 37°C. Also, transfusion reactions resulting in antibody production owing to transfused foreign red cell antigens can result in antibody-coated red cells that produce a positive direct Coombs test. This may promote a "mixed field" or weak agglutination in the forward grouping, resulting in an ABO discrepancy. These warm-reacting antibodies, which are coating the patient's red cells, will yield weaker reactions at room temperature during ABO testing. The type of discrepancy in the forward and reverse grouping caused by warm autoantibodies or transfusion reactions yielding antibody-coated red cells is shown below:

	Forward Grouping			Reverse Grouping	
	Reaction of Patient Cells with			Reaction of Patient Serum with	
	Anti-A	Anti-B	Anti-A,B	A_1 Cells	B Cells
Patient	+	+	+	++++	++++

3. Unexpected ABO isoagglutinins in the patient's serum react at room temperature with the corresponding antigen present on the reagent cells. Examples of this type of ABO discrepancy include A_2 and A_2B individuals who can produce "naturally occurring" anti-A_1, or A_1 and A_1B individuals who may produce "naturally occurring" anti-H. (For review, refer to previous sections on ABO subgroups.)

4. Unexpected alloantibodies in the patient's serum other than ABO isoagglutinins may cause a discrepancy in the reverse grouping. Reverse grouping cells possess other antigens in addition to A and B, and it is possible that other unexpected antibodies present in the patient's serum will react with these cells (see below):

	Forward Grouping			Reverse Grouping	
	Reaction of Patient Cells with			Reaction of Patient Serum with	
	Anti-A	Anti-B	Anti-A,B	A_1 Cells	B Cells
Patient	+ + + +	+ + + +	+ + + +	+	+

5. Antibodies other than anti-A and anti-B may react to form antigen-antibody complexes that may then adsorb onto the patient's red cells. For example, acriflavin is the yellow dye used in some commercial anti-B reagents. Some individuals have antibodies against acriflavin in their serum. The patient's antibody combines with the dye and attaches to the patient's red cells, resulting in agglutination in the forward grouping. The type of discrepancy in the forward grouping caused by this red cell-adsorbed, soluble, antigen-antibody complex is shown below:

	Forward Grouping			Reverse Grouping	
	Reaction of Patient Cells with			Reaction of Patient Serum with	
	Anti-A	Anti-B	Anti-A,B	A_1 Cells	B Cells
Patient	neg	+ + +	neg	+ + + +	+ + + +

6. The serum of most "cis-AB" individuals (a rare occurrence) contains a weak anti-B, which leads to an ABO discrepancy in the reverse grouping. Cis-AB refers to the inheritance of both AB genes from one parent carried on one chromosome and an O gene inherited from the other parent. This results in the offspring inheriting three ABO genes instead of two (Fig. 5-4). The designation cis-AB is utilized to distinguish this mode of inheritance from the more usual AB phenotype in which the alleles are located on different chromosomes. Usually the B antigen yields a weaker reaction with the anti-B from random donors, with mixed field agglutination typical of subgroup B_3 reported in several cases. The serum of most cis-AB individuals contains a weak anti-B, which reacts with all ordinary B red cells, yet not with cis-AB red cells. Some investigators have suggested that the B antigen in the cis-AB

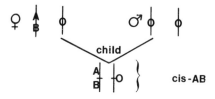

FIGURE 5-4. Cis-AB inheritance.

represents only a piece of the normal B antigen. Cis-AB blood can be classified into four categories: A_2B_3, A_1B_3, A_2B, and A_2B_x. Various hypotheses have been offered to explain the cis-AB phenotype. Many favor a crossing over of a portion of a gene resulting in unequal expression by the recombinant. However, the banding pattern of the distal end of the long arm of chromosome nine representing the ABO locus is normal.

RESOLUTION OF ABO DISCREPANCIES

Most ABO discrepancies are detected because forward and reverse groupings do not agree. Therefore, the first step in problem solving is to repeat all tests to be sure that the cell suspension is not too heavy or too light, that the red cells, reagents, and equipment are free of contamination, and that there is no sample mix-up. If repeat testing confirms the original results, then a complete work-up should be performed. This should include (1) a direct antihuman globulin test (DAT) (see Chapter 4); (2) performance of the forward grouping using red cells that have been washed three times with saline and resuspended in saline (reagents anti-A, anti-B, anti-A,B, and anti-A_1 should all be used); (3) performance of reverse grouping with three examples of A_1, A_2, and B cells, as well as group O cord cells, O screening cells, and an autologous control (patient's serum mixed with patient's red cells); and (4) incubation of all tests at room temperature for 15 to 30 minutes and, if necessary, at 4°C for 5 to 15 minutes before reading and recording results to resolve the discrepancy (Table 5-12).

Some examples of serologic reactions involving ABO discrepancies have been provided with answers for review and self-evaluation at the end of this chapter. Also, the procedure for determination of secretor status is provided at the end of this chapter. Finally, you have been briefly introduced to ABO, the first and "simplest" blood group system known to man!

ABO SUBGROUP FORMATION: A NEW THEORY

Another probable explanation of ABO subgroup formation lies in the fact that four types of glycolipids have been biochemically defined. H_1 and H_2 are unbranched straight chains and H_3 and H_4 are more complex branched chains (see Color Plate 10).

TABLE 5-12. ABO Discrepancies Between Forward and Reverse Grouping*

Patient	Forward Grouping			Reverse Grouping			Auto Control	Possible Causes	Resolution Steps
	Anti-A	Anti-B	Anti-A,B	A_1 Cells	B Cells	O Cells			
#1	neg	neg	neg	neg	neg	neg	neg	Group O newborn or elderly patient; patient may have hypogammaglobulinemia, agammaglobulinemia, or may be on immunosuppressive drugs	Check age of patient & immunoglobulin levels if possible; incubate at RT for 30 min or at 4°C
#2	4+	neg	4+	1+	4+	neg	neg	Subgroup of A; probable A_2 with anti-A_1	Use anti-A_1 lectin
#3	4+	4+	4+	2+	2+	2+	2+	(1) Rouleaux (multiple myeloma patient; any patient with reversed albumin/globulin ratio or patients given plasma expanders) (2) Cold autoantibody (probable group AB with an auto anti-I) (3) Cold autoantibody with underlying cold or RT reacting alloantibody (probable group AB with an auto anti-I & a high frequency cold antibody, e.g., anti-P_1, anti-M, anti-Le[b]	(1) Wash red cells; use saline replacement (2) Perform cold panel and autoabsorb (3) Perform cold panel, autoabsorb, & run panel on absorbed serum; select reverse cells lacking antigen for identified alloantibody; repeat reverse group on absorbed serum to determine true ABO group
#4	3+	4+	4+	1+	neg	neg	neg	Subgroup of AB; probable A_2B with anti-A_1	Use anti-A_1 lectin

							Interpretation	Recommended action
#5	4+	neg	4+	neg	4+	3+	neg	A₁ with potent anti-H	Confirm A₁ group with anti-A₁ lectin; test additional A₂, O, and A₁ cells and an O_h if available
#6	neg	neg	neg	4+	4+	4+	neg	O_h Bombay	Test with anti-H lectin; test O_h cell if available; send to reference lab for confirmation
#7	neg	neg	2+	2+	4+	neg	neg	Subgroup of A; probable A_x with anti-A₁	Perform saliva studies or absorption/elution
#8	4+	2+	4+	neg	4+	neg	neg	Group A with an "acquired B" antigen	Check history of patient for lower GI problem or septicemia; use modified BS-1 lectin if available, or acidify anti-B typing reagent to pH 6.0 by adding one or two drops of 1N HCl to 1 ml of anti-B antisera, and measure with a pH meter (this acidified anti-B antisera would only agglutinate true B antigens, *not* acquired B antigens)
#9	4+	4+	4+	2+	2+	2+	neg	Alloantibody	Perform antibody screen and panel
#10	neg	4+	4+	1+	1+	1+	1+	Group B with cold autoantibody	Enzyme treat red cells and perform autoabsorption at 4°C or perform prewarmed testing

*Absorptions should not be performed on patient cells that have been transfused within the last 3 months.

neg = negative

H_1 through H_4 correspond to the precursor structures upon which the A_1 enzyme can act to convert to blood group A-active glycolipids. Although the chains differ in length and complexity of branching, the terminal sugars giving rise to their antigenic specificity are identical. Studies on the chemical and physical characteristics of the A_1 and A_2 enzyme transferases have demonstrated that these two enzymes are different qualitatively.[7,10] Straight chain H_1 and H_2 glycolipids can be converted to A^a and A^b antigens respectively by both A_1 and A_2 enzymes, with the A_2 enzyme being less efficient. The more complex branched H_3 and H_4 structures can be converted to A^c and A^d antigens by A_1 enzyme and only very poorly by A_2 enzyme. As a result, more unconverted H antigens (specifically H_3 and H_4) are available on group A_2 red cells with only A^a and A^b A determinants being formed from H_1 and H_2 structures. In the red cells of some A_2 individuals, A^c is extremely low and A^d is completely lacking. It is feasible to expect that these are the individuals in whom one would find an anti-A_1 in the serum. This anti-A_1 antibody could really be an antibody to A^c and A^d A determinants, which these A_2 individuals lack. Also, in 22 to 35 percent of A_2B individuals, anti-A_1 can be found in the serum. Since the B enzyme transferase is usually more efficient than the A enzyme in converting H structures to the appropriate antigen, A_2 enzymes would probably fail completely when paired with a B enzyme. As a result, A_2B individuals would be far more likely to lack A^c and A^d components with subsequent production of anti-A^c and anti-A^d (anti-A_1).

Most group A infants appear to be A_2 at birth, with subsequent development to A_1 a few months later. Newborn infants, however, have been found to have a deficiency of the branched H_3 and H_4 antigens and, therefore, also the A^c and A^d antigens, possibly accounting for the A_2 phenotype. Adult cells contain a higher concentration of branched H_3 and H_4 structures and, therefore, A^c and A^d variants of the A antigen of A_1 individuals.

DETERMINATION OF THE SECRETOR PROPERTY

PRINCIPLE

Certain blood group substances occur in soluble form in secretions such as saliva and gastric juice, in a large proportion (78 percent) of individuals. Such individuals are termed "secretors" (they possess the Se gene) and secrete A, B, or H soluble antigens. These water-soluble blood group substances are readily detected in very minute quantities since they have the property of reacting with their corresponding antibodies and thereby neutralizing or inhibiting the capacity of the antibody to agglutinate erythrocytes possessing the corresponding antigen. The reaction is termed hemagglutination inhibition and provides a means of assaying the relative activity or potency of these water-soluble blood group substances.

MATERIALS

    paraffin wax
    saliva
    anti-A serum
    anti-B serum
    test tubes
    2 to 5 percent washed group A cells
    2 to 5 percent washed group B cells
    2 to 5 percent washed group O cells

PROCEDURE

1. Chew a piece of paraffin wax to stimulate secretion of saliva.
2. Collect about 2 to 3 ml of saliva in a test tube.
3. Place stoppered tube of saliva in a boiling waterbath for 10 minutes. This inactivates enzymes that might otherwise destroy blood group substances.
4. Centrifuge hard for 10 minutes.
5. Collect clear supernatant into a clean tube.
6. Add one drop of diluted antiserum to an appropriately labeled tube (anti-A, anti-B, anti-H). For dilution, titrate anti-H, anti-A, and anti-B, testing against appropriate cells at immediate spin. Select the dilution giving 2+ agglutination and prepare a sufficient quantity to complete the test.
7. Add one drop of supernatant saliva to each tube. Incubate at room temperature for 10 minutes.
8. Add one drop of the 2 to 5 percent saline suspension of washed A, B, or O cells to the appropriate tube.
9. Allow serum-saliva-cell mixture to stand at room temperature for 30 to 60 minutes.
10. Centrifuge.
11. Observe for macroscopic agglutination.

CONTROL

1. Add one drop diluted antiserum; no saliva is added.
2. Add one drop of a 2 to 5 percent saline cell suspension of appropriate blood group.
3. Incubate 30 to 60 minutes (in parallel with tests), then centrifuge and read for agglutination.

INTERPRETATIONS

1. *Nonsecretor*: Agglutination of red cells by antiserum-saliva mixture; control tube positive.

2. *Secretor*: No agglutination of red cells by antiserum and saliva mixture; control tube positive. The antiserum has been neutralized by the soluble blood group substances or antigens in the saliva, which react with their corresponding antibody. Therefore, no antibody sites in the antisera are free to react with the antigens on the reagent red cells utilized in the testing. This negative reaction is a positive test for the presence of ABH soluble antigens and indicates the individual is a secretor.

ABH SUBSTANCES IN SALIVA

ABO Group	ABH Substances in Saliva		
Secretors	A	B	H
A	much	none	some
B	none	much	some
O	none	none	much
AB	much	much	some
Nonsecretors			
A B O and AB	none	none	none

REFERENCES

1. MOURANT, AE, et al.: *The Distribution of the Human Blood Groups and Other Biochemical Polymorphisms,* ed 2. Oxford University Press, Oxford, 1976.

2. SPRINGER, GF, et al.: *Origin of anti-human blood group B agglutinins in white leghorn chicks.* J Exp Med 110:221, 1959.

3. DOBSON, A and IKIN, E: *The ABO blood groups in the United Kingdom: Frequencies based on a very large sample.* J Pathol Bacteriol 58:221, 1946.

4. KUNKEL, HG and ROCKEY, JH: $\beta_2 A$ *and other immunoglobulins in isolated anti-A antibodies.* Proc Soc Exp Biol Med 113:278, 1963.

5. LANDSTEINER, K and WITT, DH: *Observations on the human blood groups. Irregular reactions. Iso-agglutinin in sera of group 4. The factor* A_1. J Immunol 2:221, 1926.

6. DODD, BE, LINCOLN, PJ and BOORMAN, KE: *The cross-reacting antibodies of group O sera: Immunological studies and a possible explanation of the observed facts.* Immunology 12:39, 1967.

7. SCHACHTER, H, et al.: *A quantitative difference in the activity of blood group A specific N-acetylgalactosaminyl-transferase in serum from* A_1 *and* A_2 *human subjects.* Biochem Biophys Res Commun 45:1011, 1971.

8. SCHACHTER, H, et al.: *Qualitative differences in the alpha-N-acetylgalactosaminyl transferases produced by human* A_1 *and* A_2 *genes.* Proc Natl Acad Sci USA 7:220, 1973.

9. MORENO, C, LUNDBLAD, A and KABAT, EA: *Immunochemical studies on blood groups.* J Exp Med 134:439, 1971.

10. TILLEY, CA, et al.: *Human blood group A- and H-specified glycosyltransferase levels in the sera of newborn infants and their mothers.* Vox Sang 34:8, 1978.

11. SHREFFLER, DC, et al.: *Studies on genetic selection in a completely ascertained U.S. Caucasian population. I. Frequencies, age, and sex effects and phenotype associations for 12 blood group systems. Tecumseh, Michigan: pop. 10,000 West European ancestry.* American Society of Human Genetics, 1971.

12. REED, TE: *Distributions and tests of independence of seven blood group systems in a large multiracial sample from California.* Am J Hum Genet 20:142, 1968.

13. WIENER, AS: *Problems and pitfalls in blood grouping tests for non-parentage: Distribution of the blood groups.* Am J Clin Pathol 51:9, 1969.

BIBLIOGRAPHY

BEATTIE, KM, et al.: *Two chimeras detected during routine grouping test by Autoanalyzer.* Transfusion 17:681, 1977.

BEATTIE, KM, et al.: *Blood group chimerism as a clue to generalized tissue mosaicism.* Transfusion 4:77, 1964.

BIRD, GWG, et al.: *Inherited "mosaicism" within the ABO blood group system.* J Immunogenet 5:215, 1978.

BOOSE, GM, ISSITT, C AND ISSITT, P: *Weak B antigen in a family.* Transfusion 18:570, 1978.

CARTRON, J, et al.: *Study of the alpha-N-acetylgalactosaminyltransferase in sera and red cell membranes of human A subgroups.* J Immunogenet 5:107, 1978.

CARTRON, J, et al.: *Assay of alpha-N-acetylgalactosaminyltransferases in human sera. Further evidence for several types of A_m individuals.* Vox Sang 28:347, 1975.

CARTRON, J, et al.: *"Weak A" phenotypes. Relationship between red cell agglutinability and antigen site density.* Immunology 27:723, 1974.

CHENG, MS: *Two similar cases of weak agglutination with anti-B reagent.* Laboratory Medicine 12:506, 1981.

COHEN, F and ZUELZER, WW: *Interrelationship of the various subgroups of the blood group A: Study with immunofluorescence.* Transfusion 5:223, 1965.

DODD, BE and LINCOLN, PJ: *Serological studies of the H activity of O_h red cells with various anti-H reagents.* Vox Sang 35:168, 1978.

ECONOMIDOU, J, HUGHES-JONES, N and GARDNER, B: *Quantitative measurements concerning A and B antigen sites.* Vox Sang 12:321, 1967.

FINNE, J: *Identification of the blood group ABH-active glycoprotein components of human erythrocyte membrane.* Eur J Biochem 104:181, 1980.

FUDENBERG, H, KUNKEL, H AND FRANKLIN E: *High molecular weight antibodies.* Acta Haematol (Basel) 10:522, 1959.

FUJISAWA, K, FURUKAWA, K and ISEKI, S: *Chemical effects of A and B decomposing enzymes on blood group substances from red cells.* Proc Jpn Acad 39:319, 1963.

GARDAS, A and KOSCIELAK, J: *A, B and H blood group specificities in glycoprotein and glycolipid fractions of human erythrocyte membrane. Absence of blood group active glycoproteins in the membrane of non-secretors.* Vox Sang 20:137, 1971.

GIBBS, MB, AKEROYD, JH and ZAPF, JJ: *Quantitative subgroups of the B antigen in man and their occurrence in three racial groups.* Nature 192:1196, 1961.

HAKOMORI, S, STELLNER, K and WATANABE, K: *Four antigenic variants of blood group A glycolipid: Examples of highly complex, branched chain glycolipid of animal cell membrane.* Biochem Biophys Res Commun 49:1061, 1972.

HANFLAND, P: *Characterization of B and H blood group active glycosphingolipids from human B erythrocyte membranes.* Chem Phys Lipids 15:105, 1975.

HIRSCHFELD, J: *Conceptual framework shifts in immunogenetics. I. A new look at cis AB antigens in the ABO system.* Vox Sang 33:286, 1977.

HUMMEL, K, et al.: *Inheritance of cis-AB in three generations (Family Lam).* Vox Sang 33:290, 1977.

ICHIKAWA, Y: *A study of the isoagglutinin titres in the sera of Australian subjects (white).* Jpn J Med Sci Biol 12:1, 1959.

KOGURE, T and FURUKAWA, K: *Enzymatic conversion of human group O red cells into group B-active cells by alpha-D-galactosyltransferases of sera and salivas from group B and its variant types.* J Immunogenet 3:147, 1976.

KOSCIELAK, J, et al.: *Structures of fucose containing glycolipids with H and B blood group activity and of sialic acid and glucosamine containing glycolipid of human erythrocyte membrane.* Eur J Biochem 37:214, 1973.

LEVINE, P, UHLIR, M and WHITE, J: *A_h, an incomplete suppression of A resembling O_h.* Vox Sang 6:561, 1961.

LOPEZ, M, et al.: *Activity of IgG and IgM ABO antibodies against some weak A (A_3, A_x, A_{end}) and weak B (B_3, B_x) red cells.* Vox Sang 37:281, 1979.

Madsen, G and Heisto, H: *A Korean family showing inheritance of A and B on the same chromosome.* Vox Sang 14:211, 1968.

Mäkelä, O, Ruoslahti, E and Ehnholm, C: *Subtypes of human ABO blood groups and subtype-specific antibodies.* J Immunol 3:763, 1969.

Marsh, WL, et al.: *Inherited mosaicism affecting the blood groups.* Transfusion 15:589, 1975.

Mohn, JF, et al.: *An inherited blood group A variant in the Finnish population. I. Basic characteristics.* Vox Sang 25:193, 1973.

Moores, PP, et al.: *Some observations on "Bombay" bloods, with comments on evidence for the existence of two different O_h phenotypes.* Transfusion 15:237, 1975.

Morgan, WTJ: *A contribution to human biochemical genetics: The chemical basis of blood-group specificity.* Proc R Soc Lond (Biol) 151:308, 1960.

Morville, P: *Investigation on isohaemagglutination in mothers and newborn children.* Acta Pathol Microbiol Scand 6:39, 1929.

Pacuszka, T, et al.: *Biochemical, serological and family studies in individuals with cis AB phenotypes.* Vox Sang 29:292, 1975.

Poretz, RD and Watkins, WM: *Galactosyltransferases in human submaxillary glands and stomach mucosa associated with the biosynthesis of blood group B specific glycoproteins.* Eur J Biochem 25:455, 1972.

Race, C and Watkins, WM: *The action of the blood group B gene-specified alpha-galactosyltransferase from human serum and stomach mucosal extracts on group O and "Bombay" O_h erythrocytes.* Vox Sang 23:385, 1972.

Race, RR and Sanger, R: *Blood Groups in Man,* ed 6. Blackwell Scientific Publications, Oxford, 1975, pp 522–524, 531–535.

Rawson, AJ and Abelson, N: *Studies of blood group antibodies. III. Observations on the physiochemical properties of isohemagglutinins and isohemolysins.* J Immunol 85:636, 1960.

Rawson, AJ and Abelson, N: *Studies of blood group antibodies. IV. Physico-chemical differences between iso-anti-A,B and iso-anti-A or iso-anti-B.* J Immunol 85:640, 1960.

Reed, TE and Moore, BPL: *A new variant of blood group A.* Vox Sang 9:363, 1964.

Romano, EL, Mollison, PL and Linares, J: *Number of B sites generated on group O red cells from adults and newborn infants.* Vox Sang 34:14, 1978.

Romans, DG, Tilley, CA and Dorrington, KJ: *Monogamous bivalency of IgG antibodies. I. Deficiency of branched ABHI-active oligosaccharide chains on red cells of infants causes the weak antiglobulin reactions in hemolytic disease of the newborn due to ABO incompatibility.* J Immunol 124:2807, 1980.

Rubinstein, P, Allen, F and Rosenfield, RE: *A dominant suppressor of A and B.* Vox Sang 25:377, 1973.

Sabo, B, et al.: *The cis AB phenotype in three generations of one family: Serological enzymatic and cytogenetic studies.* J Immunogenet 5:87, 1978.

Salmon, C, et al.: *Quantitative and thermodynamic studies of erythrocytic ABO antigens.* Transfusion 16:580, 1976.

Schenkel-Brunner, H: *Blood-group-ABH antigens of human erythrocytes.* Eur J Biochem 104:529, 1980.

Schenkel-Brunner, H, Chester, MA and Watkins, WM: *Alpha-L-fucosyltransferases in human serum from donors of different ABO, secretor and Lewis blood group phenotypes.* Eur J Biochem 30:269, 1972.

Schenkel-Brunner, H, Prohaska, R and Tuppy, H: *Action of glycosyltransferases upon "Bombay" (O_h) erythrocytes. Conversion to cells showing blood group H and A specificities.* Eur J Biochem 56:591, 1975.

Schenkel-Brunner, H and Tuppy, H: *Enzymatic conversion of human O into A erythrocytes and of B into AB erythrocytes.* Nature 223:1272, 1969.

Schenkel-Brunner, H and Tuppy, H: *Enzymatic conversion of human blood group O erythrocytes into A_2 and A_1 cells by alpha-N-acetyl-D-galactosaminyltransferases of blood group A individuals.* Eur J Biochem 34:125, 1973.

Schmidt, P, et al.: *A hemolytic transfusion reaction due to the transfusion of A_x blood.* J Lab Clin Med 54:38, 1959.

Seyfried, H, Waleska, I and Werblinska, B: *Unusual inheritance of ABO group in a family with weak B antigens.* Vox Sang 3:268, 1964.

SOLOMON, J, WAGGONER, R and LEYSHON, CW: *A quantitative immunogenetic study of gene suppression involving A_1 and H antigens of the erythrocyte without affecting secreted blood group substances. The ABH phenotypes A_m^h and O_m^h.* Blood 25:470, 1965.

STURGEON, P, MOORE, BPL and WEINER, W: *Notations for two weak A variants: A_{end} and A_{el}.* Vox Sang 9:214, 1964.

TAKASAKI, S and KOBATA, A: *Chemical characterization and distribution of ABO blood group active glycoprotein in human erythrocyte membrane.* J Biol Chem 251:3610, 1976.

TAKASAKI, S, YAMASHITA, K and KOBATA, A: *The sugar chain structures of ABO blood group active glycoproteins obtained from human erythrocyte membrane.* J Biol Chem 253:6086, 1978.

TOPPING, MD and WATKINS, WM: *Isoelectric points of the human blood group A_1, A_2 and B gene-associated glycosyltransferases in ovarian cyst fluids and serum.* Biochem Biophys Res Commun 64:89, 1975.

TUPPY, H and SCHENKEL-BRUNNER, H: *Occurrence and assay of alpha-N-acetylgalactosaminyltransferase in the gastric mucosa of humans belonging to blood group A.* Vox Sang 17:139, 1969.

WATANABE, K, LAINE, RA and HAKOMORI, S: *On neutral fucoglycolipids having long branched carbohydrate chains: H-active I-active glycosphingolipids of human erythrocyte membranes.* Biochemistry 14:2725, 1975.

WATKINS, WM: *The appearance of H specificity following the enzymic inactivation of blood group B substance.* Biochem J 64:21, 1956.

WATKINS, WM: *Glycoproteins: Their composition, structure and function.* In GOTTSCHALK, A (ed): *Glycoproteins*, ed 2. Elsevier, Amsterdam, 1972, pp 830–891.

WATKINS, WM: *Blood group substances: Their nature and genetics.* In SURGENOR, D (ed): *The Red Blood Cell*. Academic Press, New York, 1974, p 303.

WEINER, W, et al.: *A gene, y, modifying the ABO group A.* Vox Sang 2:25, 1957.

WESTERVELD, A, et al.: *Assignment of the AK_1:Np:ABO linkage group to human chromosome 9.* Proc Natl Acad Sci 73:895, 1976.

WIENER, AS and CIOFFI, AF: *A group B analogue of subgroup A_3.* Am J Clin Pathol 58:693, 1972.

WIENER, AS and SOCHA, WW: *Macro and microdifferences in blood group antigens and antibodies.* Int Arch Allergy Appl Immunol 47:946, 1974.

WITTEMORE, NB, et al.: *Solubilized glycoprotein from human erythrocyte membranes possessing blood group A, B and H activity.* Vox Sang 17:289, 1969.

WROBEL, DM, et al.: *"True" genotypes of chimeric twins revealed by blood group gene products in plasma.* Vox Sang 27:395, 1974.

YAMAGUCHI, H: *A review of cis AB blood.* Jinrui Idengaku Zasshi 18:1, 1973.

YAMAGUCHI, H, OKUBO, Y and HAZAMA, F: *Another Japanese A_2B_3 blood group family with the propositus having O group father.* Proc Jpn Acad 42:517, 1966.

YAMAGUCHI, H, OKUBO, Y and TANAKA, M: *Cis AB bloods found in Japanese families.* Jinrui Idengaku Zasshi 15:198, 1970.

YOKOYAMA, M, STACEY, SM and DUNSFORD, I: *B_x—A new subgroup of the blood group B.* Vox Sang 2:348, 1957.

YOSHIDA, A, YAMAGUCHI, YF and DAVÉ, V: *Immunologic homology of human blood group glycosyltransferases and genetic background of blood group (ABO) determination.* Blood 54:344, 1979.

CHAPTER **6**

THE Rh BLOOD GROUP SYSTEM

JOHN CASE, F.I.M.L.S.

HISTORICAL PERSPECTIVES

In 1940 Landsteiner and Wiener[1] reported the existence of a hitherto unrecognized blood group characteristic in humans, which they chose to call the Rh factor. The name Rh derived from the fact that the antibody defining the "new" antigen had been produced by deliberately immunizing guinea pigs and rabbits with the red cells of rhesus monkeys. Sera from the immunized animals agglutinated not only rhesus monkey cells (as would be expected), but also red cells of approximately 85 percent of humans, thereby providing a means of classifying human bloods into two interesting new blood types: Rh-positive (cells agglutinated by the animal anti-rhesus sera) and Rh-negative (cells not agglutinated).

It is commonly recognized that Rh-positive indicates the presence of only one specific antigen, namely, Rh_0 (D). A lack of Rh_0 (D) is designated as Rh-negative.

It was soon realized that the Rh factor was of more than mere academic significance. Wiener and Peters[2] observed that an antibody indistinguishable in specificity from the animal anti-rhesus sera could be demonstrated in sera from some people who had suffered a hemolytic transfusion reaction on being transfused with ABO-compatible blood. Subsequently, the re-examination of an antibody reported in 1939 by Levine and Stetson[3] as having caused a severe hemolytic reaction in a woman who had been transfused with her husband's blood after giving birth to a stillborn fetus revealed that this antibody, too, was showing the same pattern of positive and negative reactions as the immune animal sera of Landsteiner and Wiener. Levine and Stetson had observed in their original investigation that the woman's serum had been incompatible with her husband's red cells, as well as with those of some 80 out of 104 random ABO-compatible donors, and they had postulated in their 1939 report that the antibody had arisen as the result of feto-maternal immunization. These authors were correct in their interpretation. In 1941 Levine and associates[4] were able to show an unmistakable relationship between hemolytic disease of the newborn (then known as erythroblastosis fetalis) and Rh blood group incompatibility between the mother and the fetus.

It is interesting to speculate that had Levine and Stetson chosen to name the blood group characteristic defined by their patient's antibody, the rhesus blood group system would have been known to us by their name today instead of by the one with which we have become so familiar. Indeed, it is questionable whether the name rhesus is an appropriate one in any case, as it is now known that the animal anti-rhesus antibodies of Landsteiner and Wiener were not in fact identical in specificity to those of human origin. This illusion-shattering revelation need cause no distress. The reader may dismiss it for the time being, as it will surface again and be explained in the section dealing with the LW antigen.

As has since often been the case when a "new" blood group antigen has been reported, human antibodies to the Rh factor were soon detected and studied by other investigators. Many proved to be identical to the antibody found to have ag-glutinated the cells of 85 percent of human bloods. Still others were not identical, yet were obviously directed at related antigens. Even by 1943, the Rh blood group system was beginning to show signs of considerably greater complexity than those (ABO, MN, and P) previously known. By that stage, four separate but related an-tibodies had been recognized. Their patterns of reactivity led to the adoption of two different systems of Rh nomenclature, each based on separate genetic presumptions made by scientists on opposite sides of the Atlantic Ocean. The two nomenclatures were to some extent irreconcilable. They have coexisted for many years, however, and are sometimes used interchangeably, although they are founded on entirely different genetic concepts. It will be recalled that the original anti-Rh agglutinated the red cells of about 85 percent of random bloods. The second, third, and fourth anti-bodies to be discovered gave, respectively, 70 percent, 30 percent, and 80 percent positive reactions.

MODE OF INHERITANCE

The mode of inheritance of blood groups has been covered comprehensively in Chapter 2. There is no purpose in presenting the principles again here, although their application to the complexities of the Rh system possibly merits a brief reminder or two. Blood group antibodies do not detect genes directly, but merely recognize gene products on the red blood cells. The gene products present on a person's red cells are always a combination of those inherited from both parents, and antibodies directed at the products of allelic genes are called antithetical antibodies. Absence of the product of any gene of a known allelic pair implies homozygosity for its allele—always supposing, of course, that there is no third allele that may occupy the particular locus on the chromosome. When there are more than two alleles, the existence of the third may be established by the results of family studies or, more tangibly, by the discovery of an antibody directed at its product. Additional alleles may be recognized as the result of similar evidence. Sometimes an allele may be an amorph, which has no detectable product. On other occasions the expression of a gene product may be altered in some way by the influence of another gene. The amount of detectable product may be suppressed, even to a point at which its specific antibody fails to recognize it altogether, or it may be enhanced to a degree that alters its characteristic behavior in serologic tests with the corresponding antibody. Examples illustrating all these principles are to be found in the Rh blood group system, as will soon be apparent.

NOMENCLATURE

In introducing the subject of Rh nomenclature it would be simpler in some ways to begin with CDE, but Rh-hr has chronologic precedence and will therefore be treated first.

Rh-hr NOMENCLATURE OF WIENER

When Wiener presented his initial theory about the inheritance of the Rh blood groups, his concepts were based on tests with only three of the first four antibodies. After making an effort to understand the differences between these known antigen/antibody reactions, Wiener postulated the following genetic theory. He believed that the Rh genes coded for a specific "agglutinogen" that gave rise to three serologic factors (or antigens) that could be demonstrated on the red cell. Antibodies could then be formed to each individual factor or to complexes of the factors (which will be described under Compound Antigens, below). Refer to Table 6-1 and Figure 6-1 for a summary of Wiener's theory.

Wiener's genetic concept was that multiple allelic genes at a single complex locus give rise to the production of "agglutinogens," each comprising a potentially infinite number of "factors." Each individual factor is detectable by its own specific antibody, and the agglutinogens present on a given sample of red cells is derived

TABLE 6-1. Wiener Nomenclature

Gene	Agglutinogen	Serologic Factors
R^0	Rh_0	Rh_0, hr', hr"
R^1	Rh_1	Rh_0, rh', rh"
R^2	Rh_2	Rh_0, hr', rh"
R^z	Rh_z	Rh_0, rh', rh"
r	rh	hr', hr"
r'	rh'	rh', hr"
r''	rh"	hr', rh"
r^y	rh_y	rh', rh"

from a knowledge of which factors compose which agglutinogens. By convention, italic type is always used to denote genes and qualifying subscript designations become superscript. If they are already used as superscript symbols in the notation for the antigen, they remain that way. (All of this will make more sense when we come to the examples.) Wiener proposed that ordinary roman type would serve for the agglutinogens, while boldface type would be adopted for the factors of which each agglutinogen is composed. Thus, the gene R^0 determines an agglutinogen named Rh_0, of which the three principal component factors are **hr'**, **Rh_0**, and **hr"**. The agglutinogen includes other factors as well, of course, but to introduce them at this stage would make incomprehensible that which is already showing a tendency toward become confusing. Note that in this example one of the factors composing the agglutinogen has exactly the same letter designation as the agglutinogen itself. Here is where the importance of using boldface type asserts itself. Rh_0 is the entire agglutinogen, while **Rh_0** is one of its component factors. It should also be noted that the capital letter R is reserved for the original Rh factor **Rh_0**, for agglutinogens that include it as a component, and for genes that determine them, while a lower case letter is employed to denote the other factors, as well as agglutinogens that do not include **Rh_0** and their respective genes. The eight main agglutinogens postulated by Wiener, with their principal component factors in parentheses, were as follows: Rh_1 (**rh'**, **Rh_0**, **hr"**), rh (**hr'**, **hr"**), Rh_2 (**hr'**, **Rh_0**, **rh"**), Rh_0 (**hr'**, **Rh_0**, **hr"**), rh' (**rh'**, **hr"**), rh" (**hr'**, **rh"**), Rh_z (**rh'**, **Rh_0**, **rh"**), and rh_y (**rh'**, **rh"**). Reversal of the letters (rh to hr) implies that the factors are reciprocally related, which is to say that their corresponding antibodies are antithetical. Thus, anti-rh' and anti-hr' are antithetical, as are anti-rh" and anti-hr".

CDE NOMENCLATURE OF FISHER AND RACE

Studying the reactions given by the first four human Rh antibodies, Fisher[5] recognized the antithetical relationship between the one that gave 70 percent of positive reactions and the one that was always positive with Rh-negative red cells. He called them anti-C and anti-c, respectively, postulating that these two antibodies were defining the antigens C and c, which were the products of an allelic pair of genes called C and c. Fisher further hypothesized that this pair of alleles shared a locus on

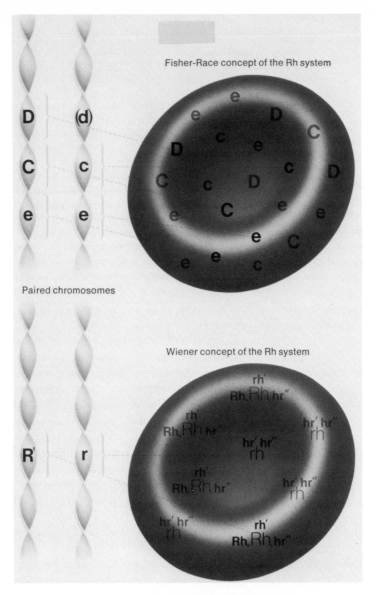

FIGURE 6-1. Fisher-Race and Wiener concepts of the Rh system. (From *Blood Group Antigens and Antibodies as Applied to the ABO and Rh Systems.* Ortho Diagnostics, Inc., with permission.)

the chromosome that was closely linked to two additional loci, each of which was shared by a further allelic pair (Fig. 6-1). Working through the alphabet, Fisher gave the designations *D* and *d* and *E* and *e* to the second and third pairs of alleles. The product of *D* he considered to be the antigen detected by the original anti-Rh, while the antigen that evidently had a 30 percent frequency was assigned as the product of the E gene. Fisher predicted that it would only be a matter of time before the two additional antibodies would be discovered that would recognize the antigens determined by d and e. In one respect he was right. The first example of anti-e was reported only 2 years later by Mourant,[6] but anti-d still awaits discovery. The fact that it has not been found in 40 years makes it seem unlikely that it ever will be. If the gene d exists at all, we must consider it to be an amorph.

It will be apparent that there are eight possible combinations of Fisher's six genes. These are, in descending order of frequency, CDe, cde, cDE, cDe, Cde, cdE, CDE, and CdE. The first three occur commonly while the last one is exceedingly rare and the one before it is seen only infrequently. If crossing over were other than a rare event, the effect would be to even out these frequencies, hence Fisher's concept that the three loci were very closely linked. As a matter of fact, in order to explain occasional crossing over as the origin of the rarer gene complexes, Fisher suggested that the locus for C/c lies between those for D/d and E/e, and this order (DCe, dce, DcE, and so on) is used by some authors in their writings.

It is now believed that Rh genes occupy many mutational sites on the chromosome, rather than three separate loci strung closely in sequence, but whether this belief ascribes greater validity to Wiener's concept than to Fisher's need not concern us. The matter is largely an academic one, as whatever the correctness of the genetic principles on which the two systems of notation were founded, the Rh-hr symbols have fallen largely into disuse. Their opponents were not confined to the printing business. Teachers consider it more convenient to explain the relationships between antigens in terms of CDE and students generally find this system easier to understand. At the same time, the various antigen combinations in capital and lower case letters are cumbersome to communicate verbally, so a shorthand system of notation based on the symbols assigned by Wiener to his agglutinogens is frequently used in conversation. Dr. Wiener always considered this device a heresy, perhaps with some justification, although common usage has lent it an odor of sanctity. A simple method of conversion from Fisher-Race to Wiener can be found in Table 6-2 and should be memorized by the student!

Table 6-3 lists, in order of frequency in whites, the eight Rh gene complexes and their products, both as antigen combinations (agglutinogens as Wiener called them) and as individual component antigens (factors). Pride of place is given to the

TABLE 6-2. Conversion from Wiener to Fisher-Race Nomenclatures*

$R^0 = Dce$	$r = (d)ce$
$R^1 = DCe$	$r' = (d)Ce$
$R^2 = DEc$	$r'' = (d)cE$
$R^z = DCE$	$r^y = (d)CE$

*R implies presence of D; r implies absence of D or (d); ^{0} implies small letters; 1 or ' implies capital C; 2 or '' implies capital E; letter z or y implies capital C and E.

TABLE 6-3. Rh Gene Complexes and Their Products*

Gene Complexes		Antigen Combinations (Agglutinogens)			Principal Antigens (Factors)		
CDE	Rh-hr	CDE	Rh-hr	Shorthand			
CDe	*(R¹)*	CDe	(Rh_1)	R_1	C(rh′)	$D(Rh_0)$	e(hr″)
cde	*(r)*	cde	(rh)	r	c(hr′)		e(hr″)
cDE	*(R²)*	cDE	(Rh_2)	R_2	c(hr′)	$D(Rh_0)$	E(rh″)
cDe	*(R⁰)*	cDe	(Rh_0)	R_0	c(hr′)	$D(Rh_0)$	e(hr″)
Cde	*(r′)*	Cde	(rh′)	r′	C(rh′)		e(hr″)
cdE	*(r″)*	cdE	(rh″)	r″	c(hr′)		E(rh″)
CDE	*(Rᶻ)*	CDE	(Rh_z)	R_z	C(rh′)	$D(Rh_0)$	E(rh″)
CdE	*(rʸ)*	CdE	(rh_y)	r_y	C(rh′)		E(rh″)

*The eight principal Rh gene complexes and their products are listed in order of frequency in the white population. The order of frequency differs substantially in blacks, with *cDe* *(R⁰)* being the most common gene complex in that group.

CDE notation, using the correct alphabetical sequence, but in each case the Rh-hr equivalents are given in parentheses for comparison. The shorthand notation for each antigen combination is also given, as these symbols are still in common use and will probably continue to be used interchangeably with their CDE counterparts.

Many Rh antigens exist besides the original five. These will be dealt with later, some in greater detail than others. Where possible, the relationships between these further determinants and the five considered so far will be clarified. Except in instances where no CDE symbol has been assigned, this system of notation will be used from this point, although on first mentioning each antigen any alternative name will be given once in parentheses.

Rh PHENOTYPES AND GENOTYPES

A phenotype is merely the expression of observed reactions when the red cells are tested with the available antisera. Deriving the genotype from these reactions necessitates making genetic presumptions based on any known allelic relationship between the antigens concerned. A person whose red cells are positive with both anti-C and anti-c is considered heterozygous for *C* and *c*, while a positive reaction with anti-C and a negative one with anti-c, or vice versa, imply homozygosity for *C*, or for *c*, respectively. The same reasoning may be applied to tests with anti-E and anti-e, but the lack of an antibody capable of recognizing any product of the *d* gene introduces a difficulty when the cells being tested are D-positive. In such cases there is no way of knowing whether the D antigen present on the cells is the product of one of the person's Rh genes or of both. Studying the reactions of the cells with anti-D sera for the effects of dosage (which provides assistance towards the determination of zygosity in the case of some blood group antigens) does not provide reliable data because the D antigen is subject to considerable variation in expression, for a number of reasons besides zygosity. Hence, the derivation of a person's "probable

Rh genotype" is necessarily founded in many cases on the known frequencies of the eight principal gene complexes and on the probability that the most common of two or more possible alternatives is applicable in each case.

With the 5 original Rh antisera, 18 reaction patterns are possible, assuming that no person's red cells can be negative with all 5 sera, nor with both of any pair of known antithetical antisera. This assumption is false, as it happens, but violators of the rule are exceedingly rare. The 18 possible reaction patterns are listed in Table 6-4, together with the approximate frequencies with which each is likely to be observed in testing populations of European or African origin. In the case of phenotypes having a frequency of 1 percent or more, the most probable genotype for each race is listed, followed by any other possible alternatives. As will be seen, there are substantial differences between the phenotype frequencies in blacks and in whites. The interpretation of a phenotype in terms of most probable genotype is accordingly influenced by the racial origin of the person whose cells have been tested. For example, a black whose cells give the reactions $C-D+E-c+e+$ will be almost equally likely to be cDe/cDe as cDe/cde, whereas a white whose cells were of the same

TABLE 6-4. Eighteen Possible Reaction Patterns with Five Principal Rh Antiserums*

Reactions with Anti-					Approximate Frequency		Most Probable Genotype		Other Possibilities (Both Groups)
C	D	E	c	e	Whites (%)	Blacks (%)	Whites	Blacks	
+	+	−	+	+	35	26	CDe/cde	CDe/cDe	Cde/cDe
+	+	−	−	+	19	3	CDe/CDe	CDe/CDe	CDe/Cde
+	+	+	+	+	13	4	CDe/cDE	CDe/cDE	CDe/cdE, Cde/cDE CDE/cde, CDE/cDe or CdE/cDe
−	+	+	+	+	12	16	cDE/cde	cDE/cDe	cdE/cDe
−	+	+	+	−	2	1	cDE/cDE	cDE/cDE	cDE/cdE
−	+	−	+	+	2	42	cDe/cde	cDe/cde or cDe/cDe	—
−	−	−	+	+	15	7	cde/cde	cde/cde	—
+	−	−	+	+	1	1	Cde/cde	Cde/cde	—
−	−	+	+	+	1	rare	cdE/cde		—
+	−	+	+	+	Each of		Cde/cdE		CdE/cde
+	−	−	−	+	these		Cde/Cde		—
−	−	+	+	−	phenotypes		cdE/cdE		—
+	+	+	−	+	occurs with		CDE/CDe		CDE/Cde
+	+	+	+	−	a frequency		CDE/cDE		CDE/cdE
+	+	+	−	−	of less		CDE/CDE		CDE/CdE
+	−	+	−	+	than 0.2%		CdE/Cde		—
+	−	+	+	−	in both		CdE/cdE		—
+	−	+	−	−	racial groups		CdE/CdE		—

*Percentages are rounded off.

phenotype would be *cDe/cde* with a probability of about 16:1. More precise interpretation of genotypes may sometimes be derived from the results of family studies.

NUMERICAL NOMENCLATURE
OF ROSENFIELD AND COLLEAGUES

No dissertation on the Rh blood group system would be complete without at least a superficial account of a third system of nomenclature. Failure to introduce this earlier, immediately after the Rh-hr and CDE notations, may appear at first to be a departure from logical sequence. It seemed important, however, to cover phenotypes first, as this third system of notation was designed expressly as a method of recording observed reactions with the various antisera.

In 1962 Rosenfield and colleagues[7] introduced a system of numerical terminology for the Rh antigens. This amounted to a considerably expanded version of a scheme proposed originally in 1944 by Murray,[8] taking into account the many additional antigens studied and categorized during the intervening years. Briefly, this system of notation assigns a number to each antigen in chronologic order of discovery or of admission into the Rh system. Thus, D is Rh1, C is Rh2, E is Rh3, c is Rh4, e is Rh5, and so on. The use of numerals enables observed reactions with one or more Rh antisera to be recorded objectively and in their entirety for future reference, innocent of any genetic interpretations or implications. Data recorded in such a fashion are eminently attuned to the digestion of a computer.

TABLE 6-5. Antigens of the Rh Blood Group System in Three Nomenclatures

Numerical	CDE	Rh-hr	Other	Numerical	CDE	Rh-hr	Other
Rh1	D	Rh_0		Rh22	CE	rh	
Rh2	C	rh'		Rh23	D^w		Wiel
Rh3	E	rh"		Rh24	E^T		
Rh4	c	hr'		Rh25			LW
Rh5	e	hr"		Rh26	"c-like"		Deal
Rh6	ce	hr	f	Rh27	cE	rh_{ii}	
Rh7	Ce	rh_i		Rh28		hr^H	
Rh8	C^w	rh^{w1}		Rh29		HR	total Rh
Rh9	C^x	rh^x		Rh30	D^{Cor}		Go^a
Rh10	ce^s	hr^v	V	Rh31		hr^B	
Rh11	E^w	rh^{w2}		Rh32		$\overline{R}^N$	
Rh12	G	rh^G		Rh33	D^{Har}	R_0^{Har}	
Rh13		Rh^A		Rh34		Hr^B	Bas.
Rh14		Rh^B		Rh35			1114
Rh15		Rh^C		Rh36			Be^a
Rh16		Rh^D		Rh37			Evans
Rh17		Hr_0		Rh38			Duclos
Rh18		Hr		Rh39	"C-like"		
Rh19		hr^S		Rh40			Targett
Rh20	e^s		VS	Rh41	"Ce-like"		
Rh21	C^G			Rh42	Ce^s	rh_i^s	

The Rh phenotype of a blood specimen, expressed in the numerical notation, begins with the letters Rh, followed by a colon and then by the numerical designations of all antigens for which the blood has been tested. A minus symbol preceding the number for a particular antigen indicates a negative test result, while the absence of a minus symbol indicates a positive. As examples, the phenotype C+D+E−c+e+ becomes Rh:1,2,−3,4,5, and C−D−E−c+e+ becomes Rh:−1,−2,−3,4,5. The recording of results obtained with additional antisera merely necessitates the addition of more numbers, with or without a preceding minus symbol, depending on whether the observed reaction is negative or positive. It is thus possible to record the results of tests for any or all of the 40 or more Rh antigens reported to exist and to do so in a concise and readily interpretable manner. (The necessary code is to be found in Table 6-5.)

The omission of a number implies that no test was performed for that determinant, and a perceptibly weaker-than-normal reaction may be indicated by placing the letter w before the number designation for the antigen in question.

QUALITATIVE AND QUANTITATIVE VARIATION OF ANTIGENS

DIMINISHED EXPRESSION OF D

The fact that red cell specimens sometimes behave variably in their reactions with anti-D sera was reported in 1946 by Stratton.[9] The collective name D^u was allocated to describe the supposed variant of the D antigen, which was characterized by positive reactions with some anti-D sera and negative or equivocal reactions with others.

The original definition is sometimes still applied to draw the distinction between "normal D" and the so-called D^u variants, although the development of more sensitive technics since 1946, not to mention the availability of more potent anti-D sera, should have called for the adoption of revised criteria. At any rate, the term D^u is commonly used to embrace a wide range of diminished D expression, ranging from cells showing strong to weak or negative reactions with different anti-D reagents to those whose D antigen is only detectable by means of an indirect antiglobulin test after incubation with potent IgG anti-D sera.

HIGH-GRADE D^u

The so-called high-grade D^u most often results from gene interaction, or from a positional effect exerted by another Rh gene. Red cells from a person of the genotype *CDe/Cde* may exhibit weakened expression of D because of a depressing effect by *Cde* on the D that is the product of *CDe*. This effect is possibly aggravated by the presence of C in both gene complexes, although it is also seen to some extent in cells from *Cde/cDe*, which are otherwise not distinguishable from those of *CDe/cde*. A somewhat similar weakening of D expression appears to accompany the presence of a recently reported low-frequency antigen of the Rh system called Targett (Rh40). In all these cases it is generally only saline-reactive anti-D sera that consistently show weak or negative reactivity. Saline anti-D is usually diluted in 6 to 8 percent albumin. Modern commercial high-protein anti-D sera, diluted in 22 to 30 percent albumin, usually show reactions that are not perceptibly weaker than those they give with any other D-positive red cells. Depending on the potency of the high-protein reagent, or on the effectiveness of the macromolecular reagent additives used by the manufacturer to accelerate the specific anti-D reaction, weak or negative to strong reactions may be obtained at the immediate-spin phase of the test, but strong macroscopic agglutination is invariably seen with high-grade D^u cells after a period of incubation at 37°C. Notwithstanding the historical precedent for including cells showing this kind of reactivity with anti-D sera within the overall definition of D^u-positive, this usage is inappropriate. Red cells showing definite macroscopic agglutination when tested directly with anti-D sera should be reported as D-positive, even when incubation of the test is required for the reaction to develop. In such cases, the designation D^u-positive may be misleading to a physician receiving the report.

LOW-GRADE D^u

Cells belonging to the low grade of D^u are not agglutinated directly by anti-D sera, at least when tests are performed in tubes, even after incubation. Agglutination may be seen in slide tests with high-protein anti-D sera, but this is always perceptibly weaker than that seen when the same serum is used to test regular D-positive cells, and the reaction may take longer to develop than the 2-minute time limit generally placed on the slide test procedure. The reliable recognition of any kind of D antigen on low-grade D^u cells is dependent on the performance of an indirect antiglobulin test after first incubating the cells with a suitable reagent anti-D serum for (usually) 15 minutes at 37°C (see Color Plate 11). The suitability or otherwise of commercial anti-D sera in tests for D^u is invariably stated by manufacturers in their package inserts.

SUBDIVISIONS OF D (D "MOSAIC")

On rare occasions, a person who is D-positive or D^u-positive may be observed to have made an alloantibody appearing to have anti-D specificity. The serum in such cases gives the clear-cut reaction pattern of anti-D, yet the red cells of the individual concerned are D-positive and do not react with the serum. The phenomenon was first reported in 1953 by Argall, Ball, and Trentelman,[10] but it soon proved to be heterogeneous. In other words, the "anti-D" antibodies made by D-positive or D^u-positive people are not invariably of identical specificity. The cells of such people are not always mutually compatible.

After studying a number of these cases, Wiener and Unger[11] postulated that the D antigen (which, to be consistent with the nomenclature these authors invariably used, we should temporarily revert to calling Rh_0 at this point) is a mosaic composed of several separate parts. Four individual determinants were recognized

MODERN BLOOD BANKING AND TRANSFUSION PRACTICES

and were given the names Rh^A, Rh^B, Rh^C, and Rh^D. The absence of one or more of these components would not necessarily be recognized on testing the cells with most anti-D sera, yet the person concerned would be susceptible to producing antibody to the missing component(s). For example, a person who lacks the Rh^A piece can produce anti-Rh^A. That antibody, naturally enough, would not be distinguishable from any other anti-D when tested with cells possessing an intact D antigen or all the pieces of the mosaic.

These portions of the D antigen were never assigned exactly corresponding names in the CDE nomenclature, but a series of examples of "partial anti-D" were studied in 1962 by Tippett and Sanger,[12] who found that they fell within six broad categories. The same six classifications also accommodated cases investigated later, although some of the original categories have proved to be subdivisible.[13] The usual system of notation is to modify the letter D in the designation for the phenotype by using a superscript symbol corresponding to the category to which the particular D antigen belongs. Thus, CD^{IV}e cells (or cD^{IV}e, etc.) belong to Category IV, CD^{VI}e cells to Category VI, and so on.

The cells of a person belonging to Tippett's Category VI usually behave like low-grade D^u, and (among whites at any rate) it is people of this category who are the ones most often found to have made "anti-D" after exposure to the necessary stimulus. That is not to say that all low-grade D^u cells belong to Category VI, nor that Category VI people are nearly as prone to making anti-D as those whose cells are truly D-negative. Most low-grade D^u cells do not, in fact, belong to Category VI. Their D^u status in most instances results from a gene coding for a quantitatively weaker expression of D, rather than for a qualitatively different D. As for the incidence of anti-D in sera from D-positive or D^u-positive people, this is still an uncommon event. Certainly it will be encountered less frequently than, for instance, anti-E or anti-c in immunized persons negative for those antigens.

In blacks, it is perhaps most likely that D-positives who make anti-D will prove to be of Category IV. Category IV includes whites also, but in blacks the variant D is generally accompanied by the presence of the low-frequency antigen Go^a (Gonzales, D^{Cor} or Rh30), and by a somewhat enhanced expression of D—at any rate, when measured by the reactivity of some anti-D sera. Another low-frequency antigen, D^w (Wiel or Rh23) is present on the cells of Category V people. A possible explanation for the presence of these low-frequency antigens is that they are replacing the missing components of D.

ENHANCED EXPRESSION OF D

The reactivity of "normal" D-positive red cells with anti-D sera covers a wide range of variation. Cells of the genotype *cDE/cDE* consistently show higher titration scores than those of *CDe/CDe*, although both possess the gene product in double dose. Sometimes no cause can be found for unusually strong expression of D, but on other occasions the cause is understood, as in the case of phenotypes resulting from partial deletion at the Rh locus.

R₀Har PHENOTYPE AND THE Rh33 ANTIGEN

Individual treatment is merited for the phenotype that results when the gene complex R^{0Har} is partnered with a gene that does not produce D, because the reactivity of different anti-D sera with these cells may be confusing. The products of R^{0Har} include a normal c antigen, considerably diminished expression of both D and e, and a low-frequency antigen called Rh33. Reactivity of the cells with anti-D sera may vary from negative with some, through weak agglutination at the antiglobulin phase with others, to strong direct agglutination with a few. Anti-D sera that directly agglutinate the cells are uncommon, but they are most often saline-reactive ones. Eluates prepared after incubating the cells with reactive anti-D sera can be demonstrated to contain anti-D, which is an indication that some form of the D antigen was present on the cells to begin with. Investigators have differed in regard to their ability to detect anti-D in eluates made after incubating the cells with nonreactive anti-D sera, but it is not inconceivable that this might be possible. There could be insufficient binding of anti-D to such a weak D antigen to produce a detectable antiglobulin reaction, yet there could certainly be enough to give a positive reaction when the eluate is subsequently tested with cells possessing a normal D antigen. Success in this regard is no doubt dependent on the many variables that influence the yield of antibody in eluates. When Rh33 cells are directly agglutinated by an anti-D serum, the reaction is ascribed to an anti-Rh33 component in that serum. This was separable from the anti-D in at least one serum, but it is more usually inseparable. Naturally, the weakened e antigen determined by R^{0Har} will not be recognized if the gene is accompanied by one that produces a normal e.

—D— AND SIMILAR PARTIAL DELETIONS

The existence of red cells lacking products of the C/c and E/e genes was first reported in 1950 by Race, Sanger, and Selwyn.[14] A striking feature of the cells, besides negative reactions with anti-C, anti-c, anti-E, and anti-e, was that some incomplete anti-D sera agglutinated them strongly in a low-protein test system, while the same examples of anti-D required a high-protein environment to give a direct agglutination reaction at all with normal D-positive red cells. The phenotype concerned was considered to be the result of homozygosity for a rare gene that was called $-D-(\bar{R}^0)$. The considerably enhanced expression of D is possibly attributable to the lack of competition from other Rh genes. Further examples of the same phenotype were soon reported, and in all but a few cases they were initially recognized as a result of studies being conducted on antibodies produced by the propositi rather than through unexpected results encountered when testing their cells. The antibody these people make is generally considered to be directed at a high-frequency antigen called Rh17 (Hr₀), which is absent from the products of $-D-$, but some examples of it have appeared to contain separable components as well, such as anti-e or anti-c. In studying members of the families, it was found that a similar but somewhat lesser enhancement of D activity was present on the cells of heterozygotes ($-D-/CDe$,

$-D-/cDE$, $-D-/cde$, and so on) and a curiously high rate of consanguinity was present among parents of the propositi.

Of similar rarity are at least two gene complexes in which the deletion is confined to the E/e locus. C^wD- and $cD-$ have each been recognized in at least two families. The D antigen produced by each was enhanced, but the respective phenotypes reflected depressed C^w and c.

·D·

Another gene complex lacking C/c and E/e genes is one that is possibly even more rare, called ·D·. In 1978 Contreras and colleagues[15] made the interesting discovery that the cells of one person formerly thought to be $-D-/-D-$ were strongly positive for an earlier reported low-frequency antigen called Evans. This person was considered to be homozygous for ·D·, a gene similar to $-D-$ except that its products include the Evans antigen. The two phenotypes are essentially similar, but the enhanced expression of D is not as marked in ·D· as in $-D-$.

SIALIC ACID-DEFICIENT RED CELLS

In a few quite uncommon instances, the red cells may exhibit a deficiency of sialic acid from their surfaces. Most notably, this occurs in the case of modification of the MN sialoglycoprotein on the cells, which may be associated with the presence of some of the low-frequency antigens of the MNSs system, or with the En(a−) phenotype. Rh-positive cells in these cases have been reported to show enhanced reactivity with anti-D sera. Rather than a stronger-than-normal D antigen, the explanation is likely to be that the removal of sialic acid reduces the negative surface charge on the cells, causing them to behave as if they were enzyme treated and making the cells more readily agglutinated. At any rate, antisera of other specificities also show increased reactivity with these cells.

OTHER ALLELES

Cᵂ ANTIGEN

In 1946 Callender and Race[16] reported a new antibody directed at an antigen called Willis. The gene of which this antigen was a determinant was found to be an allele at the C/c locus, accordingly named C^w. The C^w antigen, originally called rh^w in the Rh-hr nomenclature, but subsequently renamed rh^{w1} to accommodate the discovery of E^w (rh^{w2}), has a frequency of about 2 percent in the overall white population, but is very rare in blacks.

A curious feature of C^w-positive red cells is that they react with most anti-C sera, irrespective of whether the C antigen itself is present or not. This phenomenon is sometimes misunderstood. In ordinary circumstances, one would not expect to be able to find on a single specimen of red cells the products of more than two alleles at a given locus. Thus, if a blood gives the reactions C+c+, thereby implying heterozygosity for C and c, one would not expect to obtain a positive reaction with anti-C^w. The fact is, however, that the reactions C+c+C^w+ are not at all unusual. Red cells of the genotypes *C^{w}De/cde* and *C^{w}De/cDE* (or their less probable alternatives) give positive reactions with most anti-C sera, which must accordingly be thought of as "anti-CC^w." Although produced in response to C+C^w− cells, a majority of anti-C sera appear to contain an inseparable anti-C^w component. Pure anti-C^w has been produced in response to both transfusion and pregnancy and it sometimes occurs without a red cell-induced stimulus at all, that is, as a "naturally occurring" antibody.

OTHER ANTIGENS ALLELIC TO C AND E

Several other antigens have been reported as being products of alleles at the *C/c/C^w* or the *E/e* loci, but they are all quite uncommon. Most notably they include C^x (rh^x), E^w (rh^{w2}), and E^T. Also mentioned in the literature are C^u and E^u, which appear to be quantitative variants of C and E, respectively, perhaps analogous to D^u

COMPOUND ANTIGENS

In 1953 Rosenfield and colleagues[17] reported an antibody in the serum of a patient of the genotype *CDe/cDE* to which they originally gave the name anti-f. Cells possessing both c and e as products of the same gene (*cde, cDe,* or *cD^{u}e*) were f-positive, while those possessing c and e as products of different genes (*CDe/cDE*) and those lacking either c or e (*CDe/CDe* or *cDE/cDE,* and so on) were f-negative. The antigen was subsequently renamed ce, as it was considered to be a compound determinant of genes that produce both c and e. Wiener utilized (hr) as the designation for ce.

Anti-ce, if available, provides useful information leading to the more reliable interpretation of Rh genotypes, most especially when red cells being tested give the reactions C+D+E+c+e+. Reference to Table 6-4 will remind the reader that the most probable genotype in this situation is *CDe/cDE*. If this (or two of the five possible alternatives, *CDe/cdE* or *Cde/cDE*) were the true genotype, the cells should be ce-negative. On the other hand, a positive reaction with anti-ce would suggest *CDE/cde* as the most likely genotype, with *CDE/cDe* and *CdE/cDe* as the less likely alternatives.

Just as there is a compound antigen associated with c and e as products of the same gene, there is another associated with C and e. Ce (rh$_i$) is a product of the *CDe* and *Cde* genes. In fact, most "anti-C" antibodies produced by Rh-positive persons are predominantly anti-Ce. This can be substantiated by performing parallel titration studies, using C+Ce+ cells (e.g., *CDe/cDE*) and C+Ce− cells (e.g., *CDE/cde*). Many anti-C sera show a significantly lower titer with C+Ce− cells than with C+Ce+ cells and, at an appropriately chosen dilution, could just as usefully provide the same information as anti-ce, except that the reactions with C+D+E+c+e+ cells would be reversed. Thus, *CDe/cDE, CDe/cdE,* and *Cde/cDE* cells can be expected to be Ce-positive (ce-negative), and *CDE/cde, CDE/cDE,* and *CdE/cDe* cells will be Ce-negative (ce-positive). Of course, this ingenious approach to the more precise determination of Rh genotypes should not be applied unless previously proven C+ce− red cells are available to use for a negative control test. Such cells are not easy to find, which is a pity because they also provide the most reliable positive control for tests with anti-C itself. Anti-C blood grouping sera licensed by the Food and Drug Administration are required to be tested by manufacturers and shown to be reactive with C+Ce− cells, but there is no stipulation that this reaction must be as strong as that given by the more common C+Ce+ cells, nor would it be practical for manufacturers to meet such a requirement. In consequence, false-negative reactions with anti-C sera are not all that unusual because the weaker reactions by C+Ce− cells are sometimes missed when the positive control cells (almost invariably Ce-positive) give such reassuringly strong agglutination.

Anti-CE (-rh) and anti-cE (-rh$_{ii}$) have also been reported, but these antibodies are much rarer than the two specificities previously mentioned.

G ANTIGEN

It has been known for many years that immunized Rh-negative people sometimes make what appear to be "anti-C+D" antibodies, even when the immunizing cells are unquestionably C-negative. An explanation for this response was offered in 1958 when Allen and Tippett[18] reported an unusual phenotype in a Boston blood donor. The cells, though negative with anti-C and anti-D sera, gave positive reactions with anti-CD sera. Elution experiments after incubating the cells with anti-CD sera yielded antibodies that agglutinated both C+D− and C−D+ red cells. Accordingly, it was postulated that the cells in question possessed a "new" Rh antigen called G (rh^G), which also occurs on the cells of all normal Rh phenotypes except those lacking both C and D. Thus, only cells of the genotypes *cde/cde* and *cdE/cde* (or *cdE/cdE*) lack G, and when an Rh-negative person produces an antibody reacting with *Cde/cde* cells on being immunized with C−D+ cells, the "anti-C" component is in reality anti-G, produced in response to the G antigen that is present on all D-positive red cells, whether or not C is also present. A few rare cases have since been reported in which D-positive cells were not G-positive, but to date no example of C+G− cells has been described; perhaps it never will be. Further cells of the r^G phenotype have been reported, and a proportion of anti-C sera do in fact react with some of them. It has been suggested that these reactions are due to an inseparable component in those sera called anti-C^G (-Rh21). Some examples of r^G cells show weaker expression of the G antigen than others, and somewhat weaker G has also been recognized in a few instances on cells that otherwise appear to be *cdE/cde*.

BLACK Rh ANTIGENS

Among blacks, both quantitative and qualitative variants of the Rh antigens are legion. Not all fit neatly into the generally accepted classifications, but it would seem pertinent to review at least those likely to be of interest in the routine hospital blood bank situation.

ANTIGENS V AND VS

The first example of anti-V was reported in 1955 by DeNatale and colleagues.[19] The V (hr^v) antigen was found to be a product of the gene complexes *cde, cDe,* or *cD^{u}e.* In that respect it is similar to ce except that it occurs predominantly in blacks. The likelihood that V can be thought of as a further example of a compound antigen is reflected in its alternative name in the CDE nomenclature, ce^s.

In 1960 Sanger and associates[20] reported a further antibody that, besides reacting with all V+ cells, gave reactions also with cells of the so-called Negro Cde phenotype, which was already known to be rather different from the Cde that occurs in whites. This antibody was called anti-VS, not in recognition of its reactions with V+ cells, but merely in utilization of the initials of the patient in whose serum it was originally found. It was later considered that anti-VS was directed at the e^s component of the ce^s compound antigen, but a clear view of this relationship is obscured by the fact that not all subsequent examples of anti-VS (nor those of anti-V, for that matter) have proved to be of identical specificity. One school of thought contends that the original serum of Mrs. V.S. contained a mixture of two antibodies: anti-V and "anti-hr^H." That explanation does not, however, fully account for the diverse behavior of different examples of anti-V and anti-VS. To add further to the confusion, another antibody has been reported recently that is not the same as anti-VS (nor the same as "anti-hr^H") and reacts specifically with cells of the black Cde phenotype. This antibody has been called anti-Ce^s (-rh^s_i or -Rh42) and is considered to be analogous to anti-Ce, in the same way as anti-V (-ce^s) is analogous to anti-f (-ce). We are in very deep water here when even the experts cannot agree. Suffice for the present to accept the notion that ce^s is to c and e^s what ce is to c and e and to remain prepared for the possibility that some future inspired investigation will either prove it or disprove it.

As with C^w, the V and VS antigens are not usually represented on reagent red blood cells used for routine antibody screening; hence, these antibodies may not be detected unless a V+ or VS+ donor unit is selected for compatibility testing, or unless the serum happens for some reason to be subjected to testing against a panel that includes having the V and/or VS antigens.

BLACK Cde AND r^G

Cde/cde cells encountered in blacks show rather different phenotypic characteristics than those of whites belonging to ostensibly the same genotype. Their VS+ and Rh:42 status have already been mentioned. In addition, black Cde cells react more weakly than white Cde cells when tested with anti-C sera. This may be attributable to the predominantly anti-Ce specificity of most examples of anti-C, as black Cde cells are generally considered to be Ce-negative. This is not quite true, as a matter of fact. It is perfectly possible to absorb or dilute most "anti-C" reagents until they are functionally pure anti-Ce (i.e., until they are giving negative reactions with *CDE/cde* cells and the like, and are still agglutinating *CDe/cde* cells strongly), and these sera do still give a reaction with black Cde cells, albeit a weak one. Studies in families in which the black *Cde* gene has been inherited with various gene complexes other than *cde* have shown other interesting features. The e antigen produced is weaker than normal, and it seems that both C and c are determinants of this unusual gene, which is accordingly designated Ccde^s (r$'^s$). The reader with an inquiring mind may wonder why, if *Ccde^s* produces both c and e^s, its products do not include ce^s (V), and why cells of the black Cde phenotype are not accordingly V-positive as well as VS-positive. One would sooner nobody asked. It may be some consolation to know that cells from a person who is *Ccde^s/CDe* do react with anti-ce (-f), so the compound antigen ce is apparently produced by *Ccde^s*, even though the reaction strength suggests rather less than a normal single dose.

When the r^G phenotype is found in blacks, the G antigen present is usually weaker than that observed in the original Boston case and fewer anti-C sera are likely to show detectable reactions. Indeed, a range of G antigen reactivity has been noted, ranging down to a level at which it can only be detected by an indirect antiglobulin test after incubating the cells with anti-CD. The G antigen in this form has been called G^u by Beattie and associates.[21]

These cells in blacks, whether r^G or r^{Gu}, are VS+, a feature they share with r$'^s$ cells. In effect, these phenotypes are all essentially similar except for the differences in expression of G: r$'^s$ cells manifest the greatest amount of G (though this is rather less than is normally seen on white r$'$ cells) and r^{Gu} the least.

hr^S AND hr^B ANTIGENS

It should be understood at the outset that hr^S and hr^B are not black antigens. The cells of most e-positive people are in fact both hr^S-positive and hr^B-positive. The variant state that appears to be a predominantly black characteristic is that of being e-positive and yet negative for hr^S and hr^B. In that regard, these determinants are more similar to the components of the D antigen than to e^s, already mentioned as an antigen present on some black cells.

Not all the variant behavior among e antigens in blacks can be explained by the absence of hr^S or hr^B. There appear to be numerous subdivisions of e, most of which have remained unclassified. The matter generally comes under scrutiny only when (1) an e-positive person makes alloantibodies appearing to have anti-e specificity, (2) a red cell suspension shows discrepant reactivity with different anti-e sera, or (3) a negative anti-e test is observed when testing cells that are expected to be e-positive.

The circumstances leading to the recognition of the hr^S-negative and hr^B-negative phenotypes are worth treating briefly, as in neither case was the situation a straightforward one of "anti-e" being produced by e-positive people. Both patients, in fact, produced antibodies reacting with a high proportion of cells but not with their own. In both cases, E-positive e-negative cells were showing weaker reactions than all others. The serum of Mrs. Shabalala, a black South African woman, appeared to contain two antibodies. When the serum was absorbed with E+e− cells, the antibody remaining in the absorbed serum was plainly akin to anti-e in that it gave negative reactions with all e-negative cells and was positive with most e-positive cells. The exceptions among e-positives were almost 1 percent of blacks and about 0.17 percent of whites in the South African population, whom Shapiro[22] deemed to lack an e-like determinant he called hr^S. The second antibody originally present in the Shabalala serum, the one recovered in an eluate from the absorbing E+e− cells, reacted with virtually all cells tested except those of Mrs. Shabalala herself. It did not react with cells of homozygous −D−, however, and was named anti-Hr (-Rh18) in recognition of its similarity to anti-Hr_0 (-Rh17), the antibody homozygous −D− people make. A caret symbol surmounting the gene notation is used to designate genes that produce hr" (e) itself, but not hr^S, thus $\hat{R}^0$ or $\hat{r}$, and similarly with the agglutinogens, $\hat{R}h_0$ and $\hat{r}h$. No CDE symbol was formally conferred, but the same symbol serves, most appropriately placed over the e. Thus, $cd\hat{e}$ produces cdê, and $cD\hat{e}$ produces cDê.

The case of Mrs. Bastiaan, a woman of mixed European and African descent, was similar but not the same. Again, this was a matter of an e-positive patient making an antibody reacting with virtually all cells but giving perceptibly weaker agglutination with E+e− cells. Absorption with E+e− cells left behind an anti-e-like component, or perhaps more correctly, an anti-Ce-like component, since it consistently gave stronger reactions with cells that were C+ as well as e+ than with those that were C− and e+. Shapiro, Le Roux, and Brink[23] gave the name hr^B to the determinant absent from the e-positive cells that failed to react with the absorbed serum and used a dot to distinguish the genes and agglutinogens concerned. Thus, $\dot{R}^0$ ($cD\dot{e}$) and $\dot{r}$ ($cd\dot{e}$) determine $\dot{R}h_0$ ($cD\dot{e}$) and $\dot{r}h$ ($cd\dot{e}$), the components of which include hr" (e) but not hr^B. Again, the antibody removed by absorption with E+e− cells was directed at a high-frequency antigen now called Hr^B. There is at least a possibility that neither of these sera contained two antibodies at all, but that in each case absorption with E+e− cells merely "took the edge off" a single antibody directed at a high-frequency antigen that is produced in varying amounts by the different gene complexes (with cDE producing the least in each case). The possibility is more of a probability in the case of the Bastiaan serum, as anti-Hr^B has since been found to show the same preference for Ce that is shown by anti-hr^B, which is quite strange when the antibody was adsorbed to and eluted from cells that were Ce-negative. At a practical level in the working hospital blood bank, of course, who cares? The important point to remember here is that not all anti-e sera react reliably with ê (hr^S-negative) and with $\dot{e}$ (hr^B-negative) red cells. This could be a source of false-negative reactions.

$\bar{\bar{R}}^N$ AND ITS PRODUCTS

An Rh gene exists, with a frequency perhaps as high as 1 percent among blacks, that is similar in some ways to −D− ($\bar{R}^0$). Named $\bar{\bar{R}}^N$ to indicate the similarity, the products of this gene include weak C, weak e, and possibly just a slightly elevated D. Besides the opportunities presented for further false-negative reactions with anti-C and anti-e sera, this entity deserves mention because another product is a low-frequency antigen, and its antibody may cause hemolytic disease of the newborn. This determinant may be referred to by the same letter designation as the whole gene, which is possibly acceptable if rendered in boldface type ($\overline{\overline{\mathbf{R}}}^N$), thereby leaving the roman type form for the whole agglutinogen. It does seem better, however, to avoid confusion by using an alternative name. The designation in the numerical system of nomenclature for this low-frequency antigen is Rh32, and anti-Rh32 sometimes occurs without a known red cell-induced stimulus, most especially in autoimmune hemolytic anemia sera, often enough in the company of multiple antibodies directed at other low-frequency antigens, both inside and outside the Rh blood group system.

Rh$_{null}$ AND Rh$_{mod}$ PHENOTYPES

In 1961 Vos and coworkers[24] reported studies in Australia on a blood that was completely devoid of Rh antigens. Other examples of the same phenomenon have been recognized since, although it is still exceedingly rare. The name Rh$_{null}$ is applied to the condition, which has been found to result from two different genetic effects. In one form, the most common, the absence of Rh antigens is caused by homozygosity for an unlinked suppressor gene. There is a parallel in the ABO system in the form of the Bombay (O$_h$) phenotype, although the actual mechanism by which antigen expression is prevented is not the same. Rh$_{null}$ people of this type inherit a normal Rh gene complex from each parent in the same way as everyone else. However, the antigenic determinants of those genes do not appear on the red cells because the suppressor prevents their expression. The products of whichever of their Rh genes they pass on to each of their offspring may be demonstrably weaker than normal, but the very presence of these products in the offspring is evidence that an Rh gene was inherited from the Rh$_{null}$ parent.

The other form of Rh$_{null}$ occurs in people who are homozygous for an amorph at the Rh locus itself, which has been called $\overline{\overline{r}}$. Since these people pass $\overline{\overline{r}}$ to each of their children, members of the next generation possess only one set of Rh antigens, that determined by the Rh gene inherited from the normal parent. Refer to Figures 6-2, 6-3, and 6-4 for a comparison of these two genetic schemes with the normal situation.

As might be expected, immunized Rh$_{null}$ people may make antibodies to any or all Rh antigens. Apparently separable components may be present, but the immune response is generally considered to be directed against "total Rh" (Rh29).

The red cells in both forms of Rh$_{null}$ show bizarre morphology (stomatocytosis), when examined with the aid of a microscope (see Color Plate 12), and are functionally abnormal, probably because the Rh antigens form an integral part of the red cell membrane.[25] In most cases, an increased reticulocyte count and reduced red cell survival provide evidence of hemolytic anemia. This may be severe, but is more often sufficiently compensated for the individual to lead a normal life.

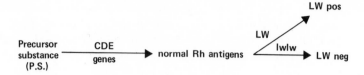

FIGURE 6-2. Normal Rh genetic pathway.

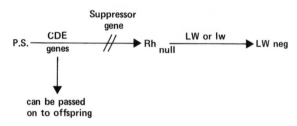

FIGURE 6-3. Suppressor Rh$_{null}$.

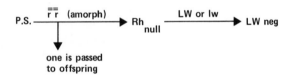

FIGURE 6-4. Amorphic Rh$_{null}$.

One other feature of Rh$_{null}$ cells is that they have been shown to give negative reactions when tested with anti-S, anti-s, and anti-U sera. This is not a consistent finding and it seems to occur mainly with antisera used in the indirect antiglobulin test procedure. It may be that the binding of antibody to the S, s, and U antigens is affected by the structural abnormality of the membrane in Rh$_{null}$ cells.

The Rh$_{mod}$ phenotype, which is really a collective entity because the reactivity of the cells with different Rh antisera varies, is believed to result from a similar genetic cause to that which gives the "suppressor type" of Rh$_{null}$. In fact, it could be the same suppressor gene showing lesser penetrance. At any rate, Rh$_{mod}$ red cells have similar morphologic abnormalities to those of Rh$_{null}$. Depending on the Rh genes actually inherited by the individual concerned, the red cells are found to give very much weaker reactions than normal with Rh antisera directed at the appropriate antigens. In fact, agglutination may be so reduced as to lead Rh$_{mod}$ cells to be mistaken for Rh$_{null}$. One case originally reported as an example of Rh$_{null}$ was subsequently reclassified as Rh$_{mod}$.

LW ANTIGEN

It is now generally accepted that the animal "anti-rhesus" sera of Landsteiner and Wiener were directed at a different antigen than the one defined by the human examples of anti-Rh_0 (anti-D). The early mistake (which Dr. Wiener never conceded) was understandable, as the antigens recognized by the immunized animal sera are present in greater amount on D-positive than on D-negative red cells. This antigen was called LW by Levine, in honor of its discoverers, Landsteiner and Wiener, and does not really belong in the Rh system. (We shall come to that in a moment.) The phenotype LW-negative occurs in humans, but rarely. People who belong to it may make anti-LW, and studies with such sera have led to the conclusion that these antibodies, and the LW-negative phenotype itself, are divisible into two kinds. The LW antigen is not completely absent from cells belonging to either form of "LW-negative," but is merely reduced in strength to different degrees. A numerical system has been applied to make the necessary distinction, but this is not wholly satisfactory, as it implies a proven qualitative rather than an apparent quantitative difference in antigen expression. The use of numbers, however, will facilitate the explanation. LW1 represents the LW antigen as it occurs on D-positive red cells, LW2 as it occurs on D-negative cells. LW4 is the phenotype representing the least expression of LW antigen, and LW3 cells (which may be D-positive or D-negative) have rather more. Immunized LW4 people make a form of anti-LW that reacts, in ascending order of strength, with LW3, LW2, and LW1 cells, while anti-LW made by LW3 people reacts, again in ascending order of strength, only with LW2 and LW1 cells. In studying families with LW members, it has been established that LW is not an Rh antigen at all. Though consistently expressed more strongly on D-positive cells, the LW antigen is a product of a gene that clearly segregates independently of Rh. Several genetic pathways have been proposed to explain why D-positive cells have more LW antigens than D-negative cells, and why the Rh_{null} phenotype is the only one that is completely LW-negative, but they need not concern us greatly. The most likely explanation, perhaps, is that the Rh antigens have to be present before the product of the *LW* gene can be expressed (just as H has to be present before A and B can be expressed) and that the presence of D somehow enhances that expression. Naturally, the absence of the *LW* gene itself (*lwlw*) results in no LW antigen (or very little), though the Rh antigens are still expressed normally.

A feature of most examples of anti-LW, and one that has sometimes provided the first clue to the specificity of the antibody, is that with cord bloods the antibodies react just as strongly with D-negative as with D-positive cord cells.

MISCELLANEOUS Rh ANTIGENS AND PHENOTYPES

In the part of this chapter devoted to Rh antigen and phenotype behavior, coverage has been confined to the basic antigens and to variants that may be expected to raise difficulties from time to time in the performance of phenotyping tests. Some phenotypes, though rare, have been covered because they represent interesting manifestations of unusual genetic effects; still others, because rare, have been denied mention at all. Table 6-5 lists all the Rh antigens that have to date been sufficiently studied as to be categorized and given names. It will be useful as a means of converting from one system of notation into another and will facilitate the interpretation and use of the numerical nomenclature. The reader who is interested in exploring further the complexities of the Rh blood group system should consult the works of Race and Sanger[26] and of Issitt.[27]

SOME PRACTICAL CONSIDERATIONS

COMPLETE AND INCOMPLETE Rh ANTIBODIES

The Rh antigens recognized, studied, and used for antigen typings by the early investigators were, like those used in testing for A and B, capable of agglutinating saline suspensions of red cells possessing the appropriate antigens. Had the antibodies not been reactive in a saline test system, it is unlikely they would have been found in the first place, as this was the test procedure invariably used in the early 1940s for hemagglutination tests.

It soon became apparent, however, that not all sera from patients who were suspected to have made Rh antibodies were giving detectable reactions in antibody detection tests. In 1944, Wiener[28] and Race[29] separately reported the existence of Rh antibodies that would not agglutinate saline-suspended red cells. These antibodies were considered to be incomplete, in that they were thought to possess only a single antigen-combining site. Thus handicapped, incomplete antibodies could bind to a specific antigen receptor on only one red cell and, since agglutination depends on the formation of intercellular bridges by antibody molecules attached to two red cells, there would be no visible evidence that an antigen-antibody reaction had taken place. Moreover, once red cells had been incubated with a serum containing incomplete antibodies directed at antigens on their surfaces, they would become unagglutinable by saline-reactive antisera of the same specificity, since their receptor sites for that antigen would not be blocked. Saline-agglutinating Rh antibodies were considered to be complete in that they possess in two antigen-combining sites needed to form intercellular bridges should the cells possess the relevant antigen.

IMMUNOGLOBULIN CLASSES IgG AND IgM

Later understanding of the structure of immunoglobulins provided greater insight into the reasons why complete antibodies agglutinate antigen-positive cells when suspended in saline and why the so-called incomplete antibodies do not. The terms "complete" and "incomplete" have persisted, even though it is now realized that nonagglutinating antibodies do in fact possess two antigen-combining sites. These antibodies belong usually to the IgG class of immunoglobulin. The inability of IgG antibodies to produce demonstrable agglutination in a saline test system results from various physical forces that hold particles apart when suspended in an electrolyte solution. The distance between red cells in saline exceeds the span between the antigen-combining sites of the IgG molecule; hence, agglutination is unable to take place (for review, refer to Chapter 3). The saline-agglutinating antibody, consisting as it does of five units similar in structure to the entire IgG molecule, is much larger than IgG and is accordingly able to bridge the distance between red cells in saline suspension. Thus, red cells possessing the antigen for which the antibody is specific can be agglutinated (again, for review refer to Chapter 3).

Most examples of Rh antibodies encountered are not saline-reactive. The exceptions are anti-E (rh") and anti-C^w, which are often found reacting in all phases of testing. "Naturally occurring" saline agglutinins have also been reported. Since the production of IgM is usually only a transient phase in the immune response, the antibodies present in sera immunized to the Rh antigens are most commonly IgG. In order to detect such antibodies reliably, a test system is required that either (1) enables the suspended red cells to come close enough to each other for the IgG molecule to be able to span the distance between antigen receptors situated on two separate cells or (2) enables IgG bound to red cells to be detected.

In 1945, without being aware that the substitution of a high-protein suspending medium for saline was bringing the red cells into closer proximity, Diamond and Denton[30] observed that incomplete Rh antibodies would agglutinate antigen-positive red cells if they were suspended in 20 to 30 percent bovine albumin. These workers had merely applied a principle outlined in 1909 by Bordet and Streng,[31] who had considered that agglutination of red cells sensitized with antibody and complement could be brought about by a substance called "conglutinin," present in bovine serum. Modern high-protein reagent antisera developed from a high-protein slide test were originally introduced as an antibody detection procedure in 1945 by Diamond and Abelson.[32]

The detection of incomplete antibodies coated to red cells was also made possible in 1945, when Coombs, Mourant, and Race[33] rediscovered the antiglobulin test procedure that was described originally in 1908 by Moreschi.[34] The antiglobulin test, which also came to be known as the Coombs' test, could be applied directly to the detection of antibody coated to the red cells in vivo, as in the diagnosis of hemolytic disease of the newborn; or indirectly to cells after prior incubation with serum, as in the detection of IgG antibodies in unknown sera, or in the detection of blood group antigens using sera containing IgG antibodies of known specificity (for review, refer to Chapter 4).

In many cases of warm autoimmune hemolytic anemia, the autoantibodies implicated in red cell destruction demonstrate specificity within the Rh system. For a more complete discussion of this subject, refer to Chapter 19.

Many cases of severe hemolytic disease of the newborn are caused by anti-Rh_0(D). Other cases of this disease have been reported in which other Rh antibodies were responsible. This subject is treated more fully in Chapter 18.

Finally, hemolytic transfusion reactions also have been attributed to all antibodies of the Rh system. These reactions are discussed more fully in Chapter 16.

TESTING FOR ANTIGENS
OF THE Rh BLOOD GROUP SYSTEM

After A and B, the most important blood group antigen in everyday blood bank routine is unquestionably D. Because it is powerfully immunogenic, this antigen can be expected to give rise to an immune response in at least 50 percent of D-negative recipients who are given a single unit of D-positive donor blood. Accordingly, the red cells of both recipients and donors are always tested for D in order to permit D-negative blood to be selected for D-negative patients. After D, the order of immunogenicity of the other Rh antigens appears to be $\bar{c} > E > C > \bar{e}$.

Since anti-D may also be formed by D-negative women as a result of feto-maternal immunization during pregnancy, testing the red cells for the D antigen has for many years been a routine in early pregnancy. Before it became a standard procedure to screen the sera of all patients for unexpected antibodies, this enabled the sera of D-negative women to be selected for screening at intervals throughout the pregnancy for the presence of anti-D and, if antibodies developed, allowed for preparations to be made for exchange transfusion to be carried out, if needed, on the infant after delivery. In more recent times, because immunization to D can be prevented in many cases by administering Rh immune globulin to Rh-negative women within 72 hours of delivering a D-positive or D^u-positive infant, testing the red cells of pregnant women for the D antigen remains an important part of routine prenatal testing.

Testing for the other antigens of the Rh system is neither justified nor practical as a matter of daily routine. Rh phenotyping may be required to assist in confirming the identity of an Rh antibody detected during screening, or perhaps when a family study is being undertaken for some reason, but this would be wasteful if practiced on all patients. It would not be feasible, in any case, to select donor blood to match the Rh phenotypes of all recipients, although donor centers commonly maintain limited supplies of phenotyped blood for issue to patients who have already become immunized.

Unlike ABO grouping tests, procedures used in testing for the Rh antigens do not possess the advantage of built-in controls. Since the vast majority of people negative for any of the Rh antigens do not regularly have antibodies directed at those antigens, there are no results of reverse grouping tests to provide confirmation of reactions obtained in testing red cells. Correct interpretation depends entirely on the antisera being of true specificity and on the care with which the tests are performed and controlled.

HIGH-PROTEIN ANTI-D BLOOD GROUPING SERA

The most abundantly available raw material for the manufacture of anti-D blood grouping sera contains antibodies in the form of IgG. Since it is important for test results to be obtained promptly and with minimal prior preparation of the test red cell suspension, manufacturers of these antisera have for 30 or more years used a concentrated solution of bovine albumin as a diluent. Most such reagents also contain a macromolecular additive (such as dextran, Ficoll, or polyvinylpyrrolidone) to accelerate the agglutination reaction and to make it possible for the tube test to be performed with red cells suspended in saline. Antisera of this kind are known generically as "high-protein" reagents and are commonly supplied as being suitable for the slide or modified tube test (or some such similar description).

If used correctly and adequately controlled, sera of this kind give strong dependable reactions with D-positive cells and clear-cut negative reactions with D-negative cells, whether used in the slide test or in the tube test procedure. Cells of the low-grade D^u phenotype may give equivocal or negative reactions on initial direct testing, but can usually be confirmed as D^u-positive by performing an indirect antiglobulin test after incubating the cells with the serum.

CAUSES OF FALSE REACTIONS

The causes of false reactions in blood grouping tests are mostly common to all blood grouping reagents. It goes without saying that the test procedure or procedures recommended by the manufacturer must be strictly followed, as all specificity and potency testing will have been carried out by those methods. Particular attention must be paid to the strength of the cell suspension, the volumes of serum and cells to be used, and the temperature and duration of incubation required. The application of more sensitive or less sensitive test procedures could lead to false reactions for which the manufacturer cannot reasonably be held responsible. An inherent source of error with high-protein antisera, however, is the proneness of these reagents to cause red cells that have become coated with immunoglobulin to agglutinate spontaneously. Thus, D-negative cells that have become coated with immunoglobulin in vivo (as in hemolytic anemia, or as a result of treatment with certain drugs) may give a false-positive test result. A control test to enable these false reactions to be recognized is essential when testing the red cells of patients. Such a control test assumes less importance in donor testing, although even normal, healthy donors sometimes have a sufficient coating of immunoglobulin on their red cells to give a false-positive test result. The extent to which false agglutination is likely to occur is dependent on a number of variables besides the amount of immunoglobulin coated to the cells. Macromolecular additives used in commercial high-protein antisera vary in molecular weight and concentration, as do total protein concentrations in different products. These antisera may therefore be expected to potentiate spontaneous agglutination to different degrees. The phenomenon is also influenced by the amount of the patient's own serum in the cell suspension and by the duration and temperature of incubation before the serum/cell is centrifuged and read. Accordingly, the Rh control test must always be performed in parallel with the anti-D test itself, using identical test conditions and an inert high-protein control reagent containing the same concentration of protein and additives that are present in the corresponding anti-D serum. Although the Rh control reagent of almost any manufacturer can be expected to provide a more reliable control test than bovine albumin alone, only that furnished by the manufacturer of the anti-D serum in use will provide a truly valid control test. If prepared correctly, this should be identical to the anti-D serum itself, except for the antibody component, and should therefore potentiate spontaneous agglutination to exactly the same extent. To repeat, the same manufacturer's reagent anti-D and Rh control must be used in Rh typing.

TESTING ON SLIDES

There is no purpose in attempting to detail the actual test procedure, as this may vary slightly from brand to brand of antiserum. The equipment required generally includes a heated Rh viewbox, which enables slides to be tilted and examined while in contact with a heated and lighted surface. The test calls for a 40 to 50 percent suspension of red cells in serum or plasma, which is equivalent to anticoagulated whole blood from a person who is not anemic. This point should be borne in mind, as the use of a significantly lower concentration of cells could lead to false results. In cases of hemorrhage, clot retraction is sometimes so efficient that it is not possible to obtain a sufficient amount of cells from the clot to make the required cell suspension. Similarly, a reduced hematocrit may necessitate centrifuging the blood specimen to enable a more concentrated cell suspension to be prepared. Almost invariably, the test requires a mixture consisting of one drop of antiserum and two drops of the heavy cell suspensions, mixed on a glass slide and spread to cover almost the whole area of the slide. The manufacturer's directions should be followed, but generally the sequence is as follows:

1. Mix anti-D serum and test cell suspension on a slide.

2. Mix Rh control reagent (supplied by the same manufacturer as the anti-D serum) and test cell suspension on a second slide.

3. Place both slides on an Rh viewbox that has been switched on for a long enough time to allow the heated surface to reach the required temperature (45 to 50°C—this brings the temperature of the reactants on the slide to 37°C).

4. Tilt the viewbox back and forth while examining the test mixture for agglutination.

5. Interpret the test and control results within 2 minutes.

If clearcut agglutination is seen in the test with anti-D serum, and the Rh control test shows no agglutination, the patient is D-positive. It should be noted here that, under the conditions of the slide test, low-grade D^u cells commonly give detectable agglutination with anti-D sera. This is invariably weaker than normal, however, and may take the full 2 minutes or longer to develop. If it is considered essential to be able to recognize D^u patients (presumably for the purpose of treating them as D-negative), it would be better not to use the slide test procedure. When there is any doubt about the test result and the specimen being tested is from a potential recipient (rather than a donor), the safest course is to treat the result as being negative.

If the test with anti-D serum shows no agglutination (in which case the Rh control test is most unlikely to show otherwise), the patient is probably D-negative, but may be D^u-positive. A D^u test may be performed if required, but this is only mandatory when testing donors (see below). The D^u test cannot be performed on a slide; a tube test must be set up.

If agglutination is observed in both the anti-D test and in the Rh control test, no valid interpretation of the test can be made. Avoid attempting an interpretation based on comparing the strength of reactivity with the anti-D serum and that with the control reagent. This could be very misleading. The next step should be to wash the cells thoroughly in saline and retest using the tube test procedure, again with a parallel Rh control test. The same high-protein reagent may be used (providing the manufacturer states that the product is suitable for use by the tube test with washed saline-suspended cells). Saline-reactive anti-D serum will only be required if the Rh control test is still positive on retesting. If the Rh control test on washed cells is negative, the presence or absence of agglutination in the anti-D test may be interpreted accordingly. If the Rh control test is still positive on washed cells, the cause is almost certainly a coating of immunoglobulin on the cells. The direct antiglobulin test is probably positive, and the patient may be suffering from autoimmune hemolytic anemia or may be taking some drug that causes immunoglobulin to coat the cells in vivo. Saline-reactive anti-D serum will be required to determine the patient's D antigen status. D^u status cannot be determined on cells having a positive DAT unless further measures are implemented.

TESTING IN TUBES

The tube test with anti-D serum is performed in very much the same way as ABO grouping in tubes. A low concentration of cells is required (usually 3 to 5 percent) and the use of too heavy a cell suspension may cause false-negative reactions. With most anti-D sera, a washed or unwashed suspension of cells in saline may be used, but the manufacturer's directions should be consulted in this matter. The macromolecular potentiator added to the antiserum by the manufacturer generally compensates for the suboptimal concentration of protein that results from the use of saline-suspended cells. Most anti-D sera require one drop of serum to be mixed with one drop of the test cell suspension, and the manufacturer's directions usually give the sequence of the test procedure as follows:

1. Mix one drop of antiserum and one drop of cell suspension in a suitably-sized tube. (The serum should always be placed in the tube first, as it is not possible to check that the serum has indeed been placed in the tube once the red cell suspension has been added.)

2. Mix one drop of Rh control reagent (from the same manufacturer as the anti-D serum in use) and one drop of the cell suspension in a second tube.

3. After mixing, centrifuge both tubes (usually at 900 to 1000 G for 30 seconds).

4. Gently resuspend the cell buttons in both tubes and read.

As with the slide test, definite agglutination in the test with anti-D serum and no agglutination in the Rh control test mean that the test cells are D-positive. Under the conditions of the tube test, low-grade D^u cells do not agglutinate directly. With some anti-D sera, so-called high-grade D^u cells or even cells possessing a slightly weaker-than-average expression of D may give weak or equivocal reactions on immediate centrifugation, but go on to show strong and definite agglutination after 5 to 15 minutes of incubation at 37°C. Naturally, such cells will give strong reactions at the antiglobulin phase of the D^u test, but this does not mean that they should be reported as D^u positive. Patients whose red cells show strong and definite direct agglutination (before the antiglobulin phase) should be regarded as D-positive and given D-positive blood. The consequence of classifying these people as D-negative (or as D^u-positive and treating them as D-negative for purposes of transfusion) will be an artificial and unjustified shortage of D-negative blood for true D-negative recipients. As many as 5 percent or more of D-positive red cell samples may require a short period of incubation before agglutinating strongly with anti-D sera, and there is no good reason to believe that such people may make anti-D if transfused with D-positive blood. Indeed, it is even debatable whether low-grade D^u people are substantially more prone in that regard, but we shall come to that in a moment.

Interpretation of the tube test is otherwise exactly the same as for the slide test. Cells showing agglutination in the Rh control test should be washed and retested, and the absence of agglutination means that the cells are probably D-negative. When the anti-D test gives a negative reaction on being centrifuged, the same mixture of serum and cells may be incubated and carried through to the D^u test if a D^u test is required. The Rh control test should be incubated and carried through in parallel, as cells having a positive direct antiglobulin test may not necessarily show direct spontaneous agglutination when mixed with high-protein Rh antisera, yet could plainly give a false-positive reaction at the antiglobulin phase of the D^u test. An alternative would be to perform a direct antiglobulin test selectively on test red cell samples giving a positive D^u test.

D^u TEST

Most high-protein anti-D sera are suitable for the detection of D^u, and the test is carried out simply by setting up the tube test incubating at 37°C (usually for 15 minutes) and then performing an antiglobulin test after washing the cells (refer to Color Plate 11). As mentioned above, the tube should always be centrifuged and examined for agglutination before proceeding to wash the cells, as cells showing direct macroscopic agglutination are most properly interpreted as D-positive.

Only bloods from donors are required to be tested for D^u, the purpose being to prevent D^u-positive donor units from being classified as D-negative and transfused to D-negative recipients. The principle is sound, as D^u-positive cells possess the D antigen, albeit a weak one, and it is at least theoretically possible for such cells to cause an immune response to D in susceptible D-negative recipients. The hazard may be more apparent than real, as no well-authenticated example of such an event has been recorded in the literature. Cases have been reported, however, in which transfusion reactions have occurred when D^u-positive blood was given to people whose sera already contained anti-D. The prevention of further similar reactions is sufficient justification for classifying D^u-positive donors as D-positive.

In the case of recipients, a D^u test is not considered essential. The premise is that, if the cells are so weakly D-positive as to require an indirect antiglobulin test for such a detection, the patient should receive D-negative blood in any case. There are two schools of thought on this point. One holds that the low-grade D^u status may be attributable to the lack of one or more components of the D antigen mosaic and that this is tantamount to being D-negative in that a form of anti-D may be formed in response to transfusion with D-positive blood. That such an immune response can occur in persons lacking parts of D in their cells is undeniable. The categories of subdivided D antigens were all discovered because people belonging to them made anti-D; but the opposing school of thought argues that most low-grade D^u cells do not in fact lack components of D. Even though some may, the production of anti-D by D^u-positive individuals is quite uncommon. Certainly, it is much less common than, for instance, immunity to E, or to c, and yet nobody seriously advocates a concerted effort to give only E-negative or c-negative blood to people whose cells lack E or c.

At any rate, some laboratories prefer to know when patients are D^u-positive, whether or not they treat them as D-negative for purposes of receiving transfusions, and perform the D^u test on all cells that do not directly agglutinate when tested with anti-D sera. The D^u test is also frequently carried out on the red cells of D-negative women who have just delivered a D-positive infant and is read microscopically as a means of recognizing and roughly quantitating any fetal D-positive cells present in the maternal circulation. If sufficient numbers of fetal D-positive cells are present, a mixed-field agglutination reaction will be seen, as only the minority population of fetal cells are showing a positive indirect antiglobulin reaction with the anti-D serum. It is important in these cases not to interpret the mixed-field reaction as indicating that the mother herself is D^u-positive, as this may result in a decision not to administer Rh immune globulin and consequently in failure to provide the patient with protection against making anti-D. Tests to distinguish adult from fetal red cells must then be performed. If the D-positive cells are of fetal origin, then an increased dose of Rh immune globulin may be indicated. Some physicians believe that D^u-positive women should be given Rh immune globulin after delivering a D-positive or D^u-positive infant in any case, for the same reason that D^u-positive recipients are sometimes transfused with D-negative blood. The administration of Rh immune globulin is not harmful to a D^u-positive patient, but it is hard to see how it could be effective in preventing immunization to any parts of the D antigen she may lack, as the antibodies in the dose will surely attach immediately to the patient's own red cells, which are present in much higher concentration than fetal red cells.

In interpreting the D^u test, the cells are D^u-positive if (1) the cells are not agglutinated directly by the anti-D serum, yet (2) are agglutinated at the antiglobulin phase of the D^u test, and (3) there is no agglutination at the antiglobulin phase of the test with Rh control reagent (or, alternatively, a direct antiglobulin test on the cells gives a negative result). The cells should be reported as simply "D^u-positive," never as "D-negative D^u-positive."

If no agglutination is observed in the antiglobulin phase of the D^u test, the cells may be reported as "D-negative D^u-negative," assuming that the test was correctly performed. The reactivity of the antiglobulin serum can be proved by adding

Coombs control cells after interpreting each negative antiglobulin test, and the performance of the anti-D serum with D^u-positive red cells can be checked periodically by running known low-grade D^u cells as a positive control.

If the indirect antiglobulin test with Rh control reagent (or the direct antiglobulin test) is positive, the test cannot be interpreted unless the positive antiglobulin test happens to be due to complement rather than immunoglobulin on the cells. If the test is only positive with antiglobulin reagents containing anticomplement, anti-IgG may be used for the D^u test and a valid test result obtained. Otherwise, if the cells are from a patient, they should be treated as D-negative; if from a donor, the blood should not be used for transfusion whatever the coating of protein present on the cells, as survival is likely to be diminished in a recipient.

In cases in which it is considered important to know the D^u status of the cells, an attempt may be made to elute enough immunoglobulin from the cells for the direct antiglobulin test to become negative. Unlike elution procedures applied when the focus of interest is antibody removed from the red cells, it is necessary in this situation to retain the red cells themselves intact for testing. Hence, techniques necessitating lysis of the cells cannot be used, and success or failure may be dependent on the amount of immunoglobulin bound and the extent of its affinity. The method that has been most usefully applied is one that involves incubating a saline suspension of the cells at 56°C for 3 minutes, then washing and retesting them.[35] A longer period at this temperature may destroy the Rh receptors, which are very susceptible to damage by heat, but in many cases it will be possible to remove enough immunoglobulin from the red cells to render the direct antiglobulin test negative. At this point, they may be tested for D^u by means of an indirect antiglobulin test with anti-D serum and a valid test result obtained.

SALINE-REACTIVE ANTI-D BLOOD GROUPING SERA

For many years, saline-reactive anti-D sera have been manufactured from raw material containing antibodies in the form of IgM. Because of the scarcity of Rh antibodies in this form, the products have been correspondingly expensive and sometimes difficult to obtain. Certainly these reagents have never been in sufficiently abundant supply to enable them to be used routinely for all testing to detect the D antigen, which would thereby avoid the main cause of false reactions with high-protein antisera.

A significant scientific breakthrough in recent years has been the development of a method whereby truly saline-reactive Rh antisera may be manufactured from chemically modified IgG antibodies.

In 1963 Pirofsky and Cordova[36] noted that IgG anti-D could be converted into a saline agglutinin by incorporating 2-mercaptoethanol into the test mixture. This was a somewhat surprising discovery, as 2-mercaptoethanol is one of the compounds that, by cleaving the disulfide bonds holding the individual units of the IgM molecule together, causes saline-agglutinating antibodies to lose their ability to agglutinate antigen-positive cells suspended in saline. These investigators suggested, however, that the reverse effect on IgG was also due in some way to disulfide reduction.

The idea was discredited in 1965 by Mandy, Fudenberg, and Lewis,[37] who repeated the experiments and concluded that the apparent conversion of IgG to give saline agglutination was a nonspecific phenomenon, possibly the result of some change brought about by 2-mercaptoethanol on the red cell membrane. The matter evidently fell into obscurity until 1977, when Romans and coworkers[38] in Canada reported success in converting IgG antibodies of several specificities into saline agglutinins by using dithioerythritol and dithiothreitol as well as 2-mercaptoethanol. These substances are all sulfhydryl compounds and are all capable of depolymerizing IgM molecules and causing them to cease behaving as agglutinins. Their effect on IgG is brought about by reduction of the disulfide bonds holding the heavy chains of the molecule together near the hinge region. This gives greater flexibility to the molecule, permitting its two antigen-combining sites to span a distance approximately 140 A greater than the native IgG molecule. The extra reach gained by the molecule enables it to form intercellular bridges between individual antigen-positive cells suspended in saline and, accordingly, to cause them to agglutinate without the need for a high-protein environment or for the presence of macromolecular additives. The change, however, is not permanent. Oxidation causes the disulfide bonds to reform, restoring the IgG molecule to its more rigid native state. Treatment with an alkylating agent, such as iodoacetamide, is needed to make the disulfide bond reduction permanent, after which the treated antibody-containing serum is dialyzed to remove the reactants and is then used to manufacture true saline-reactive antisera.

Saline-agglutinating antisera, whether made from IgM or from reduced and alkylated IgG, are suitable for testing red cells that, because they are coated with immunoglobulin, cannot be tested reliably with high-protein antisera. Both kinds, being formulated in a diluent having a total protein concentration close to that of normal human serum and lacking the need for macromolecular additives, give mainly specific reactions when used to test immunoglobulin-coated red cells. Spontaneous agglutination, if it occurs at all with the particular cell suspension being tested, will be at least equally likely to occur in the ABO test, where it should be recognized because it causes discrepancy between the results of forward and reverse grouping tests. Antisera made from IgM and those made from reduced and alkylated IgG differ somewhat in performance, so it would be appropriate to treat them separately.

IgM ANTISERA

Anti-D sera made from IgM antibodies cannot be used in the slide test procedure. The test must be performed in tubes, and a period of incubation at 37°C (usually from 15 to 30 minutes) is essential before centrifugation because the reaction takes some time to develop. This is a disadvantage when testing for D is being performed to enable donor blood to be selected for an urgently needed transfusion. Even if IgM anti-D sera were readily available and at a cost comparable with that of high-protein antisera, they would have disadvantages that would limit their usefulness in routine testing for the D antigen. Apart from the need for incubation before centrifugation, cells having weaker-than-average expression of the D antigen may tend to give weak or equivocal reactions, and the test cannot be taken to an antiglobulin phase for the D^u test as IgM antibodies are not suitable for the detection of D^u.

CHEMICALLY MODIFIED IgG ANTISERA

The overwhelming advantage of anti-D sera manufactured from reduced and alkylated IgG antibodies is that they give reactions as reliable as those of high-protein reagents, yet without the accompanying disadvantage of being prone to cause immunoglobulin-coated cells to agglutinate spontaneously. These products react reliably by the slide test procedure, give strong macroscopic reactions with a minimum of incubation in the tube test, and, since they contain IgG antibodies, can be used for the detection of D^u by the indirect antiglobulin test. Thus, these antisera may be used confidently in place of high-protein anti-D reagents in routine testing for the D antigen and will give comparably reliable test results without the need for a parallel control test on every red cell specimen tested. In most cases, the ABO test will serve as a sufficient control for spontaneous agglutination, although naturally it will still be necessary to control the D^u test in case the cells have a positive direct antiglobulin test.

FALSE REACTIONS WITH SALINE-REACTIVE ANTI-D SERA

Somewhat greater care is needed in performing hemagglutination tests with saline-reactive Rh antisera than with those containing a high concentration of protein. Owing to the lesser viscosity, the agglutinates are rather more fragile than those obtained with high-protein reagents. Accordingly, resuspension of the cell button after centrifugation needs to be done more gently than with high-protein antisera, but the necessary skill is easily acquired.

Understandably, if the red cells of a patient with strong cold agglutinins are tested unwashed there will be the possibility of a false test result. Similarly, if the patient's serum shows a tendency to promote the formation of rouleaux there may be aggregation that could be mistaken for agglutination. These potential sources of error are avoided, however, when the anti-D test is being performed in parallel with some other blood grouping test, such as ABO grouping. Except in the case of cells of group AB, one or more tubes showing a negative result in the ABO grouping provide sufficient control against spontaneous agglutination. When the test cells are group AB, a simple control can be set up using 6 to 8 percent bovine albumin or the patient's own serum.

On relatively infrequent occasions, false-negative reactions may be obtained when testing red cells that have become coated in vivo with IgG antibodies specific for the particular antigen that is being tested for. This situation arises most often when the red cells of an infant suffering from hemolytic disease of the newborn caused by anti-D are tested with a saline-reactive anti-D serum and are found to give a negative result. The cause of this phenomenon is in-vivo blocking of the D receptors by the coating anti-D protein. In rare cases, the amount of IgG anti-D present on the cells may be so great that there are not even enough free D receptors for spontaneous agglutination to occur when the cells are placed in a high-protein environment. In this event, high-protein anti-D sera will be unable to agglutinate the cells either, although the direct antiglobulin test is strongly positive and the only antibody apparently present in the maternal serum is anti-D. In such a case, elution of some of the antibody from the infant's cells (by heating at 56°C for 3 minutes and then washing, as previously described) usually enables the test for D to be performed with a saline-reactive antiserum, and identification of the eluted antibody as anti-D enables the diagnosis to be confirmed.

TESTING FOR OTHER Rh ANTIGENS

As with anti-D, antisera required for the detection of the other principal Rh antigens are available both as high-protein and as low-protein reagents. Those containing a high concentration of protein suffer from the same disadvantage as high-protein anti-D sera in that they may cause spontaneous agglutination of immunoglobulin-coated red cells. Their low-protein counterparts may be manufactured either from IgM antibodies or from reduced and alkylated IgG.

Test procedures applied in testing for the other Rh antigens are basically similar to those used in testing for D, except that there is no antiglobulin phase. Since Rh phenotyping sera are not required to be tested for specificity by the indirect antiglobulin test, it is not generally safe to apply this test method when using them. In most cases this would be necessary, as antigens expressed in normal strength are readily detected either with high-protein or with low-protein antisera. Variant antigens, such as those discussed earlier, particularly those representing comparatively weak expression of e and of C, are perhaps more reliably detected with high-protein antisera than with low-protein ones. Cells carrying some of these variant antigens may give false-negative reactions with saline-reactive antisera, not because these reagents are less potent than their high-protein counterparts but because a high-protein test system is inherently more sensitive than a low-protein test system.

REFERENCES

1. LANDSTEINER, K and WIENER, AS: *An agglutinable factor in human blood recognized by immune sera for rhesus blood.* Proc Soc Exp Biol (NY) 43:223, 1940.

2. WIENER, AS and PETERS, HR: *Hemolytic reactions following transfusions of blood of the homologous group with three cases in which the same agglutinogen was responsible.* Ann Int Med 13: 2306, 1940.

3. LEVINE, P and STETSON, HR: *An unusual case of intragroup agglutination.* JAMA 113:126, 1939.

4. LEVINE, P, et al.: *The role of isoimmunization in the pathogenesis of erythroblastosis fetalis.* AM J Obstet Gynecol 42:925, 1941.

5. FISHER, RA, cited in RACE, RR: *An "incomplete" antibody in human serum.* Nature 153:771, 1944.

6. MOURANT, AE: *A new rhesus antibody.* Nature 155:542, 1945.

7. ROSENFIELD, RE,et al.: *A review of Rh serology and presentation of a new terminology.* Transfusion 2:287, 1962.

8. MURRAY, J: *A nomenclature of subgroups of the Rh factor.* Nature 154:701, 1944.

9. STRATTON, F: *A new Rh allelomorph.* Nature 158:25, 1946.

10. Argall, CI, Ball, M and Trentelman, E: *Presence of anti-D antibody in the serum of a D^u patient.* J Lab Clin Med 4:895, 1953.

11. Wiener, AS and Unger, LJ: *Rh factors related to the Rh_0 factor as a source of clinical problems.* JAMA 169:696, 1959.

12. Tippett, P and Sanger, R: *Observations on subdivisions of the Rh antigen D.* Vox Sang 7:9, 1962.

13. Tippett, P and Sanger, R: *Further observations on subdivisions of the Rh antigen D.* Das Ärztliche Laboratorium 23:476, 1975.

14. Race, RR, Sanger, R and Selwyn, JG: *A probable deletion in a human Rh chromosome.* Nature 166:520, 1950.

15. Contreras, M, et al.: *The Rh antigen Evans.* Vox Sang 34:208, 1978.

16. Callender, ST and Race, RR: *A serological and genetical study of multiple antibodies formed in response to blood transfusion by a patient with lupus erythematosus diffusus.* Annals of Eugenics 13:102, 1946.

17. Rosenfield, RE, et al.: *A "new" Rh antibody, anti-f.* Br Med J i:975, 1953.

18. Allen, FH Jr and Tippett, P: *A new Rh blood type which reveals the antigen G.* Vox Sang 3:321, 1958.

19. DeNatale, A, et al.: *V: A new Rh antigen, common in Negroes, rare in white people.* JAMA 159:147, 1955.

20. Sanger, R, et al: *An Rh antibody specific for V and R'^s.* Nature 186:171, 1960.

21. Beattie, KM, et al.: *G^u, a variant of G.* Transfusion 11:152, 1971.

22. Shapiro, M: *Serology and genetics of a new blood factor: hr^S.* J Forens Med 7:96, 1960.

23. Shapiro, M, Le Roux, M and Brink, S: *Serology and genetics of a new blood factor: hr^B.* Haematologia 6:121, 1972.

24. Vos, GH, et al.: *A sample of blood with no detectable Rh antigens.* Lancet i:14, 1961.

25. Nicholson, GL, Masouredis, SP and Singer, SJ: *Quantitative two-dimensional ultrastructural distribution of $Rh_0(D)$ antigenic sites on human erythrocyte membranes.* Proc Natl Acad Sci USA 68:1416, 1971.

26. Race, RR and Sanger, R: *Blood Groups in Man,* ed 6. Blackwell Scientific Publications, Oxford, 1975, ch 5.

27. Issitt, PD: *Serology and Genetics of the Rhesus Blood Group System.* Montgomery Scientific Publications, Cincinnati, 1979.

28. Wiener, AS: *A new test (blocking test) for Rh sensitization.* Proc Soc Exp Biol (NY) 56:173, 1944.

29. Race, RR: *An "incomplete" antibody in human serum.* Nature 153:771, 1944.

30. Diamond, LK and Denton, RL: *Rh agglutination in various media with particular reference to the value of albumin.* J Lab Clin Med 30:821, 1945.

31. Bordet, J and Streng, O: *Le phénomène d'absorption et la conglutinine du sérum de boeuf.* Zentralbl Bakteriol [Orig A] 49:260, 1909.

32. Diamond, LK and Abelson, N: *The demonstration of Rh agglutinins—an accurate and reliable slide test.* J Lab Clin Med 30:204, 1945.

33. Coombs, RRA, Mourant, AE and Race, RR: *A new test for the detection of weak and "incomplete" agglutinins.* Br J Exp Pathol 26:255, 1945.

34. Moreschi, C: *Neue Tatsachen über die Blutkörperchen Agglutinationen.* Zentralbl Bakteriol [Orig A] 46:49 and 456, 1908.

35. Morel, PA, Bergren, MO and Frank, BA: *A simple method for the detection of alloantibody in the presence of warm autoantibody.* 30th Annual Meeting of the American Association of Blood Banks, Atlanta, 1977, Abstract S-53.

36. Pirofsky, B and Cordova, MS: *Bivalent nature of incomplete anti-D (Rh_0).* Nature 197:392, 1963.

37. Mandy, WJ, Fudenberg, HH and Lewis, FB: *On "incomplete" Rh antibodies: mechanism of direct agglutination induced by mercaptoethanol.* J Clin Invest 44:1352, 1965.

38. Romans, DG, et al.: *Conversion of incomplete antibodies to direct agglutinins by mild reduction. Evidence for segmental flexibility within the Fc fragment of immunoglobulin G.* Proc Natl Acad Sci USA 74:2531, 1977.

39. Shreffler, DC, et al.: *Studies on genetic selection in a completely ascertained U.S. Caucasian population. I. Frequencies, age, and sex effects and phenotype associations for 12 blood group systems. Tecumseh, Michigan: pop: 10,000 West European ancestry.* Am Soc Hum Genet 23:150, 1971.

Color Plate 1
The antihuman globulin (AHG) test.

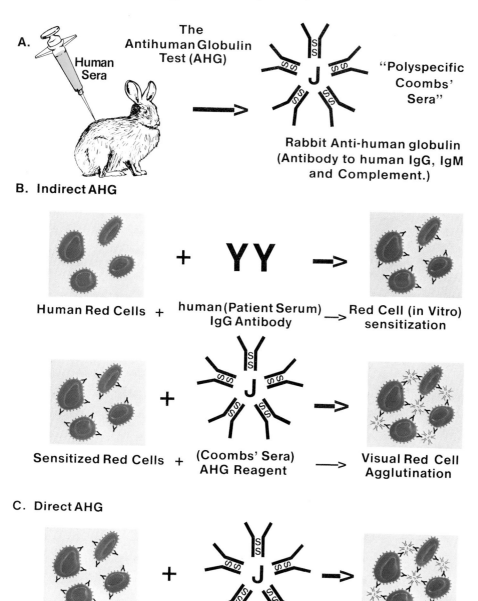

A. The Antihuman Globulin Test (AHG)

Human Sera

"Polyspecific Coombs' Sera"

Rabbit Anti-human globulin (Antibody to human IgG, IgM and Complement.)

B. Indirect AHG

Human Red Cells + human (Patient Serum) IgG Antibody → Red Cell (in Vitro) sensitization

Sensitized Red Cells + (Coombs' Sera) AHG Reagent → Visual Red Cell Agglutination

C. Direct AHG

Washed (3x's) Patient Red Cells (sensitized in Vivo) + (Coombs' Sera) AHG Reagent → Visual Red Cell Agglutination.

Color Plate 2
Agglutination reactions.

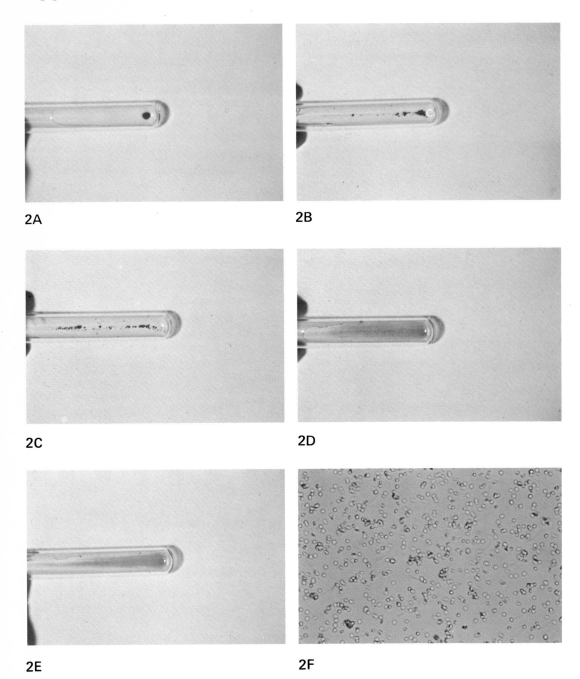

2A

2B

2C

2D

2E

2F

FREQUENCY

The antigens of the MNSs system that are most often encountered in routine laboratory testing are M, N, S, and s. Table 8-2 summarizes the relative frequencies of
these antigens as well as the frequencies of the common MNSs phenotypes. The U
antigen is found in nearly 100 percent of the white population; its frequency in blacks
ranges from 65 to 99 percent.

ANTIGENS

Structurally, the MNSs antigens are glycoproteins that form a portion of larger red
cell membrane components known as the glycophorins. Carbohydrate moieties are
attached to the protein portion that extends beyond the membrane exterior (see Color
Plate 15).

The definition of the structure of these antigens has been facilitated through
the use of sodium dodecyl sulfate (SDS) polyacrylamide gel electrophoresis (PAGE).
Red cell membranes that have been solubilized by the *anionic* detergent SDS are separated by electrophoresis into their components based on molecular weight, since
SDS renders a net negative charge onto all membrane components. Staining with
periodic acid-Schiff or Coomassie blue defines the carbohydrate or protein nature of
these constituents. By further evaluating the individual components, the exact structure of the MNSs antigens may be described. This structural analysis has resulted in
the formation of a new genetic model that may withstand the intense scrutiny under
which other models have failed.

The MN sialoglycoprotein, so named because it is rich in sialic acid residues
(*N*-acetylneuraminic acid or NANA), is a polypeptide chain of 131 amino acids
known as glycophorin A.[6] It is particularly rich in serine and threonine, amino acids
that contain alcohol groups. By inheriting an M or N gene, different amino acid sequences are expressed within this polypeptide backbone. In fact, M and N antigens
only differ by *two* amino acids, at positions one and five from the amino (NH_2) ter-

TABLE 8-2. Frequencies of Common MNSs Antigens and Phenotypes

	Antigen Frequencies (%)			Phenotype Frequencies (%)	
	White	Black		White	Black
M	80	74	MS	5	1
N	74	79	MSs	13	5
S	53	28	Ms	8	16
s	94	96	MNS	3	3
U	>99.9	65–99	MNSs	26	12
			MNs	25	37
			NS	<1	1
			NSs	5	6
			Ns	15	16

minus.[7] Whether the genes code for the entire polypeptide chain or just those two amino acids remains to be elucidated.

The Ss sialoglycoprotein (also called glycophorin B) needs to be studied in greater detail to determine its exact structure. However, it has been shown that a portion of the polypeptide chain from the amino terminus is identical to that of the N antigen; it is often designated 'N'.[8] It is not clear how 'N', S, and s are different from each other. Figure 8-1 and Color Plate 15 briefly depict these antigens.

The MNSs structures are glycoproteins and thus have a variety of sugar moieties attached to certain amino acids along the polypeptide chain, for example, sialic acid (NANA), N-acetylgalactosamine (GalNAc), and D-galactose (Gal). Interactions between the sugars and the protein chain result in a certain spatial conformation of the total structure. It has been suggested that this spatial conformation may be recognized as an antigenic determinant by certain types of antibodies.[9] Differences in amino acid sequence or in sugar-amino acid interactions may account for the diversity of antigens within this system. Perhaps the many variant antigens are the result of an amino acid substitution or an unexpected steric configuration of the basic polypeptide chain.

One other antigen must be considered at this time, as it is intimately associated with the Ss antigens. The antigen U, a very high-frequency antigen, has been incorporated into the MNSs system because of the observation that all U negatives are also negative for S and s.[5] The Ss negative phenotype occurs infrequently and most examples have occurred in the black population. It has been found that 16 percent of Ss negative individuals possess the U antigen, whereas the remainder lack U. In

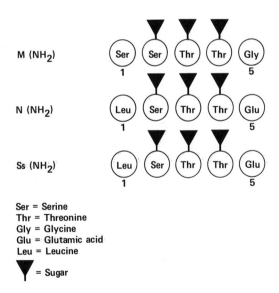

Ser = Serine
Thr = Threonine
Gly = Glycine
Glu = Glutamic acid
Leu = Leucine

▼ = Sugar

FIGURE 8-1. Amino terminal portion of the MNSs polypeptides. Note the amino acids that distinguish M from N and the similarity of Ss to N.

other words, all U-negative people are negative for Ss, but not all Ss-negative people are U negative. It is thought that U specificity lies on the Ss glycoprotein in close proximity to the S/s determinants.[10] It is also interesting to note that the U antigen is difficult to detect on Rh_{null} cells; the exact relationship between the two is unclear.

The MNSs antigens possess certain characteristics that are important both clinically and serologically. These antigens are very well developed at birth; this fact has a dual significance. All the antibodies except anti-N have been reported to cause hemolytic disease of the newborn, providing the maternal antibody was of the IgG type. In addition, the antigens have proven useful in paternity exclusion cases. Only well-developed antigens can be reliably typed on a newborn child's red cells, and the MNSs antigens fulfill this requirement.

These antigens are also selectively susceptible to enzyme treatment. Treating red cells with neuraminidase, which cleaves sialic acid residues, will abolish the reactivity of these cells with some types of anti-M and anti-N (notably the antibodies produced in humans and rabbits). The enzyme has no effect on Ss reactivity. There are other examples of anti-M and anti-N that react preferentially with desialicized red cells; these may be recognizing an alternative receptor, not affected by neuraminidase.

Treatment of cells with proteolytic enzymes such as ficin and papain has the same inhibitory effect, but cleaves off larger sections of the polypeptide chain. Because different enzymes will cleave the protein at different sites, there appears to be variability as to whether or not the antigen reactivity is completely abolished. Historically, it has been stated that all M, N, and S reactivity is lost after treatment with proteolytic enzymes, whereas s and U activity is not affected. However, it seems that S is resistant to trypsin. These findings should be kept in mind when utilizing enzyme treatment of red cells for the differentiation of multiple antibodies in a patient's serum.

Another group of antibodies is affected by the use of enzyme treatment of red cells and should be mentioned here. There are many lectins (extracts of plant seeds) that have been manipulated into demonstrating anti-M or anti-N activity. Among these are Vicia graminea (anti-N), and Iberis amara (anti-M). Vicia graminea shows anti-N specificity, but if the red cells to be tested are first treated with neuraminidase, even MM cells will react with the reagent. This suggests that the receptor for Vicia graminea is masked somewhat by the steric conformation induced by the NANA-protein interactions of the M chain, whereas in the N chain, the receptor is more accessible.

The U and s antigens do not appear to be affected by enzyme pretreatment. In fact, the antigen/antibody reactions are sometimes enhanced as a result of enzyme treatment.

In general, a double dose of M, N, S, or s demonstrates better reactivity with the appropriate antibody; this phenomenon is known as dosage. It manifests itself in this manner: an antibody will react more strongly with a cell homozygous for the corresponding antigen and will demonstrate weaker reactivity with a heterozygous cell. In fact, if the antibody itself is not extremely potent, no reactions at all may be observed in the heterozygous cell. This can lead to confounding results when attempting to resolve antibody problems. Table 8-3 demonstrates such a phenomenon.

OTHER MAJOR BLOOD GROUP SYSTEMS   **173**

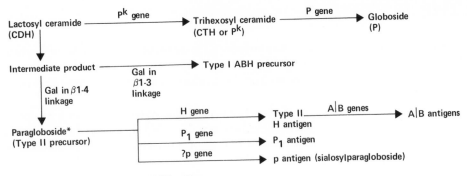

* Review the biochemistry of the ABH antigens.

FIGURE 8-2. Proposed pathway for the development of P system antigens. Note the interaction with ABH genes.

The genes of the P system code for glycosyl transferases, which attach specific immunodominant sugars to predetermined acceptor molecules. The P^k gene codes for the addition of α-galactose to ceramide dihexoside (CDH), yielding ceramide trihexoside (CTH). The P gene codes for the addition of N-acetylgalactosamine to ceramide trihexoside (CTH), yielding globoside. Thus, on the red cell, P^k serves as the precursor molecule for P antigen. The P_1 gene codes for the attachment of α-galactose onto paragloboside. It is not known whether the P_1 gene is a separate gene or not. Some theories have been suggested: (1) the P_1 gene codes for the attachment of α-galactose also, but to a different acceptor molecule, paragloboside; (2) the P_1 gene is actually a regulator or modifier that permits the P^k controlled transferase to use paragloboside as an additional acceptor. Further work must be performed before this mechanism is completely understood.

Table 8-5, summarized from Naiki and Marcus[13] and Graham,[14] compares the sugar sequences of the P antigens compared with the ABO antigens. It should be noted that sialosylparagloboside, the substance recognized as p antigen, differs from paragloboside only by the addition of a sialic acid residue. It is not yet known whether there is actually a "p gene" that codes for a sialyl transferase.

ANTIGENS

P_1 ANTIGEN

This antigen is most commonly encountered in routine testing. It is poorly developed on newborn blood cells and may take years to reach adult levels.[15] At adult levels, the antigen strength varies from one individual to another. Some people have much more P_1 antigen; these are P_1-strong individuals. There are also P_1-weak people. Any given example of anti-P_1, then, will give variable reactivity with a panel of P_1-positive cells. Keep in mind that a weak anti-P_1 antibody might not agglutinate a P_1-weak cell.

TABLE 8-5. Sugar Sequences of the P Antigens

Lactosyl ceramide	Gal (β,1-4)Glc-Cer
Trihexosyl ceramide	Gal(α,1-4)Gal (β,1-4)Glc-Cer
Globoside	GalNAc(β,1-3)Gal(α,1-4)Gal (β,1-4)Glc-Cer
Paragloboside	Gal(β,1-4)GlcNAc(β,1-3)Gal (β,1-4)Glc-Cer
P_1	Gal(α,1-4)Gal(β,1-4)GlcNAc(β,1-3)Gal (β,1-4)Glc-Cer
p	Gal(β,1-4)GlcNAc(β,1-3)Gal (β,1-4)Glc-Cer |(α2,3) NeuNAc
H	Gal(β,1-4)GlcNAc(β,1-3)Gal (β,1-4)Glc-Cer | Fucose (α,1-2)
A	GalNAc(α,1-3) Gal(β,1-4)GlcNAc(β,1-3)Gal (β,1-4)Glc-Cer | Fucose (α,1-2)
B	Gal(α,1-3)Gal(β,1-4)GlcNAc(β,1-3)Gal (β,1-4)Glc-Cer | Fucose (α,1-2)

The antigen also deteriorates rapidly on storage. This may create problems when phenotyping donor units for a patient with anti-P_1. When using reagent typing serum, fresh donor cells should be used so that false negatives are avoided.

P_1 antigen expression is diminished by the inhibitor gene InLu.[16] This gene is further described in the section on the Lutheran system. In the presence of InLu, normal P_1 antigen strength is drastically reduced.

To recapitulate antigen biochemistry, P_1 is a glycosphingolipid on the red cell. The addition of α-galactose to the ABH type-2 precursor (paragloboside) results in the production of P_1 antigen. P_1 antigen is also found on leukocytes, tissue cells, and in some secretions.[14,17,18]

P ANTIGEN (GLOBOSIDE)

This antigen occurs universally on red cells, in plasma, on leukocytes, and on tissue cells.[14,17,18] Only the P^k and p phenotypes can be shown to lack P antigen.

P^k ANTIGEN (TRIHEXOSYL CERAMIDE)

This is a rare, yet universal antigen. It is undetectable on red cells owing to its almost complete conversion to P antigen by the addition of GalNAc to CTH. It occurs on some tissue cells, some leukocytes, and in plasma. Fibroblasts of all but pp individuals possess P^k antigen.[14,17,18] It is produced by the addition of α-galactose to lactosyl ceramide.[17]

p ANTIGEN

It was historically thought that the p gene was an amorphic gene, that is, that no P group antigens were produced when a double dose of the gene was inherited. However, Tj^a-negative red cells seem to have an excess of sialosylparagloboside on their membrane, so that this substance has been designated the p antigen.[19] An antibody recognizing this determinant, that is, reacting preferentially with p cells, has also been described.[20-22] Cells of the p phenotype also demonstrate an excess of CDH and paragloboside. It is suggested that the genetic abnormality here is an absence of the α-galactosyl transferase(s) that codes for P^k and P_1.[19] Red cells that have been desialicized no longer react with anti-p.[19]

LUKE ANTIGEN

This antigen has not been well studied but seems to have some relationship to both the ABO and P systems. The exact relationship may become more clear if biochemical evaluation is pursued.

Further discussions on the antigens and antibodies are found in *Applied Blood Group Serology* by Issitt and Issitt;[15] *Blood Transfusion in Clinical Medicine* by Mollison;[18] and *Blood Groups in Man* by Race and Sanger.[23]

ANTIBODIES

ANTI-P_1

This is usually a cold-reacting, weak antibody present in the serum of two out of three P_2 individuals.[24] As such, it is an IgM saline agglutinin that can bind complement. The reactions of this antibody are often enhanced by enzyme treatment. Albumin may not affect the reactions at all, but a potent example of the antibody could react in albumin. There have been rare examples of IgG anti-P_1 and antibodies with a wide thermal range have also been described.[15] These antibodies, when found in a patient's serum, should be regarded with caution and the recipients transfused with P_2 blood. Examples of anti-P_1 that only react at 4°C have not been considered clinically significant. It has been suggested that in some circumstances crossmatch compatible blood is medically safe and economically feasible.[25] There is also evidence that some examples of anti-P_1, particularly the IgG variety and that found in anti-Tj^a, may be quite cytotoxic.[26] There have been very rare cases of transfusion reactions attributed to anti-P_1.[27,28]

ANTI-P

This is an extremely rare antibody. In its pure form, it can only be produced by individuals of the P^k phenotype, as these individuals lack P antigen; people of the p phenotype produce anti-PP_1P^k. Anti-P is usually a potent IgM hemolysin that has a wide thermal range of activity, but it may also occur as an IgG antibody. This is suggested because of the occasional examples of habitual abortion attributed to anti-P.[29]

Another type of anti-P is observed in patients with paroxysmal cold hemoglobinuria, an autoimmune disorder seen in children secondary to viral infections. (This rare disorder is discussed more completely in Chapter 19.) In most cases, the autoantibody is anti-P and it is an IgG biphasic hemolysin, that is, it binds complement to red cells at colder temperatures and then hemolyzes them at 37°C.

ANTI-P^k

This antibody has only been found as a component of anti-Tj^a by selective absorption with P_1-positive cells. It has not been reported as a pure antibody as of this writing.

ANTI-p

Only a few examples of this antibody have been reported and the antibodies have reacted either at 4°C or in the antiglobulin phase.[19-21] This antibody is neutralized by sialosylparagloboside and is most reactive with Tj^a-negative cells. Treatment of test cells with neuraminidase abolishes the reactivity, yet papain treatment seems to enhance the reaction.[20]

ANTI-Tj^a

Also known as anti-PP_1P^k, this antibody occurs consistently in the sera of p individuals, often without prior red cell stimulation. It can be IgG or IgM or a combination of the two and it is an efficient binder of complement, thus making it a potent hemolysin. Wide thermal activity is also found routinely. All in all, this is a deadly antibody. Severe hemolytic transfusion reactions, chronic abortions, and mild to severe hemolytic disease of the newborn have all been attributed to this antibody.[30-32] Owing to its cytotoxic nature, anti-Tj^a might also prove hazardous in organ transplantation, especially if the organ is not from a p donor.

COMPOUND ANTIBODIES

Many examples of compound antibodies have been reported in the literature; among them are anti-IP_1, anti-iP_1, and anti-I^TP_1. These are cold-reactive antibodies that react optimally against cells carrying all the necessary determinants. Considering the biochemical intimacy of the ABO, P, I, and Lewis systems, one should not be surprised that antigen interactions (steric or structural) could result in the production of antibodies recognizing these compound structures.

P_1 SUBSTANCES

When one recalls that ABO antibody specificity can be produced from seeds or snails, it should not be surprising that P_1 antigen exists in nature not only on the human red cell, but also in other, more exotic sources. These have a practical application in blood group serology.

The most common source of P_1 antigen other than the red blood cell is hydatid cyst fluid.[33] When an animal or human becomes infected with the tapeworm Echinococcus granulosus, cysts containing live heads (scolices) can be drained and the harvested fluid used to neutralize anti-P_1 antibodies. This fluid then is rich in P_1 substance. Its uses have included (1) neutralizing suspected anti-P_1 to confirm specificity, (2) neutralizing and therefore removing anti-P_1 from multiple antibody sera, thereby facilitating identification of the other antibodies, and (3) coating group O cells for injection into animals to stimulate anti-P_1 production.

Other sources of P_1 substance include liver flukes (Fasciola hepatica), roundworms (Ascaris), earthworms (Lumbricus), salmon and trout roe, and pigeons.[15,34,35] Perhaps there is some truth to the suggestion (made by chemists, microbiologists, and hematologists) that blood banking is part science, part witchcraft.

THE I SYSTEM

When Wiener first described the I system in 1956,[36] he named it "I" for "individuality." Little did he know just how appropriate that designation would become, for recent evidence suggests that Ii antigens may just be structures that are peculiar to each individual's red cells yet common to all red cells.[37] Heterogeneity and individuality seem to be the hallmarks of this system.

ANTIGENS

Only two antigens will be discussed in detail in this section—I and i. Both of these antigens are found on 100 percent of human red blood cells.[15] The quantity of each antigen on the red cells may vary from one individual to the next. Adults generally possess a significant quantity of I on their cells; the amount of i is virtually undetectable. Cord blood cells and the cells of newborns are, in contrast, rich in i; their concentration of I is virtually undetectable using routine techniques. The transition of i to I requires about 18 months time in the average human.[15] Very rarely are adults identified whose red cells lack detectable amounts of I antigen. These occur in approximately 1 in 10,000 persons and the individual is designated i_{adult}.[15]

This difference in Ii antigen concentration is important from a practical point of view. Cord blood cells are frequently included as part of the antibody identification process because of the fact that they are essentially I negative. Anti-I is a *very* common antibody in the routine laboratory setting and its identity is confirmed by using cord cells; adult I-negative cells (i_{adult}) are so rare that it is difficult to acquire them on a routine basis. Keep in mind, however, that this is just a practical difference. As was stated previously, all red cells contain some I and i antigen; very sensitive techniques may be necessary to demonstrate the weaker antigen.

STRUCTURE AND BIOSYNTHESIS

At this point, it is wise to review ABH biochemistry (Chapter 5), as this is intimately involved in Ii biochemistry and antigen synthesis. The reader should review the structure of type-1 and type-2 ABH glycolipids on the red cell membrane and in the secretions. Ii antigen specificity appears to reside on the same glycolipid chains that determine ABO specificity. As with the ABO antigens, oligosaccharides determine this specificity. If ABO antigens are stripped off the red cell with enzymes, enhanced I activity results, which indicates that I activity is located within or below the ABO structure. Bombays have been shown to possess the greatest concentration of I antigen of all adults.[38]

As described in the ABO chapter, ABH antigens exist as either straight or branched glycosphingolipid chains. Evidence suggests that the linear chain glycolipid structures form the i antigen, while the branched chains define the I antigen.

The transition in Ii status from newborn to adult is felt to be a reflection of changes in antigen density on the membranes of their respective red cells. Newborn red cells are more endowed with straight chain glycosphingolipids and as the child matures, branched glycosphingolipids begin to develop and eventually predominate.[39] This evolution of glycolipid structure thus accounts for the decrease in i and the increase in I as a baby matures.

It is also generally accepted that there is no one I or i antigen, that, in fact, the diversity of antibodies we call "anti-I" or "anti-i" may be recognizing any single sugar, combination of sugars, or perhaps even the entire chain.[14]

INHERITANCE

The next issue to address, once we understand the heterogeneous nature of these antigens, is the inheritance of these structures. In the past, single genes resulting in either I or i were proposed. These I or i genes would code either directly or indirectly (through a transferase mechanism) for the production of these antigens. Since we now know that numerous sugars may constitute the structures we call i or I,[40] it seems unlikely that numerous transferases are involved. Rather, it seems more likely that there is no single I or i gene.[37] The many glycosyl transferases that attach these sugars, when present or absent, result in different sugar sequences; these would be recognized as "I" or "i" antigens by the many antibodies we call anti-I and anti-i. This too may explain the heterogeneity of both the antigens and antibodies of this system. Another possible theory to consider is that an I gene does exist and that it codes for a "branching" enzyme that promotes the branching of red cell glycosphingolipids.[40]

OTHER SOURCES OF Ii

Not only are Ii antigens present on red cells, they also exist on other cells and as soluble antigens in plasma and secretions. Ii antigens have been found on the membranes of leukocytes and platelets.[18,41] It is quite likely that they exist on many tissue cells as well, as do the ABH antigens.

Both I and i are found in plasma and serum in both adults and newborns.[15] Ii substances have also been found as glycoproteins in secretions such as saliva.[42] Human milk (colostrum) is also rich in I.[15]

One last interesting point is that mitotically active cells, such as immature blood cells, have increased i activity.[18] In certain disease states in which marrow stress occurs and immature blood cells are released prematurely, these cells will show increased concentration of i antigen.[43,44] Reactive lymphocytes observed in infectious mononucleosis also seem to possess increased i antigen.[41]

OTHER ANTIGENS

Mention must be made of the other antigens described in the literature that are associated with the I system. These include I^F, I^D, I^T, $I_{intermediate}$, i_1, and i_2. At the time these antigens were described, the structure of Ii was unknown. Perhaps these are simply additional examples of the heterogeneous nature of I and i.

ANTIBODIES

The antibodies of the I system are consistently IgM, naturally occurring saline-reactive agglutinins. Most examples are weak and difficult to detect at temperatures used in routine serologic testing. Some may react at room temperature, but these are often undetected since room temperature incubation is no longer required in compatibility testing. Rarely, a very potent example may react at greater than room temperature; these antibodies should be evaluated closely because they may create transfusion problems. These antibodies may also bind complement at room temperature; antiglobulin reactivity may then be observed because of complement-coating of the test cells. Albumin and enzymes are known to enhance the reactivity of these antibodies, a fact that is useful in antibody identification and autoadsorption procedures. These antibodies have also been found to be extremely cytotoxic to lymphocytes and to agglutinate leukocytes.[45] Whether this has any clinical significance has yet to be determined.

ANTI-I

This antibody is perhaps the result of an ancient curse on all blood bankers. Using sensitive techniques, it can be demonstrated in the serum of most normal, healthy individuals as an autoantibody. In this capacity, it is a totally harmless antibody. However, when found in the serum of a patient who requires transfusion, this antibody can create havoc. If the antibody is strong enough to react at room temperature, complement may be bound and numerous weak incompatibilities will be observed in the antiglobulin phase. The dedicated blood banker must then (1) identify the antibody and confirm that this is, indeed, an auto-anti-I, (2) prove that no other significant alloantibodies are present and being masked by the autoantibody, and (3) eliminate the autoantibody via autoadsorption or prewarmed techniques to provide compatible crossmatches. (See Chapter 19 for further discussion of these methods.)

A potent auto-anti-I may be observed in patients with some autoimmune disorders. This autoantibody differs from the previously described autoantibody. (Refer to Chapter 19.)

Individuals who are the i_{adult} type will often produce an "allo-anti-I" that reacts at a wider thermal range and is a more potent antibody than auto-anti-I. This antibody could conceivably reduce the survival of transfused red blood cells and may warrant the use of other I-negative blood if transfusion is necessary.

ANTI-i

Anti-i is rarely found and seems to occur secondary to some viral disorders, particularly Epstein-Barr virus and cytomegalovirus.[46-49] When present in serum, it will react preferentially with cord cells. Its role in hemolytic anemias is discussed in Chapter 19.

OTHER ANTIBODIES

Bearing in mind the intimate relationship between the structures of the ABH, I, Lewis, and P systems, one should not be surprised that antibodies have been described that recognize compound structures made up of antigens from one or more systems. Examples of this phenomenon include anti-IP$_1$, anti-ILe^{bH}, anti-IH, and numerous others. Of importance here is that they are usually cold-reactive antibodies that react preferentially with cells carrying all the determinants being recognized. Table 8-6 depicts the typical reactivity of the more commonly encountered antibodies of this system.

RELATIONSHIP TO DISEASE

This topic is completely discussed in Chapter 19. The antibody usually associated with cold agglutinin disease and atypical pneumonia (pleuropneumonia-like organism or mycoplasma pneumoniae induced) is anti-I. Anti-i is associated with infectious mononucleosis. In cases of paroxysmal cold hemoglobinuria, although the antibody implicated is usually auto-anti-P, a rare example has been auto-anti-IH induced.

TABLE 8-6. Reactivity of Common Antibodies of the I System

Serum Antibody	Test Cells						
	A₁ Adult*	A₂ Adult*	B Adult*	O Adult	O Cord	Oₕ†	Oᵢ Adult†
Anti-I	+	+	+	+	weak or negative‡	+	negative
Anti-i	weak or negative	weak or negative	weak or negative	weak or negative	+	weak or negative	+
Anti-IH	negative or weak positive	+	less positive than A₂/O	+	negative or weak positive	negative	negative
Anti-H	weak or negative	+§	+¶	+	+	negative	+

*These cells would be tested only if ABO compatible with the serum being evaluated.
†Rare cells that are helpful if available; they are not necessary, however, in most cases.
‡Very potent examples of anti-I may need to be diluted before specificity can be determined.
§Weaker than O cells; O cells give strongest reaction.
¶Weaker than A₂ cells.
Note: Anti-H is included here for comparison. This anti-H is typical of the antibody that may be formed by A₁ and A₁B individuals (review Ch. 5).

THE KELL SYSTEM

The Kell system was first described in 1946[50] during the evaluation of a woman whose serum contained a new antibody resulting in hemolytic disease in her newborn child. Her antibody agglutinated approximately 9 percent of random bloods, those of her child, and those of her husband and was apparently the result of a previous transfusion of her husband's blood. The antigen, designated Kell (K), was subsequently matched in 1949[51] with its hypothetical partner, Cellano (k), and a new blood group system evolved.

Allen and associates described a new antigen Kpᵃ (Penney) in 1957,[52] as well as its genetic partner Kpᵇ (Rautenberg) in 1958.[53] These antigens were found to be related to the system and were thus incorporated into it. In 1958 Giblett[54] described the Jsᵃ (Sutter) antigen. Jsᵇ (Matthews) was described in 1963 by Walker and associates.[55] These antigens were found to be antithetical partners and subsequently incorporated into the Kell system.[56]

Since these early discoveries, many more antigens have been found and incorporated into this blood group system. There are now at least 20 antigens included in the Kell system; the majority of these are high frequency, that is, they occur in greater than 99 percent of the random population. The antigens of particular interest are K, k, Kpᵃ, Kpᵇ, Jsᵃ, Jsᵇ, Kx, and KL. The Kell_null phenotype, designated K₀, which lacks the high-frequency antigen Ku, as well as the other Kell system antigens, is also of interest. These will be described fully in subsequent sections.

ANTIGENS

Some of the antigens of the Kell system are listed in Table 8-7 with their frequencies. In addition, Table 8-8 enumerates the frequencies of the phenotypes most commonly encountered in the laboratory.[15]

Very little is known about the structure of these antigens. It is presumed that glycoproteins constitute at least a portion of the antigenic determinant.[57] There is also some question as to the significance of the carbohydrates attached to the protein backbone, and an "immunodominant sugar" mechanism may be playing a role in the development of Kell antigen specificity.[57] This latter concept is supported by the fact that certain polysaccharide metabolites produced by an Escherichia coli species have inhibited anti-Kell activity in vitro.[58]

These antigens in general are very well developed at birth, as is evidenced by the severity of hemolytic disease of the newborn caused by the antibodies. With one exception (Kx), the antigens seem to be restricted to the red cell membrane. Kx is also found on the membranes of macrophages and neutrophils, the phagocytic cells of the body.[59]

KELL

This antigen warrants special consideration in that the most common Kell system antibody encountered in the blood bank is anti-Kell. This is due to the immunogenicity of the Kell antigen. It has been rated as second only to the $Rh_0(D)$ antigen in that respect. In other words, when Kell-negative individuals are challenged by the antigen, either by transfusion or pregnancy, they are quite likely to form the antibody in response to that challenge. Fortunately, the frequency of the Kell anti-

TABLE 8-7. Antigens of the Kell System*

Name	Rosenfield's	Frequency (%)
K (Kell)	K1	9.0 (w)
k (Cellano)	K2	99.8 (w)
Kp^a (Penney)	K3	2.0 (w)
Kp^b (Rautenberg)	K4	99.9 (w)
Ku (Peltz)	K5	>99.0 (w)
Js^a (Sutter)	K6	20.0 (b)
Js^b (Matthews)	K7	99.0 (b)
K^w†	K8	5.0 (w); 18.0 (b)
KL (McLeod, Claasen)	K9	>99.9
Ul^a (Kahula)	K10	2.6 (Finns)
Côté	K11	>99.9
K$_x$‡	K15	>99.9
Wk^a (Weeks)	K17	0.3 (w)

*Alleles (known to date): K/k; Kp^a/Kp^b; Js^a/Js^b; Côté/Weeks.
†Inclusion in Kell system questionable.
‡Included in Kell system but produced by an independent X-linked gene.
w = white; b = black

TABLE 8-8. Phenotype Frequencies of Kell System

	White (%)	Black (%)
kk	91	96.5
Kk	8.8	3.5
KK	0.2	<0.1
Js(a+b−)	0.1	1.1
Js(a+b+)	0.1	18.4
Js(a−b+)	>99.9	80.5
Kp(a+b−)	<0.1	
Kp(a+b+)	2	
Kp(a−b+)	98	

gen is so low (9 percent) that donor bloods are rarely Kell positive; therefore, the chance of a Kell-negative recipient being transfused with a Kell-positive donor unit is also small. The same explanation holds true for immunization via pregnancy. If this were not the case, anti-Kell would be detected in the sera of many more patients.

PENNEY AND SUTTER

Because of the extremely low frequency of these antigens, they do not pose many problems to the blood bank technologist. It is of interest that these antigens (as well as K) are believed to be mutations of their high-frequency counterparts, Cellano, Kp^b, and Js^b. This hypothesis will be discussed further in the section on Inheritance and Biosynthesis. In addition, the frequency of Js^a is much greater in the black population; the antigen occurs in 20 percent of blacks versus less than 1 percent of whites.

CELLANO, RAUTENBERG, AND MATTHEWS

These antigens are all of very high frequency. Their significance lies in the fact that the rare individuals who lack one of these *could* develop the appropriate antibody upon transfusion or pregnancy. Fortunately, this is a rare occurrence because most people possess the antigens. In the event that blood lacking one of these antigens is required, it is best to seek out (1) siblings or (2) a rare donor file in which names of rare donors are kept for just such a need. Also, if Js^b-negative blood is required, it is helpful to select black donors, since the black population carries a greater proportion of Js^b-negative individuals.

THE K_0 PHENOTYPE

These rare individuals were first described by Chown and associates.[60] They are the null phenotype of the Kell system, that is, they lack all the known Kell antigens, particularly the high-frequency antigens. The danger here is that upon transfusion or pregnancy, they can develop antibodies to any or all the Kell antigens they are exposed to; this would make finding compatible blood virtually impossible. For example, they could simultaneously develop anti-Cellano and anti-Kp^b; finding blood negative for both of these antigens is unlikely. These individuals also lack the antigen Ku, which is considered a universal antigen present on all cells with normal Kell phenotypes. Anti-Ku may also be formed by the K_0 individual who is Ku negative, and this antibody is only compatible with other K_0 cells. Keep in mind that K_0 is not an antigen; it designates a phenotype. The K_0 individual is considered Ku negative, as well as negative for all the other antigens previously described.

Kx

There is one exception to the previous statement about K_0. It has been shown that K_0 cells are rich in Kx antigen, and this is the *only* Kell system antigen they possess. This finding gives support to the notion that Kx is a precursor substance that is acted upon by Kell genes to produce the appropriate antigens. It stands to reason that if one lacks the Kell genes (as does the K_0) there is no conversion of precursor; therefore, the precursor builds up and is strongly detectable. In normal Kell phenotypes, the majority of red cell Kx is converted to the antigens we are familiar with (e.g., K, k, Kp^a, Kp^b). Consequently, only trace amounts of Kx are detectable on these cells. This, too, lends support to the precursor theory. Kx is believed to be an erythrocyte membrane protein to which are added the substances that dictate Kell group specificity. The fact that K_0 cells are rich in Kx proves that this antigen is controlled by a genetic locus separate from the Kell group. This will be discussed further under Inheritance and Biosynthesis. Not only is Kx present (weakly) on red cells, but it is also found in significant concentrations on the membranes of neutrophils and monocytes.[59] Lack of this Kx membrane protein leads to significant hematologic changes that will be discussed later.

KL

This antigen is also a universal antigen of the Kell system, but is lacking on K_0 cells. It is also lacking on cells of the McLeod phenotype, that is, red cells that lack Kx (this unusual entity was alluded to above and will be discussed later). Thus, it appears that KL is a substance produced by the Kell genes from Kx protein. Its role in the biosynthetic scheme is not clear; however, it could possibly be an intermediate product between Kx and the completed Kell system antigens.[23]

INHERITANCE AND BIOSYNTHESIS

The inheritance of the Kell system antigens appears to be extremely complicated; in fact, it has been likened to the inheritance of the Rh system. It is not known which chromosome dictates the production of these antigens; however, several facts are known. The Kell genes appear closely linked to the genes controlling the ability to taste phenylthiocarbamide (PTC).[61] This may be a useful investigative tool in the future.

The Kell antigens are produced from a precursor substance (Kx) that is coded for by the X chromosome.[59] This Kx substance is then converted, perhaps by enzymatic (transferase) action, to the various antigens recognized in the system.[62] The location of the gene or genes that code for this conversion process is not known, but probably is on an autosome. The transferases would be the result of the Kell genes, although this mechanism has not yet been confirmed.

It is believed that, like the Rh antigens, the Kell antigens are controlled by an inherited gene complex or by one gene that codes for several antigenic determinants. This parallels the Fisher-Race and Wiener theories of inheritance. This is based on the observation that antigens are passed as a complex or cluster. Figure 8-3 illustrates a possible inheritance scheme.

It has been suggested that the original Kell gene is the one that codes for k, Kp^b, and Js^b and that the others are single mutations of that gene.[63] This hypothesis is supported by the fact that, given the many possible genotypes that could occur within the Kell system, some have never been described. This may be true because to create these complexes would require two or three mutations within one gene, a situation not likely to occur.[63] Table 8-9 lists the genotypes possible, given the six common alleles, K and k, Kp^a and Kp^b, and Js^a and Js^b. Those indicated with an asterisk are the genotypes that have been described in the literature. The others have not been described as of this writing.

In general, all the autosomal genes, other than k^0, are inherited as codominant alleles. Expression of the K_0 phenotype requires homozygous k^0 inheritance. Inheriting two k^0 genes results in the complete shut-down of Kell activity and in no antigen production. There is then an accumulation of Kx.

The inheritance of an X-linked gene, X^1k, is mandatory for the production of Kx, for without this protein, the other Kell antigens cannot be properly synthesized. Inheritance of a variant of this X^1k gene may result in the abnormal McLeod phenotype, which will be discussed shortly. Other variants of X^1k result in abnormal

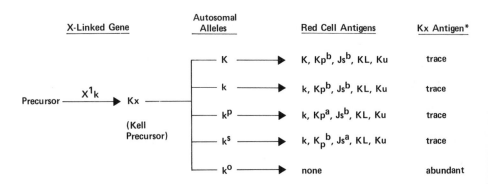

* In addition, inheritance of X^1k results in the presence of significant amounts of Kx on the monocytes and neutrophils. Other Kell antigens are not found on these cells.

FIGURE 8-3. Proposed scheme for the production of Kell system antigens. For simplification, other Kell system antigens have been excluded from this scheme (e.g., K11, K17, U1ª).

MODERN BLOOD BANKING AND TRANSFUSION PRACTICES

TABLE 8-9. Possible Genotypes of Kell System

k, Kp^b, Js^b *	K, Kp^b, Js^b *
k, Kp^a, Js^b *	K, Kp^a, Js^b
k, Kp^b, Js^a *	K, Kp^b, Js^a
k, Kp^a, Js^a	K, Kp^a, Js^a

*These genotypes have been identified via family studies.

leukocytes (monocytes and neutrophils) leading to impaired bactericidal function and a pathologic state known as chronic granulomatous disease (CGD). To summarize, this implies that normal Kx production is required for (1) normal Kell antigens, (2) normal red cells, and (3) normal phagocytic leukocytes. This has been perhaps the most exciting discovery associated with the Kell system.

ANTIBODIES

GENERAL CHARACTERISTICS

The vast majority of Kell system antibodies are red cell stimulated, either by transfusion or pregnancy. In addition, they are usually warm-reacting, IgG antibodies that react optimally in the antiglobulin phase. Although exceptions do occur, it is very unusual to detect a Kell system antibody in any phase other than the AGT. Albumin and enzymes do not generally affect the reactivity of these antibodies; they neither enhance the reactions nor degrade the antigens. The antibodies may react in these phases, however.

These antibodies generally are not efficient at binding complement; thus they are not hemolytic in vitro or in vivo. Exceptions to this, however, have been reported. Red cell destruction caused by these antibodies would be mediated by extravascular hemolysis via the macrophages in the spleen which ingest immunoglobulin-coated red cells. These antibodies are quite significant, when present in a patient's serum. Numerous examples of transfusion reactions and hemolytic disease of the newborn have been attributed to the Kell system; therefore, they must be regarded with a great deal of respect. In fact, anti-Kell has been found to be the most common antibody implicated in non-ABO hemolytic transfusion reactions where the antibody was detectable but missed in serologic testing.[64]

Anti-Kell is the most commonly encountered of the Kell group antibodies because of the potency of the antigen. It is most commonly encountered as an antiglobulin-reactive antibody, although reactions may be observed at room temperature, at 37°C, and in enzyme testing. Most examples are IgG, but IgM "naturally occurring" examples have been described.[58]

The other antibodies of the Kell system occur infrequently. Anti-Kp^a and anti-Js^a pose no problem in that so few donors are positive for these antigens. They could, however, be a serious consideration in hemolytic disease of the newborn and transfusion reactions. The antibodies to high-frequency antigens are problems in that it may be difficult to acquire antigen-negative blood. Anti-Kp[b] has also been found coating the cells of patients with warm autoimmune hemolytic anemia.

THE McLEOD PHENOTYPE AND CGD

These rare phenomena are associated with a lack of the gene coding for Kx production. There are four alleles postulated at the Xk locus, which is the site of control of this gene. Normal individuals inherit the X[1]k gene and produce Kx antigen on their leukocytes and red cells. The erythrocyte Kx is subsequently converted to Kell antigens unless an individual has inherited the k[0] gene. The alternative genes at this locus have been designated X[2]k, X[3]k, and X[4]k. Table 8-10, modified from Marsh,[57] summarizes the effects of the various Xk alleles.

The McLeod phenotype results from a lack of Kx on the erythrocyte membrane. One effect is that normal Kell antigens cannot be synthesized. Some synthesis occurs, but the resulting antigens react very weakly, if at all, with appropriate antisera.[65] Consequently, these individuals type very weakly positive for their particular antigens. These cells are also morphologically abnormal and appear in Wright-stained blood smears as acanthocytes. As is the fate of most morphologically abnormal red cells, these cells are sequestered in the spleen and destroyed by local macrophages. The result of this red cell destruction is that individuals with the McLeod phenotype suffer from a chronic, compensated hemolytic anemia.[65]

Chronic granulomatous disease (CGD) comprises a group of heterogeneous disorders that demonstrate a common feature: an inability of the leukocytes to effectively destroy certain microorganisms.[66] There has been an association made be-

TABLE 8-10. Effects of Xk Alleles

Allele	Kx on Red Cells	Kx on Leukocytes	Morphologic, Serologic, and Clinical Results
X[1]k	weak	abundant	normal Kell antigens normal red cell morphology normal leukocyte function
X[2]k	absent	absent	weakened Kell antigens (McLeod phenotype) hemolytic anemia (acanthocytes) type II CGD—impaired bacterial killing
X[3]k	weak	absent	normal Kell antigens normal red cell morphology type I CGD—impaired bacterial killing
X[4]k	absent	abundant	weakened Kell antigens (McLeod phenotype) hemolytic anemia (acanthocytes) normal leukocyte function

(Modified from Marsh.[57])

tween two types of CGD (type I and type II) and the Kell System.[67] In these two disorders, which are both sex-linked and restricted to males, there is a proven lack of Kx antigen on the membranes of the neutrophils and monocytes.[67] There is also a deficiency in the enzyme NADH-oxidase, a membrane enzyme of importance in the generation of hydrogen peroxide (H_2O_2) within the phagolysosome of these phagocytic cells.[68] If the neutrophil cannot successfully generate H_2O_2, it cannot kill microorganisms via the myeloperoxidase-peroxide-halide killing mechanism.[69]

Many organisms produce H_2O_2 during their own metabolic processes and these organisms actually precipitate their own destruction. Others, such as Staphylococcus species produce an enzyme known as catalase, which degrades H_2O_2 to harmless metabolites. These organisms are not killed by CGD neutrophils and may subsequently produce overwhelming, even fatal, infection in affected children. It may be interesting to speculate whether Kx antigen and NADH-oxidase are portions of the same protein or whether one is an integral portion of the other.

In summary, it is apparent that the Kell system plays an important role in normal homeostasis. It seems to be necessary for normal erythrocyte structure and normal leukocyte function.

THE DUFFY SYSTEM

The first identified example of a Duffy system antibody occurred in the serum of a multiply-transfused hemophilia patient, Mr. Duffy. This antibody was described in 1950 by Cutbush, Mollison, and Parkin.[70] The antigen recognized by it was named Duffy ^{a}(Fy^a) and the antibody, anti-Fy^a. Numerous examples soon followed this initial report. In 1951 an antibody recognizing its hypothetical allele, Fy^b, was reported by Ikin and colleagues.[71]

Studies utilizing anti-Fy^b with red cells from whites showed an unusual phenomenon that was reported in 1965 by Chown, Lewis, and Kaita.[72] They demonstrated that some red cells from whites that appeared to be negative for the Fy^b antigen were, in fact, very weakly positive. This was confirmed with adsorption and elution studies, and the antigen was designated Fy^x. It was believed that this antigen differed from Fy^b only quantitatively, but the exact relationship has yet to be elucidated.

Since 1970 three new and interesting Duffy antibodies have been described. Their interest lies in the fact that they have contributed much to the understanding of the genetics of the system and its relationship to the Rh system. They also seem to clarify the relationship observed between the Duffy system and malaria. The antibodies are anti-Fy3, anti-Fy4, and anti-Fy5; the antigens they recognize have been designated Fy:3, Fy:4, and Fy:5. These will be described in greater detail, but for now, let us discuss the antigens of interest in the routine blood bank setting.

FREQUENCY

In large-scale donor testing, the Duffy antigens have shown an intriguing disparity of distribution between white and black populations. Table 8-11 illustrates this dis-

TABLE 8-11. Distribution of Duffy Phenotypes

	Frequency (%)	
Phenotype	White	Black
Fy(a+b−)	18	14
Fy(a+b+)	49	2
Fy(a−b+)	33	19
Fy(a−b−)	0*	65†

*Essentially 0 percent.
†This frequency is reported in American blacks. The frequency in African blacks has been much higher, on the order of 90 percent.

parity. The frequency of white Fy(a−b−) individuals is indeed quite low, with only a handful having been described thus far in the literature. This finding has demonstrated another odd coincidence. Of the many thousands of black Fy(a−b−) patients transfused annually with blood containing one or both Duffy antigens, there have been essentially no cases of antibody production reported. The extremely rare exception will be discussed later. However, in contrast to this, the few white (or non-black) Fy(a−b−) individuals identified thus far have been found because their serum contained an antibody reacting against all Fy(a+) and Fy(b+) bloods. This observation led to the hypothesis that black and white Fy(a−b−) phenotypes arose by two different genetic mechanisms.

ANTIGENS AND ANTIBODIES

Fy^a AND Fy^b (Fy^x)

These antigens appear early in fetal life and are well developed on fetal red cells, even prior to birth. They are probably protein in nature, and proteolytic enzymes commonly used in blood banks, particularly papain and ficin, will destroy the antigen sites. Enzyme-treated cells will give no reaction with the appropriate antibody. Homozygosity of the gene will result in increased expression on the red cell; however, not all antibodies will detect this dosage effect. Compared with the Rh_0 (D) and Kell antigens, Fy^a and Fy^b do not appear strongly antigenic. As was stated earlier, Fy^x appears to be a weak form of Fy^b. It reacts with some examples of anti-Fy^b but it will absorb and elute all examples of the antibody.

The antibodies to these antigens are usually immune IgG agglutinins. They usually require antiglobulin testing to be demonstrable and they may bind complement occasionally. Both have been implicated in hemolytic transfusion reactions. Anti-Fy^a has been responsible for a number of cases of hemolytic disease of the newborn; anti-Fy^b has that same potential.

Generally, anti-Fy^a is seen much more frequently in the laboratory than anti-Fy^b; the latter occurs in sera of multiple specificities rather than as a single antibody.

These antibodies tend to occur more frequently in whites than in blacks. To date, there has been no report of the existence of anti-Fy^x and attempts to selectively absorb out anti-Fy^x from anti-Fy^b have been unsuccessful.

Fy:3 AND ANTI-Fy3

The Fy:3 antigen is one that seems to occur on all bloods except Fy(a−b−). It was first described in 1971[73] as the result of isolation of the corresponding antibody. An interesting feature is that, unlike Fy^a and Fy^b, this antigen is not deteriorated by enzyme treatment.

The antibody, anti-Fy3, reacts with all Fy^a-positive and Fy^b-positive bloods but is not reactive with Fy(a−b−) cells. It is not, however, a combination anti-Fy (a+b) (see Table 8-12). Reactions are best seen in the antiglobulin phase and enhanced reactivity is observed after enzyme treatment of the test cells. Anti-Fy3 is an IgG antibody, is immune stimulated, and has the potential to cause a hemolytic transfusion reaction. Hemolytic disease of the newborn has been caused by the antibody. It has been consistently observed in the serum of non-black Fy(a−b−) individuals.

Fy:4 AND ANTI-Fy4

The frequency of the Fy:4 antigen is quite high in blacks. Prior to the discovery of Fy:4 it was thought that blacks of the Fy(a−b−) type had inherited two amorphic Fy genes. It is now believed that these people have inherited Fy4 genes instead, as they consistently type Fy:4 positive. The frequency among whites is low: approximately 5 percent. Again, like Fy:3, this antigen resists degradation by proteolytic enzymes.

The antibody was first described in 1973[74] in the serum of a multiply-transfused Fy (a+b+) child. This antibody reacts with all Fy(a−b−) bloods, some Fy^a positive bloods and some Fy^b positive bloods. It does not, however, react with Fy(a+b+) (see Table 8-12). As is anti-Fy3, this antibody is an immune, IgG type immunoglobulin, with the potential to cause transfusion reactions and hemolytic disease of the newborn, although no cases have yet been described.

The reason it reacts with some, but not all, Fy(a+b−) and Fy(a−b−) bloods is as follows: Genetically, some Fy(a+b−) are Fy^{a}Fy^a and some are Fy^{a}Fy4. The latter type would produce Fy:4 antigen and react with the antibody. The same mechanism holds true with Fy(a−b+) cells.

Fy:5 AND ANTI-Fy5

The Fy:5 antigen appears to be the result of interaction between normal Rh genes and normal Fy genes (Fy^a, Fy^b, Fy^x). This theory was given credence by the reactions observed when the first example of the antibody was tested.[75] Initially, it was thought to be anti-Fy3, because it reacted with all Fy^a-positive or Fy^b-positive bloods, but failed to react with Fy (a−b−) bloods. Then, two observations were made that excluded anti-Fy3. First, the antibody reacted with a white Fy(a−b−) Fy:−3. Second,

TABLE 8-12. Reactivities of Anti-Fy3, Anti-Fy4, and Anti-Fy5

Cells	Reaction					
	Anti-Fy3		Anti-Fy4		Anti-Fy5*	
	AGT	Enz	AGT	Enz	AGT	Enz
Fy(a+b−)	+	+	some +	some +	+	+
Fy(a+b+)	+	+	0	0	+	+
Fy(a−b+)	+	+	some +	some +	+	+
Fy(a−b−) black	0	0	+	+	0	0
Fy(a−b−) white	0	0	0	0	+	+†

*Reactivity with anti-Fy5 implies that the common Rh antigens are present.
†Fy(a−b−) individuals who are genetically Fy4Fy4 would not produce Fy:5 antigen and would be unreactive with anti-Fy5. Fy(a−b−) whites (who produce anti-Fy3) apparently have normal Fy genes but are unable to express them. These individuals are capable of producing Fy:5 antigen and will react with the antibody.

the antibody would not react with Rh_{null} cells that had normal Fy antigens. These two tests showed that if an individual lacks either the common Fy genes (i.e., one who has the Fy4Fy4 genotype) or the common Rh genes (an Rh_{null}), that individual cannot produce Fy:5 antigen and has the ability to produce anti-Fy5. This is further strengthened by the observation that deletion cells (i.e., D−/D−) carry less Fy:5 antigen than normal Rh cells.

As was true of the previous two antibodies, anti-Fy5 is an IgG immune antibody. It reacts best in the Coombs phase and in enzymes, and the antigen is not destroyed by enzyme treatment.

With regard to antigen frequency, the Fy:5 antigen is found on most red cells of whites. Because of the increased incidence of the Fy4 gene in blacks, the Fy:5 antigen is not as widespread in that race. Table 8-12 summarizes the typical reactivities of anti-Fy3, anti-Fy4, and anti-Fy5.

GENETICS AND BIOSYNTHESIS

The Fy genes have been shown to be located on autosome 1 in man, as are the Rh genes. A number of studies have provided the evidence for this. They are not located closely enough to the Rh genes to be linked; therefore, any relationship between the two systems is syntenic.

There is a great deal of speculation as to how the antigens are produced. A very interesting and plausible *theoretical* model is described by Issitt and Issitt[15] and is summarized in Figure 8-4. In Figure 8-4 it can be noted that most "normal" individuals produce Fy precursor (FyPS) from a basic precursor by the action of a hypothetical "F" gene. Racial differences become apparent at this point. Most whites

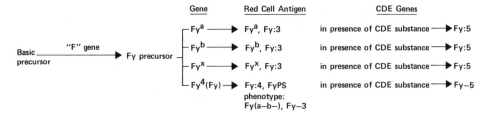

FIGURE 8-4. A proposed model for the inheritance and synthesis of the Duffy antigens.

have Fy^a, Fy^b, or Fy^x genes that convert this FyPS to the appropriate antigen. Another mechanism, possibly utilizing the same genes, results in the simultaneous production of Fy:3 antigen. In blacks, most of whom have the Fy4Fy4 genotype, only Fy:4 antigen is produced, which is structurally very similar to FyPS and the other Fy antigens. Because the other Fy genes are not present, these individuals do not produce Fy:3 antigen. Their phenotype is Fy(a−b−), Fy:−3, Fy:4. It is believed that these individuals do not produce the antibodies to the antigens they lack (anti-Fy^a, anti-Fy^b, anti-Fy3) because FyPS is such a similar structure that these antigens are not recognized as foreign.

Alternatively, as demonstrated in Figure 8-5, there are a few rare individuals who cannot make Fy precursor. These are designated genetically as the hypothetical "f" person. They may have normal Fy^a and Fy^b genes, but are unable to utilize them because these genes cannot convert the basic precursor to Duffy antigen. This pathway seems to accommodate the white who is Fy(a−b−) Fy:−3 and who can and does produce anti-Fy3. This individual has no Fy precursor and all Fy antigens are recognized as foreign.

It has long been known that Fy^a and Fy^b are alleles at the same locus of the Fy gene. There is now a strong suspicion that Fy:3 and Fy:4 are alleles at a different locus on the same gene. The exact location of the Ff genes that are involved in the production of Fy precursor is unknown, but it is believed to be independent of the Fy^a, Fy$^{b/x}$, Fy3, and Fy4 genes. The fact that the f individual is able to pass on to offspring Fy^a and Fy^b genes seems to confirm this.

But how does Fy:5 fit into this scheme? As is shown in Figures 8-4 and 8-5, any individual who possesses a normal CDE phenotype and has the Fy^a or Fy^b gene, even the Fy(a−b−) f type, will produce the Fy:5 antigen. The exceptions are the Fy:4 type Fy(a−b−), who has neither Fy^a nor Fy^b genes, and the Rh$_{null}$ individual who has no CDE antigens (Fig. 8-6). This, of course, is all speculation, but it does seem to explain the racial differences and antibody-forming potential of the Fy phenotypes.

One last and very interesting aspect of this system has been elucidated in recent work by Miller and coworkers.[76] It seems that, in order to invade a red cell, the malaria parasite (Plasmodium knowlesi) requires Fy^a or Fy^b antigen as the "doorway" to enter that cell. Many blacks have also been reported to be resistant to Plasmodium vivax. It is very intriguing that in Africa, where malaria is endemic, almost 100 percent of the native population lacks both these antigens, that is, they

(Lack of F)

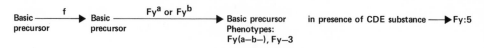

FIGURE 8-5. Theoretical model of inheritance for the non-black Fy(a−b−).

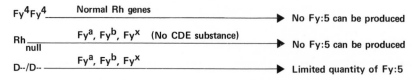

FIGURE 8-6. Proposed model to explain the inability to produce Fy:5 antigen.

are Fy(a−b−). It seems that Africans have developed a natural defense system against this parasite, one that has persisted through natural selection. The decreased incidence of Fy(a−b−) in American blacks may be the result of two factors: interracial mating throughout the centuries and a lack of need for this defense system (owing to the lack of malaria in this country). This interesting relationship is still being evaluated by other investigators, because there are some discrepancies that cannot be explained.

THE KIDD SYSTEM

The Kidd system was first described in 1951[77] in an infant suffering from hemolytic disease of the newborn caused by maternal anti-Jk^a. The Jk^b antigen was subsequently described in 1953.[78] An apparently universal antigen (Jk3) was included in 1959.[79] There have been no additional antigens described within this system.

In terms of inheritance, there is very little information available. The genes coding for Jk^a and Jk^b exist as alleles and they are expressed in a codominant fashion. Rare individuals have been described who lack both these antigens and have been named the Kidd$_{null}$ or Jk(a−b−). It is thought that this phenotype may arise from one of two mechanisms: homozygous inheritance of an amorphic Jk gene or inheritance of a suppressor gene that prevents Jk^a/Jk^b expression on the red cell.

ANTIGENS

Table 8-13 summarizes the frequencies of the antigens and phenotypes in a white population. The distribution among blacks tends to be more heavily weighted in favor of the Jk^a antigen.

Very little is known about the nature and structure of the Kidd antigens. They are very well developed at birth, which contributes to the incidence of hemolytic dis-

TABLE 8-13. Phenotypes of the Kidd System

Phenotype	Frequency (%)	Antigen Frequency (%)
Jk(a+b−)	28	Jk3 = >99.9
Jk(a+b+)	49	Jk(a+) = 77
Jk(a−b+)	23	Jk(b+) = 73
Jk(a−b−)*	very rare	

*Described most frequently in people of Oriental and Philippine origin.

ease of the newborn, and they are enzyme-insensitive. In fact, enzyme treatment of test cells results in enhanced reactivity with the appropriate antibody. The antigens also demonstrate a dosage effect when tested with the corresponding antibody. At this time, there is no evidence to suggest that Jk^a and Jk^b exist on any cell other than erythrocytes.

ANTIBODIES

The antibodies of this system present certain problems that contribute to their significance. These antibodies are IgG, immune, antiglobulin-reactive for the most part, although IgM examples have been reported. Because the antigens are poor immunogens, the antibodies tend to be weak and occur in the sera of patients with multiple antibodies. They are rarely pure and potent.

Activity of these antibodies tends to be enhanced after enzyme treatment of the test cells. In addition, the antibodies bind complement well and may, in fact, be difficult to detect if fresh serum is not used.

The antibody produced by Jk(a−b−) individuals is rather unique. It is named anti-Jk3 and has all the serologic properties of anti-Jk^a plus anti-Jk^b. Anti-Jk3 reacts with all cells except Jk(a−b−), but it is not separable into components. Compatible blood for patients having the antibody is generally acquired through a rare donor file or by testing siblings. The determinant recognized by this antibody appears on neutrophils as well as red blood cells.[80]

Finally, these antibodies tend to be very labile on storage. They deteriorate rapidly, and this fact has two important ramifications. When typing donor units for either antigen with old antisera, false negatives may be encountered, particularly if the donor cells are heterozygous, that is, Jk(a+b+). More importantly, these antibodies tend to disappear from a patient's plasma very rapidly. Because of this, they have been nicknamed the "treacherous Kidds." These antibodies are notorious for causing delayed hemolytic transfusion reactions and are the antibodies most often implicated in delayed hemolytic transfusion reactions where the antibody was undetectable in pretransfusion testing.[64]

After a period of time, the Kidd antibodies diminish in titer and become undetectable by routine serologic methods. Even enhancement methods may not demonstrate the antibodies. Consequently, if previous records are unavailable to verify the former existence of the antibody, the patient may inadvertently be crossmatched and transfused with Kidd-positive blood. This second exposure to the antigen elicits an "anamnestic response," a rapid, secondary rise in antibody titer that is potent and sustained. This example illustrates the crucial nature of keeping meticulous records and making patients aware of possible transfusion complications if they develop antibodies. It has been suggested that patients with problematic antibodies, such as the Kidds, wear or carry some type of warning statement so that physicians and technologists can be made aware of their particular problems.

THE LUTHERAN SYSTEM

This system has been recognized since 1945, when the first example of anti-Lu[a] was described.[81] With the discovery of anti-Lu[b], a new blood group system evolved.[82] Since that time, nearly 20 antigens have been incorporated into the Lutheran system, although many have not been well investigated. As with the Kell system, most of these factors occur as high-frequency antigens. This section will focus on Lu[a] and Lu[b].

ANTIGENS

The frequencies of the common Lutheran phenotypes are listed in Table 8-14, as are the antigen frequencies. As is evident from the table, most individuals possess the Lutheran antigens. There is a group of individuals who lack all expression of these antigens; these rare people are the Lutheran null phenotype or Lu(a−b−). The antigens of this group are probably glycoprotein[62] and are poorly developed at birth, requiring several years to evolve.[83] Their immunogenicity is questionable and studies in which Lu[a]-negative volunteers were transfused with Lu[a]-positive blood have yielded conflicting results. In some instances anti-Lu[a] was produced in the recipient, but in many cases it was not.

The antigens may also demonstrate some dosage; this is not as dramatic as that seen in the MN system. Enzyme treatment does not generally affect the antigens, neither enhancing nor diminishing the reactivity with the appropriate antibody.[62]

TABLE 8-14. Frequencies of Lutheran Phenotypes

Phenotype	White (%)	Black (%)
Lu(a+b−)	0.1	0.1
Lu(a+b+)	7.0	5.2
Lu(a−b+)	92.9	94.7
Lu(a−b−)	very rare	

ANTIBODIES

Anti-Lu^a is found infrequently in a random population, possibly as a result of the low frequency of the antigen. Most examples are IgM, saline-reactive agglutinins, but occasionally a warm-reacting IgG or IgA antibody may occur. It has been reported that this antibody gives a characteristic, loose mixed-field type of agglutination.[15]

There is no solid evidence that anti-Lu^a has caused hemolytic disease of the newborn or a hemolytic transfusion reaction; however, a potent example of the antibody should be considered carefully. Complement may be bound by anti-Lu^a.

Anti-Lu^b has been reported to occur as both an IgG and an IgA antiglobulin-reactive antibody, although it occurs rarely as an IgM saline-reactive antibody.[15] Decreased red cell survival and transfusion reactions have been attributed to this antibody.[83,84] A rare case of hemolytic disease of the newborn has also been described.[85] In conclusion, anti-Lu^b should be regarded as a significant antibody. It, too, may demonstrate the agglutination pattern described for anti-Lu^a. This antibody may also bind complement.

Anti-Lu3 is an antibody produced by the rare Lu(a−b−) individual. It recognizes all Lutheran-positive cells and is only nonreactive with other Lu(a−b−) cells. This antibody is usually IgG or IgA and could be quite capable of destroying incompatible red cells.

INHERITANCE AND BIOSYNTHESIS

Very little is known about the genetics of this system, although much has been postulated. It has been determined that Lutheran genes are *linked* to the gene controlling secretor status.[86] The location of the Lutheran genes is not known. As are most other blood group genes, Lutheran genes are inherited in a codominant fashion, that is, if inherited, the antigen will be expressed on the red cell. The exception to this is the Lutheran null phenotype.

There are two types of Lu(a−b−) that have been described. These have been designated as either "dominant" or "recessive" according to the mode of inheritance. These differ in several respects and are only distinguishable by using special techniques and family studies.

The recessive Lutheran null results from homozygous inheritance of the silent Lu allele. This amorphic gene results in no antigen production, and the individual subsequently lacks all Lutheran antigens. This individual, upon transfusion or pregnancy, is capable of forming anti-Lu3 as well as any other Lutheran system antibody.

Dominant Lutheran null individuals are unique. They inherit a gene that has been named InLu (for Lutheran inhibitor). This is an extremely rare and dominant gene; only one needs to be inherited in order for its effects to be demonstrated. This InLu gene is a *suppressor* that prevents normal Lutheran antigen synthesis. In other words, even in the presence of normal Lu^a and Lu^b genes, the individual's phenotype is Lu(a−b−). Adsorption and elution techniques have demonstrated traces of

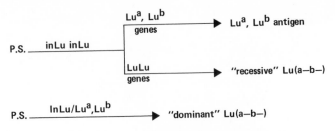

FIGURE 8-7. A proposed mechanism for the inheritance and formation of Lutheran types.

the Lutheran antigens on these cells, but the antigens are undetectable by routine methods. These individuals will not produce anti-Lu3 because they do possess traces of Lutheran antigen on their cells.[18] InLu also suppresses P_1, i, and Au^a antigen production.[16]

Figure 8-7, modified from Issitt and Issitt's *Applied Blood Group Serology*,[15] demonstrates a proposed inheritance scheme. There is no information regarding the production of these antigens, however, so this scheme must be regarded as a *possible* model.

REFERENCES

1. LANDSTEINER, K and LEVINE, P: *Further observations on individual differences of human blood.* Proc Soc Exp Biol Med 24:941, 1927.
2. WALSH, RJ and MONTGOMERY, C: *A new human isoagglutinin subdividing the MN blood groups.* Nature 160:504, 1947.
3. LEVINE, P, et al.: *A new blood factor, s, allelic to S.* Proc Soc Exp Biol Med 78:218, 1951.
4. WIENER, AS, UNGER, LJ and GORDON, EB: *Fatal hemolytic transfusion reaction caused by sensitization to a new blood factor U.* J Am Med Soc 153:1444, 1953.
5. GREENWALT, TJ, et al.: *An allele of the S(s) blood group genes.* Proc Natl Acad Sci 40:1126, 1954.
6. TOMITA, M and MARCHESI, VT: *Amino acid sequence and oligosaccharide attachment of human erythrocyte glycophorin.* Proc Natl Acad Sci USA 72:2964, 1975.
7. WASNIOWSKA, K, DRZENIEK, Z and LISOWSKA, E: *The amino acids of M and N blood groups are different.* Biochem Biophys Res Comm 76:385, 1977.
8. FURTHMAYR, H: *Structural comparison of glycophorins and immunochemical analysis of genetic variants.* Nature 271:519, 1978.
9. JUDD, WJ, ISSITT, PD and PAVONE, BG: *The Can serum: Demonstrating further polymorphism of M and N blood group antigens.* Transfusion 19:7, 1979.
10. DAHR, W, ISSITT, PD, MOULDS, J, et al.: *Further studies on the membrane glycoprotein defects of S−, s− and En(a−) erythrocytes.* Hoppe Seylers Z Physiol Chem 359:1217, 1978.
11. STOLTZ, JF, STREIFF, F and GENETET, B: *Demonstration of M antigen on human lymphocytes by liquid phase electrophoresis.* Vox Sang 26:467, 1974.
12. MARSH, WL, ØYEN, R, NICHOLS, ME, et al.: *Studies of MNSsU antigen activity on leukocytes and platelets.* Transfusion 14:462, 1974.
13. NAIKI, M and MARCUS, DM: *Human erythrocyte P and P^k blood group antigens: Identification as glycosphingolipids.* Biochem Biophys Res Commun 60:3, 1974.
14. GRAHAM, H: *An overview of the biochemistry of the Lewis, ABH and P systems.* In *A Seminar on Antigens on Blood Cells and Body Fluids,* 33rd Annual Meeting of the American Association of Blood Banks, 1980.

15. Issitt, PD and Issitt, CH: *Applied Blood Group Serology*. Spectra Biologicals, Division of Becton Dickinson Company, Oxnard, California, 1976.

16. Crawford, MN, Tippett, P and Sanger, R: *Antigens Au^a, i, and P$_1$ of cells of the dominant type of Lu(a−b−)*. Vox Sang 26:283, 1974.

17. Marcus, DM and Kundu, S: *Immunochemistry of the P blood group system*. In Sandler, G and Nusbacher, J (eds): *Immunobiology of the Erythrocyte, Progress in Clinical and Biological Research*. Alan R. Liss, Inc., New York, 1980.

18. Mollison, PL: *Blood Transfusion in Clinical Medicine*. Blackwell Scientific Publications, Oxford, 1979.

19. Schwarting, GA, Marcus, DM and Metaxas, M: *Identification of sialosylparagloboside as the erythrocyte receptor for an anti-p antibody*. Vox Sang 32:257, 1977.

20. Issitt, CH, et al.: *Another example of an antibody reacting optimally with p red cells*. Br J Haematol 34:19, 1976.

21. Engelfriet, CP, et al.: *Haemolysins probably recognizing the antigen p*. Vox Sang 23:176, 1972.

22. Metaxas, MJ, Metaxas-Buehler, M and Tippett, P: *A "new" antibody in the P blood group system*. Communications of the 14th Congress of the International Society of Blood Transfusion, Helsinki, 1975.

23. Race, RR and Sanger, R: *Blood Groups in Man*. Blackwell Scientific Publications, Oxford, 1975.

24. Henningsen, K: *Investigations on the blood factor P*. Acta Pathol Microbiol Scand 26:639, 1949.

25. Cronin, CA, Pohl, BA and Miller, WV: *Crossmatch compatible blood for patients with anti-P$_1$*. Transfusion 18:728, 1978.

26. Levine, P: *Comments on hemolytic disease of newborn due to anti-PP$_1$P^k (anti-Tj^a)*. Transfusion 17:573, 1977.

27. Moureau, P: *Les reactions post-transfusionnelles*. Rev Belge Sci Med 16:258, 1945.

28. Wiener, AS and Unger, LJ: *Isoimmunization to factor P by blood transfusion*. Am J Clin Pathol 14:616, 1944.

29. Furukawa, K, et al.: *Examples of blood groups P and P^k in Japanese families*. Jpn J Hum Gen 12:137, 1974.

30. Yamaguchi, H, et al.: *Rare blood type p and p^k in Japanese families*. Proc Jpn Acad 50:764, 1974.

31. Levine, P and Koch, E: *The rare human isoagglutinin, anti-Tj^a, and habitual abortion*. Science 120:239, 1954.

32. Levene, C, et al.: *Hemolytic disease of the newborn due to anti-PP$_1$Pk (anti-Tj^a)*. Transfusion 17:569, 1977.

33. Cameron, GL and Staveley, JM: *Blood group P substance in hydatid cyst fluids*. Nature 179:145, 1957.

34. Effler, D, Roland, F and Redding, RA: *The P blood group system in pigeon breeders and pigeon breeders' disease*. Chest 70:719, 1976.

35. Cooper, EL, Lemmi, CAE and Moore, TC: *Agglutinins and cellular immunity in earthworms*. In *Biomedical Perspectives of Agglutinins of Invertebrate and Plant Origins*. Ann NY Acad Sci 234:34, 1974.

36. Wiener, AS, et al.: *Type-specific cold auto-antibodies as a cause of acquired hemolytic anemia and hemolytic transfusion reactions: Biologic test with bovine red cells*. Ann Intern Med 44:221, 1956.

37. Ginsburg, V, McGinnis, MH and Zopf, DA: *Biochemical basis for some blood groups*. In Sandler, G and Nusbacher, J (eds): *Immunobiology of the Erythrocyte, Progress in Clinical and Biological Research, Vol 43*. Alan R. Liss, Inc., New York, 1980.

38. Moores, PP, et al.: *Some observations on "Bombay" bloods with comments on evidence for the existence of two different O$_h$ phenotypes*. Transfusion 15:237, 1975.

39. Beattie, KM: *Perspectives on some usual and unusual ABO phenotypes*. In *A Seminar on Antigens on Blood Cells and Body Fluids*, 33rd Annual Meeting of the American Association of Blood Banks, 1980.

40. Kóscielak, J: *Chemistry and biosynthesis of erythrocytic membrane glycolipids with A, B, H and I blood group activities*. In Mohn, JF, et al. (eds): *Human Blood Groups*. Karger, Basel, 1977.

41. PIERCE, SR: *A review of erythrocyte antigens shared with leukocytes.* In *A Seminar on Antigens on Blood Cells and Body Fluids,* 33rd Annual Meeting of the American Association of Blood Banks, 1980.

42. FEIZI, T, et al.: *Immunochemical studies on blood groups. XLVII. The I antigen complex-precursors in the A, B, H, Le^a, and Le^b blood group system—hemagglutination inhibition studies.* J Exp Med 133:39, 1971.

43. GIBLETT, ER and CROOKSTON, M: *Agglutinability of red cells by anti-I in patients with thalassemia major and other hematological disorders.* Nature 201:1138, 1964.

44. HILLMAN, RS and GIBLETT, ER: *Red cell membrane alteration associated with "marrow stress."* J Clin Invest 44:1730, 1965.

45. LALEZARI, P and MURPHY, GB: *Cold-reacting leukocyte agglutinins and their significance.* In Curtoni, ES, Mattiuz, PL and Tosi, RM (eds): *Histocompatibility Testing.* Munksgaard, Copenhagen.

46. JENKINS, WJ, KOSTER, HG, MARSH, WL, et al.: *Infectious mononucleosis: An unsuspected source of anti-i.* Br J Haematol 11:480, 1965.

47. ROSENFIELD, RE, SCHMIDT, PJ, CALVO, RC, et al.: *Anti-i, a frequent cold agglutinin in infectious mononucleosis,* Vox Sang 10:631, 1965.

48. HOROWITZ, CA, MOULDS, J, HENLE, W, et al.: *Cold agglutinins in infectious mononucleosis and heterophile-antibody-negative mononucleosis-like syndromes.* Blood 50:195, 1977.

49. BERLIN, BS, CHANDLER, R and GREEN, D: *Anti-"i" antibody and hemolytic anemia associated with spontaneous cytomegalovirus mononucleosis.* Am J Clin Pathol 67:459, 1977.

50. COOMBS, RRA, MOURANT, AE and RACE, RR: *In vivo iso-sensitization of red cells in babies with haemolytic disease.* Lancet i:264, 1946.

51. LEVINE, P, et al.: *A new human hereditary blood property (Cellano) present in 99.8 percent of all bloods.* Science 109:464, 1949.

52. ALLEN, FH and LEWIS, SJ: *Kp^a (Penney), a new antigen in the Kell blood group system.* Vox Sang 2:81, 1957.

53. ALLEN, FH, LEWIS, SJ and FUDENBERG, H: *Studies of anti-Kp^b, a new antibody in the Kell blood group system.* Vox Sang 3:1, 1958.

54. GIBLETT, ER: *Js, a "new" blood group antigen found in Negroes.* Nature 181:1221, 1958.

55. WALKER, RA, et al.: *Js^b of the Sutter blood group system.* Transfusion 3:94, 1963.

56. MORTON, NE, et al.: *Genetic evidence confirming the localization of Sutter in the Kell blood group system.* Vox Sang 10:608, 1965.

57. MARSH, WL: *The Kell blood groups and their relationship to chronic granulomatous disease.* In *Cellular Antigens and Disease,* 30th Annual Meeting of the American Association of Blood Banks, 1977.

58. MARSH, WL, et al.: *Naturally occurring anti-Kell stimulated by E. coli enterocolitis in a 20-day-old child.* Transfusion 18:149, 1978.

59. MARSH, WL, et al.: *Kx antigen of the Kell system and its relationship to chronic granulomatous disease: Evidence that the gene is X-linked.* Transfusion 15:527, 1975.

60. CHOWN, B, LEWIS, M and KAITA, H: *A "new" Kell blood group phenotype.* Nature 180:711, 1957.

61. CONNEALLY, PM, et al.: *Linkage relations of the loci for Kell and phenylthiocarbamide.* Hum Hered 26:267, 1976.

62. MARSH, WL: *Recent developments relating to the Duffy and Lutheran blood groups.* In *A Seminar on Recent Advances in Immunohematology,* 26th Annual Meeting of the American Association of Blood Banks, 1973.

63. CHOWN, B: *XIIIth John G. Gibson II Lecture.* Published by Columbia-Presbyterian Medical Center, College of Physicians and Surgeons, New York, 1964.

64. TASWELL, HF, PINEDA, AA and MOORE, SB: *Hemolytic transfusion reactions: Frequency and clinical and laboratory aspects.* In *A Seminar on Immune-Mediated Cell Destruction,* 34th Annual Meeting of the American Association of Blood Banks, 1981.

65. WIMER, BM, et al.: *Haematological changes associated with the McLeod phenotype of the Kell blood group system.* Br J Haematol 36:219, 1977.

66. BRIDGES, RA, BERENDES, H and GOOD, RA: *A fatal granulomatous disease of childhood.* Am J Dis Child 97:387, 1959.

MODERN BLOOD BANKING AND TRANSFUSION PRACTICES

67. MARSH, WL, URETSKY, SC and DOUGLAS, SD: *Antigens of the Kell blood group system on neutrophils and monocytes: Their relation to chronic granulomatous disease.* J Pediatr 87:1117, 1975.

68. SEGAL, AW and PETERS, TJ: *Characterization of the enzyme defect in chronic granulomatous disease.* Lancet i:1363, 1976.

69. KLEBANOFF, SJ and WHITE, LR: *Iodination defect in the leukocytes of a patient with chronic granulomatous disease of childhood.* N Engl J Med 280:460, 1969.

70. CUTBUSH, M, MOLLISON, PL and PARKIN, DM: *A new human blood group.* Nature 165:188, 1950.

71. IKIN, EW, et al.: *Discovery of the expected hemagglutinin, anti-Fy^b.* Nature 168:1077, 1951.

72. CHOWN, B, LEWIS, M and KAITA, H: *The Duffy blood group in Caucasians: Evidence for a new allele.* Am J Hum Gen 17:384, 1965.

73. ALBREY, JA, et al.: *A new antibody, anti-Fy^3, in the Duffy blood group system.* Vox Sang 20:29, 1971.

74. BEZHAD, O, et al.: *A new anti-erythrocyte antibody in the Duffy system: Anti-Fy4.* Vox Sang 24:337, 1973.

75. COLLEDGE, K, PEZZULICH, M and MARSH, WL: *Anti-Fy5, an antibody disclosing a probable association between the Rhesus and Duffy blood group genes.* Vox Sang 24:193, 1973.

76. MILLER, LH, et al.: *Erythrocyte receptors for (Plasmodium knowlesi) malaria: The Duffy blood group determinants.* Science 189:561, 1975.

77. ALLEN, FH Jr, DIAMOND, LK and NIEDZIELA, B: *A new blood group antigen.* Nature 167:482, 1951.

78. PLANT, G, et al.: *A new blood group antibody, anti-Jk^b.* Nature 171:431, 1953.

79. PINKERTON, FJ, et al.: *The phenotype Jk(a−b−) in the Kidd blood group system.* Vox Sang 4:155, 1959.

80. MARSH, WL, ØYEN, R and NICHOLS, ME: *Kidd blood group antigens of leukocytes and platelets.* Transfusion 14:378, 1974.

81. CALLENDER, ST and RACE, RR: *A serological and genetical study of multiple antibodies formed in response to blood transfusion by a patient with lupus erythematosus diffusus.* Annals of Eugenics (Cambridge) 13:102, 1946.

82. CUTBUSH, M and CHANARIN, I: *The expected blood-group antibody, anti-Lu^b.* Nature 178:855, 1956.

83. GREENWALT, TJ and SASAKI, T: *The Lutheran blood groups: A second example of anti-Lu^b and three further examples of anti-Lu^a.* Blood 12:998, 1957.

84. CUTBUSH, M and MOLLISON, PL: *Relation between characteristics of blood group antibodies in vitro and associated patterns of red cell destruction in vivo.* Br J Haematol 4:115, 1958.

85. SCHEFFER, H and TAMAKI, HT: *Anti-Lu^b and mild hemolytic disease of the newborn: A case report.* Transfusion 6:497, 1966.

86. MOHR, J: *A search for linkage between the Lutheran blood group and other hereditary characters.* Acta Pathol Microbiol Scand 28:207, 1951.

BIBLIOGRAPHY

ALLEN, FH and ROSENFIELD, RE: *Notation for the Kell blood groups.* Transfusion 1:305, 1961.

ANSTEE, DJ: *Blood-group MNSs-active sialoglycoproteins of the human erythrocyte membrane.* In Sandler, G and Nusbacher, J (eds), *Immunobiology of the Erythrocyte, Progress in Clinical and Biological Research.* Alan R. Liss, Inc., New York, 1980.

BEATTIE, K and ZUELZER, WW: *The frequency and properties of pH-dependent anti-M.* Transfusion 8:254, 1965.

CRAWFORD, MN, et al.: *The phenotype Lu(a−b−) together with unconventional Kidd groups in one family.* Transfusion 1:228, 1961.

DARNBOROUGH, J, et al.: *A "new" antibody, anti-Lu^{a}Lu^b, and two further examples of the genotype Lu(a−b−).* Nature 198:796, 1963.

Greenwalt, TJ, Sasaki, T and Steane, EA: *The Lutheran blood groups: A progress report with observations on the development of the antigens and characteristics of the antibodies.* Transfusion 7:189, 1967.

Judd, WJ, et al.: *Antibodies that define NANA-independent MN system antigens.* Transfusion 19:12, 1979.

Marsh, WL: *The Kell blood group.* In *Advances in Immunohematology, Vol 4.* Spectra Biologicals, Division of Becton Dickinson Company, Oxnard, California, 1976.

Marsh, WL, et al.: *Chronic granulomatous disease and the Kell blood groups.* Br J Haematol 29:247, 1975.

McGinnis, MH and Miller, LH: *Malaria, erythrocyte receptors and the Duffy blood group system.* In *Cellular Antigens and Disease,* 30th Annual Meeting of the American Association of Blood Banks, 1977.

Mourant, AE, Kopec, AC and Domaniewska-Sobczak, K: *The Distribution of the Human Blood Groups and Other Biochemical Polymorphisms.* Oxford University Press, Oxford, 1976.

Shreffler, DC, et al.: *Studies on genetic selection in a completely ascertained U.S. Caucasian population. I. Frequencies, age and sex effects and phenotype association for 12 blood group systems. Tecumseh, Michigan: Population: 10,000 West European ancestry.* Am J Hum Genet, 1971.

White, WL, Miller, GE and Kaehry, WD: *Formaldehyde in the pathogenesis of hemodialysis-related anti-N antibodies.* Transfusion 17:443, 1977.

Young, MD, et al.: *Experimental testing of the immunity of Negroes to Plasmodium vivax.* J Parasitol 41:315, 1955.

CHAPTER 9

MISCELLANEOUS
BLOOD GROUP SYSTEMS

DENISE HARMENING PITTIGLIO, PH.D., MT(ASCP)

In the category of miscellaneous blood groups, some 300 blood group antigens have been described that may or may not represent independent blood group systems. In light of this, it would be quite ludicrous to try to present all these miscellaneous antigens. As a result only the more commonly studied blood group systems will be briefly presented, dependent on the information currently available. All the other antigens will be grouped into various categories or headings for simplicity.

THE SEX-LINKED BLOOD GROUP SYSTEM: Xg^a

The Xg^a blood group was discovered in 1962.[1] It is unique in that it is believed to be the only blood group antigen produced under the control of a gene located on the X chromosome. Many family studies have confirmed that the inheritance of Xg^a occurs on a sex-linked basis: therefore, a difference in the frequency of the Xg^a antigen is noted between the sexes. Approximately 89 percent of females are Xg(a+), while 66 percent of males are Xg(a+).[2]

Several examples of anti-Xg^a have been described. Most of these antibodies are only reactive in the antihuman globulin phase of in vitro testing and appear to be IgG immunoglobulins. The majority of Xg^a antibodies possess the ability to bind complement, but have not been demonstrated to produce in vitro hemolysis. Most Xg^a antibodies are the result of red cell stimulation, but have not been implicated in transfusion reactions or hemolytic disease of the newborn. Therefore, Xg^a antigen does not appear to be an efficient immunogen.

THE WRIGHT BLOOD GROUP SYSTEM: Wr^a AND Wr^b

The Wright blood group system was discovered in 1953 and is composed of two allelic antigens: Wr^a, a low frequency antigen occurring in less than 0.1 percent of the random population, and Wr^b, a high-incidence antigen occurring in 99.9 percent of the random population.

Although the antigen Wr^a is extremely rare, the antibody anti-Wr^a has been reported quite frequently. Two types of Wr^a antibody exist. The first is an IgM antibody that is naturally occurring. It is frequently found in the serum of individuals who have never been pregnant nor transfused. The second type is an IgG antibody that is only reactive in the antihuman globulin phase of in vitro testing. The IgG anti-Wr^a is a red cell stimulated antibody that has been reported to cause moderately severe hemolytic disease of the newborn as well as severe transfusion reactions.

Anti-Wr^a is also commonly found in the sera of patients suffering from autoimmune hemolytic anemia. The serum of one in every two or three patients studied with autoimmune hemolytic anemia contains anti-Wr^a.

The Wr^a antigen is rare and has only been detected in the white population and has not been reported in the black race. Only one example of an antibody that appeared to have anti-Wr^b specificity has been described.[4]

THE CARTWRIGHT BLOOD GROUP SYSTEM: Yt^a AND Yt^b

The Cartwright blood group system was discovered in 1956.[5] It is believed to be composed of two antigens: Yt^a, a high-frequency antigen occurring in 99.7 percent of the random white population, and Yt^b, a low-frequency antigen occurring in 8 percent of the random white population. Three phenotypes have been described, with virtually the same frequencies in both the white and the black populations: $Yt(a+b-)$ occurs at 91.9 percent; $Yt(a+b+)$ occurs at 7.8 percent; and $Yt(a-b+)$ occurs at 0.3 percent. The phenotype $Yt(a-b-)$ has not been reported.[6]

The Yt^a antigen is poorly developed at birth and, therefore, cord bloods are usually Yt^a negative. However, the Yt^a antigen is an efficient immunogen, and, consequently, the antibody anti-Yt^a is not that uncommon in spite of the rare $Yt(a-b+)$ phenotype.[7]

The Yt^b antigen appears to be a poor immunogen. Therefore, anti-Yt^b is rare and has only been reported in patients who have been transfused a great deal and have produced multiple antibodies.[8]

Both anti-Yt^a and anti-Yt^b are only reactive in the antihuman globulin phase of in vitro testing and appear to be IgG immunoglobulins. These antibodies are usually red cell stimulated and have not been implicated in hemolytic disease of the newborn.

THE DIEGO BLOOD GROUP SYSTEM: Di^a AND Di^b

The Diego blood group system was discovered in 1955 when the antibody to the Di^a antigen was described. Di^b was described in 1967 when the antibody anti-Di^b was reported. The Di^a antigen is extremely rare in the white population, but more frequent in individuals of Mongolian background. The Di^a antigen is therefore useful as a genetic marker for mongolian derivation and is significant in anthropologic studies. South, Central, and North American Indians have been shown to have a high incidence of Di^a. In the Chinese people, Di^a is found in 2 to 5 percent of the population. In the Japanese people, Di^a is found in 3 to 12 percent of the population. Di^b is a high-frequency antigen in whites. Both Di^a and Di^b are only reactive in the antihuman globulin phase of in vitro testing and appear to be IgG immunoglobulins. Although both antibodies have been implicated in causing hemolytic disease of the newborn, anti-Di^b has only been reported to cause mild forms of the disease. Both anti-Di^a and anti-Di^b are usually red cell stimulated.

THE SCIANNA BLOOD GROUP SYSTEM: Sm(Sc:1) AND Bu^a(Sc:2)

In 1962 the antibody to the Sm antigen was reported. In 1963 an antibody to the Bu^a antigen was described; however, the investigators were not aware that this was an allele to Sm. As a result, the original names tend to remain, since both antibodies were already named in the literature before it was realized that these were detecting antithetical antigens. Sm(Sc:1) is a high-incidence antigen in whites, occurring in approximately 100 percent of the population. Bu^a(Sc:2) is a low-incidence antigen, occurring in less than 1 percent of the random population, and has not been found in the black race.[9] Both anti-Sc1 and anti-Sc2 are rare antibodies. Most anti-Sm antibodies are red cell stimulated and react only in the antihuman globulin phase of in vitro testing. Some anti-Bu^a antibodies react in the saline phase and are naturally occurring, while others only react in the antihuman globulin phase and are red cell stimulated. Neither anti-Sm nor anti-Bu^a has been implicated in hemolytic disease of the newborn or in transfusion reactions.

THE DOMBROCK BLOOD GROUP SYSTEM: Do^a AND Do^b

The Dombrock blood group system was discovered in 1965 when the antibody to the Do^a antigen was described.[10] Do^b was defined in 1973 when the antibody anti-Do^b was reported.[11] The Do^a antigen can be found in 67 percent of the white population; however, it appears to have a lower incidence in the black race as well as in the population of American Indians. Do^b antigen can be found in approximately 83 percent of the white population. Three phenotypes have been described in the Dombrock system with the followng approximate frequencies: Do(a+b−) occurs at 17.2 percent; Do(a+b+) occurs at 49.5 percent; and Do(a−b+) occurs at 33.3 percent. The phenotype Do(a−b−) has not been reported.

Both anti-Do^a and anti-Do^b are only reactive in the antihuman globulin phase of in vitro testing and appear to be IgG immunoglobulins. These antibodies are usually red cell stimulated and their reactivity appears to be enchanced when enzyme-treated red cells are utilized. Anti-Do^a has been implicated in a mild case of hemolytic disease of the newborn. Neither anti-Do^a nor anti-Do^b has been implicated in transfusion reactions. The occurrence of these antibodies is very infrequent. Both anti-Do^a and anti-Do^b have been shown to demonstrate "dosage."

THE COLTON BLOOD GROUP SYSTEM: Co^a AND Co^b

The Colton blood group system was discovered in 1967 when the antibody to the Co^a antigen was described.[12] Co^b was defined in 1970 when the antibody anti-Co^b was reported.[13] Co^a is a high-frequency antigen occurring in 99.7 percent of the random white population. Co^b can be found in 9.7 percent of the random white population. Three phenotypes have been described in the Colton system with the following approximate frequencies: Co(a+b−) occurs at 90.3 percent; Co(a+b+) occurs at 9.4 percent; and Co(a−b+) occurs at 0.3 percent. The phenotype Co(a−b−) has been described in two patients with monosomy-7.[14] Although they are rarely found, both anti-Co^a and anti-Co^b are usually red cell stimulated. Some of these antibodies are only reactive in the antihuman globulin phase of in vitro testing, while others only react with enzyme-treated red cells. Both anti-Co^a and anti-Co^b appear to be IgG immunoglobulins. Anti-Co^a has been implicated in a mild case of hemolytic disease of the newborn and has been suspected in causing transfusion reactions.

TABLE 9-1. High-Titered Low-Avidity Antibodies (HTLA)* and Human Leukocyte Antigen (HLA) Related Systems

Antigen	Blood Group System or Nomenclature	Approximate Percentage of Population Positive	General Characteristics
Yk^a†	York	92	White cell determinants expressed on RBCs and in plasma
Cs^a†	Cost-Sterling	98	
Kn^a†	Knops	99	white cell determinants expressed on RBCs and in plasma
McC^a†	McCoy	>99	Antibody found more often in whites / Antibody found more often in blacks
Ch^a	Chido	98	Determinants on the C4d fragment present in plasma which is coded for by the HLA locus / Demonstrated to be "high-titer low-avidity" antibodies; Ch^a and Rg^a (C4) adsorb onto red cell membrane
Rg^a	Rogers	98	
Bg^a	Originally called DBG (Donna, Bennett, Goodspeed antigen)		Correlation with HLA has been demonstrated / HLA-B7 = Bg^a / HLA-Bw17 = Bg^b / HLA-A28 = Bg^c / Therefore these anti-HLA and anti-Bg antibodies are synonymous
Bg^b	Ho antigen		
Bg^c	Ot antigen		
	Also grouped together as the Bg antigens		

*Holley (Hy) and Gregory (Gy^a) have been placed in the HTLA category by some immunohematologists.
†Demonstrated to be "high-titer low-avidity" antibodies.

TABLE 9-2. High-Incidence Antigens

Antigen	Blood Group System or Nomenclature	General Characteristics	Approximate Percentage of Population Positive
Vel:1 Vel:2	Vel	Antibodies are usually IgM, complement binding, some IgG, usually red cell stimulated, HDN not reported, Vel antigens not well developed at birth	100
Gy^a Hy	Gregory Holley	Antibody usually IgG, AHG reactive only, red cell stimulated, implicated in transfusion reactions, antigens not well developed at birth, HDN not reported	100
Sd^a	Sid	Soluble antigen found in saliva and urine of Sd(a+) individuals; the amount of Sd^a present on red cells varies greatly from person to person; rare "super-Sid" or Sd(a++) red cells exist, which possess a high concentration of Sd^a antigen and have been termed "Cad;" the Cad or super-Sid red cell characteristic is the only known form of inherited polyagglutination (see Chapter 21); antibody is usually IgM, complement binding, few are IgG; most antibodies are "naturally occurring;" almost all adult serum contains anti-Cad or anti-Sd(a++); rarely implicated in transfusion reactions; HDN not reported; agglutination pattern is unique and shows a very refractile mixed-field clumping with tight agglutinates in a sea of free cells; antibody neutralizable with fresh urine	96
Ge:1 Ge:2 Ge:3	Gerbich	Most antibodies are IgG, a few are IgM, some are red cell stimulated, others are "naturally occurring," antibodies have been implicated in causing a mild HDN	100
En^a	En^a antigen	Antibody is usually IgG reacting in all phases of in vitro testing, most are red cell stimulated, antibody has been implicated in transfusion reactions, suspected in causing HDN, En^a-negative individual's red cells have reduced sialic acid as well as reduced or depressed M and N antigens	100
Lan	Langereis	Antibody is usually IgG, most reactive in only AHG phase, some reactive in both albumin and AHG phases, most are red cell stimulated and have been implicated in causing transfusion reactions, implicated in causing a mild HDN	100
Pr(Sp)	Pr(Sp) antigen	Antibodies are usually IgM, some are IgA, some are IgG, most are "naturally occurring" antibodies, Pr(sp) antigens are destroyed by enzyme treatment, most antibodies present as high-titered cold autoagglutinins (see Chapter 19)	100

THE AUBERGER BLOOD GROUP SYSTEM: Au^a

In 1961 the Au[a] antigen was described.[15] Approximately 82 percent of all Europeans are Au(a+); American frequencies have not been well established. The Auberger antigen is well developed at birth and its expression is not only dependent on the Au[a] gene but also on the inheritance of the Lutheran genes (see Chapter 8). It appears that the inheritance of the Lutheran In(Lu) gene is responsible for the dominant Lu(a−b−) phenotype and also suppresses the expression of the Au[a] antigen. The anti-Au[a] antibodies are rare and appear to react only in the antihuman globulin phase of in vitro testing.

MISCELLANEOUS ANTIGENS

For simplicity some of the other miscellaneous antigens are listed in Tables 9-1 and 9-2. Numerous other antigens have been described in the category of high-incidence antigens found in Table 9-2. The inquisitive student should refer to other texts, such as *Applied Blood Group Serology* by Issitt and Issitt[6] and *Blood Groups in Man* by Race and Sanger,[2] for further discussion. The low-incidence antigens are also discussed in these texts.

REFERENCES

1. MANN, J, et al.: *A sex-linked blood group.* Lancet i:8, 1962.
2. RACE, RR and SANGER, R: *Blood Groups in Man,* ed 5. FA Davis, Philadelphia, 1968.
3. HOLMAN, C: *A new rare human blood group antigen (Wr^a).* Lancet ii:119, 1953.
4. ADAMS, J, et al.: *An antibody in the serum of a Wr(a−) individual, reacting with an antigen of very high frequency.* Transfusion 11:290, 1971.
5. EATON, BR, et al.: *A new antibody, anti-Yt^a, characterizing a blood group antigen of high incidence.* Br J Haematol 2:333, 1956.
6. ISSITT, P and ISSITT, C: *Applied Blood Group Serology.* Spectra Biologicals, Oxnard, California, 1976, pp. 216–218.
7. GILES, CM, BEVAN, B and HUGHES, RM: *A family showing independent segregation of Bu^a and Yt^b.* Vox Sang 18:265, 1970.
8. BETTIGOLE, R et al.: *Rapid in vivo destruction of Yt(a+) red cells in a patient with anti-Yt^a.* Vox Sang 14:143, 1968.
9. LEWIS, M, KAITA, H and CHOWN, B: *Scianna blood group system.* Vox Sang 27:261, 1974.
10. SWANSON, JL, et al: *A "new" blood group antigen, Do^a.* Nature 206:313, 1965.
11. MOLTHAN, L, et al.: *Enlargement of the Dombrock blood group system: The finding of anti-Do^b.* Vox Sang 24:382, 1973.
12. HEISTO, H, et al.: *Three examples of a red cell antibody, anti-Co^a.* Vox Sang 12:18, 1967.
13. GILES, CM, et al.: *Identification of the first example of anti-Co^b.* Br J Haematol 19:267, 1970.
14. DE LA CHAPELLE, A, et al.: *Monosomy-7 and the Colton blood groups.* Lancet ii:817, 1975.
15. SALMON, C, SALMON, D, LIBERGE, G, et al.: *Un nouvel antigène de group sanguine erythrocytaire présent chez 80% des sujets de race blanche.* Nouv Rev Franc Haematol 1:649, 1961.

CHAPTER 10

DONOR SELECTION AND COMPONENT PREPARATION

PATRICIA A. WRIGHT, MT(ASCP)SBB

WHOLE BLOOD DONOR SELECTION

For the purpose of insuring reasonable safety to the donor and subsequently to the recipient, the following guidelines or standards for the selection of blood donors have been established. With little exception, these guidelines have been adopted by all blood banks and transfusion services as the minimal required standards of practice.

REGISTRATION INFORMATION AND GENERAL REQUIREMENTS

According to the Code of Federal Regulations (CFR) 21 CFR 606.160, "Records shall be maintained concurrently with the performance of each significant step in the collection, processing, compatibility testing, storage, and distribution of each unit of blood and blood components so that all steps can be clearly traced."[1]

To insure that the donor can be "identified and recalled,"[2] information must be recorded on a registration or medical health/history form each time a donor presents himself for donation (Fig. 10-1). This information must be kept on file, generally in the blood bank, for no less than 5 years, and includes the following:

1. Date of donation.

2. Donor's name (first, last, and middle initial).

3. Address and phone number. If the donor has a job outside the home it is helpful to have both home and business addresses and phone numbers.

4. Sex.

5. Date of birth and/or age: Between 17 and 66 (up to the 66th birthday) is the accepted age range. There are two general exceptions: (a) Parental permission may be required of donors considered by law to be minors. Check individual state laws. (b) Donors beyond their 66th birthday require an evaluation and approval by the blood bank physician. Evidence of this evaluation must be made a part of the permanent donation record.

6. Donor consent: Donors must sign a statement giving the blood bank personnel permission to draw the unit and to use it as they deem necessary. This consent should be "informed." Donors should have the procedure explained and their

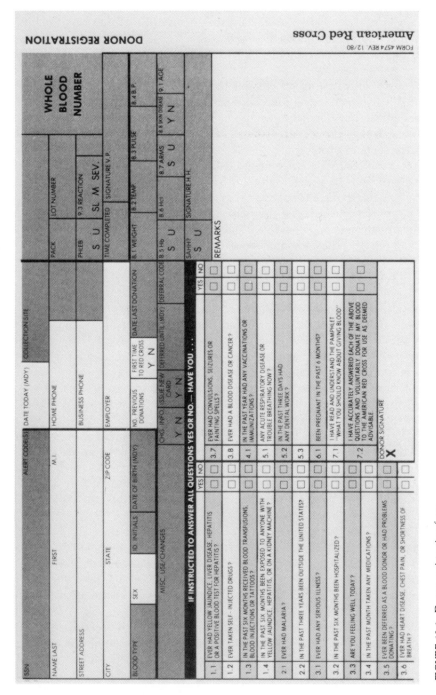

FIGURE 10-1. Donor registration form.

questions answered, and/or they should be given a pamphlet explaining the process, which they should be advised to read carefully.

Though not required by AABB standards, it may be useful to have the following additional information about the donor:

1. Additional identification: (a) Social Security number or (b) driver's license number.

2. Time of last meal: It is preferable that a donor not be fasting at the time of donation. If it has been longer than approximately 4 hours since the last meal, it is recommended that the donor be given something to eat and drink before donating.

3. Race: It may prove useful later to know the racial origin of the donor when screening for some phenotypes.

4. Intended recipient/replacement credit/donor group: Since blood donations are generally directed to a donor group or for a particular patient, it is important to obtain the patient/credit information, which will ensure proper crediting. Even if the donor is rejected or deferred, the information may still be useful or necessary. The following information should be obtained: (a) patient's name and hospital, (b) patient's identification/hospital number, and (c) donor group name.

PHYSICAL EXAMINATION

A brief physical examination is required. This examination must be done on the day of donation and generally is performed at the time of donation along with the medical history. The physical examination is primarily designed to ensure the donor's safety, to rule out or defer a donor whose physical condition is such that the donation of a unit of blood at this time could be detrimental.

The following guidelines are considered the "standard of practice":

1. General appearance: The donor should appear to be in general good health. If the donor shows signs of being under the influence of alcohol or drugs, appears to be extremely nervous, or has the symptoms of a cold, he should be deferred.

2. Skin lesions: The antecubital area of both arms is to be inspected for evidence of habitual drug use and for the presence of skin eruptions, such as poison ivy, rash, or psoriasis, which, if present in that area, are cause for deferment. The venipuncture site must be free of any lesions or infections in order to avoid possible contamination of the donor unit.

3. Weight: The donation of a unit of blood should not exceed approximately 10 percent of the donor's blood volume. This means that for the standard donation of 450 ± 45 ml plus a maximum of 30 ml in pilot tubes, the donor must weigh at least 110 lb (50 kg). Donors who weigh less than 110 lb can be drawn, provided the amount of blood drawn and the amount of anticoagulant used are proportionately reduced.

Standard blood bags contain a predetermined volume of anticoagulant which is calculated to effectively anticoagulate 450 ± 45 ml donor blood (refer to Chapter 1). As little as 405 ml of blood can be drawn into standard bags without requiring a change in the anticoagulant volume. This will generally accommodate donors who weigh from 100 to 110 lb. However, it is required that the amount of blood drawn be accurately determined. If the amount of blood to be withdrawn is less than 405 ml, the following formulas can be used.

(a) To calculate amount of blood to be drawn:

$$\frac{donor's\,wt}{110} \times 450 = amount\,allowable$$

Example. Donor's weight is 90 lb:

$$\frac{90}{110} \times 450 = 368.18\,ml\,allowable\,to\,draw$$
$$plus\,30\,ml\,for\,pilot\,tubes$$

(b) To calculate amount of anticoagulant to remove from primary bag when less than 405 ml of blood is collected:

$$63\,ml - \frac{donor's\,wt}{110} \times 63\,ml = amount\,to\,remove$$

Example. Donor's weight is 90 lb:

$$63\,ml - \left[\frac{90}{110} \times 63\right] = 11.45\,ml$$

4. Temperature: Not to exceed 37.5°C (99.6°F). NOTE: If using a regular glass thermometer, do not perform the finger or ear stick for hemoglobin/hematocrit procedure while the thermometer is in the donor's mouth. (The donor could involuntarily bite down and break the thermometer.)

5. Pulse: Between 50 and 100 with no irregularity. Pulse should be taken for at least 30 seconds, and if in doubt extend to 1 minute. Pulse rates that exceed these limits should be further evaluated to determine the donor's suitability. Increased pulse rates may be caused by such factors as anxiety, fear, or recent physical exercise. If the pulse rate exceeds 100 beats per minute, allow the donor to relax for 10 to 15 minutes, then repeat. Decreased pulse rates (below 50) may be normal for athletes or other persons who have a high tolerance to exercise. Irregularities must be evaluated by a qualified person (physician or a qualified designee).

6. Blood pressure: The systolic pressure should be from 90 to 180 mm Hg; the diastolic pressure from 50 to 100 mm Hg. Blood pressures outside these ranges or a pulse pressure (difference between systolic and diastolic pressure) less than 30 or more than 90 must be evaluated by the blood bank physician before the donor can be drawn.

7. Hemoglobin (Hgb)/Hematocrit (Hct): (a) Female—12.5 g per dl (38 percent Hct); (b) Male—13.5 g per dl (41 percent Hct). Although determination of either Hgb or Hct is acceptable, the preferred procedure is a hemoglobin determination.

The most widely used procedure for screening large numbers of donors is the copper sulfate method. This method uses the principle that when a drop of whole blood is dropped into a solution of $CuSO_4$, which has a given specific gravity, the drop will maintain its own density for approximately 15 seconds. The density of the drop is directly proportional to the amount of hemoglobin in that drop. If the drop is denser than the specific gravity of the solution, the drop sinks to the bottom; if not, it will float on top. The specific gravities of the $CuSO_4$ solutions, which correspond to the minimum hemoglobin levels for men and women, are 1.055 and 1.053, respectively. This is not a quantitative test; however, it is a quick, easy, and quite accurate technique to screen donors for possible anemia. If a donor fails this procedure or there is a question concerning the results, it is advisable to confirm the results with a microhematocrit.

Hemoglobin levels can also be determined using the spectrophotometric method. This method is very accurate but it is more expensive, harder to perform, and not suited to a large mobile operation.

MEDICAL HISTORY

The Code of Federal Regulations states "donor suitability...shall be determined... by means of a medical history, a test for hemoglobin level and...physical exam."[3] The medical history must be performed on the day of donation and is generally performed at the same time as the physical examination. One form is generally used for everything: registration, physical examination results, and the medical history (see Fig. 10-1). The interview should be conducted in a somewhat secluded place, which allows fewer distractions and permits privacy. The interviewer should be familiar with the questions in order to observe the donor during the medical review. It is helpful to be aware of the donor's body postures and facial expressions. Be ready to elaborate on a question if the donor seems not to understand it. Try to make the donor comfortable and ease the anxiety, particularly for first-time donors.

The questions should start with the more general areas and progress to the more specific. They should be designed to require "yes" or "no" answers that can be elaborated.

1. Have you ever been a blood donor before? If yes—when? Have you ever been rejected as a blood donor? If yes—why?

The time interval between whole blood donations is 8 weeks (56 days). Be sure to include the possibility of apheresis donations (plasma, platelets, leukocytes). The donor must wait 48 hours after an apheresis donation before donating whole blood.

Previous causes for rejection may alert the interviewer to problems requiring more in-depth questioning.

2. Have you ever had yellow jaundice, hepatitis, or liver disease? Ever had a positive blood test for hepatitis? Taken self-injected drugs? Within the last 6 months have you been in contact with someone who has hepatitis? Received a transfusion or injection of blood or blood products? Had a tattoo? (Ear piercing and acupuncture, if not performed by a physician, should require further questioning concerning procedure.) If the answer to any of these questions is yes, the donor should be further questioned as to when, where, and how.

All the above questions are considered "hepatitis" questions. They are included because the laboratory tests for the hepatitis agent are not 100 percent effective at eliminating units that are capable of transmitting hepatitis. The medical history can not completely eliminate the potential hazard either; however, the combination of the increased sensitivity of laboratory tests, the emphasis on the use of volunteer donors, and the medical history has caused a significant reduction in the incidence of transfusion-transmitted hepatitis.

Permanent rejection must be given if the donor

(a) Gives a history of viral hepatitis;

(b) Has had a positive test for hepatitis B surface antigen (HBsAg);

(c) Indicates present or past drug addiction (injectable);

(d) Was the donor of the only unit involved in a case of post-transfusion hepatitis.

A 6-month deferral must be given if the donor

(a) Has had "close" contact with someone who has hepatitis. "Close contact" is generally defined as sharing the same household, kitchen, and bathroom facilities. It also includes any person who is institutionalized (e.g., prison, psychiatric hospital, institution for the retarded). It does not routinely apply to hospital personnel performing normal duties, with the possible exception of dialysis personnel. Guidelines regarding the selection and deferment of these personnel must be defined by the blood bank physician.

(b) Has received a transfusion or injection of blood or blood products, a skin allograft, or a tattoo. Ear piercing and acupuncture may be included, depending upon the procedure used.

Donors who have received hepatitis B immune globulin (HBIG) are deferred for 12 months following injection.

3. Have you ever had malaria? Traveled outside the United States in the last 3 years? Are you a visitor or an immigrant from an area outside the United States? Have you been on anti-malarial therapy?

(a) Active malaria is cause for deferment, since malaria can be transmitted through the transfusion of red cell products.

(b) Donors who have had malaria are acceptable 3 years after cessation of therapy, provided they have remained asymptomatic. These same requirements must be met by visitors/immigrants from areas considered by the Center for Disease Control (CDC), Malaria Programs, to be endemic for malaria, and by persons who have been on prophylactic therapy.

(c) Travelers to endemic areas are deferred for 6 months after leaving the endemic area, provided they have remained asymptomatic and were not taking preventive medication.

(d) The malaria qualification can be exempted if the donation is for plasma products (free of intact red cells) only.

4. Have you ever had a serious illness? Been hospitalized, or had major surgery in the last 6 months?

A yes answer to any of these questions requires further investigation and evaluation. A person who has had major surgery should be deferred for 6 months following surgery to ensure that recovery is complete and because of the possibility of having received blood or blood products during surgery.

Prospective donors who have undergone minor surgery can be accepted once healing is complete. Although a determination of "major" and "minor" may have to be made by a physician, the following are generally accepted as "minor" procedures:

tonsillectomy, appendectomy, hemorrhoidectomy, closed reduction of a fracture, hernia repair, minor gynecologic procedures, varicose vein stripping, and removal of skin lesions.

5. Have you any history of heart, lung, liver, or kidney disease? Have you ever had chest pain? Suffered shortness of breath? Have you had tuberculosis?

(a) A history of cardiovascular disease or coronary or rheumatic heart disease will generally be cause for deferral, although some of these donors may be acceptable after evaluation by the blood bank physician.

(b) Active pulmonary tuberculosis is cause for deferral. Donors who have had tuberculosis that has been successfully treated and is now nonactive are acceptable.

(c) Donors with positive skin tests but no other indications of disease are acceptable.

(d) "A history of inflammatory or degenerative disease which could cause organ dysfunction"[4] is cause for deferral. Chronic conditions need to be evaluated by a physician.

6. Have you had any unexplained weight loss recently? How much? A recent weight loss that cannot be explained by diet or normal changes in eating or exercise habits could indicate an undiagnosed illness. It should be evaluated and further investigated.

7. Have you ever had any convulsions or seizures or been told you had epilepsy? Any history of fainting spells? Persons known to have epilepsy or seizures other than febrile convulsions in early childhood will generally be deferred for their own protection. The removal of a unit of blood could precipitate an attack. A statement of frequent fainting spells needs to be carefully checked because it may be the way a person describes seizures or may be a symptom of cardiovascular disease.

8. Have you ever had a blood disease? Cancer? History or evidence of cancer, leukemia, or lymphoma is generally cause for permanent deferral. There may be exceptions for some cancer if it is minor, and after evaluations are approved by the blood bank physician. There are no exceptions with leukemia and lymphomas.

9. Do you have a tendency to bleed a long time from a cut or after a tooth is pulled? Do you bruise easily or frequently for no apparent reason? These problems may indicate a clotting disorder. The prospective donor should be evaluated by the blood bank physician before being accepted.

10. Are you in general good health? How do you feel today? The prospective donor should be in general good health and free of any acute respiratory disease or infection. Donors who have active cold or flu symptoms are to be deferred until the symptoms are gone (CFR 640.3 [b] [4]). This question can be used as a "lead-off" question to help the donor relax or can be used in the middle to make sure the donor is paying attention to the questions. It is the only question requiring a "yes" answer.

11. Have you had a tooth extraction in the last 3 days? This has become an optional question (ARC, AABB, CFR). There may be some risk of "bacterial embolization"[5] following oral surgery. Some state laws may still require the question. Be sure to check local and state regulations.

12. Have you been pregnant in the last 6 weeks? A prospective donor is deferred for at least 6 weeks following a full-term delivery or termination of pregnancy

in the third trimester. An abortion (usually performed in the first trimester) is not of itself cause for deferral.

13. Are you currently taking or have you recently taken any drugs or medications? What? When? Why? A recent history of medication frequently indicates an underlying serious illness that could be cause for deferment or rejection. Any time a prospective donor gives an affirmative answer to this question, further investigation and evaluation is indicated. It is a good idea to have a list of drugs and medications (generic and brand names) that cause deferral or rejection available in the blood bank. Some of the fairly common medications that do not routinely disqualify a donor are oral contraceptives, mild analgesics, minor tranquilizers, psychic energizers, vitamins, diet pills, hormones, and marijuana (if the donor is not currently under the influence). Aspirin and aspirin-containing medications are acceptable provided the prospective donor is not being evaluated for a plateletpheresis procedure (aspirin causes a decrease in platelet function for up to 5 days).

14. Have you had any shots or immunizations within the last year? Most shots and immunizations are not cause for deferral as long as the donor is symptom free (this includes toxoids, killed virus, bacterial, or rickettsial vaccines).

The following are exceptions to this rule:

(a) Smallpox: acceptable after 2 weeks or the scab has fallen off.

(b) Measles (rubeola), rabies, mumps, oral polio (Sabin), yellow fever, animal serum products (attenuated virus vaccines): acceptable after 2 weeks.

(c) Rubella (German measles): acceptable after 4 weeks from last injection.

(d) HBIG: requires 1-year deferral.

APHERESIS DONOR SELECTION

The donor selection requirements for an apheresis donor are generally the same as for a whole blood donor. Under normal conditions, an apheresis donor must meet all the criteria for a whole blood donor. In addition, the following criteria are specific for the potential apheresis donor and need to be investigated before continuing with the procedure.

MEDICAL HISTORY

1. Has the donor had a history of donor reactions, particularly to previous apheresis procedures? Possible adverse reactions to the hydroxyethyl starch (HES), steroids, or heparin? Must be determined and carefully evaluated.

2. A history of bleeding problems and/or thrombocytopenia. May be critical if a procedure using heparin is to be performed. Defer women donors from heparin procedures during menses.

3. Allergies to beef or pork. They are generally the source of heparin.

4. Indication or history of fluid retention problems. This may be a significant problem if using HES and/or steroids in the apheresis procedure.

5. Underlying medical condition, which may be aggravated by steroids (e.g., hypertension, tuberculosis, diabetes mellitus).

6. Donors weight may be more critical because some procedures have larger volumes of blood outside the body (extracorporeal) during the procedure.

7. Medications: Any medication which might increase the donor's risk or decrease the effectiveness of the product—*most* particularly, aspirin (or aspirin-containing substances). Donor should be free of aspirin ingestion 2 to 5 days before platelet or leukapheresis.

PHYSICAL EXAMINATION AND LABORATORY TESTS

As with the medical history, under normal circumstances the apheresis donor must meet all the minimum physical examination requirements of a whole blood donor. Depending on which apheresis procedure is being used, the following additional laboratory tests must be performed before each donation:

(a) Hemoglobin/hematocrit

(b) Serum protein

(c) Platelet count (not less than 150,000 per microliter)

(d) White cell count and differential

(e) Partial thromboplastin time (PTT), if using heparin

In addition, the following should be performed after donation:

(a) Hemoglobin/hematocrit

(b) Platelet count

(c) White cell count

Protein electrophoresis should be performed every 4 months if the donor is a regular, biweekly plasma donor.

WHOLE BLOOD COLLECTION

Once the donor has been registered and has successfully passed the physical examination and medical history requirements, the next step is the actual collection of the donor unit. The following criteria must be met to be in compliance with the Code of Federal Regulations and/or AABB standards.

1. The personnel performing the phlebotomy procedure must be well trained and under the supervision of a "qualified, licensed physician."[6]

2. The blood must be drawn in an aseptic manner, using a sterile, closed system and a single venipuncture.

(a) The phlebotomy site on the donor's arm(s), usually the antecubital area, must be free of any skin lesions or rashes that could cause contamination of the unit or infection of the donor.

(b) The venipuncture site must be thoroughly cleaned and disinfected. Although sterilization is not possible, a surgical preparation is used to provide maximum protection. Table 10-1 lists two acceptable methods that are in use by most blood banks.

TABLE 10-1. Arm Preparation Methods

Method I

1. Scrub vigorously for 30 seconds using a 15% aqueous solution of soap ("green soap"). Scrub area should be an area of at least 2 × 2 inches around the intended venipuncture site. The scrub is designed to remove dirt, oils, and loose skin cells.

2. Remove the soap using an alcohol (70%) and acetone (10%) solution (9:1 ratio). Apply solution in a concentric spiral motion, starting in the center and moving outward. Do not go back toward the center. Allow to dry.

3. Apply a tincture of iodine solution (3% iodine in 70% alcohol). Use the same concentric motion as with the alcohol. Allow to dry.

4. Remove the iodine with alcohol and acetone solution as in step 2. The iodine should be removed; it is no longer needed in order to maintain the cleanliness of the area and, if left on, may cause skin irritation.

5. Site is ready for venipuncture. Cover with sterile gauze until ready for needle insertion.

Method II

1. Scrub the site (2 × 2 inches) for 30 seconds using an aqueous iodophor scrub solution (0.7%). Iodophor is a PVP-iodine or poloxamer iodine complex. Remove excess foam. Area need not be dry before proceeding.

2. Apply iodophor complex and let it stand for 30 seconds. Use the previously stated concentric motion when applying the solution. Removal of the iodophor solution is not necessary. The iodine is complexed and will generally not cause skin irritation.

3. Site is ready for venipuncture. Cover with a sterile gauze until ready for needle insertion.

3. Some system must be established that will uniquely and positively identify each donor unit, subsequent products prepared, the medical history/donor registration form, and all pilot tubes. The system may use numbers, letters, other symbols, or various combinations. However, it must provide a positive donor identification that is traceable. The numbers (ID system) must be applied to the bags, donor registration/medical history form, and pilot tubes *before* proceeding with the phlebotomy.

4. The following anticoagulants have been approved by the Food and Drug Administration (FDA) (see 21 CFR 640.4[d] and Chapter 1 for specific formulas).[7]

(a) Acid citrate dextrose (ACD)

(b) Heparin

(c) Citrate phosphate dextrose (CPD)

(d) Citrate phosphate dextrose adenine (CPDA-1)

5. According to the CFR the pilot samples to be used for donor processing must be firmly attached to the container prior to the phlebotomy. They must be filled at the time the donor unit is being drawn, usually immediately following the collection of the unit. The procedure must be performed by the individual who drew the unit. The AABB standards also note that samples to be used for compatibility testing must be prepared from the integral tubing in such a manner as to allow individual separation without contamination of the unit.

6. The following procedures should be followed in phlebotomy and pilot tube collection (*do not at any time during the phlebotomy procedure leave the donor unattended*).

(a) Make the donor comfortable. Confirm the donor's identification.

(b) Select and locate the desired vein. Marking may be necessary if the vein is deep and does not visually distend.

(c) Prepare the site and cover with a sterile gauze pad.

(d) Set up and check the bag and scale unless this was previously done.

(e) Place a clamp on the tubing between the needle and the primary bag.

(f) Give the donor something to squeeze. Instruct him to clench his fist several times and then hold a tight fist.

(g) Use a tourniquet or blood pressure cuff (maximum 60 mm Hg) to increase the distension of the vein.

(h) Perform venipuncture using the thumb of your free hand, placed below the prepared site and pulling the skin taut. With the needle at a 45 degree angle to the skin, make a quick, clean puncture. Once in the skin, reduce the angle of the needle to about 10 to 20 degrees, orient the line of the vein, and make a second push through the vein wall. Thread the needle up the vein about ½ inch to aid in securing the needle.

(i) Release the clamp on the tubing; check to make sure the flow is fairly rapid and steady.

(j) Tape the needle and tubing lightly to the arm. This will help prevent accidently pulling the needle out. Cover with a sterile gauze.

(k) Reduce the tourniquet/blood pressure cuff to approximately 40 mm Hg.

(l) Continue to monitor the donor for signs of a reaction. Continue to observe flow rate and periodically mix the blood to insure contact with the anticoagulant. Mixing is not required if vacuum equipment is being used.

(m) Remind the donor to stop squeezing.

(n) When the primary unit has tripped the preset scale, clamp off (or tie knot in) tubing. The volume/weight conversion for whole blood is 1.053 g/1.055 g. A unit of whole blood should weigh from 425 to 520 g plus the weight of the bag, anticoagulant, and the empty pilot tubes.

(o) Collect the pilot tubes before removing the needle from the donor's arm. The most convenient system is one with an inline needle; however, it is not mandatory.

(p) Release the tourniquet/blood pressure cuff.

(q) Permanently clamp/seal the donor tubing close to the needle.

(r) Remove the needle from the donor's arm, apply pressure to the site (over the gauze), and instruct the donor to raise his arm, elbow straight, and have him continue pressure over the site. Once the bleeding has stopped (approximately 2 minutes), have the donor lower his arm. Check for bleeding and place a bandage over the site.

(s) Strip the tubing to ensure that the blood is completely mixed with anticoagulant. Stripping forces the blood in the tubing toward and into the blood bag so it too can be mixed with anticoagulant. Allow the tubing to refill, being careful to avoid any bubbles. Separate the tubing into *segments* at approximately 3-inch intervals, making sure that the lot number is present on each segment. The seal between each segment should be clean and allow for easy separation. These segments are to be used for compatibility testing.

(t) Place the units in storage. All units except those that will be used for platelet production are to be stored at 1 to 6°C or placed into a container for transportation, which will gradually reduce the temperature toward 4°C. Those units destined for platelet production are to be stored at 20 to 24°C until the platelets have been removed.

7. Before allowing the donor to leave the area, instruct him in postphlebotomy care. The following are some examples of instructions that should be given.

(a) Increase fluid intake for the next few hours (up to 24 hours). Have something to eat and/or drink before leaving the donor area. Remain in the area for at least 10 minutes.

(b) Do not drink any alcoholic beverages before the next meal.

(c) Do not smoke for the next ½ hour.

(d) Leave the bandage on for a few hours.

(e) Do not use strong pressure or try to lift or carry heavy objects with the donating arm for a few hours.

(f) If bleeding occurs from the phlebotomy site, reapply direct pressure until it stops.

(g) If you feel dizzy or faint, sit down with head lowered between your knees. If the symptoms continue, return to the blood bank or see your doctor.

(h) Refrain from very strenuous activity or hazardous work for a few hours.

DONOR REACTIONS

Although the majority of donations proceed without any complications, occasionally a donor will have an adverse reaction to the donation. Most reactions are of the vasovagal type. The reactions may be the result of psychologic influences, such as the sight of blood, excitement, fear, or apprehension, or may be a neurophysiologic response to the actual donation. The reactions can be roughly grouped into three categories: mild, moderate, and severe.

MILD REACTIONS

Mild reactions are the most frequently encountered type. They can be generally defined as reactions in which the donor exhibits signs of shock, but does not lose consciousness. The symptoms generally include one or more of the following:

1. Nervousness, anxiety
2. Complaints of being warm
3. Pallor and sweating
4. Increased or rapid and thready pulse
5. Increased respirations leading to hyperventilation

6. Decreased blood pressure
7. Nausea and possible vomiting

General treatment for mild reactions includes the following:

1. Stop the donation: remove the tourniquet and needle from the donor's arm.
2. Have donor rebreath in a paper bag. This will counter the effects of hyperventilation by increasing the amount of CO_2 in the air the donor is breathing.
3. Loosen any tight clothing, particularly a tie or shirt buttoned around the neck.
4. Ensure that the donor has a clear airway.
5. Raise the feet (approximately a 45-degree angle) above the head. The angle and height can be reduced to about 15 to 20 degrees as the donor recovers.
6. Apply a cold towel to the forehead and neck and use aromatic spirits of ammonia if necessary.
7. Talk to the donor as the treatment is being given to reassure and to reduce the stress and anxiety of the donor. These may be the primary cause of the reaction.
8. If the donor does not quickly respond and recover, additional medical help should be summoned.
9. *Do not leave the donor!*

MODERATE REACTIONS

Moderate reactions can be described as reactions in which the symptoms are a progression of the kind found in mild reactions, but the donor also loses consciousness. In addition to the symptoms already described, the donor will also exhibit:

1. Periods of *unconsciousness* (which may be repetitive).
2. *Decreased* pulse rate.
3. Rapid shallow respirations and hyperventilation.
4. Continued decrease in blood pressure (hypotension) (systolic pressure may drop as low as 60 mm Hg).

The recommended counter measures for moderate reactions include:

1. Proceeding with the appropriate measures listed for treatment of mild reactions.
2. Frequent checking of blood pressure, pulse, and respirations until they return to normal.
3. Administering oxygen (95 percent O_2; 5 percent CO_2).
4. Removing the donor from the general area by use of screens or actual removal to another room.

SEVERE REACTIONS

To reach the classification of a severe reaction, convulsions are added to the previously listed symptoms. Convulsions or seizures can be caused by cerebral ischemia associated with vasovagal syncope (reduced blood flow to the brain owing to the deepening shock symptoms); by marked hyperventilation (severe CO_2 depletion can cause convulsions/tetany); or by epilepsy. These severe reactions can be further categorized by the symptoms they produce.

1. Hyperventilation tetany: This is the earliest stage of convulsions caused by hyperventilation.

(a) The donor has not lost consciousness, but may complain of stiffness or tingling in the fingers.

(b) The fingers and thumb may spasm and assume an unnatural position.

(c) The symptoms will progress to deeper, more pronounced convulsions if CO_2 intake is not increased.

The recommended counter measures for severe reactions include the following:

(a) Remain calm; do not alarm other donors if possible.

(b) Have the donor rebreath air from a paper bag.

(c) *Do not leave donor*; however, help should be summoned as the reaction may progress to a more severe state.

2. Mild convulsions:

(a) Short lapse of consciousness.

(b) Voice fade out.

(c) Slight involuntary movement of the arms and legs.

3. Severe convulsions:

(a) Rigid body and tightly clenched teeth.

(b) Temporary loss of breathing activity followed by a rasping or stertorous type breathing.

(c) Violent, rhythmic muscle contractions.

The recommended counter measures are as follows:

(a) Gently restrain to prevent the donor from injury. It may be necessary to move the donor from the couch to the floor.

(b) Summon help immediately. Remain calm and stay with the donor.

(c) Place padded tongue blades between teeth to help prevent damage to the donor's teeth and tongue. However, *do not force* anything between the teeth.

(d) Insure an adequate airway.

(e) Administer 95 percent O_2, 5 percent CO_2 if necessary.

(f) Maintain observation of donor until fully recovered and released by the blood bank physician.

CARDIAC AND RESPIRATORY PROBLEMS

If the donor develops respiratory difficulties or appears to be having cardiac problems, call for medical assistance immediately. If the donor goes into cardiac arrest, administer cardiopulmonary resuscitation until medical help arrives.

HEMATOMAS

Hematomas are not an uncommon complication of the phlebotomy process. They can occur if the needle is not seated properly and there is leakage of blood into the tissue or if the needle goes through the vein and punctures the back wall. If a hematoma develops, remove the tourniquet and the needle. Apply pressure to the venipuncture site and raise the arm for 5 to 10 minutes. Make sure the bleeding has completely stopped, then apply a bandage. If the arm is stiff or sore, a cold (ice) pack can be used over the dressing. Caution the donor that a "black and blue" area will develop. If it is sore or uncomfortable, the donor may apply ice packs. If the arm becomes painful, the donor should see a doctor or return to the donor center. The discoloration will last a while and will gradually change colors from black and blue to purple to reddish brown to yellow.

A report of any adverse reaction should be kept in the blood bank as a part of the donor record.

DONOR PROCESSING

All donor units collected must be processed to some degree prior to their being made available for crossmatching and transfusion. According to the CFR (21 CFR 640.5) "all laboratory tests shall be made on a pilot sample . . . taken . . . at the time of collecting . . . ."[8] Although there are some minor differences between the AABB standards and the CFR as to which tests should be performed, the following tests are considered by most blood bankers to be standard. The routine performance of these procedures will satisfy both AABB and FDA requirements.

ABO GROUPING

Accurate determination of the ABO group must be performed (Fig. 10-2). This will require two different tests, which must be in agreement. According to the AABB standards the required tests are a red cell antigen determination (forward grouping) and a plasma antibody determination (reverse grouping). The CFR, however, allows an option of two different test methods (i.e., forward and reverse) or two tests using antisera of different lot numbers. The standard procedure is to use both the forward grouping and reverse grouping procedures.

Rh TYPING

The Rh type must be determined using anti-Rh_0 (D) antiserum (Fig. 10-2). If the test (the "test" being a rapid tube test) is positive, the unit is designated as "Rh positive." If the test is negative, a test for the D variant (D^u) must be performed. If both are negative, the unit is designated as "Rh negative." The D-negative D^u-positive unit must be labeled as such or as "Rh positive."

ANTIBODY SCREEN

Although not *required*, the AABB strongly recommends the performance of a test to detect the presence of unexpected antibodies in the serum of the donor. The procedure must be one that will detect antibodies reactive at 37°C. The actual procedure

MODERN BLOOD BANKING AND TRANSFUSION PRACTICES

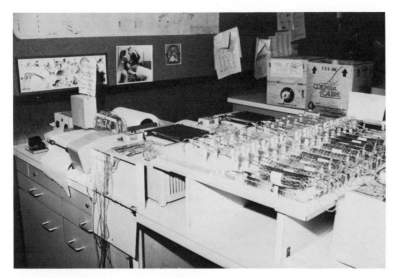

FIGURE 10-2. ABO and Rh testing using a *Technicon Auto Analyzer.*

or phases that are used for the test vary widely. The trend is to eliminate the 22°C phase, but to keep both a 37°C (with or without high protein) and an antiglobulin phase. The AABB recommends that whole blood units found to contain unexpected antibodies be "processed into components which contain minimal amounts of plasma."[9] It is not, in the opinion of this author, advisable to use this plasma in the production of platelet concentrates or cryoprecipitate. The routine use of an antibody screening procedure in donor blood processing completely eliminates the requirement or need for a minor crossmatch (21 CFR 606.151).

SEROLOGIC TEST FOR SYPHILIS (STS)

Although this test is listed as a requirement for donor processing by the FDA (21 CFR 640.5), it is not listed in the AABB standards. However, many state and municipal laws do require the STS of all donor units (Fig. 10-3).

HEPATITIS B SURFACE ANTIGEN

All donor units must be tested for hepatitis B surface antigen (HBsAg) by a method approved by the FDA or a documented equivalent method. The methods currently approved are radioimmunoassay (RIA) (Fig. 10-4), enzyme-linked immunosorbent assay (ELISA), and reverse passive hemagglutination (RPHA). In an emergency, blood and blood products can be released before HBsAg testing is completed, provided the test is performed and the results transmitted to the transfusion service as soon as possible. Records of the early release and the subsequent test results must be maintained. Also, a notification procedure, should the test be positive, must be documented.

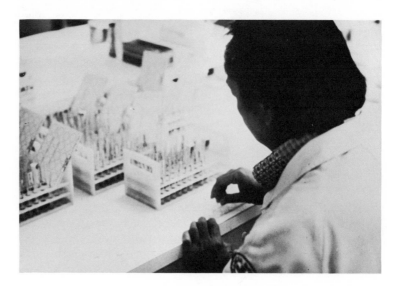

FIGURE 10-3. Serologic test for syphilis using an 18-mm circle card test by Hynson, Westcott and Dunning.

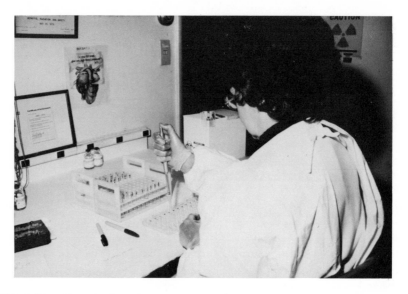

FIGURE 10-4. Hepatitis testing by radioimmunoassay technique.

MODERN BLOOD BANKING AND TRANSFUSION PRACTICES

LABELING

Once all testing is completed, the whole blood or components must be labeled (Fig. 10-5). The label should include the following information:

1. Classification of the donor (volunteer or paid).
2. Name of the component.
3. Type and quantity of anticoagulant used.
4. Amount of blood collected.
5. Donor or whole blood number.
6. Name and address of the collecting facility.
7. Required storage temperature for the specific component.
8. ABO and Rh type.
9. Test method used and interpretation of results for HBsAg and STS testing.
10. Interpretation of tests for unexpected antibodies (if performed).
11. Expiration date and time (if appropriate).

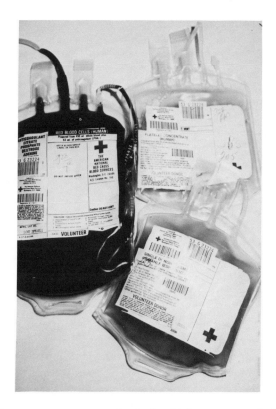

FIGURE 10-5. Blood components: concentrated red cells, platelet concentrate, fresh-frozen plasma (to be frozen).

REPEAT TESTING

If the blood collecting facility is separate from the transfusion facility, the latter is required to perform some repeat testing prior to issuing the blood or component for transfusion. The tests that must be repeated are

1. ABO type on all whole blood (WB) and concentrated red cells (CRC)
2. Rh type on all Rh-negative WB and CRC

These tests are to be performed on a "segment" sample from the attached integral tubing.

COMPONENT PREPARATION

CONCENTRATED RED CELLS

The concentrated red cells (CRCs) or packed red cells are one of the products resulting from the removal of most of the plasma from whole blood (WB). Their oxygen carrying capacity is equal to that of whole blood, with approximately 50 percent of the volume.

In today's era of component transfusion therapy, CRCs are the primary product of choice when replacement red cells are needed. They are used for elective transfusion to reduce anemia, to replace blood loss during surgery, and even to combat massive blood loss in trauma.

The use of concentrated red cells for routine transfusions has several advantages.

1. The same O_2 carrying capacity in a reduced volume helps to reduce the possibility of volume overload, particularly in the patient with a compensated anemia.

2. With the reduction in plasma, there is a significant reduction in the level of isoagglutinins (anti-A and anti-B). It allows the transfusion of ABO group-compatible red cells (i.e., O cells to an A recipient).

3. If the plasma is removed just before transfusion, there is a significant reduction in the level of acid, citrate, ammonia, and potassium, producing a much better product for cardiac, renal, or liver disease patients. The improvement is not nearly so dramatic when the cells are packed at the time of collection and stored as CRC.

The actual production of CRC can be performed at any time during the normal dating period by sedimentation or centrifugation. The amount of plasma to be removed is approximately 250 ml. The final hematocrit of the products should be between 70 percent and 80 percent. The hematocrit of a unit of concentrated red cells, collected in CPDA-1, must not exceed 80 percent. If it does, the cells cannot be stored for 35 days. A procedure for gauging hematocrit during production should be established. If CRCs are prepared in a closed system, the expiration date is not affected. If the system must be entered (opened to remove the plasma), the expiration date is reduced to 24 hours from the time of packing.

The following is a general procedure for CRC production using centrifugation:

1. Weigh and balance each unit.

2. Place the balanced units in a centrifuge. The centrifuge of choice is a swinging bucket type. It produces a better pack and a better plasma/cell interface. The refrigerated centrifuges should be calibrated every 6 months and checked each day of use for correct speed and temperature. Quality control documents should be maintained.

3. Centrifuge for specified time and speed. Although the average speed is approximately 3600 RPMs for about 5 minutes, each centrifuge must be calibrated individually and used accordingly to ensure a quality product. Also, the speed and time will change depending on the plasma product(s) to be prepared. (The AABB *Technical Manual* has data on centrifuge calibrations as well as procedures for performing them on your equipment.[10])

4. When the centrifuge has come to a complete stop, remove the unit carefully and place on an expressor.

5. Express the plasma into the attached satellite bag. An easy method of hematocrit estimation is to express the plasma until the plasma/cell interface reaches the shoulder of the bag (top corner). Another method could be to establish maximal and minimal amounts of plasma (by weight), which can be removed.

6. When the desired amount of plasma has been removed, seal the tubing using a dielectric sealer or metal clips.

7. Separate the plasma and CRC and store the CRC appropriately at 4°C. Plasma can be stored at 4°C, 22°C, or −30°C, depending on the product desired.

The AABB requires that the hematocrits of the CRCs produced be checked periodically and records of the results be maintained. The Red Cross Blood Service Directives (BSDs) require that at least 4 units per month be checked, and that 90 percent of those sampled be within control.

LEUKOCYTE-POOR RED CELLS

Leukocyte-poor or buffy-poor red blood cells are products in which at least 70 percent of the original white cells have been removed and at least 70 percent of the original volume of red cells remain. They are of great value in transfusing patients who have febrile reactions to regular red cell transfusions. Multiply-transfused, multiparous, immunosuppressed, and immunodeficient patients, as well as patients with leukemia or aplastic anemia, are all potential candidates for "leuko-poor" transfusions.

There are several acceptable techniques for preparing leukocyte-poor red cells. The particular technique used may depend on the patient's needs, the equipment available in the blood bank, and the cost. The following is a brief summary of the acceptable techniques.

1. Inverted centrifugation. This is the easiest and least costly of the methods. It requires a minimum of equipment and can be performed within 15 to 20 minutes. The drawback is that, although it removes better than 80 percent of the leukocytes, approximately 20 percent of the red cell volume is sacrificed.

(a) Centrifuge a fresh unit (0 to 5 days old) of whole blood upside down. Use a "hard" spin 3600 to 4200 RPM for 5 to 6 minutes at 1 to 6°C. Use of a multiple-bag system will allow preparation in a closed system.

(b) Hang the centrifuged unit and allow the cells to drain by gravity into the satellite bag. Measure the amount of cells in the bag by weight. A simple scale is adequate.

(c) Calculate the amount of cells needed in the final product (minimum is 70 percent):

ml in WB unit (450 ml) × hematocrit (0.40—females; or 0.43—males) = 180 ml RBCs in WB unit.

ml of RBCs in WB (180) × percentage of RBC to transfer (.70) = 126 ml RBCs.

ml of RBCs to transfer (126) × ml/g conversion (1.08) = 136 g

(d) Allow the calculated volume of RBCs to drain. Clamp off tubing. Seal using dielectric sealer or clips. Label final product.

(e) Be sure to confirm whole blood number on the satellite bag before disconnecting from the whole blood bag.

If the unit was prepared in an open system, indicate expiration date and time, 24 hours from the time of entry. If prepared in a closed system, the expiration date of the original whole blood may be used. Caution should be used, however, since the hematocrit may be above 80 percent. Leukocyte-poor preparations should be transfused as soon as possible.

2. Double Centrifugation: A similar centrifugation procedure allows for the harvesting of platelet concentrates (PLT) and fresh frozen plasma (FFP), as well as the leukocyte-poor preparation. The advantages and disadvantages are the same as in the inverted spin method. The procedure is as follows:

(a) Using a freshly drawn unit (less than 6 hours old) perform a routine "light" spin (3200 RPMs for about 2 to 3 minutes).

(b) Separate the platelet-rich plasma and further process into platelet concentrates and fresh frozen plasma.

(c) Recentrifuge the CRC in an inverted position and follow the previously described procedure, removing 70 to 80 percent of the cells. The use of a quadruple bag will allow all products to be prepared in a closed system.

3. Nylon filtration: This procedure is not frequently used because it requires the blood to be drawn in heparin and the procedure to be performed within 1 hour of collection, and although it removes most of the granulocytes and platelets, it leaves all of the lymphocytes. The finished product must be transfused within 24 hours because the preparation is in an open system.

4. Filtration of a unit of whole blood through a 40μ microaggregate filter may also produce a leukocyte-poor product. This may be a particularly effective method to use on stored units that are greater than 5 days old.

5. Freezing/deglycerolizing/saline washing: All these techniques can produce a leukocyte-poor product. The advantages that these techniques have over the techniques previously discussed are that the glycerolizing/deglycerolizing process removes 90 to 98 percent of the leukocytes and all the plasma, making the product also useful for patients who have plasma protein antibodies. The disadvantages are the 24-hour expiration date owing to the open system, the special equipment necessary, and the greatly increased cost. These techniques are the method of choice for

transfusion to a patient with paroxysmal nocturnal hemoglobinuria (PNH) or to an IgA-deficient patient with anti-IgA antibodies in his plasma or serum (refer to Chapter 16). Caution must be used when saline washing alone. Although plasma removal is acceptable, not all automated systems are approved for leukocyte removal using this procedure.

FROZEN/DEGLYCEROLIZED RED CELLS

In the last 10 years frozen red blood cells have come into widespread use. They provide a red cell product that is almost free of leukocytes, platelets, and plasma. They have an extended (3 years or more) shelf-life in the frozen state, which has made long-term storage of rare units possible and autotransfusions more plausible.

There are many procedures for freezing and deglycerolizing red cells. The author directs the reader to the AABB *Technical Manual*, the American Red Cross BSD on red cell freezing and deglycerolizing, and manufacturer's directions on the use of their equipment. This section will briefly describe some of the general procedures.

Red blood cells can be frozen by three methods. The first method, high glycerol concentration using approximately 40 percent weight/volume, increases the cryoprotective power of the glycerol, allowing a slow, uncontrolled freezing process. The freezer used is generally a mechanical freezer that provides for storage at a temperature of at least −65°C. This particular procedure is probably the most widely used, because the freezer does not require a constant supply of liquid N_2, which is expensive, and because the products require less delicate handling. It does require a larger volume of wash solution for deglycerolizing. The second method uses a low glycerol concentration, approximately 14 percent weight/volume. In this method, the cryoprotection of the glycerol is minimal and a very rapid, more controlled freezing procedure is required, so liquid nitrogen (N_2) is routinely used. The frozen units must be stored at about −150°C, which is the temperature of liquid N_2 vapor. Because of the minimal amount of protection by the glycerol, temperature fluctuations during storage can cause red cell destruction. The third method uses the red blood cells' ability to reversibly agglomerate in a high sugar concentration. A 79.2 percent weight/volume concentration of glycerol with dextrose, fructose, and EDTA is used. This method like the high glycerol method previously described uses a slow, mechanical freezing and storage process.

The deglycerolizing processes depend on the method used to glycerolize cells. The high glycerol and low glycerol methods use similar equipment but slightly different solutions and volumes.

1. High glycerol method (40 percent wt/vol)
   (a) 150 ml 12 percent NaCl; equilibrate for 5 minutes.
   (b) Wash with 1000 ml of 1.6 percent NaCl.
   (c) Continue wash with 1000 ml of 0.9 percent NaCl and 0.2 percent dextrose; this also functions as final suspending media.
   (d) Use batch wash or continuous flow equipment.

2. Low glycerol method (14 percent wt/vol)
   (a) First wash is 300 to 350 ml of 15 percent mannitol in 0.45 percent NaCl or 3 to 3.5 percent NaCl.
   (b) Continue wash with 1000 to 2000 ml 0.9 percent NaCl or 0.8 percent NaCl plus 0.2 g/dl of dextrose.
   (c) Use automated or manual batch washing only.
3. Agglomeration
   (a) In a pH of 5.2 to 6.1, red cells will agglomerate (reversible reaction).
   (b) First wash is a 50 percent dextrose plus a 5 percent fructose solution.
   (c) Cells agglomerate and rapidly settle to the bottom of the bag; solution is removed.
   (d) Second wash is a 5 percent fructose only; cells again agglomerate and settle to the bottom; solution is removed.
   (e) Final wash solution is 250 ml of normal saline (0.85 percent NaCl).
   (f) The only equipment that can be used is the cytoagglomerator.

The quality control procedures necessary for red cell freezing include all the standard procedures for monitoring refrigerators, freezers, water baths, dry thaw baths, and centrifuges. They also include procedures to ensure good red cell recovery (80 percent), good viability (70 percent survival, 24 hours after transfusion), and adequate glycerol removal (less than 1 percent residual intracellular glycerol).

1. Red cell recovery can be easily determined by estimating the recovered red cell mass (the final volume × final hematrocrit = volume of RBC in unit). Compare that against the initial (prefreeze) red cell mass.

2. Post-transfusion survival should be studied when the program is first being established; however, if one is using a standard procedure with data already published in the literature, these survival studies are not mandatory.

3. Glycerol must be removed to a level of less than 1 percent residual. The published procedures, if followed, should accomplish this. It is important to perform this check on each unit before releasing it for transfusion. The procedures are very simple.
   (a) Measure the osmolarity of the unit using an osmometer. The osmolarity should be about 420 mOsm. Maximum allowable is 500 mOsm.
   (b) Perform a simulated transfusion. Place one segment, approximately 3 inches, of deglycerolized cells into 7 ml of a 0.7 percent NaCl. Mix centrifuge and check for hemolysis. Compare to standard hemoglobin color comparator. If the hue exceeds the 7 level, hemolysis is too great and the unit is not transfusable as is.

4. Tests after deglycerolizing include confirmation of ABO and Rh and a direct antiglobulin test (DAT), which must be negative.

5. Tests before deglycerolizing may include:
   (a) Direct antiglobulin test (DAT). Unit with a positive DAT should not be used.
   (b) Sickle test. Cells that carry the sickle trait do not survive routine freezing and deglycerolizing procedures. It is recommended that cells known to carry sickle trait not be routinely used in a frozen red cell program. If for some reason the cells must be frozen, there is a special deglycerolizing procedure that may be used.[11] If

there is a high percentage of black donors in the area, it may be worthwhile to prescreen units before freezing.

6. Accurate and complete records must be maintained for all phases of the glycerolizing/deglycerolizing procedures.

PLATELET CONCENTRATES

Platelet concentrates are one of the primary products of routine conversion of whole blood into concentrated red cells. They have widespread use for a variety of patients, such as actively bleeding patients who are thrombocytopenic (< 50,000/microliter blood) owing to decreased production or decreased function; cancer patients, during radiation and chemotherapy because of an induced thrombocytopenia (< 20,000/ microliter); and thrombocytopenic, preoperative patients (< 60,000/microliter). Prophylactic platelet transfusions are not generally indicated or recommended in disseminated intravascular coagulation (DIC) or idiopathic thrombocytopenic purpura (ITP). In both cases there is an induced thrombocytopenia that is due to increased destruction—in ITP probably owing to an autoantibody and in DIC owing to systemic consumption.

Platelet concentrates prepared from whole blood are generally referred to as "random donor" platelets, to distinguish them from "single donor" platelets produced by apheresis. The random donor platelet concentrate contains at least 5.5×10^{10} platelets and can be stored in two ways. Platelets stored at 1 to 6°C ("cold") have a volume of 20 to 30 ml and a shelf-life of 48 hours. The more common platelet storage temperature is 20 to 24°C. These "warm" platelets can be stored for 72 hours, but require suspension in 50 to 65 ml of plasma. Since December 1981, a new plastic bag has made it possible to store "warm" platelets for 5 days.

The units used for the preparation of platelet concentrates must have been drawn by a single, nontraumatic venipuncture. Platelet concentrates must be prepared within 6 hours of collection.

The following is a general procedure for the preparation of random donor platelet concentrates with storage at 22°C:

1. Maintain the whole blood at 20 to 24°C before and during platelet preparation.

2. Set the centrifuge temperature at 22°C. The RPMs and time must be specifically calculated for each centrifuge. It will generally be a short (2 to 3 minutes), light (3200 RPMs) spin. This setting should separate out most of the RBCs but leave the majority of platelets suspended in the plasma.

3. Platelet preparation is to be done in a closed, multiple bag system.

4. Express the platelet-rich plasma into one of the satellite bags. Enough plasma must remain on the CRC to maintain a 70 to 80 percent hematocrit. The hematocrit estimation methods stated in the CRC procedure can be employed here.

5. Seal the tubing between the CRCs and the plasma. Disconnect the CRCs and store them at 4°C.

6. Recentrifuge the platelet-rich plasma at 22°C using a heavy spin (approximately 3600 RPMs for 5 minutes). This will separate the platelets from the plasma.

7. Express the majority of the plasma into the second satellite bag, leaving approximately 50 to 65 ml on the platelets. The volume is important to maintain the pH (above 6.0) during storage.

8. Seal the tubing between the bags and separate. Make some segments for both the platelets and the plasma. These segments can be used for testing purposes.

9. The separated plasma can be frozen as fresh-frozen plasma (FFP), or stored as liquid recovered plasma. Be sure to record the volume of plasma suspending the platelets on the platelet bag.

10. Allow the platelet concentrate to lie undisturbed for 1 to 2 hours at 20 to 24°C. Be sure that the platelet button is covered by the plasma. Platelets should be resuspended. Gentle manipulation can be used to accomplish this.

11. Store on a rotator, allowing constant, gentle agitation during storage. Temperature must be monitored at 20 to 24°C.

12. Shelf-life is 72 hours or 5 days from time of collection, depending on the plastic bag used. If the system is opened, transfusion must be within 6 hours. The volume and expiration date and time must be on the label.

In the preparation of "cold" (1 to 6°C) platelet concentrates, the procedure remains the same with the exception of the following:

1. A suspending plasma of 20 to 30 ml is sufficient. The platelet metabolism and the lactic acid buildup are slower, so the pH buffering needed is not as great (step #7).

2. The concentrates are stored at 1 to 6°C and do *not* require constant agitation (step #11).

3. Shelf-life is 48 hours from time of collection. If the system is entered, the concentrate must be transfused within 24 hours (step #12).

The disadvantage of platelets stored at 1 to 6°C is that they do not maintain function or viability as well as 22°C platelets. They will act to produce immediate hemostasis but they will not continue to circulate after transfusion.

The quality control measures that must be checked and recorded are

1. Platelet count (minimum = 5.5×10^{10})

2. pH (minimum = 6.0)

3. Volume (50 to 65 ml—ARC requirement for "warm" platelets)

These determinations should be performed regularly (ARC-BSDs require a minimum of 4 units per month). The CFR and AABB require that 75 percent of all units tested must meet the minimal standards. Records must be maintained on all quality control procedures that are performed. Temperature monitoring must be performed during whole blood transport, platelet preparation, and platelet storage, and records must be maintained.

SINGLE DONOR FRESH-FROZEN PLASMA

Fresh-frozen plasma (FFP) is a frequent by-product of concentrated red cells and platelet concentrate production. It is fresh plasma obtained from a single, uninterrupted, nontraumatic venipuncture. The plasma is placed in a freezer within 6 hours of collection and stored at −18°C or colder. The product is red cell free and contains all the plasma clotting factors, factors V and VIII included. The shelf-life of FFP is

12 months in the frozen state ($-18°C$) and 24 hours after thawing when maintained at 1 to 6°C. After 24 hours, FFP may no longer be considered a source of *labile* clotting factors, but is still acceptable for use as single donor plasma (see below).

The use of FFP is indicated in patients who are actively bleeding and present multiple clotting-factor deficiencies. Examples include massive blood replacement with banked blood, trauma, surgery, liver disease, and DIC, as well as cases in which a specific disorder cannot or has not yet been identified. Specific deficiencies such as factor VIII or fibrinogen deficiencies are more appropriately treated with cryoprecipitate. Deficiencies of factors II, VII, IX, and X would be better treated using the prothrombin complex concentrates.

A single unit of FFP should contain 150 to 250 ml of plasma. The specific volume must be written on the label. It should also contain approximately 400 mg of fibrinogen, and about 1 unit of activity per milliliter of each of the other factors.

If FFP is to be prepared from whole blood, as part of the production of platelet concentrates, follow the procedure outlined in the platelet concentrate section. At step #9, after the platelet concentrate has been separated from the plasma:

1. Weigh plasma and determine the volume. Record the volume on the bag.

2. Place the plasma in a protective container and freeze. The plasma must be frozen in such a way that evidence of thawing can be determined. Freezing some sort of indentation into the bag, which is visible as long as the plasma remains frozen, is an easy way to accomplish this. The container is important because the plastic bag becomes quite brittle when frozen at low temperatures and can crack or break quite easily.

3. The plasma must be placed in a freezer within the 6-hour time allotment. The lower the temperature of the freezer and the greater the air circulation around the plasma, the faster the freeze. Freezing at $-65°C$, packing units between dry ice, or using an ice-ethanol bath can all be used to speed up the freezing process.[12]

4. Be sure to tuck in the tubing segments and the transfusion parts ("ears") of the bag to help prevent breakage.

5. The label on the FFP must include all the standard information required (see 21 CFR 640.35 for the specifics).

6. FFP is rapidly thawed, in a 37°C water bath, prior to issue.

FFP can also be produced directly from whole blood, without preparing platelet concentrates. The procedure changes to eliminate the platelet production section, and the general volume of the FFP will be greater.

There is not any specific testing of fresh-frozen plasma required as part of a quality control program. Determination of specific factor levels is not required. Records must be maintained on the production process to ensure that the product was prepared within the time frames required and that it was prepared, frozen, and stored at the appropriate temperatures.

SINGLE DONOR PLASMA

Recovered plasma or single donor plasma and single donor plasma liquid can be prepared directly from whole blood, or as a by-product of platelet concentrate or cryoprecipitate production. The products can be used as volume expanders or for treatment of stable clotting factor deficiencies. Because of the availability of hepatitis-free volume expanders, single donor plasma is not generally used for that purpose. Probably most recovered plasma is used for the manufacture of plasma fractionation products, such as plasma protein fraction (PPF), normal serum albumin (NSA), and immune serum globulin (ISG).

If recovered plasma is produced from whole blood, the plasma can be removed from the cells at any time during the normal dating period and up to 5 days after expiration (26 and 40 days after collection for CPD and CPDA-1, respectively). If single donor plasma is being prepared, the plasma is to be stored at $-18°C$ and must be placed in a freezer within 6 hours of its transfer to the final container. The shelf-life is 5 years in the frozen state. FFP that is not used within the 12-month dating period can be converted to single donor plasma. Single donor plasma liquid is collected in the same manner, but stored at 1 to 6°C rather than being frozen. Liquid plasma must be used within the 26 to 40 days stated earlier.

The production procedure is similar to that for platelets and FFP, and quality control measures are limited to production and storage temperatures.

CRYOPRECIPITATED ANTIHEMOPHILIC FACTOR

Cryoprecipitate is a cold-precipitated concentration of factor VIII, antihemophilic factor (AHF). It is prepared from fresh-frozen plasma that is thawed slowly at 4°C. The product contains most of the factor VIII and part of the fibrinogen from the original plasma.[13] It contains at least 80 units of AHF activity and approximately 250 mg of fibrinogen. Other factors of significance found in cryoprecipitated antihemophilic factor (Cryo) are factor XIII and von Willebrand factor. Cryo has a shelf-life of 12 months in the frozen state and must be transfused within 6 hours of thawing. Like FFP, Cryo is to be thawed quickly at 37°C. Cryoprecipitate is indicated in the treatment of classic hemophilia (hemophilia A), von Willebrand's disease, and factor XIII deficiency, and is a source of fibrinogen for hypofibrinogenemia.

The whole blood donor requirements and preparation requirements for cryoprecipitate are the same as those for platelets and FFP.

1. The venipuncture must not be traumatic.

2. The whole blood can be cooled before and during production, since platelets are not generally prepared from the units. The volume of plasma required to remain on the CRC and the platelet concentrate will reduce the amount of plasma available for cryo production significantly enough to reduce the final AHF activity in the precipitate. The CFR requires a minimum of 200 ml plasma.

3. The plasma must be frozen within 6 hours of collection.

4. The second stage of cryo preparation begins by allowing the frozen plasma to thaw slowly in the refrigerator at 1 to 6°C. This requires approximately 14 to 16 hours in a standard blood bank refrigerator. The end point is achieved when the plasma has reached a "slushy" stage.

5. Hard spin the plasma in a 4°C refrigerated centrifuge.

6. Express the supernatant plasma into the attached satellite bag. The cryo concentrate will be a small, white mass in the original plasma bag. Leave only 10 to 15 ml plasma in the bag.

7. Refreeze the cryoprecipitate immediately. It should be no longer than 1 hour from the time the plasma reaches the slushy stage until the cryoprecipitate is refrozen. Exposure of the plasma to elevated temperatures or a delay in refreezing the cryoprecipitate will cause a significant drop in final factor VIII activity. Be sure that the centrifuge temperature is 4°C. It may also be wise to chill the centrifuge cups.

8. The final product should be placed in a protective container because of the brittle nature of the plastic bags at freezer temperatures.

9. Labeling requirements are the same as for other products (see the donor processing section).

Quality assurance requirements mandate that routine measurements of the volume and percentage of AHF activity of the final product be performed. The volume should not exceed 25 ml and the CFR requires that 75 percent of all units tested show a minimum of 80 AHF units. Records must be maintained of all quality assurance testing that is performed.

REFERENCES

1. US Department of Health and Human Services, Food and Drug Administration: *The Code of Federal Regulations, 21, CFR 600-799*. US Government Printing Office, Washington DC, 1981, p 31.

2. WIDMANN, FK (ED): *Technical Manual*, ed 8. American Association of Blood Banks, Washington, DC, 1981.

3. US Department of Health and Human Services, Food and Drug Administration, op cit, p 113.

4. WIDMANN, FK, op cit, p 5.

5. American Red Cross Blood Services: *Guidelines for Conducting a Blood Donor Health History Interview, ARC Form #1767*. American Red Cross, Washington, DC, 1979.

6. WIDMANN, FK, op cit, p 8.

7. US Department of Health and Human Services, Food and Drug Administration, op cit, p 111.

8. Ibid, p 115.

9. WIDMANN, FK, op cit, p 15.

10. WIDMANN, FK, op cit, p 411.

11. MERYMAN, HT and HORNBLOWER, M: *Freezing and deglycerolizing sickle-trait red blood cells.* Transfusion 16:627, 1976.

12. WIDMANN, FK, op cit, p 44.

13. Ibid, p 47.

BIBLIOGRAPHY

OBERMAN, HA (ed): *Standards for Blood Banks and Transfusion Services*, ed 10. American Association of Blood Banks, Washington, DC, 1981.

American Red Cross Blood Services: *Guidelines for the Nursing Management of Reactions and Complications Associated with Blood Donors, ARC Form #1783*. American Red Cross, Washington, DC, 1972.

BORUCKI, DT (ed): *Blood Component Therapy: A Physician's Handbook*, ed 3. American Association of Blood Banks, Washington, DC, 1981.

MILAM, JD, et al.: *Donor Room Procedures: Workshop Manual*. American Association of Blood Banks, Washington, DC, 1977.

KATZ, AJ: *Fundamentals of a Pheresis Program: Workshop Manual*. American Association of Blood Banks, Washington, DC, 1979, Ch 3.

CHAPTER 11

COMPATIBILITY TESTING

BARBARA G. McKEEVER, M.S., MT(ASCP)SBB

Pretransfusion testing includes a series of procedures performed to assure the best possible results of blood transfusion. Each of the following are critical for safe transfusion therapy and must be considered in a comprehensive review of the process utilized to select blood for a patient:

1. Identification of the patient and donor and collection of appropriate samples for testing

2. Verification of current and previous testing results
3. Preliminary testing of the donor sample
4. Preliminary testing of the patient sample
5. Selection of appropriate donor units
6. Compatibility testing or crossmatching
7. Reidentification of the patient prior to infusion of the blood selected

No testing procedure can prevent sensitization of the recipient to foreign red cells, avoid a delayed transfusion reaction caused by the rapid rise in titer of an antibody present in subdetectable amounts in the pretransfusion serum, or guarantee normal survival of transfused cells in the patient's circulation. The potential benefits of transfusion should be weighed against the potential risks anytime this form of therapy is anticipated. While adverse responses to transfusion cannot always be avoided, results are much more likely to be favorable if pretransfusion testing is carefully performed and results of in vitro testing show no incompatibility between donor and patient.

IDENTIFICATION PROCEDURES AND COLLECTION AND PREPARATION OF SAMPLES

PATIENT SAMPLES

The most common cause of transfusion accidents is misidentification of the patient or donor involved in the transfusion. Honig and Bove[1] found that 38 of 44 fatal acute hemolytic transfusion reactions reported to the Food and Drug Administration during 1976 to 1978 were caused by ABO incompatible transfusions. Thirty-three of 37 cases in which error could be defined resulted from confusion in identification of the patient when the blood sample was obtained for testing, a mixup of samples during handling in the laboratory, or error in identification of the patient when the transfusion was initiated.

Clearly, clerical error remains the single greatest threat to safe transfusion therapy. Collection of samples and actual infusion of products is often not directly controlled by technical personnel who appreciate the possible consequences of failure to properly identify the recipient and the donor unit. Therefore, exact procedures for performance of these tasks must be established and utilized by all staff responsible for these duties.

In order to prevent collection of samples from the wrong patient, the blood request form must be used to confirm the patient's identity before phlebotomy is performed. The request form must state the intended recipient's full name and unique hospital identification number.[2] Other information such as age, address, sex, and name of requesting physician can be used to further verify patient identity, but is not required on the form. Printing must be legible and indelible, so nameplate impressions or computer program transmittals are preferable to hand-written forms.

The phlebotomist should ask a coherent patient to state his full name and spell his last name. If the age or home address is printed on the form, the patient might also be asked to state this information. Occasional errors result from two patients with the same name being mistaken for one another. The patient should not be told the information and asked for his assent (e.g., Are you Mr. Jones?). Some patients may answer in the affirmative to any direct question. If the patient is a very young child or is incoherent, some other reliable professional individual should be asked to verify his identity by visual comparison of the patient and the requisition form.

After verbal confirmation of identity, the patient's wristband identification must be compared with the requisition form. In most facilities, the same nameplate or program will have been used to generate both, so information should be identical. Any discrepancies must be completely resolved before the sample is taken. Nameplates on the wall or bed labels must never be used to verify identity, since the patient specified may not occupy the bed or space intended. If blood must be taken from a patient whose identity is unknown, some positive identifier must be attached to the patient prior to collection of samples. This may be a temporary tie tag or a wrist or ankle band, but it should not be removed until proper identification has been attached to the patient and verification of identity is made by blood bank staff.

After satisfactory identification has been accomplished, blood samples should be drawn using careful technique to avoid mechanical hemolysis. Serum from hemolyzed samples cannot be used for testing, since hemolysis caused by activation of complement by antigen-antibody complexes will be masked. Clotted and anticoagulated samples should be obtained. About 15 ml of blood is ample for all testing procedures; however 5 ml of clotted blood is usually sufficient if no serologic problems are encountered.

Tubes must be labeled while still at the patient's bedside. Labeling of tubes prior to blood collection requires extra care in verification of identity before and after filling. If imprinted labels are used, they must be compared with the patient's wristband and requisition form before use. Labels should be attached to the tubes in a tamper-proof manner that will make obvious removal and reattachment after samples are taken impossible. Prelabeled labels or nongummed labels held on with tape should not be used. All writing must be legible and indelible, and each tube must be labeled at least with the patient's full name, hospital identification number, and the date of sample collection.[3] The phlebotomist may initial or sign the label and add any additional pertinent information as required by standard procedure.

Blood samples should not be taken from intravenous tubing lines. If possible, samples should be obtained from a site distant from the infusion site for other fluids to avoid contamination with materials that cause confusing serologic results.

Patient samples should be tested as soon as possible after collection. Fresh serum, obtained from samples less than 48 hours after collection, must be used for antibody screening and compatibility testing according to federal regulations.[4] Plasma may be used, according to AABB standards, for these procedures but fibrin clots that interfere with interpretation of results may form after plasma is mixed with saline-suspended red cells. Activation of complement is also prevented in plasma-containing substances such as EDTA or CPDA that bind free calcium and magnesium ions to prevent clotting. Detection of complement components bound to red cells by antigen-antibody complexing may be necessary to demonstrate the presence of some antibodies in patients' sera. Alternatively, in vitro binding of complement by clinically insignificant cold auto-antibodies may cause positive antiglobulin results when serum is used for testing.

If testing cannot be performed within a short period after collection, samples should be refrigerated. With respect to serum specimens, Garratty[5] showed that at least 60 percent of normal serum complement activity was necessary to accurately detect weak examples of some complement-binding antibodies. An average activity of 40 percent of normal was found in serum samples stored for 48 hours at room temperature, while 90 percent of activity was retained in samples stored for 72 hours at 4°C. Sera should not be frozen before testing, since some develop anticomplementary properties.

Patient red cells can be obtained from either clotted or anticoagulated samples. They can be washed prior to use to remove plasma or serum that may interfere with some testing procedures. A 2 to 5 percent saline suspension of red cells is used for most serologic testing procedures; however, the manufacturer's directions should be consulted for the proper cell concentration to use for typing tests performed with licensed reagents. A method for preparing a button of washed red cells suitable for performing one test is given in Appendix 1 of this chapter.

DONOR SAMPLES

Samples for donor testing must be taken at the same time as the full donor unit. Depending on the method used for testing, either or both clotted and anticoagulated samples are obtained. The donor information and medical history card, the pilot samples for processing, and the collection bag must be labeled with the same unique number code prior to filling, and the numbers verified again immediately after filling. The donor number is used to identify all records of testing and eventual disposition of all component parts of the unit of blood.

Donor pilot samples should be refrigerated if testing is not completed within 24 hours of collection. Clotted samples and samples stored in EDTA should not be used for testing beyond 72 hours following collection. Preparation of samples for testing depends largely on methods utilized. Red cells obtained from either clotted or anticoagulated samples can be used for manual typing tests and either serum or plasma can be safely used for serum grouping and antibody screening.

Samples for compatibility testing must contain CPDA-1 anticoagulant-preservative solution when the blood for transfusion contains CPDA-1.[6] When stored in other media, some red cell antigens do not retain their full reaction strength throughout the allowable 35-day storage period for blood collected into CPDA-1. Clotted samples or samples collected in anticoagulants such as EDTA for processing are not acceptable for compatibility testing, since incompatibilities with patients' sera may not be detected if impotent red cells are used for testing.

Ideal samples for compatibility testing can be prepared from the tubing through which the donor was bled. After blood in the tubing has been stripped into the collection bag and thoroughly mixed with CPDA-1, the tubing is allowed to re-fill and is then sealed or clamped at intervals. Each segment of tubing should bear the unique identification number printed on the tubing at intervals by the manufacturer to allow positive identification of the segments with that donor bag after separation for testing. Whereas pilot tubes bear the inherent risk of number mixups since they cannot be made an integral part of the collection bag, segments provide a positive means of sampling a given unit of blood.

Donor cells can be obtained from integral segments in a number of ways that permit several procedures to be performed from the same segment. One technique that works well for sampling is to use a lancet to make a tiny hole in the segment through which a single drop of blood can easily be expressed. The hole is essentially self-sealing, so the rest of the blood in the segment remains uncontaminated. Alternatively, the end of the segment can be cut open next to the cell pack and an applicator stick used to remove cells, or a drop expressed by squeezing the tubing. The segment should be stored with the cut end down in a test tube to minimize contamination. The contents of the segment should preferably not be emptied into a test tube for storage, since contamination and loss of positive identity are unavoidable.

Donor and recipient samples must be stored for a minimum of 7 days following transfusion.[7] The samples should be refrigerated, carefully labeled, and adequate in volume so that they can be re-evaluated if the patient experiences an adverse response to the transfusion. Red cell suspensions should not be stored beyond 1 working day, since some antigens deteriorate rapidly in saline.

VERIFICATION OF CURRENT AND PREVIOUS TESTING RESULTS

A record of all results obtained in testing patient and donor samples should be maintained. Some large donor collection and transfusion services keep this information on a computerized retrieval system for ready access.

The same unique identification number should ideally be assigned each time a patient is admitted for treatment. The number can then be used as a means of positive identification for comparing results of previous and current testing. Verification of previous results helps to establish that the current samples were collected from the correct individual. Any discrepancies between previous and current results must be thoroughly investigated before transfusion is initiated. A new sample should be collected from the patient if necessary to resolve the problem.

In addition to ABO and Rh typing results, notations concerning unusual serologic reactions and the identity of unexpected antibodies in the patient's serum should be included in the file. While blood should never be selected for a patient based solely on results of previous testing, the information can prove valuable if suitable units must be located in an emergency.

Files on donor testing results can be maintained using the last name and birthdate, social security number, or any other coding system that allows reliable discrimination between two individuals of the same name. No donor product can be labeled based on results of previous testing; however, results of ABO and Rh typing tests can be filed and used to verify that results of current testing are correct and that no mislabeling of pilot samples has occurred. Laboratory staff can also be alerted when individuals donate who have previously had positive results in antibody screening tests or tests for hepatitis or syphilis.

PRELIMINARY TESTING OF THE DONOR SAMPLE

According to the Code of Federal Regulations (CFR),[8,9] ABO grouping, Rh typing (including a test for D^u), and tests for hepatitis B and syphilis must be performed on a sample of blood taken at the time of collection of the unit of blood from the donor. A screening test for unexpected antibodies to red cell antigens is not required by the CFR, but is required by AABB standards on samples from donors revealing a history of prior transfusion or pregnancy.[10]

Testing is usually performed by the collecting facility and results must be clearly indicated on all product labels. The transfusing facility is required by AABB standards[11] to repeat the ABO cell grouping on all units and Rh typing (including a test for D^u) on units labeled Rh negative received from other collecting facilities. Repetition of other testing is not recommended.

Depending on the number of samples that must be tested, donor processing can either be done manually on slides or in test tubes, or by using automated instruments like the AutoAnalyzer or Groupamatic. A microplate system can also be utilized to manually process large numbers of samples efficiently when an automated instrument is unavailable. All testing must be performed using in-date, licensed reagents, according to manufacturers' directions and protocol established in the written standard operating procedure of the facility.

ABO GROUPING

At least two procedures must be used to confirm the correct ABO group of each donor sample.[12] Cell grouping is performed using potent anti-A and anti-B. Bloods that test as negative with these reagents must also be tested with anti-A,B to assure detection of some weak subgroups of A and B. Serum grouping is performed using known A_1 and B cells. A pool of cells from five group-A donors can be used instead of known A_1 cells selected by typing with anti-A_1 lectin. Use of A_2 cells is optional, but is helpful in resolving grouping discrepancies caused by the presence of anti-A_1 in A_2 or weaker subgroups of A. Results of cell and serum grouping should be interpreted separately and then compared for agreement. All discrepancies must be satisfactorily resolved before labeling the donor unit.

Rh TYPING

Rh typing can be performed using "slide and rapid tube" anti-D or chemically modified anti-D and appropriate diluent controls. If a negative result is obtained, the test for D^u must be performed, since D^u-positive bloods can stimulate the production of anti-D in Rh-negative recipients. If the test for D^u is positive, a direct antiglobulin test must be performed on the donor red cells. If the direct antiglobulin test is positive, the donor unit cannot be used for patient transfusion and the Rh typing result is invalid.

No additional tests for other Rh antigens, such as C or E, need to be performed. Blood is labeled Rh-positive if positive results are obtained in testing the red cells for Rh_0 (D) or D^u. Blood is labeled Rh-negative if results of testing for Rh_0 (D) and D^u are negative.

ANTIBODY SCREENING

Screening of all donor samples for unexpected antibodies to red cell antigens is still performed in most facilities, even though requirements limit the need for screening to samples from donors with a history of prior exposure to red cells. The clerical effort and labeling complications involved in sorting those who have such a history from those who do not precludes selective screening in most large processing centers. Screening procedures should be aimed at detecting only high-titer, potent antibodies that may be capable of causing destruction of patient red cells carrying the corresponding antigens. Such antibodies are rare. Only a few reports of transfusion reactions caused by passively infused donor antibodies are available.[13-16] As early as 1959, Mollison[17] noted that antibodies in donor units were unlikely to cause harm to recipients because of rapid dilution of small amounts of donor plasma in the recipient's circulation.

Current standards do not stipulate testing methodology, but state only that the procedure must permit detection of "antibodies active at 37°C."[18] Incubation of the serum-cell mixture for 30 minutes at 37°C prior to washing and the performance of an antiglobulin test is adequate to detect antibodies that may be significant to recipients.

If large numbers of samples must be processed, serum from several donors can be pooled for testing.[19] Kitagawa, Lee, and Bezhad[20] found that 22 different antibodies were detected equally well in either serum or plasma. Pooled screening cells provide adequate sensitivity for testing donor samples.[21] Addition of albumin or LISS is costly and probably unnecessary, since donor antibodies that are so weak that they require potentiation to be demonstrable do not present a threat to recipients. Antiglobulin serum that contains anti-IgG and anticomplement can be used; however, a reagent that contains predominantly anti-IgG activity is satisfactory.[21,22]

Donor units that contain antibodies can be safely used for transfusion as packed red cells.[23] Unless the antibodies are of extremely high titer, there is no need to type the red cells of recipients for the corresponding antigens.

TESTS FOR HEPATITIS B AND SYPHILIS

Post-transfusion hepatitis is a serious complication of blood transfusion. A sensitive test for the presence of hepatitis B surface antigen (HBsAg) must be performed on all donor samples, using methods employing techniques such as radioimmunoassay (RIA), reverse passive hemagglutination (RPHA), or coupled enzyme systems.[24]

Tests for other varieties of hepatitis (notably non-A, non-B, or "hepatitis C") are not currently required, but may be mandatory in the future if suitable methodology can be developed and evidence indicates that such testing is necessary for recipient safety.

A donor found to have a positive test for HBsAg must be permanently deferred from further blood donations, since current testing procedures may not always identify individuals whose blood is still infectious. Blood from the donor must not be used for transfusion, and the unit and pilot samples should be destroyed by autoclaving or incineration.

A serologic test for syphilis (STS) must be performed on all donor samples.[25] Tests used to screen blood donors include the VDRL (Venereal Disease Research Laboratory), RPR (rapid plasma reagin) test, and ART (automated reagin test). Since these tests are not specific for the causative agent of syphilis, samples that are reactive should be further evaluated by a specific test such as the FTA (fluorescent treponemal antibody). Donors whose samples are FTA reactive may be contacted by local health agencies for treatment and follow-up according to applicable state law.

Donor blood that is STS reactive is likely to be noninfectious, but cannot be used for transfusion. Blood from donors who have had a previously reactive STS, but who test as seronegative on a subsequent occasion, can be safely utilized for transfusion.

PRELIMINARY TESTING OF THE PATIENT SAMPLE

ABO grouping, Rh typing, and antibody screening of the patient's serum can be performed in advance of, or concurrently with, compatibility testing. An accurate medical history, including information on medications and recent blood transfusions, may help to explain any unusual results encountered.

ABO GROUPING

Determination of the patient's correct ABO group is the most critical pretransfusion serologic test. ABO grouping can be performed on slides or in tubes; however, tube tests offer greater sensitivity. Testing is performed in a manner similar to that described for donors, using potent licensed reagents according to manufacturers' directions. If cell and serum grouping results do not concur, additional testing must be conducted to carefully resolve the discrepancy. Useful information on resolving ABO grouping discrepancies has been presented in Chapter 5, and other excellent reviews are available.[26,27] If the patient's ABO group cannot be satisfactorily determined and immediate transfusion is essential, group O packed red cells should be utilized.

Rh TYPING

Rh typing is also performed as described for testing donor samples. Tube or slide tests should be performed according to manufacturers' directions for using the reagent selected. Suitable diluent controls must be run in parallel with Rh-typing tests performed on patient samples, to avoid incorrect designation of Rh-negative patients as Rh-positive. If the diluent control is positive, the result of the Rh-typing test is invalid. A direct antiglobulin test should be performed on the patient's red cells in such a case, to determine if uptake of autoantibodies (or alloantibodies, if the patient has been recently transfused) is responsible for the positive control. If a positive direct antiglobulin test is found, accurate Rh typing can sometimes be performed using saline-active or chemically modified Rh-typing serum with an appropriate diluent or 8 percent albumin control.[28] Alternatively, the presence or absence of the Rh_0 (D) antigen can be assessed by examining the ability of the patient's red cells to adsorb anti-D, according to the technique of Beattie.[29]

The test for D^u is optional when testing recipients, since those typing as Rh_0 (D) negative in direct testing should probably receive Rh-negative blood, especially if they are females of child-bearing age. Some patients who type as D^u positive are still at risk of forming anti-D if transfused with Rh-positive blood, although the incidence of sensitization appears to be much lower than that found with true Rh-negative individuals.

ANTIBODY SCREENING

The incidence of unexpected antibodies in the patient population is low. Giblett[23] found an incidence of 1.64 percent positive results in testing sera from 43,000 patients. Spielmann and Seidl[30] reported an incidence of 0.78 percent positive results in their study, which included over 55,000 recipients' samples.

Correct ABO grouping results are much more critical to assuring safe transfusion than antibody screening. Most antibodies, other than anti-A and anti-B, do not cause severe hemolytic transfusion reactions. Therefore, the vast majority of patients would not suffer grave consequences if transfused with blood from ABO group compatible donors, without the benefit of antibody screening tests.

Detection of unexpected antibodies is important, however, for the selection of donor red cells that are likely to survive maximally in the patient's circulation. Even weakly reactive antibodies that are capable of complexing with their antigens at 37°C can cause decreased survival of transfused incompatible red cells. Since large numbers of antibody molecules are present in the patient's circulation compared with the number of red cells in a unit of blood, incompatible donor cells are highly vulnerable to destruction by patient antibodies. The subject of destruction of incompatible transfused red cells has been extensively reviewed by Mollison.[31]

Antibody screening offers several advantages over direct compatibility testing for detection of antibodies:

1. Testing is performed using selected red cells that are known to carry optimal representation of important blood group antigens. The antigenic content of screening cells is known, while the antigenic content of donor red cells is largely unknown.

2. Testing can be performed well in advance of the anticipated transfusion, allowing ample time for identification of specificity if a positive result is found and location of suitable donor units.

Methods used to detect antibodies in patients' sera must demonstrate all significant coating, hemolyzing, and agglutinating antibodies active at 37°C. Incubation of screening tests at room temperature or below is not advocated, since antibodies that react only at lower temperatures in vitro are incapable of complexing with their antigens in vivo. Standards stipulate the necessity of performing an antiglobulin test, the best method for demonstrating potentially dangerous IgG antibodies.[32]

Single donor screening cells offer increased sensitivity over pooled cell preparations. Therefore, they are preferred for screening patients' sera, when detection of even weak reactivity is important. In a screening cell product made from cells pooled from two donors, 50 percent of the cells lack any antigen that is lacking from one donor's phenotype. These cells will be incapable of reacting with the corresponding antibody in a patient's serum, and many unagglutinated cells in the screening test may lead to falsely negative interpretation. Single donor screening cells are supplied as sets of individual cell samples from two or more donors whose red cell phenotypes have been carefully matched so that they complement each other. If an antigen is lacking from one cell sample, it is present on the other. Ideally, one sample in each set should carry the products of homozygous genes for antigens such as Jk^a and c. Antibodies to these antigens sometimes fail to react with cell samples carrying a single dose of the corresponding antigen.

Polyspecific reagents that contain adequate levels of anticomplement as well as high levels of anti-IgG activity are preferable for patient antibody screening and compatibility testing.[33] Detection of complement components bound to red cells by complexing of antigens and antibodies may be necessary to demonstrate the presence of some weakly reactive antibodies.[34] Wright and Issitt[35] found that over 50 percent of antibodies in the Kidd and Duffy blood group systems were detected better when reasonable levels of anticomplement were present in the antiglobulin serum utilized.

The sensitivity of antibody detection tests can be further augmented by increasing the amount of serum added to the test,[36-38] increasing the length of incubation time at 37°C,[39,40] or adding albumin to the test.[41,42] Screening cells can also be treated prior to use with proteolytic enzyme solutions such as 0.1 percent papain or ficin to enhance their ability to detect some antibodies.[43,44] Other antibodies cannot be detected using enzyme pretreated cell samples, however, so these cells cannot be used as the only means of screening patients' sera.

Increased sensitivity is especially important when screening the sera of patients who have already formed at least one antibody, since they have proven their capability of producing antibodies in response to red cell antigens, and other specificities may also be present.[45,46] Patients who have been recently transfused and those who have experienced previous unexplained adverse reactions to blood transfusion are also candidates for more sensitive antibody screening procedures. These patients may have formed antibodies that are too weak to be demonstrable using routine testing procedures. Re-exposure to the corresponding antigens on donor red cells may cause a rapid rise in antibody titer and subsequent destruction of circulating incompatible cells.[47-49]

Antibody screening tests should demonstrate the presence of all potentially significant antibodies in the patient's serum and rapidly indicate the need for further studies. All antibodies encountered should be identified, so that a logical decision can be made as to whether there is a need to select antigen-negative units for transfusion by typing donor red cells for the offending antigen. Apparently compatible direct tests between patient serum and donor red cells may be unreliable in the presence of some antibodies, since the status of the corresponding antigens on donor red cells is unknown.

TESTING PROTOCOLS

SELECTION OF APPROPRIATE DONOR UNITS

In almost all cases, blood of the patient's own ABO and Rh type should be selected for transfusion. On occasions when blood of the patient's type is unavailable or some other reason precludes its use, units selected must lack any antigen against which the patient has a significant antibody. It is completely acceptable, however, to use blood that does not contain all of the antigens carried on the patient's own red cells (e.g., group A or B blood can be safely given to a group AB recipient). Whenever non-ABO-group-specific transfusions must be given, packed red cells should be used rather than whole blood containing plasma antibodies that are incompatible with the patient's red cells. Group O red cells can be safely used for all patients; however, conservation of a limited supply of group O blood should dictate its use for patients not of group O only in special circumstances.

Rh-negative blood can be given to Rh-positive patients; however, good inventory management again should dictate use of this limited resource for Rh-negative recipients. Rh-positive blood should not be given to Rh-negative female patients who are still of childbearing age. Transfusion of Rh-negative male patients and females beyond menopause with Rh-positive blood is acceptable as long as no preformed anti-D is demonstrable in their sera. About 50 percent of these patients may respond to such a transfusion by producing anti-D;[50] however, this outcome must sometimes be weighed against the alternatives of not transfusing at all if the supply of Rh-negative blood has been exhausted, or of depriving another young female recipient, if she should need transfusion after the Rh-negative blood supply has been used for an earlier transfusion. If the formation of anti-D is unlikely to be of great significance, such as in an Rh-negative elderly surgical patient, use of Rh-positive blood is judicious in the opinion of many workers.

When an unexpected antibody is found in the patient's serum during antibody screening, the decision to select units of blood by phenotyping the red cells of donors with commercial antiserum or by straight-forward compatibility testing with the patient's serum must be based on the in vitro reaction characteristics of the antibody and its specificity. There is no need to provide antigen-negative red cells for patients whose sera contain antibodies that are reactive only below 30°C, since these antibodies are incapable of causing significant red cell destruction in vivo. Significant or potent examples of anti-P_1, anti-Le^a, anti-Le^b and other typically cold-reactive antibodies in patients' sera can be utilized to select appropriate donor units that are "crossmatch compatible" in tests conducted at 37°C.

Potent examples of IgG, warm-reactive antibodies in patients' sera can also be utilized to select suitable donor units by direct testing. Commercially prepared typing reagents must be utilized to select blood for patients whose sera contain weak examples of antibodies active at 37°C, antibodies that react well only with cell samples carrying homozygous representation of the corresponding antigens, and for patients whose sera no longer exhibit demonstrable in vitro reactivity, but previously were known to contain clinically-significant IgG antibodies, such as anti-Jk[a], anti-K, or anti-E.

Donor units should be selected so that the red cells are of appropriate age for the patient's needs. Fresher units should be selected, if maximal survival of transfused cells is required; however, it should be remembered that a minimum of 70 percent of the red cells are viable in 35-day-old blood collected in CPDA-1.

Packed red cell units should be selected if the patient does not require volume, but only increased oxygen-carrying capacity. Whole blood should be reserved for those occasions when the patient genuinely needs volume expansion, such as in major trauma or surgery. Even in these cases, however, support with appropriate crystalloid solutions and blood components usually produces results equal or superior to those achieved by transfusion of whole blood.

Donor units should be visually examined prior to compatibility testing for unusual appearance, correct labeling, and hermetic seal integrity. Donor units showing abnormal color change, turbidity, clots, incomplete or improper labeling information, or leakage of any sort should be returned to the collecting facility.

COMPATIBILITY TESTING

Since its introduction in 1908 by Ottenberg, the direct compatibility test, or crossmatch, between donor and patient blood samples has been viewed as absolutely necessary for safe blood transfusion. The crossmatch is the most commonly performed testing procedure in most hospital blood banks and consumes a majority of the total work effort in this section of most hospital laboratories.[51]

It is important to note that direct crossmatching preceded antibody screening as part of patient pretransfusion testing by several decades. Selected red cells were first used in some laboratories[17,23] during the late 1950s to screen sera from donors. Separate antibody screening of patients' sera was not popularized as an adjuvant to crossmatching until the early 1960s, when phenotyped red cells for this purpose were marketed commercially. By that time, direct crossmatching was firmly entrenched as a routine procedure that was necessary to assure recipient well-being. As early as 1964, however, Grove-Rasmussen[52] questioned the need for an antiglobulin test as part of the crossmatch when antibody screening tests were negative.

Considering that over 99 percent of significant antibodies in patients' sera will be detected by adequate antibody screening procedures, what then is the value of performing direct compatibility testing between patient and donor samples? Two main functions of the compatibility test can be cited:

1. It is a final check of ABO compatibility between donor and patient.
2. It may detect the presence of an antibody in the patient's serum that was

not detected in antibody screening because the corresponding antigen was lacking from the screening cells.

In addition, direct compatibility testing is still required by AABB standards[53] and is included as part of the Current Good Manufacturing Practices for Blood and Blood Components, cited in the Code of Federal Regulations.[54] Therefore, compatibility testing prior to actual transfusion must continue to be performed, although much effort has been directed toward reduction of the complexity of testing procedures. Elimination of advance compatibility testing for patients undergoing surgical procedures in which blood is unlikely to be used has been implemented successfully in many facilities, using the "type and screen" approach first described by Boral and Henry in 1977[55] and discussed more completely later in this chapter.

MAJOR AND MINOR COMPATIBILITY TESTS

Traditional compatibility testing procedures have been divided into two parts: the major compatibility test consisting of mixing the patient's serum with donor red cells, and the minor test consisting of mixing the donor's plasma with patient red cells. As the names imply, the major test is much more critical for assuring safe transfusion that the minor test.

The minor compatibility test need only be performed if antibody screening has not been performed on the donor sample.[56] The minor compatibility test is not recommended, since it takes some attention away from the major test, and therefore, it is no longer performed in most facilities.

METHODS

Many different procedures can be used for compatibility testing. The objective of testing, to select donor units able to provide maximal benefit to the patient, should be kept in mind, however, when developing the test protocol. Detection of in vitro incompatibilities that are not likely to be duplicated in vivo or use of enormously complicated protocols that require several tubes for each unit tested results in delay of service to the patient and does not improve the quality of the eventual transfusion. For this reason, incubation of tests at room temperature has been eliminated in many facilities, and a simple compatibility test of "one tube" per unit has become the standard. A sample procedure for a one-tube compatibility test is given in Appendix 2 of this chapter.

For the major test, a 2 to 5 percent suspension of donor red cells in saline should be prepared from a sample taken from an integral segment on the unit selected. The cells may be washed at least one time to eliminate plasma that may cause interference in test results. The ratio of serum to red cells should be at least 2:1, or equivalent to 2 drops of serum to 1 drop of a 3 percent red cell suspension dispensed from droppers of equal size. Albumin may be added prior to incubation at 37°C to enhance reactivity of some antibodies. Low ionic strength solution (LISS) can also be added in place of albumin to facilitate complexing of antigens and antibodies and is especially useful for emergency compatibility testing requiring shortened incubation times. The antiglobulin test must be performed,[57,58] and for greatest sensitivity, a reagent containing both anti-IgG and anticomplement should be selected.

An autocontrol, consisting of the patient's own cells and serum, should be tested in parallel with the compatibility test. Results of the autocontrol help to clarify possible explanations for positive results in the compatibility test.

Tubes should be carefully labeled so that the contents can be identified at any stage of the procedure. After centrifugation of tubes, the supernatant should be examined for hemolysis that must be interpreted as a positive result. Results should be read against a white or lighted background, and a magnifying mirror or hand lens can be used to facilitate reading, if desired. The button of cells should be gently resuspended. Violent shaking or tapping of the tubes may yield falsely negative results, since fragile agglutinates may be disrupted. A jagged button edge is indicative of a positive result, while a smooth button edge and swirling free cells indicate the absence of a demonstrable antigen-antibody interaction. After the button has been completely resuspended, the contents of the tube should be examined and positive results graded according to a scale used by all technologists in a facility. Uniform grading of reactions allows retrospective analysis of results by supervisory staff, as well as comparison of serial results obtained on samples collected from the same patient. Results can be examined microscopically for verification, if desired. Review Color Plate 2 for the grading of typical agglutination reactions.

All results must be immediately recorded in a permanent ledger using a logical system that allows them to be easily recalled, and actual observations, as well as interpretations, must be recorded. All work should be signed or initialed by the technologist. If an incompatibility is found, the record should clearly show the location of results of follow-up studies and additional testing performed.

RESULTS OF THE MAJOR COMPATIBILITY TEST

The primary objective of the major compatibility test is to detect the presence of antibodies, including anti-A and anti-B, in the recipient's serum that could destroy transfused red cells. A positive result in the major compatibility test requires explanation and the patient *should not be transfused* until the cause of the incompatibility has been fully elucidated. Results of the autocontrol and antibody screening test should be reviewed when the compatibility test result is positive to identify patterns that may help to elucidate the cause of the problem.

A positive result in the major compatibility test may be caused by:

1. *Incorrect ABO grouping of the patient or donor.* ABO grouping should be immediately repeated, especially if strong incompatibility is noted in a reading taken after immediate spin. Samples should be used for retesting that bear undisputable identity with the original patient sample and the donor bag.

2. *An alloantibody in the patient's serum reacting with the corresponding antigen on donor red cells.* The autocontrol tube will be negative unless the patient has been recently transfused with incompatible cells. If the antibody screening test is positive, panel studies should allow identification of antibody specificity and selec-

tion of units lacking the offending antigens for compatibility testing. Chapter 12 provides further discussion of antibody detection and identification as well as examples for study.

a. If red cells of all donors tested are incompatible with the patient's serum and the antibody screening test is positive, suspect either an antibody directed against an antigen of high incidence or multiple antibodies in the patient's serum. Consult a reference laboratory, if unable to identify specificity. *Note:* The patient's ABO compatible brothers and sisters may lack the antigen(s) to which the patient has been sensitized and may be excellent potential donors in an emergency.

b. If the antibody screening test is negative and only one donor's cells are incompatible, an antibody in the patient's serum may be directed against an antigen of relatively low incidence that is present on that donor's red cells. Panel studies of the patient's serum will usually be noninformative, and identification of the antibody is academic in any case if other compatible units are easily located.

c. If the antibody screening test is negative, the patient's serum may contain an antibody, such as anti-A_1, reacting with an antigen in the ABO blood group system. Check the serum grouping result to confirm the presence of an unexpected reaction with known A_1 cells.

3. *An autoantibody in the patient's serum reacting with the corresponding antigen on donor red cells.* The autocontrol tube will be positive. The antibody screening test is also positive in most cases as are the results of testing the patient's serum with the cells of numerous donors. Most autoantibodies have specificity for antigens of relatively high incidence. Panel studies may reveal specificity of the autoantibody; however, the far greater concern is to assess whether underlying alloantibodies are also present. Techniques for management of patients with autoantibodies include autoadsorption of the patient's serum to remove autoantibody activity. Compatibility testing should then be performed using the autoadsorbed serum. Chapter 19 provides further discussion of autoantibodies and their serologic activity.

4. *Prior coating of the donor red cells with protein, resulting in a positive antiglobulin test.* If one isolated positive result is obtained, a direct antiglobulin test should be performed on the donor's red cells. Donor cells that demonstrate a positive DAT will be incompatible with *all* recipients tested in the antiglobulin phase, because the cells are already coated with immunoglobulin and/or complement.

5. *Abnormalities in the patient's serum.*

a. Imbalance of the normal ratio of albumin and gamma globulin (A/G ratio) may cause red cells to stick together on their flat sides, giving the appearance of stacks of coins when viewed microscopically. This rouleauxing property of the serum will affect all tests, including the autocontrol. Strong rouleaux may mimic true agglutination; however, clumps are refractile. Rouleaux are usually strongest after 37°C incubation, but do not persist through washing prior to the antiglobulin test. Problems with rouleaux can often be resolved using the saline replacement technique[59] or by adding albumin to the tests.

b. The presence of high-molecular weight dextrans or other plasma expanders may cause falsely positive results in compatibility and other tests. All tests including the autocontrol are generally affected equally. Saline replacement may be useful to resolve the problem.

6. *Contaminants in the test system.* Dirty glassware, bacterial contamination of samples, chemical or other contaminants in saline, fibrin clots, and overcentrifugation may produce positive compatibility test results.

RESULTS OF THE MINOR COMPATIBILITY TEST

A positive result in the minor compatibility test may be caused by:

1. *Incorrect ABO grouping of the patient or donor.* See explanation in remarks under major compatibility test.

2. *An antibody in the donor plasma reacting with the corresponding antigen on patient red cells.* Unless the antibody is exceptionally potent, it is not likely to be of consequence to the recipient.

3. *Prior coating of the patient's red cells with protein, resulting in a positive antiglobulin test.* Either the autocontrol or a direct antiglobulin test performed on the patient's red cells will also reveal this information.

Contaminants mentioned as causing positive major compatibility test results may similarly affect resutls of the minor compatibility test.

COMPATIBILITY TESTING FOR TRANSFUSION OF PLASMA PRODUCTS

For transfusion of a large volume of plasma, a compatibility test between the donor plasma and patient red cells may be performed. The purpose for testing is to detect ABO incompatibility between donor and patient, and therefore an immediate spin reading, without incubation or the performance of an antiglobulin test, is sufficient.

COMPATIBILITY TESTING IN SPECIAL CIRCUMSTANCES

In selected instances, standard methods for compatibility testing may require alteration. Because these procedures may be performed infrequently, it is especially important that they be documented in the written procedure manual.

TRANSFUSION OF NON-GROUP-SPECIFIC BLOOD

When units of ABO group other than the patient's own have been transfused, additional units should be selected after analysis of a new post-transfusion patient sample for the presence of unexpected anti-A and anti-B in the recipient's serum. Selection of additional units should always be based on this parameter. For example, if a group A patient has been given a large number of units of group O blood, anti-A and anti-B may be demonstrable in his plasma. Group O units should therefore be used for additional transfusions. The decision to revert to the patient's own type should be based on results of compatibility testing and analysis of serum grouping results, carried through to the antiglobulin test.

INTRAUTERINE TRANSFUSIONS AND TRANSFUSION OF THE NEONATE

Blood for intrauterine transfusion must be selected to be compatible with maternal antibodies capable of crossing the placenta. Unless the ABO group and Rh type of the infant are known from prior amniocentesis, group-O, Rh-negative red cells should be selected. These group-O, Rh-negative cells must lack any other antigens against which the mother's serum contains antibodies, (e.g., anti-Kell, anti-Jk^a, etc.). Compatibility testing is performed using the mother's serum sample.

Blood for neonatal exchange or regular transfusion should similarly be compatible with any maternal antibodies that have entered the infant's circulation. Blood of the infant's ABO and Rh type can be utilized, if ABO and Rh are not involved in feto-maternal incompatibility as judged from studies of maternal and cord samples. Compatibility testing can be performed using the maternal serum or, alternatively, using the infant's serum or cord serum *and* an eluate prepared from the infant's red cells. Refer to Chapter 18 for additional information on hemolytic disease of the newborn (HDN).

MASSIVE TRANSFUSIONS

When amounts of blood infused approach or exceed the patient's total blood volume, the compatibility testing procedure may be abbreviated to an immediate spin test for ABO compatibility. A pretransfusion patient sample should be used for compatibility testing for up to 48 hours following the initiation of massive transfusion. After 48 hours, a new sample must be obtained for further testing, to detect newly formed antibodies in the patient's circulation. At no time is interdonor compatibility testing warranted.

If the patient is known to have an antibody that may be clinically significant, all units infused should be tested and found to lack the offending antigen. The antibody in the patient's serum may not be demonstrable because of dilution with large volumes of plasma and other fluids; however, a rapid rise in antibody titer and subsequent destruction of donor red cells may occur, if antigen-positive units are infused after the patient has stabilized.

EMERGENCIES

Urgent need for transfusion may preclude the performance of the usual testing protocol. There are several approaches that can be utilized in these circumstances. Some technologists use an "emergency" compatibility testing procedure that employs a shortened incubation time, often with addition of low ionic strength solution (LISS) to speed antigen-antibody complexing. Others maintain that regular procedures should be used in all circumstances, and blood should be issued, if necessary, prior to completion of the standard compatibility testing procedure. They feel that there is greater danger in utilizing an unfamiliar procedure under pressure than in releasing blood without completed testing. While both lines of reasoning have merit, the ideal compromise may be to develop regular testing procedures that are concise, so that they can be used in emergency and routine situations alike. Whatever the approach, the protocol for handling emergencies must be decided in advance of the situation and be familiar to all staff in the transfusion service. Adequate pretransfusion samples should be collected prior to infusion of any donor blood to perform compatibility testing, antibody screening, and identification studies, if necessary.

If blood must be issued in an emergency, the patient's ABO and Rh type should be determined, so that group compatible blood can be given. In extreme emergencies, group O packed cells can be utilized. If the patient is Rh negative and large amounts of blood are likely to be needed, a decision should be made rapidly as to whether inventory and the situation demand transfusion of Rh-negative blood. Conversion to Rh positive is best made immediately if the patient is female beyond childbearing age or male. If amounts exceeding supply must be given to an Rh-negative female of childbearing age, available Rh-negative units are better given at the end of the episode, when the patient is stabilizing, so that Rh-negative red cells will be predominantly retained in the circulation. Injections of Rh immune globulin to prevent formation of anti-D may be appropriate after the crisis has been resolved. This product is discussed in detail in Chapter 18.

Accurate records must be maintained of all units issued in the emergency. A conspicuous tie tag or label must be placed on each unit, if compatibility testing is not completed prior to release of units, and the physician must sign a release authorizing and accepting responsibility for using incompletely tested products. Compatibility testing should be completed according to the chosen protocol, and any positive result reported immediately to the patient's physician and the blood bank director.

SPECIMENS WITH PROLONGED CLOTTING TIME

Difficulties may be encountered in testing blood samples from patients who have prolonged clotting times caused by coagulation abnormalities induced by disease or medications. A fibrin clot may spontaneously form when partially clotted plasma is added to saline-suspended screening or donor red cells. Complete coagulation of these samples can often be prompted by addition of thrombin. One drop of thrombin, 50 units per milliliter, to 1 ml of plasma, or the amount of dry thrombin that will adhere to the end of an applicator stick is usually sufficient to induce clotting.[60]

A small amount of protamine sulfate can be added to counteract the effects of heparin in samples of blood collected from patients on this anticoagulant.[60]

LIMITATIONS OF COMPATIBILITY TESTING PROCEDURES

As mentioned in the introduction to this chapter, no current testing procedure can guarantee that transfused red cells will enjoy normal survival, or that the patient will not have some type of adverse response to the transfusion. In some cases, however, even limited survival of donor cells will suffice to maintain a patient until he can begin to produce his own cells. Certainly no patient should be denied a transfusion if he needs one to survive, and donor cells that appear "incompatible" by in vitro testing procedures may, in fact, survive quite well in vivo. "Biological compatibility tests" using red cells labeled with radioactive chromium or phosphorus can sometimes be used to measure the likelihood of successful transfusion, when standard in vitro testing procedures are inconclusive.[61] Other procedures such as the in vitro macrophage assay show promise as better predictors of red cell survival than current methodology.[62]

REIDENTIFICATION OF THE PATIENT PRIOR TO TRANSFUSION

The final link in the chain of events leading to safe transfusion is re-establishment of the identity of the intended recipient and selected donor product. The same type of careful approach used to identify the patient prior to collection of samples must be used to verify that the patient is indeed the same person who provided the blood for testing. In addition, the actual product and accompanying record of testing must be verified as relating to the same donor number.

After compatibility testing is completed, two records must be prepared in addition to laboratory testing records.[63] The first is a statement of compatibility to be maintained as part of the patient's permanent record if the blood is transfused. The second is a label or tie tag that must be attached to the product stating the identity of the intended recipient, the results of compatibility testing, and the donor number. This identification must remain on the unit throughout the transfusion.

The original blood request form can be conveniently used to accomplish one or both of these record-keeping requirements. A multipart form is used in some facilities to record the entire "history" of pretransfusion testing and infusion of the unit. Useful information might include the initials or signature of the phlebotomist taking the samples, the donor numbers and summary of results of compatibility testing, the initials or signature of the technologist performing the testing, and the signatures of the persons who verify identity of the patient prior to infusion and who start the infusion. One copy of the form can be placed on the patient's chart after the transfusion is completed and the other returned to the blood bank, if desired, for filing. The last copy of the form might be printed on heavier stock and perforated so that it can be torn off and attached to the unit in the laboratory. The most important feature of this system is that the patient's name plate impression is used, rather than a hand-written transcription, for all forms used to identify the patient-donor combination. Other useful systems employing numbered strips or other unique coding systems that can be attached to the patient's wristband when samples are collected and to the compatibility form and donor unit have been marketed commercially. Bar-coded identification symbols verified by portable laser scanner devices may be the system of choice in the near future for linking sample, patient, and donor products.

Whatever system is used, the information should be verified at least twice before the infusion of the product actually takes place. A copy of the original blood requisition form, left on the patient's chart after samples are collected, can be used as the request form for release of the units from the blood bank. This allows another check of the nameplate impressions on all forms to be made.

Before blood is taken from the blood bank to the patient treatment area, the person releasing and the person accepting the units should verify agreement between the donor numbers and ABO and Rh types on the compatibility form and the products themselves.

Before transfusion is initiated, a reliable professional must once again verify identity of the patient and donor products. A system of positive patient identification by comparison of wristband identification and compatibility forms must be strictly followed. This is the most critical check and yet the most fallible, since the transfusion may take place in the operating suite or emergency room, where the person responsible for identification may also be involved with numerous other duties and where confusion may contribute to misidentification.

THE FUTURE OF COMPATIBILITY TESTING

Perhaps if this book is revised in the future, the present chapter will be deleted or at least retitled. Traditional compatibility testing has outlived its usefulness in the opinion of some workers[64] who have eliminated it entirely from the spectrum of testing procedures performed for most patients. Oberman, Barnes, and Friedman[65] showed that elimination of compatibility testing, other than immediate spin readings for verification of ABO compatibility between donor and patient, had a low level of risk in emergency situations, if the patients' sera had been screened and found to lack unexpected antibodies. If this is true in emergency situations, then the same applies to routine situations.

Following the original publication of the type and screen by Boral and Henry in 1977, numerous articles have appeared[66-69] that advocate elimination of advance compatibility testing for surgical patients who are unlikely to require transfusion. Based on negative antibody screening results, the risk of incompatible transfusion caused by antibodies not detected by the antibody screening procedure is extremely low.[51] Compatibility testing is still performed when blood is actually ordered for transfusion; however, a great deal of faith is placed on the antibody screening procedure in such instances, since the compatibility test is completed, in some cases, after the donor unit has been partially or completely infused. The immediate spin confirmation of ABO compatibility is universally retained as a safeguard of the most basic and most vital measure of compatibility. Standard advance compatibility testing is generally still performed on patients whose sera demonstrate positive antibody screening results, since these patients have proven their capability of forming red cell antibodies.

The type and screen has eliminated a great deal of unnecessary blood inventory waste caused by units being held for patients when the likelihood of transfusion was almost nonexistent. In addition, this approach has greatly reduced the workload in many transfusion services, contributing to incredible savings in cost of technologist time and reagents.

While the type and screen approach has enjoyed great popularity, an alternative philosophy was presented by Rosenfield and coworkers[70] in their publication of the LIP (low ionic polycation) test for antibody detection. These workers would abolish antibody screening in favor of a highly sensitive compatibility testing procedure. The authors admitted that the presence of some potent antibodies might go unrecognized using this approach, but questioned the need to know of the presence of all antibodies in a patient's serum, as long as the donor cells selected for infusion were compatible.

Whatever the outcome of deliberations on the subject, a healthy environment for the development of new approaches for assuring safe transfusion therapy has been created. Until regulations are revised, compatibility testing will continue to be practiced, but one hopes that expedient procedures will be selected that focus attention on critical considerations for patient safety rather than blind adherence to established practices.

REFERENCES

1. HONIG, CL and BOVE, JR: *Transfusion-associated fatalities: Review of Bureau of Biologics Reports, 1976–1978.* Transfusion 20:653, 1980.

2. *Standards for Blood Banks and Transfusion Services,* ed 10. American Association of Blood Banks, Washington DC, 1981, p 25, F1.000.

3. Ibid, F2.110.

4. *Code of Federal Regulations, (CFR), Title 21, Food and Drugs.* Office of the Federal Register, National Archives and Records Service, General Services Administration, revised April 1, 1982, Section 606.151 (b).

5. GARRATTY, G: *The effects of storage and heparin on the activity of serum complement with particular reference to the detection of blood group antibodies.* Am J Clin Pathol 54:531, 1970.

6. *CFR,* op cit, Section 640.4(g)(5).

7. *Standards for Blood Banks and Transfusion Services,* op cit, p 30, H2.000.

8. *CFR,* op cit, Section 640.5(a–c).

9. Ibid, Section 610.40(a).

10. *Standards for Blood Banks and Transfusion Services,* op cit, p 14, B5.410.

11. Ibid, B5.600.

12. *CFR,* op cit, Section 640.5(b).

13. BOWMAN, HS, et al.: *Experimental transfusion of donor plasma containing blood group antibodies into incompatible normal human recipients. II. Induction of isoimmune hemolytic anemia by a transfusion of plasma containing exceptional anti-CD antibodies.* Br J Haematol 7:130, 1961.

14. Pineda, AA, Taswell, HF and Brzica, SM: *Delayed hemolytic transfusion reaction. An immunologic hazard of blood transfusion.* Transfusion 18:1, 1978.

15. Franciosi, R, Awer, E and Santana, M: *Interdonor incompatibility resulting in anuria.* Transfusion 7:297, 1967.

16. Zettner, A and Bove, JR: *Hemolytic transfusion reaction due to interdonor incompatibility.* Transfusion 3:48, 1963.

17. Mollison, PL: *Factors determining the relative clinical importance of different blood group antibodies.* Br Med Bull 15:92, 1959.

18. *Standards for Blood Banks and Transfusion Services,* op cit, p 14, B5.420.

19. *Standard Operating Procedure, American Red Cross Blood Services, Blood Services Directive 6.14, December 1979.*

20. Kitagawa, S, Lee, CL and Bezhad, O: *Donor antibody screening using plasma in place of serum.* Transfusion 19:60, 1979.

21. McKeever, BG: *Antibody screening and identification.* In Treacy, M (ed): *Pre-Transfusion Testing for the '80's.* American Association of Blood Banks, Washington, DC, 1980, p 34.

22. Graham, HA, et al.: *Antiglobulin Testing 1977: A Position Statement.* Ortho Research Institute of Medical Sciences, 1977.

23. Giblett, ER: *Blood group alloantibodies: An assessment of some laboratory practices.* Transfusion 17:299, 1977.

24. *CFR,* op cit, Section 610.40(a).

25. Ibid, Section 640.5(a).

26. Beattie, KM: *ABO grouping discrepancies.* In Henn, RL (ed): *A Seminar on Problems Encountered in Pre-Transfusion Tests.* American Association of Blood Banks, Washington, DC, 1972, pp 129–165.

27. Treacy, M: ABO *Grouping—A crucial problem.* In Treacy, M(ed): *Pre-Transfusion Testing for the 80's.* American Association of Blood Banks, Washington, DC, 1980, pp 1–12.

28. White, WD, Issitt, CH and McGuire, D: *Evaluation of the use of albumin controls in Rh typing.* Transfusion 14:67, 1974.

29. Beattie, KM: *Laboratory evaluation and management of antibody specificities in warm autoimmune hemolytic anemia.* In Bell, CA (ed): *A Seminar on Laboratory Management of Hemolysis.* American Association of Blood Banks, 1979, pp 105–134.

30. Spielmann, W and Seidl, S: *Prevalence of irregular red cell antibodies and their significance in blood transfusion and antenatal care.* Vox Sang 26:551, 1974.

31. Mollison, PL: *Blood Transfusion in Clinical Medicine,* ed 6. Blackwell Scientific Publications, Oxford, 1979, pp 483–556.

32. *Standards for Blood Banks and Transfusion Services,* op cit, p 27, G1.300.

33. Engelfriet, CP and Giles, CM: *Working party on the standardization of antiglobulin reagents of the expert panel of serology.* Vox Sang 38:178, 1980.

34. Petz, LD and Garratty, G: *Antiglobulin sera—past, present and future.* Transfusion 18:257, 1978.

35. Wright, MS and Issitt, PD: *Anticomplement and the antiglobulin test.* Transfusion 19:688, 1979.

36. Beattie, KM: *Control of the antigen-antibody ratio in antibody detection and compatibility test.* Transfusion 20:277, 1980.

37. Wright, J: *Variation on a theme by Coombs.* Can J Med Tech 29:191, 1967.

38. Hughes-Jones, NC, et al.: *Optimal conditions for detecting blood group antibodies by the antiglobulin test.* Vox Sang 9:385, 1964.

39. Issitt, PD and Issitt, CH: *Applied Blood Group Serology,* ed 2. Spectra Biologicals, Oxnard, California, 1975, p 41.

40. Steane, EA: *The interaction of antibodies with red cell surface antigens: Kinetics, noncovalent bonding and hemagglutination.* In Dawson, RB (ed): *Blood Bank Immunology.* American Association of Blood Banks, 1977, pp 61–63.

41. Stroup, M and MacIlroy, M: *Evaluation of the albumin antiglobulin technic in antibody detection.* Transfusion 5:184, 1965.

42. RECKEL, RP and HARRIS, J: *The unique characteristics of covalently polymerized bovine serum albumin solutions when used as antibody detection media.* Transfusion 18:397, 1978.

43. MOULDS, JJ: *Multiple antibodies and antibodies to high incidence blood group factors.* In Dawson, RB (ed): *Troubleshooting the Crossmatch.* American Association of Blood Banks, Washington, DC, 1977, pp 67–84.

44. McKEEVER, BG, op cit, pp 409–50.

45. ISSITT, PD: *On the incidence of second antibody populations in the sera of women who have developed anti-Rh antibodies.* Transfusion 5:355, 1965.

46. ISSITT, PD, et al.: *Three examples of Rh-positive good responders to blood group antigens.* Transfusion 13:316, 1972.

47. DAVEY, RJ, GUSTAFSON, M and HOLLAND, PV: *Accelerated immune red cell destruction in the absence of serologically demonstrable alloantibodies.* Transfusion 20:348, 1980.

48. VAN LOGHEM, JJ, et al.: *Increased red cell destruction in the absence of demonstrable antibodies.* Transfusion 5:525, 1965.

49. SNYDER, EL, et al.: *Hemolytic anti-hr" (e) detectable solely by an automated polybrene technique.* Transfusion 18:79, 1978.

50. MOLLISON, PL: *Blood Transfusion in Clinical Medicine,* op cit, p 314.

51. WALKER, RH: *Is crossmatching utilizing the indirect antiglobulin test necessary for patients with a negative antibody screen?* Presented in part at the University of Michigan, June 1977.

52. GROVE-RASMUSSEN, M: *Routine compatibility testing: Standards of the AABB as applied to compatibility tests.* Transfusion 4:200, 1964.

53. *Standards for Blood Banks and Transfusion Services,* op cit, p 27, G1.200, G1.300.

54. CFR, op cit, Section 606.151(c).

55. BORAL, LI and HENRY, JB: *The type and screen: A safe alternative and supplement in selected surgical procedures.* Transfusion 17:165, 1977.

56. CFR, op cit, Section 606.151(d).

57. Ibid, Section 606.151(c).

58. *Standards for Blood Banks and Transfusion Services,* op cit, p 27, G1.300.

59. GREEN, TS: *Rouleaux and autoantibodies (or things that go bump in the night).* In Treacy, M (ed): *Pre-Transfusion Testing for the '80's.* American Association of Blood Banks, Washington, DC, 1980, p 93.

60. *Tests for serologic incompatibility (crossmatching).* In Widman, FK (ed): *Technical Manual.* American Association of Blood Banks, Washington, DC, 1981, p 216.

61. MOLLISON, PL: *Blood Transfusion in Clinical Medicine,* op cit, pp 26–32.

62. SCHANFIELD, MS: *Human immunoglobulin (IgG) subclasses and their biological properties.* In Dawson, RB (ed): *Blood Bank Immunology.* American Association of Blood Banks, Washington, DC, 1977, p 106.

63. *Standards for Blood Banks and Transfusion Services,* op cit, p 30, H1.110, H1.120, H1.200.

64. ROUAULT, C: *Appropriate pre-transfusion testing.* In Treacy, M (ed): *Pre-Transfusion Testing for the '80's.* American Association of Blood Banks, Washington, DC, pp 125–132.

65. OBERMAN, HA, BARNES, BA and FRIEDMAN, BA: *The risk of abbreviating the major crossmatch in urgent or massive transfusion.* Transfusion 18:137, 1978.

66. ROUAULT, C and GRUENHAGEN, J: *Reorganization of Blood Ordering Practices.* Transfusion 18:448, 1978.

67. MINTZ, PD, NORDINE, RB and HENRY, JB: *Expected hemotherapy in elective surgery.* NY State J Med 76:532, 1976.

68. HENRY, JB, MINTZ, PD and WEBB, W: *Optimal blood ordering for elective surgery.* JAMA 237:451, 1977.

69. HUANG, ST, et al.: *Type and hold for better blood utilization.* Transfusion 20:725, 1980.

70. ROSENFIELD, RE, et al.: *Augmentation of hemagglutination by low ionic conditions.* Transfusion 19:499, 1979.

APPENDIX 1

PREPARATION OF WASHED "DRY" BUTTON OF RED CELLS FOR SEROLOGIC TESTS

1. Transfer a small amount of red cells using an applicator stick into a 10 × 75 mm or 12 × 75 mm test tube filled with saline. Tube should be prelabeled to identify contents.

2. Centrifuge at high speed, until red cells are collected into a tight button at the bottom of the tube.

3. Decant saline by quick inversion of the tube over a receptacle. Flick last drop of saline from cells by giving tube a quick shake while still in inverted position.

4. Add serum directly to "dry" button of cells. Method can be utilized for antibody screening or identification procedures, compatibility testing, and cell typing using a tube technique.

APPENDIX 2

MODEL ONE-TUBE PER DONOR UNIT COMPATIBILITY TESTING PROCEDURE

Note: No minor side compatibility test is performed.

1. Into an appropriately labeled, 10 × 75 mm or 12 × 75 mm test tube, dispense 1 drop of a washed, 2 to 5 percent suspension of donor red cells. (Alternatively, prepare a washed "dry" button of donor red cells, using the technique in Appendix 1.)

2. Add 2 or 3 drops of serum to the tube to achieve an approximate 2:1 ratio of serum to red cells. (Droppers used to dispense red cells and serum should be of equivalent size.)

3. Centrifuge at a speed and for a time that has been previously shown to give clear-cut differentiation between positive and negative results (15 seconds in a Serofuge is usually adequate).

4. Observe supernatant for hemolysis that must be considered indicative of an antigen-antibody interaction. Resuspend cell button by *gentle* manipulation of the tube. Grade all positive results. Record observations.

5. Add 2 drops of 22 percent bovine albumin to the tube (may be omitted, if desired). Mix and incubate for 30 minutes at 37°C. *Note:* If LISS is added to tests at this stage in place of albumin, decrease incubation time to 15 minutes.

6. Centrifuge, as above, observe supernatant, resuspend cells, and record results.

7. Wash 3 to 4 times using an automated instrument or manual washing technique. Decant saline completely from last wash.

8. Add 1 to 2 drops of antiglobulin serum to tube. (Follow manufacturer's directions for use of reagent selected.) Centrifuge, resuspend cells, and record results. Tubes must be examined macroscopically and microscopically.

9. Add 1 drop IgG presensitized red cells (Coombs control cells) to each negative test. Centrifuge and examine. Test must be *positive* or results of procedure are invalid, and test must be repeated.

CHAPTER 12

DETECTION AND IDENTIFICATION OF ALLOANTIBODIES

ANNA J. BALDWIN, MT(ASCP)SBB

Antibody detection and identification are two of the most interesting and challenging areas in all immunohematology, particularly for the student. They are the "icing on the cake" for the student who is learning blood banking principles and procedures. Most patients do not possess alloantibodies in their serum, however, and students should keep this fact in mind. Most daily blood banking consists of ABO and Rh testing, antibody screening (usually negative), and compatibility testing. Also, medical technology students should not, after performing a handful of antibody identifications, consider themselves experts in this endeavor. Many patient antibody problems are complex, requiring a great deal of time and expertise on the part of the investigator. This expertise is obtainable by each student, given the time, desire, and experience in blood banking.

    This chapter attempts to introduce the student to the methods in current use for antibody detection. A method of approaching antibody problems, some typical examples, and further studies that can be performed are discussed. This chapter is not designed to be a step-by-step protocol for performing these tests. This area is better left to the instructor in the academic or clinical setting who can personally guide the student and suggest alternative paths of investigation for each specific unknown sample.

ANTIBODY DETECTION

Nearly all patients whose blood is tested in a blood bank laboratory will have an antibody screen performed on their sera. This antibody detection usually encompasses testing the patient's serum against two or three reagent group O screening cells and an autocontrol (patient serum X patient cells). Screening cells are commercially prepared cell suspensions from *individual* donors that are phenotyped for most common antigens. They may be used individually or, in some cases, pooled (as for donor testing). Group O donors are selected so that reactions will not be masked by ABO incompatibility between patient and reagent.

Testing is done under a variety of conditions; however, there are very few requirements as to which methodology is to be used. Generally, testing consists of the following:

1. An immediate spin phase (not required)
2. Room temperature incubation (no longer routinely performed)
3. 37°C incubation (with or without enhancement media)
4. An antiglobulin phase (required)

The immediate spin (IS) phase has essentially replaced room temperature incubation, which is neither required nor advocated. A major ABO incompatibility (e.g., O patient, B donor) should be detected in most circumstances by a simple IS test. However, even this procedure is not required and need not be performed.

Testing at 37°C is required as the preliminary step of the Coombs phase (antiglobulin test). In addition, some clinically significant antibodies are readily detectable after 37° incubation. Again, there are no regulations on how to perform this test. Examples include the following:

1. 30 minutes, no enhancement (saline only)
2. 15 to 30 minutes, bovine albumin (22 percent, 30 percent, polymerized)
3. 5 to 15 minutes, low ionic enhancement media

Obviously, there is a great deal of flexibility in this procedure; however, performance of the antiglobulin test is mandatory.[1] Even so, there is some flexibility here. Most institutions use polyspecific antiglobulin serum as the concluding step in antibody screening, while others have switched to monospecific anti-IgG serum. There is a twofold rationale for the use of monospecific serum:

1. There is still a great deal of controversy regarding the necessity of an anticomplement component in antiglobulin serum. Some workers feel that clinically significant antibodies that are *only* detectable by the anti-complement and not by the anti-IgG of polyspecific Coombs' serum are rare.
2. Interference from naturally occurring cold agglutinins in patient's sera is to-

tally eliminated. The advantages of this approach will become obvious with the first complement-binding cold autoantibody encountered by the student.

ANTIBODY IDENTIFICATION

Now that we have reviewed the many ways of performing antibody screening, we must ask the question, "What should be done when an antibody is detected?" If time permits, the antibody screen may be repeated to ensure that the test was performed correctly. Also, if the original test incorporated polyspecific antihuman serum (Coombs' serum), a repeat test using monospecific anti-IgG may provide helpful information.

It is suggested that the investigator consider the following questions:

1. In what phase(s) did the reaction(s) occur?
2. Is the autocontrol negative or positive?
3. If all screening cells reacted, were the reactions
   (a) In the same or different phases?
   (b) The same or different strengths?
4. Are the cells truly agglutinated, or are rouleaux present?
5. Is hemolysis present?

Figure 12-1 illustrates some of the results that may be observed in antibody screening.

The next step of the procedure involves performing an antibody identification or panel. The manufacturers who market antibody screening cells also market these panels. A panel consists of 8 to 16 individual group-O donor cell suspensions and an accompanying antigenic profile on each of these cells. Some manufacturers also include pooled cord cells as part of their panel.

The antigenic profile usually *states* whether the donor cell is positive or negative for the following antigens:

D, C, E, c, e, occasionally V, VS, f, C^w (the probable Rh genotype is also given)
M, N, S, s
Fy^a, Fy^b
Jk^a, Jk^b
K, k, occasionally Kp^a, Kp^b, Js^a, Js^b
Lu^a, Lu^b
Le^a, Le^b
P_1
Xg^a

Other blood groups may be included on each individual profile; in addition, rare cells are also noted, particularly cells lacking a high-frequency antigen (U, Vel, Yt^a) or possessing a low-frequency antigen (Wr^a, Co^b, Kp^a).

cell	IS	37°	AGT (poly)
SC I	neg	neg	neg
SC II	neg	neg	2+
auto	neg	neg	neg

1. Single alloantibody
2. Two alloantibodies, antigen only present on cell II
3. Probable IgG antibody

cell	IS	37°	AGT
SC I	neg	1+	3+
SC II	neg	neg	1+
auto	neg	neg	neg

1. Multiple antibodies
2. Single antibody (dosage)
3. Probably IgG

cell	IS	37°	AGT
SC I	1+	neg	neg
SC II	2+	neg	neg
auto	neg	neg	neg

1. Single or multiple alloantibodies
2. Probably IgM antibodies

cell	IS	37°	AGT
SC I	2+	neg	1+
SC II	3+	1+	2+
auto	neg	neg	neg

1. Multiple antibodies, warm and cold
2. Potent cold antibody binding complement in AGT

cell	IS	37°	AGT
SC I	neg	neg	1+
SC II	neg	neg	1+
auto	neg	neg	neg

1. Single warm antibody, present on both cells
2. Antibody to high-frequency antigen
3. Complement binding by a cold antibody not detected at IS

FIGURE 12-1. Examples of reactions that may be observed in antibody detection tests.

Figures 12-2 and 12-3 illustrate a typical antibody screening cell profile and panel sheet. The panel cells are tested in the same manner as the original screen of the patient's serum and all results are noted in the spaces provided on the panel sheet. It is also helpful to acquire a complete patient history that includes previous transfusion, pregnancy, medications, and other helpful information including age, sex, and diagnosis. This may facilitate interpreting the results of the panel. It is also extremely important that the reaction strengths be graded accurately, as this may aid in recognizing dosage and multiple antibodies.

When all reactions have been recorded and the test completed, an interpretation can be attempted. A rapid and simple method for interpreting panels is the so-called "ruling-out" or "crossing-out" method. This involves exclusion of possible antibodies based on their nonreactivity with panel cells possessing the appropriate antigen. To state this another way, if the patient's serum is nonreactive with a panel cell in *all* phases of testing, then antibodies directed against the antigens on that cell are probably *not* present in the serum being tested.

Figure 12-4 shows a panel in which anti-rh" (E) has been identified and all other antibodies ruled out by crossing-out. Cell 1 is negative in all phases, so that one would go *across* that line and cross out all antigens that this cell possesses (i.e., c, e, f, M, S, s, P_1, Tj^a, Le^b, Lu^a, k, Kp^b, Js^b, Fy^a, Fy^b, Jk^b). Cell 2 eliminates N, K, Xg^a. Cell 3 eliminates C, V. The student should complete the exercise for verification of this conclusion. Cells 4, 5, and 10 cannot be used because they show reactivity. Reactions need not be present in all phases; one phase is sufficient in this case. (Note that this figure also demonstrates dosage, which the student should recognize.)

This method is quite applicable when only one antibody is present or if simple multiple specificities are present, such as anti-K and anti-D. When only a few panel

---

Dade®

Search-Cyte®
Reagent Red Blood
Cells 5±1%

Lot No.: CE5-257

Mfg. Date: 3 Feb 82

Exp. Date: 26 Mar 82

Antigenic Constitution Matrix*

Vial No.	Rh-hr	Donor Code	Special Typings	D	C	E	c	e	f	Cw	V	M	N	S	s	P1	Tja	Lea	Leb	Lua	Lub	K	k	Kpa	Kpb	Jsa	Jsb	Fya	Fyb	Jka	Jkb	Xga
CE5-1 257	R₁r (CDe/cde)	F686BA	Co (b+)	+	+	0	+	+	+	0	0	0	+	+	+	+	+	0	+	0	+	+	+	0	+	0	+	+	+	+	+	+
CE5-2 257	R₂r (cDE/cde)	F826BA	Co (b+)	+	0	+	+	+	+	0	0	0	+	+	+	+	+	0	0	0	+	0	+	0	+	0	+	+	+	+	0	+

(column groups: Rh-hr = D C E c e f Cw V; MNS = M N S s; P = P1; Tja; Lewis = Lea Leb; Lutheran = Lua Lub; Kell = K k Kpa Kpb Jsa Jsb; Duffy = Fya Fyb; Kidd = Jka Jkb; Sex Linked = Xga)

Additional Comments: All antigen typings listed are confirmed using two sources of antiserum except for the following which are confirmed with one source: f, Tj*, Lu*, Js*, Jk*, Xg*, Vel, Yt*, Ge, Di*, Di*, V*, and Co*. These are confirmed with a second serum source when available.

Unless otherwise indicated, both Search-Cyte Cells are positive for the following antigens: Tj^a, Lu^b, k, Kp^b, Js^b, I, Ge, U, Yt^a, Vel and Di^b.

Unless otherwise indicated, both Search-Cyte Cells are negative for the following antigens: f, C^w, V, Lu^a, Kp^a, Js^a, M9, V^w, Wr^a and Di^a.

American Dade
Division of
American Hospital Supply Corporation
Miami FL USA 33152

U.S. License No. 179

FIGURE 12-2. Antigen profile of antibody screening cells.

MODERN BLOOD BANKING AND TRANSFUSION PRACTICES

Dade®
Data-File
Antigenic Constitution Matrix*

Lot No.: DC-258
Mfg. Date: 6 Jan 82
Exp. Date: 26 Feb 82

Data-Cyte® Reagent Red Blood Cells 3±1%

Name _____ Pt. I.D. No. _____
Age _____ Sex _____ Race _____ Date Drawn _____
Blood Group _____ Most Probable Rh Genotype _____ Direct Antiglobulin _____
Interpretation _____
Technologist _____ Date Tested _____

Vial No.	Rh-hr	Donor Code	Special Typings
1	rr (cde/cde)	E968	
2	rr (cde/cde)	F411BM	
3	r′r (Cde/cde)	E714BA	
4	r″r (cdE/cde)	E427BA	
5	R₂r (cDE/cde)	F688BM	U–
6	rr (cde/cde)	7468	
7	R₁R₁ (CDe/CDe)	D570	
8	R₁R₁ (CDe/CDe)	F333BM	Bg–
9	R₁R₁ʷ (CDe/CʷDe)	F516BA	
10	R₂R₂ (CDE/cDE)	F781HM	
11	R₁R₁ (CDe/CDe)	E715BA	Bg–
Auto			
SCI†			
SCII†			

†Search-Cyte® Reagent Red Blood Cells

Additional Comments: All antigen typings listed are confirmed using two sources of antiserums except for the following which are confirmed with one source: I, Tjᵃ, Jsᵃ, Jsᵇ, Kpᵃ, Vel, Yᵗᵃ, Gₑ, bᵇ, Dʷ, Vʷ, and Coᵃ. These are confirmed with a second serum source when available.
** The S antigen on this cell is variable and may show variable positive or negative reactions with different sources of antisera.

FIGURE 12-3. Antigen profile of a typical panel.

Dade®

Data-File Antigenic Constitution Matrix*

Lot No.: DC-258
Mfg. Date: 6 Jan 82
Exp. Date: 26 Feb 82

Data-Cyte® Reagent Red Blood Cells 3±1%

Name ______ Pt. I.D. No. ______
Age ______ Sex ______ Race ______ Date Drawn ______
Blood Group ______ Most Probable Rh Genotype ______ Direct Antiglobulin ______
Interpretation ______
Technologist ______ Date Tested ______

Vial No.	Rh-hr	Donor Code	Special Typings	Rh-hr								MNS				P		Lewis		Lutheran		Kell						Duffy		Kidd		Sex Linked
				D	C	E	c	e	f	C^w	V	M	N	S	s	P_1	Tj^a	Le^a	Le^b	Lu^a	Lu^b	K	k	Kp^a	Kp^b	Js^a	Js^b	Fy^a	Fy^b	Jk^a	Jk^b	Xg^a
1	rr (cde/cde)	E958		0	0	0	+	+	+	0	0	+	0	+	+	+	+	0	+	+	+	0	+	0	+	0	+	+	+	0	+	0
2	rr (cde/cde)	F411BM		0	0	0	+	+	+	0	0	0	+	0	+	+	+	0	+	0	+	+	+	0	+	0	+	0	+	0	+	+
3	r′r (Cde/cde)	E714BA		0	+	0	+	+	+	0	+	0	+	0	+	0	+	0	+	0	+	0	+	0	+	0	+	0	+	0	+	+
4	r″r (cdE/cde)	E427BA		0	0	+	+	+	+	0	0	+	+	0	+	$+^s$	+	+	0	0	+	0	+	0	+	0	+	+	+	0	+	0
5	R_2r (cDE/cde)	F688BM	U−	+	0	+	+	+	+	0	0	0	+	0	0	$+^w$	+	+	0	0	+	0	+	0	+	0	+	0	0	+	0	+
6	rr (cde/cde)	7468		0	0	0	+	+	+	0	0	+	+	+	+	+	+	0	0	0	+	0	+	0	+	+	+	0	+	+	0	+
7	R_1R_1 (CDe/CDe)	D570		+	+	0	0	+	0	0	0	+	0	+	0	0	+	+	0	+	+	0	+	0	+	0	+	0	+	+	+	+
8	R_1R_1 (CDe/CDe)	F333BM	Bg−	+	+	0	0	+	0	0	0	+	0	+	+	0	+	0	+	0	+	+	0	0	+	0	+	+	0	+	+	+
9	$R_1R_1^w$ (CDe/C^wDe)	F516BA		+	+	0	0	+	0	+	0	+	+	0	+	$+^w$	+	0	+	0	+	0	+	0	+	0	+	0	+	0	+	+
10	R_2R_2 (CDE/cDE)	F781HM		+	$+^w$	+	+	0	0	0	0	+	0	$+^{**}$	+	+	+	0	+	0	+	0	+	0	+	0	+	+	+	+	+	+
11	R_1R_1 (CDe/CDe)	E715BA	Bg −	+	+	0	0	+	0	0	0	+	0	+	+	$+^{vw}$	+	0	+	0	+	0	+	+	+	0	+	0	+	+	+	+
Auto																																
SCI†																																
SCII†																																

Vial No.	Saline			High Protein			CC	Brom
	I.S			37	AGT			
1	0			0	0			
2	0			0	0			
3	0			0	0			
4	0			$+^w$	1+			
5	0			$+^w$	1+			
6	0			0	0			
7	0			0	0			
8	0			0	0			
9	0			0	0			
10	0			1+	2+			
11	0			0	0			
Auto								
SCI†								
SCII†								

Lot No.								
	A_1 cells							
	A_2 cells							
	B cells							
	Cord							

†**Search-Cyte® Reagent Red Blood Cells** Lot No.

Additional Comments:* All antigen typings listed are confirmed using two sources of antiserums except for the following which are confirmed with one source: f, Tj^a, Lu^a, Js^a, Jk^b, Xg^a, Vel, Yt^a, Ge, Di^b, Di^a, V^w, and Co^b. These are confirmed with a second serum source when available.

** The S antigen on this cell is variable and may show variable positive or negative reactions with different sources of antisera.

FIGURE 12-4. Single antibody.

cells are nonreactive, the number of antibodies that can be eliminated decreases. Figure 12-5 demonstrates such a situation. In this case, it is helpful to see whether any one pattern is evident (i.e., if all the reactive cells are positive for a particular antigen). This is exemplified in Figure 12-5, where anti-Jk^b can be identified. In this situation, several more Jk^b-negative cells (from other panels) should also be tested in order to "rule out" other clinically significant antibodies, such as anti-C, anti-Kell, and anti-Fy^a, which could not be ruled out in the original panel. In addition, some laboratories may routinely use different media to "rule out" or "rule in" identifiable antibodies (e.g., low ionic strength media or enzymes). However, in all media used to identify antibodies there should be three positive panel cells and three negative panel cells in order to establish a 95-percent confidence level for this procedure.[2]

COMPLEX ANTIBODY PROBLEMS

If a definite antibody pattern is not evident, then several possibilities exist, such as multiple and high-frequency antibodies. These possibilities especially should be considered when all panel cells react. Figure 12-6 is an example of the presence of multiple antibodies (anti-Le^a, anti-K, and anti-Fy^a). In this example it is helpful to note that two of the antibodies react at immediate spin, while the third does not. Multiple antibody specificities are often more complex than this figure implies.

Figure 12-7 shows the typical reactivity of an antibody to a high-frequency antigen. In this situation, one would see reactions with all cells tested except the autocontrol. Resolving this type of problem is *very* difficult since a battery of reagent cells lacking high-frequency antigens must be acquired and tested. A review of high-frequency antigens is found in Chapter 9. A phenomenon that may mimic a high-frequency antibody is rouleau formation. This phenomenon, which results from serum protein abnormalities, is observed in IS, room temperature (if performed), and 37°C phases of testing. It should *not* appear in the antiglobulin phase, because washing removes *all* the serum. Macroscopically, rouleaux mimic agglutination and should be seen in all tubes, including the autocontrol. Microscopically, the characteristic "stack-of-coins" conformation should be clearly visible. Color Plate 2 depicts the appearance of rouleaux and agglutination microscopically for the purpose of comparison.

If rouleaux are noted, the addition of a drop or two of saline to the tube can be used to ascertain whether there is any true antigen-antibody activity. Rouleaux would disperse; a true reaction would not show dispersal. For strong rouleaux, saline replacement techniques are available.

Another difficult situation to evaluate is the presence of autoantibodies. Usually, an autoantibody will react with all or most of the panel cells. Reactivity in the autocontrol should alert the student to this possibility. A discussion of autoantibodies and their serologic activity can be found in Chapter 19. One note of caution to the student: a positive autocontrol does not automatically indicate autoantibodies. As an example, if a patient were recently transfused and suffered a delayed hemolytic transfusion reaction, the donor cells still present in the patient's circulation

Dade®
Data-File
Antigenic Constitution Matrix*

Lot No.: DC-258
Mfg. Date: 6 Jan 82
Exp. Date: 26 Feb 82

Date-Cyte® Reagent Red Blood Cells 3±1%

Name _____ Pt. I.D. No. _____
Age _____ Sex _____ Race _____ Date Drawn _____
Blood Group _____ Most Probable Rh Genotype _____ Direct Antiglobulin _____
Interpretation _____
Technologist _____ Date Tested _____

Vial No.	Rh-hr	Donor Code	Special Typings	Vial No.	Saline	High Protein (37 / AGT)
1	rr (cde/cde)	E958		1	0	0 / 1+
2	rr (cde/cde)	F411BM		2	0	0 / 1+
3	r'r (Cde/cde)	E714BA		3	0	0 / 1+
4	r"r (cdE/cde)	E427BA		4	0	0 / 1+
5	R₂r (cDE/cde)	F688BM	U–	5	0	0 / 0
6	rr (cde/cde)	7468		6	0	0 / 0
7	R₁R₁ (CDe/CDe)	D570		7	0	0 / 1+
8	R₁R₁ (CDe/CDe)	F333BM	Bg–	8	0	0 / 1+
9	R₁R" (CDe/C"De)	F516BA		9	0	0 / 1+
10	R₂R₂ (cDE/cDE)	F781HM		10	0	0 / 1+
11	R₁R₁ (CDe/CDe)	E715BA	Bg–	11	0	0 / 1+
Auto				Auto		
SCI†				SCI†		
SCII†				SCII†		

Antigen column groups (across): Rh-hr (D, C, E, c, e, f, Cw, V); MNS (M, N, S, s); P (P1, Tja); Lewis (Lea, Leb); Lutheran (Lua, Lub); Kell (K, k, Kpa, Kpb, Jsa, Jsb); Duffy (Fya, Fyb); Kidd (Jka, Jkb, Xga)

Lot No. ____

Lot No.	A₁ cells	A₂ cells	B cells	Cord

†**Search-Cyte® Reagent Red Blood Cells**

Additional Comments: All antigen typings listed are confirmed using two sources of antiserums except for the following which are confirmed with one source: I, Tja, Lua, Jsa, Jkb, Xga, Vel, Yta, Gea, Dib, Dia, Wra, and Coa. These are confirmed with a second serum source when available.
**The S antigen on this cell is variable and may show variable positive or negative reactions with different sources of antisera.

FIGURE 12-5. Single antibody.

Name _____ Pt. I.D. No. _____

Age _____ Sex _____ Race _____ Date Drawn _____

Blood Group _____ Most Probable Rh Genotype _____

Interpretation _____ Direct Antiglobulin _____

Technologist _____ Date Tested _____

Dade®
Data-File
Antigenic Constitution Matrix*

Lot No.: DC-258
Mfg. Date: 6 Jan 82
Exp. Date: 26 Feb 82

Data-Cyte® Reagent Red Blood Cells 3±1%

Vial No.	Rh-hr	Donor Code	Special Typings
1	rr (cde/cde)	E958	
2	rr (cde/cde)	F411BM	
3	r'r (Cde/cde)	E714BA	
4	r"r (cdE/cde)	E427BA	
5	R₂r (cdE/cde)	F688BM	U −
6	rr (cde/cde)	7468	
7	R₁R₁ (CDe/CDe)	D570	
8	R₁R₁ (CDe/CDe)	F333BM	Bg −
9	R₁R₁ʷ (CDe/CʷDe)	F516BA	
10	R₂R₂ (cDE/cDE)	F781HM	
11	R₁R₁ (CDe/CDe)	E715BA	Bg −
Auto			
SCI†			
SCII†			

†Search-Cyte® Reagent Red Blood Cells

Additional Comments: All antigen typings listed are confirmed using two sources of antisera except for the following which are confirmed with one source: I, Tjᵃ, Luᵇ, Jsᵃ, Jsᵇ, Jkᵃ, Xgᵃ, Vel, Ytᵃ, Ge, Diᵃ, Diᵇ, Vᵂ, and Coᵇ. These are confirmed with a second serum source when available.
** The S antigen on this cell is variable and may show variable positive or negative reactions with different sources of antisera.

Lot No. _____

Lot No.		
A₁ cells		
A₂ cells		
B cells		
Cord		

FIGURE 12-6. Multiple antibodies.

Dade®
Data-File
Antigenic Constitution Matrix*

Lot No.: DC-258
Mfg. Date: 6 Jan 82
Exp. Date: 26 Feb 82

Data-Cyte® Reagent Red Blood Cells 3±1%

Name _____ Pt. I.D. No. _____
Age _____ Sex _____ Race _____ Date Drawn _____
Blood Group _____ Most Probable Rh Genotype _____ Direct Antiglobulin _____
Interpretation _____
Technologist _____ Date Tested _____

Vial No.	Rh-hr	Donor Code	Special Typings	D	C	E	c	e	f	Cʷ	V	M	N	S	s	P₁	Tjᵃ	Leᵃ	Leᵇ	Luᵃ	Luᵇ	K	k	Kpᵃ	Kpᵇ	Jsᵃ	Jsᵇ	Fyᵃ	Fyᵇ	Jkᵃ	Jkᵇ	Xgᵃ	Vial No.	Saline	High Protein	CC	Brom
1	rr (cde/cde)	E958		0	0	0	+	+	+	0	0	0	0	+	+	+	+	0	+	0	+	0	+	0	+	+	0	+	+	0	+	0	1				
2	rr (cde/cde)	F411BM		0	0	0	+	+	+	0	0	0	+	0	+	+	+	+	0	0	+	0	+	0	+	0	+	0	0	+	+	+	2				
3	r'r (Cde/cde)	E714BA		0	+	0	+	+	+	0	0	+	0	0	+	0	+	0	+	0	+	0	+	0	+	0	0	0	0	+	+	0	3				
4	r'r (cdE/cde)	E427BA		0	0	+	+	+	+	0	0	0	+	0	+	0	+	0	+	0	+	0	+	0	+	0	+	0	0	+	+	0	4				
5	R₂R (cDE/cde)	F688BM	U–	+	0	+	+	+	+	0	+	+	0	0	+	+	+	0	0	0	+	0	+	0	0	0	0	0	0	+	5				
6	rr (cde/cde)	7468		0	0	0	+	+	+	0	0	0	+	0	0	+	+	0	+	0	+	0	+	0	+	0	+	+	0	+	0	6				
7	R₁R₁ (CDe/CDe)	D570		+	+	0	0	+	0	0	0	+	0	0	+	+	+	0	+	0	+	0	+	0	+	0	+	+	0	+	7				
8	R₁R₁ (CDe/CDe)	F333BM	Bg–	+	+	0	0	+	0	0	0	0	+	0	+	+	+	0	+	0	+	0	+	0	+	+	+	+	+	8				
9	R₁R₁ˣ (CDe/CʷDe)	F516BA		+	+	0	0	+	0	+	0	+	0	0	+	0	+	0	0	+	0	+	0	+	0	0	+	0	+	9				
10	R₂R₂ (cDE/cDE)	F781HM		+	0	+	0	0	0	0	0	0	+	0	+	+	+	0	0	+	0	+	0	+	+	0	+	+	+	10				
11	R₁R₂ (CDe/cDe)	E715BA	Bg –	+	+	0	0	0	0	0	+	0	0	+	+	+	0	+	0	+	0	+	0	+	+	+	+	+	11				
Auto																																	Auto				
SCI¹																																	SCI¹				
SCII¹																																	SCII¹				

Lot No. _____

¹Search-Cyte® Reagent Red Blood Cells

Additional Comments:* All antigen typings listed are confirmed using two sources of antiserums except for the following which are confirmed with one source: I, Tjᵃ, Luᵃ, Jsᵃ, Xgᵃ, Vel, Ytᵃ, Gₑ, Dⁱ, Dⁱ, Ytᵇ, and Coᵇ. These are confirmed with a second serum source when available.
** The S antigen on this cell is variable and may show variable positive or negative reactions with different sources of antisera.

Lot No.	
A₁ cells	
A₂ cells	
B cells	
Cord	

FIGURE 12-7. Antibody to high-frequency antigen.

would become coated with antibody. This could result in a positive autocontrol as well as a positive direct antiglobulin test (DAT). The patient's *own* cells would not be coated, but the specimen being tested would of necessity be a mixture of patient *and* donor cells, resulting in positive reactions. The antibody or antibodies in the patient's serum are *allo*antibodies, in spite of the positive autocontrol.

Finally, one must be aware of the possible presence of the so-called "high-titer, low-avidity" antibodies or HTLA. This subject is also reviewed in Chapter 9 but is mentioned here for the purpose of completeness. These antibodies will show reactivity with all or most panel cells in the antiglobulin phase, but the reactions tend to be weak and questionable and often are *not* reproducible. Confirming the presence of these antibodies also requires the use of rare cells, as well as titration studies to demonstrate their titer and avidity characteristics.

PHENOTYPING THE PATIENT

Once an antibody has been identified, the technologist must ensure that the patient indeed lacks the corresponding antigen. Phenotyping the patient for all antigens against which he demonstrates antibodies is the final step of the identification process. Unless the patient is suffering from an autoimmune hemolytic anemia, he should lack the offending antigen(s). Commercially prepared reagent antisera are readily available for this purpose.

It should be noted that phenotyping patient cells with an antiglobulin-reactive typing serum (e.g., commercial anti-Fy[a], anti-Jk[a]) in the presence of a positive DAT presents problems. These coated cells would type positive for the antigen regardless of whether it is present or not and therefore, the results would be invalid. There are, however, elution procedures that can be performed to remove the coating antibody; this may then render the cells capable of being typed with these AGT-reactive typing sera.

If blood is being sought for the patient, the donor units to be transfused also should be phenotyped for the offending antigen(s), particularly when the antibody in the patient's serum is a clinically significant one reactive at 37°C. It is not always necessary to phenotype donors when the patient's antibody is not considered clinically significant. Crossmatch-compatible blood may be adequate for issue (review Chapter 11).

ADDITIONAL METHODS OF RESOLUTION

Finally, some comments need to be made about how to approach inconclusive panel studies. There are many procedures that can be incorporated when an initial antibody identification does not present clear-cut specificities. These include the following:

ENZYME PRETREATMENT OF PANEL CELLS. This is known as the two-stage enzyme technique. As the name suggests, reagent cells are first incubated with a proteolytic enzyme solution that cleaves proteins from the red cell membrane. The cells are then washed to remove the enzyme and used for testing. Enzyme pretreatment makes some antigens more accessible to their corresponding antibodies but destroys others (review Chapters 5 through 9). Also note that enzymes strongly enhance *most* cold autoantibodies, particularly auto-anti-I.

ONE-STAGE ENZYME TECHNIQUE. Adding a proteolytic enzyme directly to the serum-cell mixture will have essentially the same effect as pretreating the cells, but the end-result may not be as sensitive. Also, some antibody activity may be lost by the action of the enzyme on the immunoglobulin molecule itself.

ACIDIFICATION OF THE SERUM. This procedure may enhance some antibodies, particularly anti-M. A pH of 6.5 is obtained by mixing a $^1/_{10}$ volume of 0.2 N HCl with one volume of serum.[3]

INCUBATION AT ROOM TEMPERATURE OR COLDER. If weak reactions are noted on IS and in the antiglobulin phase, a weak cold-reactive alloantibody may be present. Its activity may be enhanced by allowing the tubes to incubate at room temperature for approximately 15 minutes. If this procedure is not conclusive, incubating at 15 to 18°C may provide conclusive identification. It even may be necessary to incubate at 4°C in some cases, but these 4°C-reactive antibodies are not considered clinically significant; their identification may be purely academic. An autocontrol must be tested simultaneously at colder temperatures as a means of distinguishing cold alloantibodies from cold autoantibodies.

INCREASED SERUM: CELL RATIO. Instead of using two drops of serum, the panel is repeated with four drops per tube. Enhanced reactivity may then be demonstrated, because a greater concentration of antibody is now available for binding to red cells. HTLA antibodies usually do *not* show increased reactivity with this procedure.

USE OF RARE CELLS. Manufacturers of panels occasionally include rare cells in their kits (U neg, Tj^a neg, k neg, Yt^a neg, I neg, null phenotype cells). These may be kept in the liquid state well beyond their expiration dates and used if all panel cells react. Although antibodies to high-frequency antigens are uncommon, they do occur. If the serum reactions suggest such an antibody, a panel of "high-incidence negative" cells should be tested. These cells may also be frozen in liquid N$_2$ and maintained for long periods of time, if such equipment is available.

NEUTRALIZATION. Certain antibodies may be neutralized when reacted with antigen-specific substances. The serum will no longer react with panel cells bearing the corresponding antigen. This practice is useful in confirming a specificity or in removing an unwanted antibody that may be masking other antibodies. Lewis and P_1 blood group substances are commercially available (Ortho Diagnostics Systems) and are easy to use. Other "homemade" neutralizing substances include hydatid cyst fluid—P_1 antigen; urine (fresh)—Sd^a antigen; saliva—ABO antigens; plasma—Chido and Rogers; and human milk—Ii.

REFERENCE LABORATORIES. These laboratories perform a vital service in that they can (usually) identify the more complex antibody problems, or confirm a hospital laboratory's results. They are well equipped with rare sera and cells and, on occasion, may not charge a fee for their services. In addition, they may also be a source of rare bloods for patients who require such donor bloods. The American Red Cross and the American Association of Blood Banks provide numerous reference laboratories throughout the United States.

REFERENCES

1. *Standards for Blood Banks and Transfusion Services*, ed 10. American Association of Blood Banks, Washington, DC, 1981.
2. *Detection and identification of red blood cell antibodies.* In WIDMANN, FK (ed): *Technical Manual*, ed 8. American Association of Blood Banks, Washington, DC, 1981, p 185.
3. Ibid, p 192.

CHAPTER 13

QUALITY CONTROL AND REGULATORY REQUIREMENTS

P. ANN HOPPE, MT(ASCP)SBB, AND MARY ANN TOURAULT, M.A., MT(ASCP)SBB

Excerpts from John Judd's poem *Blood Banking: Past, Present and Future*,[1] are a good introduction to the subject of quality control:

Many years ago . . .
The crossmatch at RT,
And no QC.
Plenty of discovery:
ABO, MN and P.
Albumin and anti-Rh(D).
No mention of QC.
Things were very elementary!

And then . . .
FDA and BoB!
At last: "QC."
C3 in AHG,
Let's find that alloantibody.
JCAH and CAP,
More and more QC.
We sought to avoid calamity.

But wait . . .
Enough jocularity
Concerning this controversy
In immunohematology.
Let us the data see.
Facts, not someone's fancy,
Beyond dispute are necessary,
And undoubtedly some QC.

Entire books have been written on the subject of quality control that include detailed descriptions of the many tests that may be done to assure perfection in every area of the blood bank. However, it has been difficult to find a clear statement as to which procedures should or *must* be done, since experts are often sharply divided in their recommendations. One well-known authority clearly states that it is your responsibility to pick and choose those procedures that apply to your situation.[2] Similarly, another states that "these methods should not be considered by blood bankers (or regulatory and accrediting agencies) as mandatory or necessarily the most desirable procedures for all facilities."[3] Methods abound, but direction is lacking.

This chapter outlines the requirements of the Food and Drug Administration (FDA) that assure a safe and potent product. This is not a technical manual; test procedures will not be described in detail. Consult the references provided for methodology. This chapter discusses (1) the inspection process, which ensures that blood product standards are met; (2) quality control program design with respect to blood bank reagents; (3) the background of blood bank regulation; and (4) summaries of pertinent sections of the federal regulations for blood and blood components.

Although there are occasional discrepancies between the requirements of professional organizations such as the American Association of Blood Banks (AABB) and the FDA, all blood bank staff should be aware that FDA requirements impose a legal obligation.[4] The AABB Standards represent the informed opinion of highly respected blood bank experts and frequently incorporate information that may precede changes in the FDA regulations.

OVERVIEW OF REGULATIONS AND THE INSPECTION PROCESS

Blood banks are inspected by federal and state agencies and a number of peer review organizations. The federal agencies are the Food and Drug Administration (FDA), the Health Care Financing Administration (HCFA), the Centers for Disease Control (CDC), and the Occupational Safety and Health Administration (OSHA). The major peer review groups are the American Association of Blood Banks (AABB), College of American Pathologists (CAP), Joint Commission for Accreditation of Hospitals (JCAH), and American Osteopathic Association (AOA).

The Bureau of Biologics (now Office of Biologics, National Center for Drugs and Biologics) after 17 years of operation as the Division of Biologics Standards of the National Institutes of Health, was transferred to the Food and Drug Administration on July 1, 1972, by the Secretary of the Department of Health, Education, and Welfare (now the Department of Health and Human Services). The Office of Biologics is the part of the FDA that is responsible for establishing and maintaining the safety, purity, and potency of biologic products for human use. These products include viral and bacterial vaccines, toxins, antitoxins, therapeutic sera, allergenic extracts, human blood for transfusion, and products prepared or derived from human blood. These biologic products must be licensed if they are shipped interstate. Certain in-vitro diagnostic products are also subject to the licensing provisions of the Public Health Service Act.

The amount of regulatory control exercised by state health departments varies. Some states license both laboratories and workers; other states license neither, but may require inspection. Presently there are 17 states that have regulatory blood bank programs; 12 of these 17 states conduct inspections. These inspections are performed annually and, depending on the state, failure to "pass" an inspection could result in loss of licensure or loss of Medicare funding. Some states have agreed to accept professional organizations' inspections every other year. For example, eight states accept the AABB's inspection: Arizona, Connecticut, Illinois, New Jersey, Maryland, Wisconsin, Massachusetts, and Georgia.

The terms used for the on-site review process by the different agencies partially reflect their goals: FDA inspects; CDC examines; and HCFA surveys. Prior to a 1979 interagency agreement, CDC had inspectional jurisdiction if laboratories received 100 or more blood samples in interstate commerce. The interstate laboratories are now the inspectional responsibility of HCFA and must be licensed under the Clinical Laboratories Improvement Act of 1967 (CLIA). There are very few blood bank laboratories affected by CLIA—only 11 throughout the United States in 1981. However, if laboratories are CLIA licensed, they must participate in the CDC proficiency testing program or one that is deemed equivalent. Many unlicensed facilities voluntarily participate in one or more of the CDC proficiency testing programs. The CDC monitors 500 to 600 laboratories annually to ensure the uniform application of federal standards throughout the United States by the state agencies, JCAH, AOA, and CAP. The CDC examination focuses on quality control.

OSHA monitors the safety of workers and conducts inspections independently of all other laboratory inspections to ensure that safety regulations are being met. OSHA will not inspect a federal facility unless the inspection is requested, the facility does not have a safety and health committee, or OSHA receives a complaint. These inspections are usually unannounced and uninvited. An executive order was published in 1980 with recommended guidelines for federal facilities.

HCFA-FDA AGREEMENT ON BLOOD BANK INSPECTION

The goal of the *Memorandum of Understanding* between HCFA and the FDA was to reduce the number of federal agencies monitoring the same facilities. Of the approximately 7050 blood banks and transfusion services in the United States, HCFA surveys 4650 that do not draw blood from donors or routinely make components other than red blood cells, and FDA continues to inspect the approximately 2400 blood banks collecting blood or making components on a routine basis. FDA inspects blood banks on a 2-year cycle to determine compliance with the *Code of Federal Regulations*. The FDA inspection is based upon a blood bank checklist that follows the unit of blood from collection to infusion (see Appendix of this chapter). A set of instructions accompanies the checklist.*

HCFA adopted the FDA regulations that apply to transfusion services, and HCFA inspectors and state health department personnel are using the FDA blood bank inspection checklist. HCFA accepts the inspectional findings of JCAH and AOA, as their inspections have been deemed equivalent by HCFA. HCFA has contracts with state agencies to perform surveys and has 10 regional laboratory consultants who perform spot checks of the laboratories by doing a comparison survey on 5 percent of them.

PEER REVIEW

The AABB inspects approximately 2500 institutions every 2 years. Membership and participation in the AABB's inspectional program is voluntary and nonmember institutions may also request inspections. Failure to pass an AABB inspection results in loss of accreditation. The inspection program of the AABB is designed to be primarily educational and to motivate its members to strive for the highest attainable level of performance in all aspects of the discipline—medical, technical, scientific, and administrative.

The JCAH inspects blood banks as part of its total laboratory inspection. It inspects approximately 4500 hospitals on a 2-year cycle, and failure to pass results in loss of accreditation. Medical technologists joined the JCAH teams in November 1978, markedly increasing the thoroughness of the laboratory inspection. JCAH inspection reports may include comments on the facility's spaciousness and ambience; in addition, they may recommend topics for in-service education programs. The FDA inspection report lists only the problems found during the inspection. JCAH assesses the relationship of the blood bank to the areas of the hospital that it supplies in terms of the adequacy of the products, service, and staff, whereas FDA concentrates on *product* quality and donor safety.

The CAP is also responsible for accreditation of clinical laboratories. The primary objective of the CAP is to improve the quality of clinical laboratory services

---

*The checklist and instructions can be obtained by writing to Office of Biologics, HFB-630, Food and Drug Administration, 8800 Rockville Pike, Bethesda, MD, 20205.

and to ensure the accuracy and reliability of clinical test results. There are approximately 1900 clinical laboratories accredited by CAP; 80 percent of these are in hospitals. Membership is voluntary, with inspections occurring every 2 years. As with AABB and JCAH, failure to pass a CAP inspection results in loss of accreditation.

The AOA surveys osteopathic hospitals. It has adopted the HCFA regulations, and its inspection program has been deemed equivalent by HCFA. The primary objective of the AOA survey is to ensure compliance with standards adopted and promulgated by the AOA. Presently, there are 156 hospitals accredited by the AOA.

INSPECTORS

The inspections and surveys of the various groups are performed by a wide variety of personnel. The FDA has a staff of trained investigators who have backgrounds in science, as well as courses in blood bank inspection and on-the-job training. Many FDA investigators perform other food, drug, medical device, and cosmetic inspections in addition to blood bank and plasmapheresis inspections.

HCFA does not have a staff of surveyors. It contracts with state surveyors who have a baccalaureate degree with a major in biologic or chemical science with some laboratory experience. HCFA does have 10 regional laboratory consultants who validate laboratory surveys to ensure that interpretations by state agencies are correct. The majority of the regional laboratory consultants are medical technologists or have a degree in a related field.

The CDC has 10 medical technologists who examine laboratories. The OSHA inspections are done by safety engineers or industrial hygienists. The AABB inspections are performed by physicians and medical technologists. The JCAH inspections are done by teams composed of an administrator, a physician, a nurse, and a medical technologist. The CAP inspection includes at least one physician and, if the institution is large, the heads of the various laboratory sections as well. The AOA has a team consisting of a pathologist, a clinician, and a hospital administrator.

QUALITY CONTROL PROGRAM DESIGN

Quality control in some institutions has become an end in itself. Blood bank directors are sometimes heard to boast of having "two full-time technologists doing nothing but quality control." This boast is usually coupled with a long lament about the ridiculous "government regulations" that make extensive control necessary. Not only is much of the currently practiced quality control self-inflicted, but it has in some instances become undesirably isolated from the routine work.

In conducting a performance check on reagents, for example, the system chosen should verify not only that the reagent works, but that the person using the reagent performs the test properly. A titer performed with anti-A_1 by the quality control specialist tells you much less than a simple positive control performed in actual use. For example, such a test once revealed that anti-A_1 completely failed to agglutinate group A_1B cells by the sedimentation technique recommended by the manufacturer and used routinely in the testing laboratory, although the titer value with group A_1B cells was acceptable when tests were centrifuged. It is important to make the controls as much a part of the routine laboratory function as possible. The underlying assumption of all quality control is that the "test" is representative of "real" samples. It is also important to examine the data recorded and look for trends that may indicate subtle, but important changes, or may reveal the beginning of a problem even before values exceed acceptable limits.

No information should be kept just to satisfy inspectors. If any benefit is to be gained from the "exercise," there must be a systematic procedure for collating and reviewing the data collected. An integral part of quality control is being able to determine what went wrong; this requires good records, and that is the reason the FDA requires that every step in the manufacture of a product be recorded. The written record must be made concurrently with the work and must be indelible, legible, and signed and dated by the person performing the test. In the most simple terms, the contents of the necessary record must include *what, when,* and *who.*

The goal of every blood bank is the safe and effective transfusion of blood products to patients. Accuracy is always insisted upon because it is essential to safe transfusion. Errors can be prevented only by daily adherence to systems that ensure correct results from beginning to end. The purpose of quality control tests is to help identify deviation from expected results—and to prevent errors in final results. This is accomplished by continuously confirming that equipment, reagents, and components meet certain performance criteria.

Technical procedures should be eliminated if they do not contribute to transfusion safety. In interior decorating "less is more"; in quality control "least is best." Quantities that do not vary need not be tested. Daily checking of the speed of a hematocrit centrifuge is no longer an FDA requirement, for example, because experience showed that speed did not vary significantly. Many quality assurance procedures have been proposed empirically and do not correlate with enhanced safety; examine the reasons for every test performed.

Myhre[6] has summarized the ideal in the following "goals" for quality assurance systems:

1. Check each function or component just after it fails, and no other time.
2. Check only those functions or components which can fail.
3. Test every variable at its weakest limits of reactivity.
4. Do not test anything that does not fail.*
5. Keep records of everything forever.
6. Do not keep records on anything that does not need it.

With these goals and the FDA requirements in mind, take a critical look at what is done in your laboratory and simplify procedures wherever possible. A well-functioning quality assurance program benefits everyone. Clinicians have accurate information for decision making, patients are spared the cost of repeated tests or inappro-

---

Authors' note: The FDA disagrees in some cases.

priate therapy, and laboratory workers take pride in being part of a group that is respected for its quality of service.

PERSONNEL

The single most important element of quality control in the blood bank can be summed up in one word—personnel. It has long been recognized that the person performing the tests, recording the results, and interpreting the results is the key to attaining a high and consistent level of quality work. For example, each blood bank has a method of assuring that the reagents used each day are potent and specific, and that the test results are recorded and kept for the inspectors who will visit the laboratory in the future. It is more important to quality patient care, however, to have an alert and thinking person who recognizes that even though the quality control checks an hour ago were perfect, something is now wrong because suddenly 10 out of 10 patients have incompatible crossmatches, or all donors are e(hr") negative. These are extreme examples, and even a mildly alert person would note that something had gone awry. However, it is the truly "suspicious" technologist who is highly prized, because problems much more often manifest themselves in subtle ways. The technologist who questions the "funny looking" component unit or the reaction that is slightly stronger (or weaker) than the expected one, contributes the most to blood bank quality.

Although competency evaluation or proficiency testing programs are considered by some to be an essential part of quality control programs, they will not be considered here because the FDA has no requirement for such programs. The FDA provides for maximal flexibility in staffing and leaves the responsibility for personnel with each blood bank director by simply requiring that personnel have capabilities, training, and knowledge commensurate with their assigned functions.

ERRORS OF IDENTITY

Although everyone agrees that blood bank errors may have fatal consequences, little has been done to identify and eliminate the primary causes of the preventable transfusion fatalities. Mix-ups in patients, samples, and blood units continue despite all that has been written about quality control in the blood bank. Quality control programs do not prevent fatalities—careful people do. In reviewing all the transfusion-related fatalities reported to the FDA from 1977 through 1981, one finds no deaths that are *clearly* attributable to antibodies other than anti-A and anti-B. In no cases were these ABO mismatches the result of documented reagent failure or esoteric subgroups, but rather they were the consequence of gross carelessness in identifying recipients, samples, or blood products for transfusion.

Our primary focus, then, should be the elimination of clerical errors and identification mix-ups. Because each transfusion service is unique, there is no magic formula that can be prescribed. We spend endless hours agonizing over which centrifuge to purchase, and testing and selecting reagents and test tubes, yet all this is a fruitless expenditure of time and energy if the unit of blood intended for Mr. Jones is transfused to Mr. Johnson. Many possible solutions have been suggested. The FDA has sometimes been criticized for collecting data on fatalities, yet "not doing anything about them." It is a popular misconception that the FDA can arbitrarily decide what to regulate. The FDA has a narrow range of regulatory authority and does not regulate the practice of medicine: in most instances, the actual infusion of a unit of blood is considered the practice of medicine.

The prevention of errors requires a constant awareness by all personnel involved in the process. Whenever a discrepancy is noted in blood bank records, the source of error should be identified and corrective action initiated to preclude a recurrence. Any careless errors in identifying samples or patients must be seriously investigated, even when good fortune prevents an adverse effect on the patient. Many of the preventable transfusion-related fatalities involve more than a single mistake. Frequently, there is a whole series of errors involving several check points—all of which were designed to prevent errors, but failed.

The FDA requires that the method of collecting and identifying the blood samples of patients and donors ensures positive identification. The FDA regulations do not include specific directives as to how to achieve positive identification except to specify that a donor number or symbol must be applied to the donor sample container prior to collecting the sample. The minimal precautions employed in most laboratories for patient sample collection include the following:

1. Label tubes for one patient at a time.
2. Identify the patient by wristband, matching both name and hospital number. Confirm identification verbally, if possible.
3. Initial and date each sample as collected.

Crossmatches should be performed using donor samples from integrally attached segments of plastic tubing. Unlike pilot tube samples, red cells from these segments are sterile, well-preserved, and an integral part of the unit of red blood cells that will be transfused.

BLOOD BANK REAGENTS

Although much blood bank quality control effort is directed toward reagent performance, there is no evidence that this is an appropriate use of resources. Reagent failure is very rare. The major source of reported reagent failure is, in fact, technologist failure—failure to read and follow the manufacturer's directions. Quality control begins with ensuring that all the staff are familiar with the current package insert for each product in use.

All licensed reagents must meet FDA standards prior to distribution. The occasional problems found during use are not readily detected by any amount of prepurchase testing. It is important, however, that the blood bank worker understand the limits of the regulations and be aware of the total regulatory mechanism so that intelligent judgment can be made concerning reagent control. Published standards are just one part of regulatory oversight. Of equal or greater importance are the license application and data review process, annual inspections of licensed manufacturers, enforcement of labeling requirements, provision of reference sera as potency standards, and Office of Biologics' quality assurance testing and protocol review procedures prior to lot release.[7,8]

UNLICENSED PRODUCTS

One should be aware that not all blood bank reagents are licensed. Written standards do not exist for the unlicensed products, and consequently, larger differences in quality and potency may be found among manufacturers and from lot-to-lot.

Unlicensed products can be quickly recognized by the absence of a U.S. license number on the vial label. The unlicensed products include all products sold only for quality control purposes, such as antiglobulin control cells, special antisera, AB sera, and Rh diluents; potentiating media, which include bovine serum albumin and low ionic strength solutions; enzymes; and phytohemagglutinins, such as anti-A_1 lectin and anti-H lectin. These products do not fit the definition of a biologic product because of their origins or uses and hence do not require a license to permit interstate shipment. They are subject to the labeling requirements of 21 CFR 809.10, but their labeling does not require review and approval by the FDA prior to use. There are no uniform product standards for these reagents and samples are not tested by the FDA. If problems are encountered with these reagents, however, they should be reported to the FDA, which will investigate all complaints and determine whether labeling claims are met.

LICENSED PRODUCTS

Since 1902, the Public Health Service Act (Section 351) has required licensing of biologic products shipped in interstate commerce for sale, barter, or exchange. A biologic product is defined as a virus, therapeutic serum, toxin, antitoxin, or analogous product applicable to the prevention, treatment, or cure of diseases or injuries to man. Licensed blood bank diagnostic products include blood grouping sera, antihuman globulin sera, and reagent red blood cells. The regulations for blood grouping sera and reagent red blood cells are published as Additional Standards in 21 CFR Part 660. Additional standards for antihuman globulin sera have not been published as final regulations, but guidelines are available that include all test methods currently used by the Office of Biologics and manufacturers to determine the potency and specific reactivities of antiglobulin products. The quality of all licensed products is dependent primarily upon the manufacturer's adherence to approved procedures, which are specified in his license application. Such procedures have been demonstrated to consistently yield products meeting FDA criteria.

Reagent manufacturers are required to perform on each product lot all tests required by the Additional Standards and applicable guidelines. To obtain release of each lot from the Office of Biologics, the manufacturer submits samples and a test protocol showing that he has performed all tests required by the Additional Standards, guidelines, and his license application. Office of Biologics personnel review the manufacturer's protocol and confirm sterility; they often test the product prior to lot release, but the extent of testing varies widely. Testing by the FDA is not required.

BLOOD GROUPING SERA

The potency of all major ABO and Rh sera is controlled by the FDA through the use of lyophilized serum standards. About 85 percent of all blood grouping sera lots are ABO or Rh products for which there are reference sera; the manufacturer must perform parallel tests with each lot of product to demonstrate that the potency of his antiserum is at least equal to the corresponding reference serum. Consumers must recognize, of course, that titration scores do not always give an accurate picture of the "best" reagent because the salutary effect of special additives may be lost in the diluted serum. We do not recommend that the consumer perform titration studies because the titer results ensure only a minimal potency; they do not necessarily reflect performance when used according to the manufacturers' directions. The reference sera can only be supplied to licensed manufacturers.[5]

The use of reference sera to control potency ensures that variations in test conditions have a minimal influence on the test results. Even when procedures are prescribed in great detail, differences in technique and cell selection significantly influence serial dilution titration values, making a comparison of titers or scores found in different laboratories inconclusive. The use of a serum standard reduces the importance of such variations, however, because the product must always equal or exceed the reference serum in parallel tests. Since the manufacturer has done the critical comparison for each lot, laboratories gain little or nothing by their arbitrary selection of sera based on titer values. What one really wants to know is whether the sera will detect cells having weak phenotypic expression of the antigen. For additional information on potency test requirements, consult the *Code of Federal Regulations* and the recommended references.

CHEMICALLY MODIFIED SERA

It is especially important to realize that chemically modified reagents usually do not have normal hemagglutination slopes and a meaningful evaluation of potency by traditional titration techniques cannot be done. Furthermore, with these products saline diluents give falsely low titration values; high protein diluents give falsely high titration values. These products are exempt from the potency requirements of 21 CFR 660.25(a)(5) and are evaluated on an individual basis by the Office of Biologics.

SPECIFICITY REQUIREMENTS

Specificity tests performed by the reagent manufacturer must include at least four positive and four negative phenotypes. In addition, the manufacturer must confirm the absence of contaminating antibodies reactive with the following red cell antigens: A, B, H, Le^a, Le^b, Le^c, Le^d, I, K, k, Kp^a, Kp^b, Js^b, P$_1$, D, C, E, c, e, C^w, M, N, S, s, U, Lu^a, Lu^b, Jk^a, Jk^b, Fy^a, Fy^b, Xg^a, Do^a, Do^b, Yt^a, Yt^b, Lan, Co^a, Co^b, M^g, Wr^a, and Sd^a. If these tests are not done, the package insert must disclose an absence of testing for these antigens in the Specific Performance Characteristics section.

In addition, anti-D for D^u tests must be tested with cde, Bg^a-positive cells; anti-C must be tested with C-positive, rh$_i$-negative (Ce) cells; anti-c must be tested with c-negative, E-positive cells; anti-e must be tested with e-negative, C-positive cells; anti-CD and anti-CDE must be tested with cde G+ cells if recommended for detection of G antigen; and anti-A,B must be tested with 3 A$_x$ cells if the manufacturer claims it will detect weak A subgroups.

PERFORMANCE CHECKS

It should be obvious that even all the required tests listed above will not ensure the absence of antibodies reactive with low-incidence antigens, serum proteins, leukocyte factors, drugs, chemicals, or polyagglutinable cells. Likewise, the required daily performance checks done in blood banks are very unlikely to detect these contaminants. There is no cost-effective way to ensure perfection. The primary objective of the required performance checks is to confirm (1) that labeling errors have not occurred; (2) that the reagent has not been damaged by adverse conditions during shipment, storage, or previous use; and (3) that the techniques utilized are effective.

The extent of testing required by consumers is defined in the current *Good Manufacturing Practices for Blood and Blood Components,* which states that "representative samples of each lot of the following reagents or solutions shall be tested on a regularly scheduled basis by methods described in the Standard Operating Procedures Manual to determine their capacity to perform as required." The frequency of testing prescribed for blood bank reagents is "each day of use." The proper interpretation of this regulation is that at least once daily a vial of each of the reagents in use be tested with known positive and negative control samples. (Anti-A and anti-B do not require negative controls because the results of serum grouping tests provide confirmation that the antisera are specific.) Control samples should be selected to document both the reactivity and specificity of the reagent under the conditions of routine use in the blood bank. Whenever possible, these tests should be designed to demonstrate reasonable reactivity of the test sera with antigens at the lower extremes of phenotypic expression. Hence, group A$_2$B cells are better controls for anti-A than group A$_1$ cells. Likewise, the performance check for serum (reverse) grouping cells will be more discriminating if done with weak antibodies rather than with undiluted reagent antisera.

These required quality control tests should all be performed, interpreted, and evaluated by the personnel who will be using the reagents. If the "known" samples give the expected results, it is reasonable to assume that the reagent is satisfactory. More elaborate testing is not required. We also do not believe it should be recommended, or that it is routinely valuable. Valuable additions to control procedures include the following:

1. Make maximal use of your eyes and ears. Do reactions appear normal? Does the centrifuge sound right? Is the antiserum cloudy? Are the reagent red cells brown? Is the supernatant hemolyzed?

2. Standardize techniques.
   (a) Grade reactions consistently.
   (b) Make accurate cell suspensions (a measured concentration prepared daily can serve as a visual reference for all workers).
   (c) Control the size of drops.
   (d) Time tests accurately.
   (e) Wash antiglobulin tests thoroughly and check with IgG sensitized cells.
   (f) Follow the *Standard Operating Procedures (SOP)*.

EXPIRATION DATES OF BLOOD GROUPING SERA

Blood grouping sera are remarkably stable, often giving satisfactory results even after many years of storage. There is no limit on the age of source material used to manufacture these products. However, the dating period assigned to finished liquid products by manufacturers is no more than 2 years from the date of manufacture, which is defined as the date of the last valid potency test (1 year storage by the manufacturer is allowed plus 2 years market dating). In the event that the product is not sold prior to expiration, it can be "re-manufactured" simply by repeating the required potency test. The appropriate positive control on the day of use, therefore, is a worthwhile precaution in anticipation of the rare loss of potency that has occasionally been observed.

REAGENT RED BLOOD CELLS

The regulations require a daily performance check for reagent red blood cell products (21 CFR 606.65[c]). The intent is not to measure subtle changes in antigen strength, but rather to detect major flaws in product reactivity. There is no sterility requirement for this product, and hemolysis caused by contamination is occasionally reported. Although all licensed products contain antibiotics to retard bacterial growth, some molds thrive in these media. In addition, because occasional errors in donor phenotyping occur, consumers should be aware that reagent red blood cell phenotypes are not confirmed by the Office of Biologics. There is no lot release mechanism for reagent red blood cells because of the very short product shelf-life and the huge number of donors involved. Only red cell products that are used diagnostically are licensed. As noted earlier, reagent red blood cells that are sold for quality control use only (e.g., antiglobulin test control cells) are not licensed products.

EXPIRATION DATES

Commercially available products now have approved dating periods of up to 84 days. Although traditionally we have worried about the loss of reactivity of certain "labile" antigens, such as Lewis, $\overline{c}$, and P_1, a larger concern is the varying degree of stability in stored cells from different donors. These differences are not predictable and it is not possible to pretest donors because pretests would greatly increase the product cost. In a recent dramatic example, a reagent red cell donor sample showed almost total loss of agglutinability within 3 weeks. The most extensive comparison of manufacturers' products will not predict or eliminate this kind of problem; only a daily awareness of "expected" control results is helpful.

ANTIGEN PROFILES OF ANTIBODY SCREENING CELLS

The Additional Standards for Reagent Red Blood Cells require that each lot of group O cells recommended for detection of unexpected antibodies include the following common antigens: D, C, E, c, e, K, k, Fy^a, Fy^b, Jk^a, Jk^b, Le^a, Le^b, P_1, M, N, S, and s. Conspicuously absent from this list are antigens such as C^w, Kp^a, Lu^a, f, V/VS, Js^a, Do^a, and Xg^a, which are not low-frequency antigens, but which cannot be provided routinely on screening cells. Even the three-cell screening products fail in most cases to provide these additional antigens.

Some of the three-cell products are superior in that cells homozygous for antigens such as Fy^a, Fy^b, Jk^a, and Jk^b may be routinely included. However, if "type and screen" procedures are used to replace compatibility tests with the donor's cells, the technologist must be acutely aware of product limitations.

POOLED ANTIBODY SCREENING CELLS

Pooled group O cells recommended for the detection of unexpected antibodies may contain equal portions of cells from only two donors. Control cells, ABO cells for serum (reverse) grouping, and cord cells, however, may be produced from pools of red cells from large numbers of donors. Rarely, a manufacturing error has led to a minor population of unwanted cells in such a product (e.g., 2 percent group AB in a group O cord cell).

Because pooled products for antibody screening often combine a heterozygous cell with a cell lacking the antigen, for example, Fy(a+b+) and Fy(a−b+) or Jk(a+b+) and Jk(a−b+), these products are usually a poor choice for antibody screening tests on patients. Weak examples of Kell, Duffy, and Kidd system antibodies are known to be poorly detected with such pooled cells.

ANTIHUMAN GLOBULIN SERA

Because several varieties of antihuman globulin sera are currently marketed, it is very important to read the package insert for reactivity claims. The Office of Biologics requires that each product be appropriately tested and labeled for its content of demonstrable anti-IgG, anti-C3b, anti-C3d, and anti-C4. If the product does not contain adequate anti-C3d, it cannot be recommended for direct antiglobulin tests. If the product is recommended for indirect antiglobulin tests and contains only anti-IgG, the manufacturer must include a warning in the package insert explaining that some rare antibodies may not be detected. The best evidence available indicates that on rare occasions clinically significant antibodies are not detected with anti-IgG; however, the use of low ionic strength (LISS-AGT) tests converted to antiglobulin reduces the likelihood of missing such an antibody.

If the product claims to be "polyspecific," that is, suitable as a general-purpose reagent for both direct and indirect tests, it must contain at least anti-IgG and anti-C3d. The Office of Biologics provides potency reference standards to manufacturers for both the anti-IgG and the anti-C3d components. Consumer controls for polyspecific sera should include a daily test with IgG-sensitized cells and with normal, unsensitized cells to confirm that product reactivity and specificity are satisfactory. Monospecific anticomplement sera should be tested with cells coated with the specific component being evaluated.

MONOCLONAL ANTIBODIES PREPARED BY HYBRIDOMA TECHNOLOGY

There are now licensed anticomplement sera prepared with mouse hybridoma cells. These products are very potent and of high quality. The use of these products, however, requires particular attention to the manufacturer's directions because they are more likely to "prozone," that is, give falsely weak or negative reactions owing to antibody excess. The length of incubation prior to centrifugation is particularly critical; extending the time beyond recommended limits *decreases* the reaction strength observed in many cases.

PROBLEM REPORTING

If you encounter defects in blood bank reagents or equipment you should notify the FDA as well as the manufacturer. Call or write the Office of Biologics.*

REGULATIONS

The FDA's regulations define acceptable limits of operation and requirements for laboratory controls, record-keeping, facilities, and equipment. They apply to any facility that collects or processes blood or components; they are designed to ensure the uniform safety, effectiveness, and reliability of blood and blood products. A copy of the federal regulations may be ordered by writing to the U.S. Government Printing Office[†] and requesting Title 21, Parts 600-799 of the *Code of Federal Regulations.* This book or its applicable sections must be available in every blood bank laboratory and laboratory workers must be familiar with its contents as they relate to their particular functions. Amendments to the regulations are published throughout the year in the *Federal Register.* New rules or significant changes in rules are published first as proposals for comment. Public comment plays a very significant role in shaping the final rules. A practical and economical way to keep informed of these changes is to subscribe to the *AABB Federal Register Excerpts Program.*

---

*Office of Biologics, 8800 Rockville Pike, Bethesda, MD 20205, Quality Assurance Branch (HFB-630), 301-443-5410, or the Division of Blood and Blood Products (HFB-200), 301-496-4396.
†Superintendant of Documents, U.S. Government Printing Office, Washington, D.C., 20402

The essential regulatory elements have been paraphrased here for ready reference by the technologist. Please be aware that the *Code of Federal Regulations* is a dynamic document; revisions occur every year and it is necessary to consult the latest edition for completely accurate information. This chapter reflects regulations in effect in 1981.

STANDARD OPERATING PROCEDURES

One of the best methods of ensuring the quality of blood bank products is strict adherence to standard procedures that have been approved by the facility's medical director. The FDA requires that written standard operating procedures be maintained and include all steps to be followed in the collection, processing, compatibility testing, storage, and distribution of blood and blood components for transfusion and further manufacturing. The procedures must be available to personnel for use in the areas where the procedures are performed.

The required elements for Standard Operating Procedures (SOP) are in Title 21, *Code of Federal Regulations* (21 CFR), Part 606.100, and are listed below:

1. Criteria for donor suitability.

2. Methods of performing donor qualifying tests and the acceptable ranges, e.g., blood pressure, pulse, temperature, and hemoglobin.

3. Solutions and methods used to prepare the phlebotomy site.

4. Method of accurately relating the units to the donor.

5. Blood collection procedure.

6. Method of component preparation.

7. All tests performed on blood products.

8. Pretransfusion tests on blood product recipients.

9. Investigation of adverse donor and recipient reactions.

10. Storage temperatures.

11. Expiration dates.

12. Criteria for reissue of returned blood.

13. Procedures for tracing a unit of blood or blood component from the donor to its final disposition.

14. Quality control procedures.

15. Schedules and procedures for equipment maintenance and calibration.

16. Labeling procedures.

17. Procedures for plasmapheresis, plateletpheresis, and leukapheresis if per-

formed, including precautions to be taken to ensure reinfusion of the donor's own cells.

18. Procedure for preparing recovered plasma, including details of separation, pooling, labeling, storage, and distribution.

19. Procedure for reviewing all records pertinent to a lot (each unit of blood is a lot) before release or distribution of a lot or unit of final product. Results of investigations of an unexplained discrepancy or failure of a lot or unit to meet any specifications must be recorded.

20. A facility may utilize current SOP of the American Association of Blood Banks, American National Red Cross, or other organizations as long as the requirements are consistent with, and are as stringent as, the federal requirements.

EQUIPMENT

Part 606.60 (b) of the *Code of Federal Regulations* summarizes the minimal requirements for control of blood bank equipment (Table 13-1).

WHOLE BLOOD

Whole Blood* is defined as blood collected from donors for transfusion. The regulations are in 21 CFR, Parts 640.1 through 640.9. These basic requirements also apply to Red Blood Cells, which are separated from Whole Blood.

COLLECTION

1. Manufacturing of Whole Blood, including donor examination, blood collection, laboratory tests, labeling, storage, and issue, must be under the supervision and control of the same licensed establishment unless prior approval has been obtained from the Office of Biologics. (Licenses are required only for interstate shipment.)

2. If blood is collected in an open system, a periodic sterility test must be performed.

3. Donor suitability determination and blood collection must be performed by a physician or by trained persons under his supervision. Medical history, hemoglobin level, and physical examination must be done on the day of collection; the SOP manual must be followed.

4. Donors may not serve as a source for whole blood more than once in 8 weeks and donors must be in good health as indicated by the following:

(a) Normal temperature.

(b) Normal blood pressure.

---

*All the FDA-recognized names for blood products will probably be changed in the near future. The new, simplified names are used here for clarity.

TABLE 13-1. Minimal Requirements for Control of Blood Bank Equipment

Equipment	Performance Check	Frequency	Frequency of Calibration
Temperature Recorder	Compare against thermometer	Daily	As necessary
Refrigerated centrifuge	Observe speed and temperature	Each day of use	As necessary
Hematocrit centrifuge			Standardize before initial use, repairs, or adjustments, and annually; timer every 3 months
General lab centrifuge			Tachometer every 6 months
Automated blood-typing machine	Observe controls for correct results	Each day of use	
Hemoglobinometer	Standardize against cyanmethemo-globin standard	Each day of use	
Refractometer	Standardize against distilled water	Each day of use	
Blood container scale	Standardize against container of known weight	Each day of use	As necessary
Water bath	Observe temperature	Each day of use	As necessary
Rh view box	Observe temperature	Each day of use	As necessary
Autoclave	Observe temperature	Each day of use	As necessary
Serologic rotators	Observe controls for correct results	Each day of use	Speed as necessary
Laboratory thermometers			Before initial use
Electronic thermometers			Monthly
Vacuum blood agitator	Observe weight of the first container of blood filled for correct results	Each day of use	Standardize with container of known mass or volume before initial use, and after repairs or adjustments

(c) Hemoglobin level of 12.5 g (in the near future the requirement will be 12.5 g for females and 13.5 g for males).

(d) Freedom from acute respiratory diseases.

(e) Freedom from any infectious skin disease at the phlebotomy site and generalized skin disease that could contaminate the blood.

(f) Freedom from any disease transmissible by blood transfusion, as far as can be determined by history or examination.

(g) Freedom from arm scars indicative of drug addiction.

(h) Freedom from a history of viral hepatitis or close contact with an individual having viral hepatitis within 6 months.

(i) Freedom from having received within 6 months blood or blood products that may transmit hepatitis.

5. Blood from therapeutic bleedings may be used for transfusion only if the container label conspicuously indicates the donor's disease.

6. Blood from donors known to have been immunized to human blood cell antigens may be used if the container label conspicuously indicates the antibody present.

7. FDA-approved blood containers and anticoagulant must be used.

8. Each unit of blood must be related to the donor by number or other symbol.

9. The site of phlebotomy must be prepared by a method that gives maximal assurance of a sterile container of blood.

10. Blood samples for laboratory tests must be collected at the time of filling the final container by the person who collects the unit of blood and the sample containers must bear the donor's identification before filling.

11. The containers for pilot samples accompanying a unit of blood shall be attached to the container before collection, in a tamper-proof manner that will conspicuously indicate removal and reattachment. (This means that if plastic containers are used, the segments for laboratory tests should remain attached until used.)

12. Immediately after collection, blood should be stored between 1 and 6°C unless platelets are to be prepared. Red blood cells must be placed between 1 and 6°C immediately after the platelets are separated.

REQUIRED TESTS

All tests must be made on a sample taken at the time of collection. The following tests are required of the facility that collected the blood:

1. Serologic test for syphilis (will be deleted in the near future).

2. The ABO group must be determined by two different methods and units may not be issued until grouping tests are in agreement. (The two methods should be cell and serum grouping.)

3. Rh testing—If the test using anti-D(Rh$_0$) is negative, the results must be confirmed by further testing, which should include tests for the D(Rh$_0$) variant (D^u).

4. HBsAg test—The requirements for hepatitis B surface antigen are in 21 CFR Part 610.40 and are summarized below:

(a) Each donation of blood, plasma, or serum to be used in preparing a biologic product shall be tested for the presence of hepatitis B surface antigen by a test of third generation sensitivity.

(b) In emergency situations, a test method of second generation sensitivity may be used. In dire emergency situations, blood and blood products may be issued without any HBsAg testing provided that the product is labeled accordingly and the HBsAg test is performed as soon as possible after issuance of blood and/or blood product.

(c) Only licensed reagents may be used.

(d) If the radioimmunoassay method is used, the collection facility may perform the complete test or may have another facility count the radioactivity of the samples. The second facility must meet the Clinical Laboratory Improvement Act (CLIA) standards and must participate in the Office of Biologics (OB) proficiency testing.

(e) Written results of the completed test must be in the possession of the collection facility prior to issuance of blood, plasma, or serum, except for emergency situations and source leukocytes.

(f) Blood, plasma, or serum reactive for the hepatitis B surface antigen may not be used in manufacturing injectable biologic products, except for the hepatitis B vaccine. Plasma collected from known HBsAg-positive persons should not be retested for HBsAg; this is an unnecessary risk to laboratory staff.

DATING PERIODS

Consult 21 CFR, Part 610.53 for information on the dating periods for blood and blood products.

RED BLOOD CELLS

In addition to the requirements for Whole Blood described above, specific regulations for Red Blood Cells are found in 21 CFR Parts 640.10 through 640.18 and are summarized below:

1. Separation may be performed anytime within the dating period for the source blood and must be done by a method that does not increase the temperature of the cells.

2. Enough plasma must be left with the cells to ensure optimal cell survival. (For CPDA-1 this means that the hematocrit cannot exceed 80 percent.)

3. If an airway is required, it must exclude microorganisms and maintain a sterile system.

4. When possible, the final container should be the original blood container. If a different container is used, it must be identified by number so as to relate it to the donor.

PLATELETS

Platelets are defined as platelets collected from a single donor and suspended in a portion of the original plasma. Platelets may be collected by whole blood collection, plasmapheresis, or plateletpheresis. The phlebotomy must be performed by a single uninterrupted venipuncture with minimal damage to the donor's tissue.

The platelet regulations are in 21 CFR Parts 640.20 through 640.27 and are summarized below:

1. Platelets may not be pooled prior to completion of the processing tests (i.e., ABO, Rh, STS, and HBsAg).

2. Tests must be performed on a properly labeled sample collected at the same time as the platelets.

3. Storage at room temperature (20 to 24°C), prior to separation of the platelets, should be maintained and monitored. If whole blood must be transported prior to separation, all reasonable efforts should be made to maintain it as close as possible to 20 to 24°C.

4. Plasma for preparation of platelets must be separated within 6 hours after collection of the whole blood.

5. The time and speed of centrifugation must have been demonstrated to produce an unclumped product, without visible hemolysis, that yields a count of not less than 5.5×10^{10} platelets per unit in at least 75 percent of the units tested.

6. The original plasma in which the platelets are suspended should have a pH of not less than 6.0.

7. Final containers must be colorless and transparent to permit visual inspection, be hermetically sealed, and be identified by number or symbol so as to relate them to their respective donors.

8. Platelets stored at room temperature (20 to 24°C) must be continuously agitated. Agitation is optional if storage is at 1 to 6°C.

9. Each month of preparation, units from four different donors must be tested for platelet count and pH at the end of their dating period. If the platelet count and pH do not meet the requirements, immediate corrective action must be taken and a record maintained of the corrective action.

10. All manufacturing of platelets must be performed at the same establishment except that quality control testing (cell count and pH) may be performed by a clinical laboratory that meets the requirements of CLIA (1967). The test results must be received by the manufacturer within 10 days of platelet preparation.

11. There is an emergency provision to allow plateletpheresis of donors not meeting all the criteria if a physician has determined that the recipient must be transfused with the platelets from a specific donor. The procedure must be performed under supervision of a qualified, licensed physician who is aware of the health status of the donor, and the physician must certify in writing that the donor's health permits plateletpheresis.

CRYOPRECIPITATE

Cryoprecipitate is defined as a preparation of antihemophilic factor that is obtained from a single unit of plasma collected and processed in a closed system. The source material is plasma, which may be obtained by whole blood collection, by plasmapheresis, or as a by-product of cytapheresis.

The regulations for cryoprecipitated AHF are in 21 CFR Parts 640.50 through 640.57, and can be summarized as follows:

1. Whole blood donors must meet the criteria for donor suitability.

2. Plasmapheresis donors shall meet the criteria for blood donor suitability except for the malaria restriction. Donors excluded from whole blood donations because of malaria may be plasmapheresed because the malarial parasite is not found in plasma.

3. Donors who have been immunized with red blood cells within the last 6 months are excluded.

4. Tests must be performed on a properly labeled sample of blood collected at the time of collecting the source blood.

5. Plasma must be placed in the freezer within 6 hours after blood collection and stored at −18°C or colder.

6. Diluents may not be added prior to freezing.

7. The container must be colorless, transparent, hermetically sealed, and identified by a number to relate it to the donor.

8. The product must be prepared by a procedure that has been shown to produce an average of no less than 80 units of antihemophilic factor per final container. Four representative units of cryoprecipitated AHF must be tested each month of preparation.

9. A U.S. Standard Antihemophilic Factor (Factor VIII) preparation may be obtained from the Office of Biologics to use as a quality control reference.

10. The quality control tests may be performed by an outside clinical laboratory that meets the CLIA standards. Results must be received by the manufacturer within 30 days of preparation of cryoprecipitate. Immediate corrective action must be taken and documented if the average potency level per container is less than 80 units of antihemophilic factor.

PLASMA

There are several types of plasma: Plasma; Plasma, Fresh Frozen; Plasma, Liquid; Plasma, Platelet Rich; Recovered Plasma; and Source Plasma. Recovered plasma is not licensed and is not used for transfusion. There are currently no published standards specifically for this product. As with all products, it must be made and labeled in accordance with the Good Manufacturing Practices (21 CFR, Part 606). Source Plasma is not for transfusion; it is used for further manufacture only. It must be made in accordance with 21 CFR, Parts 640.60 through 640.76.

Plasma is defined as the fluid portion of one unit of blood, collected and separated in a closed system and intended for intravenous use. Plasma may be obtained from a unit of whole blood or by plasmapheresis. The regulations for plasma are in 21 CFR, Parts 640.30 through 640.35. These regulations are summarized in Table 13-2 and below:

1. Whole blood donors must meet the donor suitability criteria for blood donation.

2. Plasmapheresis donors shall meet the criteria for Source Plasma donor suitability, except that the malaria exemption does not apply.

3. Donors who have been immunized with red blood cells within the last 6 months are excluded.

4. Whole blood intended for Plasma; Plasma, Fresh Frozen; and Plasma, Liquid, must be stored between 1 and 6°C until the plasma is removed. Whole blood intended for Plasma, Platelet Rich must be stored at room temperature (20 to 24°C) until the plasma is separated. The red cells must be stored between 1 and 6°C immediately after the plasma is separated.

5. Plasma must be separated from the red cells within 26 days after phlebotomy (40 days for CPDA-1 anticoagulant) and stored at −18°C or colder within 6 hours after transfer to the final container.

6. Plasma, Fresh Frozen must be prepared from blood collected by a single, uninterrupted venipuncture. The plasma must be separated from the red cells, placed in the freezer within 6 hours after phlebotomy, and stored at −18°C or colder.

7. Plasma, Liquid must be separated from the red cells within 26 days after phlebotomy (40 days if CPDA-1 anticoagulant) and stored between 1 and 6°C within 4 hours after filling the final container.

8. Plasma, Platelet Rich must be prepared by a single, uninterrupted venipuncture. Plasma must be separated from the red cells within 6 hours after phlebotomy. The time and speed of centrifugation must be shown to produce a product with at least 250,000 platelets per microliter. Plasma shall be stored at 20 to 24°C (room temperature) or 1 to 6°C immediately after filling the final containers. The plasma must be continuously agitated if stored at room temperature.

TABLE 13-2. Summary of Requirements for Plasma Products

Product	Time Limits For Separation from Red Cells	Dating	Time Limits for Placing at Correct Storage Temperature	Storage
Plasma	26 days for whole blood in ACD & CPD (40 days for CPDA-1)	5 yr from date of collection	Freeze within 6 hr after transfer to final container	−18°C
Plasma, fresh-frozen	6 hr (must be placed in freezer)	1 yr from date of collection	Immediately after separation	−18°C
Plasma, liquid	26 days for whole blood in ACD & CPD (40 days for CPDA-1)	26 days from date of collection (40 days if CPDA-1)	Refrigerate within 4 hr after transfer to final container	1–6°C
Plasma, platelet-rich	Within 6 hr	72 hr from time of collection if stored at room temperature; 48 hr if at 1–6°C	Immediately after filling final container	20–24°C or 1–6°C

MODERN BLOOD BANKING AND TRANSFUSION PRACTICES

9. When platelets are removed, the remaining plasma may be labeled as Plasma, Fresh Frozen if placed in a freezer within 6 hours after phlebotomy.

10. If Cryoprecipitate is removed, or if both Platelets and Cryoprecipitate are removed, the remaining plasma may be labeled Plasma or Plasma, Liquid.

11. The final container must be transparent, colorless, hermetically sealed, and identified by number to relate it to the donor.

12. Frozen products must be stored in a manner to show evidence of thawing during storage. One way this may be accomplished is by making an indentation when freezing the plasma; subsequent thawing and refreezing will remove the indentation and alert personnel that the storage temperature has been inadequate.

STORAGE AND DISTRIBUTION

The FDA requirements for storage of blood and blood products mandate that products be stored at certain temperatures. It is the blood bank's obligation to demonstrate that this has been done by maintaining a daily log of temperature readings. Recording thermometers and elaborate alarm systems are not required by the FDA. If a recording thermometer is used, it must be verified daily by comparison to a standard thermometer because recording thermometers are subject to mechanical failure and human error in adjustment and maintenance. A written record of the temperature observed confirms that this was done. Medicare certification, however, does require an alarm system. Any significant discrepancies in reading between the recorder and thermometer should be investigated and corrected.

INSPECTION

Whole blood, red blood cells, and plasma must be inspected visually during storage and immediately prior to issue. This inspection of blood for transfusion requires observing the plasma layer for clarity. Recently transported units may require a rest period to permit the red blood cells to separate from the plasma prior to inspection and reissue. Inspection should include observation for icteric appearance, hemolysis, purplish color, or floating debris that may indicate bacterial colonies. Examine the red blood cells for clots, fibrin, white particles, and gas formation. Visual inspection is often performed in a cursory manner because problems are rarely encountered. However, bacterial contamination is extremely serious, and visual inspection can help prevent the use of infected units. There have been occasions on which blood has been inadvertently frozen before delivery to hospitals; a careful final inspection could prevent use of a severely damaged product that would not function as intended. Inspection should also ensure that the product has adequate seals and proper labels.

A record must be kept of the final disposition of all blood products. If units are discarded because they fail to pass inspection, the specific reason and mode of disposal should be recorded.

The Good Manufacturing Practices require that you review all manufacturing records before releasing blood. Transfusion centers receive blood already tested by a blood bank and the blood bank is responsible for the quality control testing and record review for the blood or component sent to the transfusion center. This final review can be an excellent safeguard, but it is often ineffective because it is not taken seriously. This final review at the blood center level ought to ensure, for example, that HBsAg-positive units (and all components that have been prepared from them) are physically collected, quarantined, and double-checked for identity before the blood processed each day is declared ready for distribution. At the hospital level all tests performed on the patient and donor should be reviewed for accuracy and completeness before the blood is placed on the "crossmatched" shelf, ready for issue.

If blood has been removed from storage under the control of the licensed establishment, it may not be reissued unless the following conditions are met:

1. The seals have not been broken (must be tamper-proof).
2. A segment (or pilot tube) is properly attached. In an emergency situation, the unit may be entered for a crossmatch sample and used within 6 hours.
3. The blood has been stored continuously at 1 to 6°C and shipped between 1 and 10°C.
4. The blood is held for observation and checked for hemolysis.

Blood may be shipped before testing is completed when such issue is essential to ensure arrival of the blood by the time it is needed for transfusion. The blood must be shipped directly to the physician or medical facility, the records must fully explain the reason for the shipment, and the labels must indicate which testing has not been completed.

LABELING

The general labeling requirements for blood products are in 21 CFR 606.120. Amendments to these requirements were recently proposed to centralize all labeling requirements for blood products and to include provision for using a uniform label. Uniform labels have deleted a number of items formerly required to appear on the container label, and this information has been moved to the instruction circular. Labeling requirements can be summarized as follows:

1. Labeling operations must be separated physically or spatially from other operations to prevent mix-ups.
2. Labels must be held upon receipt pending review and proofing against an approved final copy to ensure accuracy regarding identity, content, and conformity with the approved copy.
3. Labels for different products must be stored in a manner to prevent mix-ups, and obsolete labels must be destroyed.
4. Necessary checks in labeling procedures to prevent errors in translating test results to container labels must be utilized.
5. Labels must be clear and legible. Labels of the collection and initial processing facility may not be altered or obscured except to change the proper name when blood components have been removed. Labels must include the following:

(a) Proper name must be in a prominent position and printed in solid red.

(b) Appropriate donor classification of paid or volunteer donor must be printed in solid red in no less prominence than that of the proper name of the product.

(c) Name and address of the manufacturer, and, if licensed, the license number of the manufacturer.

(d) Donor or lot number relating the unit to the donor.

(e) Expiration date, including the day and year and, if it is a factor, the hour.

(f) The statement: "This product may transmit an agent of hepatitis."

(g) The recommended storage temperature.

(h) Reference to an instruction circular, which shall be available for distribution.

(i) Quantity of product for whole blood, plasma, platelets, and partial units of red cells; the labeled volume of product in container must be accurate within ±10 percent.

(j) Name and quantity of source material, where applicable.

(k) Caution: "Federal law prohibits dispensing without prescription."

(l) The statement: "See circular of information for indications, contraindications, cautions, and methods of infusion."

(m) The statement: "Properly identify intended recipient." This must be printed in solid red.

(n) ABO and Rh groups must be designated conspicuously if the product is intended for transfusion.

(o) If the test with anti-D is positive, label as Rh positive; if D^u test is positive, label as Rh positive. If D and D^u tests are negative, label as Rh negative. If D^u test is not performed on D-negative units, label must so indicate.

(p) Products intended for transfusion must bear machine-readable symbols for the following if they are shipped to another institution.

> Proper name.
> Type of anticoagulant (whole blood and red cells only).
> Collection center identifier.
> Unit number.
> ABO and Rh blood group of donor.

(q) Labels may be color coded or on white paper with solid black print, except Rh negative, which is white print on black background. If a color scheme is used: blood group A—yellow; blood group B—pink; blood group O—blue; and blood group AB—white. Ink colors must match OB color samples.

In addition to the above general information, whole blood and red blood cells labels must have:

1. Volume of anticoagulant, and the name of the anticoagulant preceding the proper name of the product.

2. If tests for unexpected antibodies are positive, and the blood product is intended for transfusion, the label must contain the name of the antibody unless the plasma is completely removed.

3. Red blood cells labels must include hour of expiration if prepared in an open system.

4. Recovered plasma labels must have the date of collection of the oldest material in the container (in lieu of an expiration date). They must also contain the statements: "Caution: For manufacturing use only" or "Caution: For use in manufacturing noninjectable products only" and "Not for use in products subject to license under Section 351 of the Public Health Service Act," if the recovered plasma does not meet the requirements for manufacturing into licensed products.

5. Blood and blood components not suitable for transfusion must be prominently labeled "Not for transfusion" and the reason stated, unless labeled as in the preceding section.

6. If blood or blood components are shipped prior to completion of tests, the name of the intended recipient should not be on the label, but a special label or tie-tag must be attached to the container with the following information:

> The statement: "Emergency use only."
> Results of any required tests completed.
> List of the required tests that have not been completed.

7. Autologous infusion: In addition to the information required for labeling whole blood or red blood cells, autologous units must have a special label or tie-tag with information adequately identifying the patient (e.g., name, blood group, hospital, and identification number), date of donation, and the statement: "For autologous use only." If a donor fails to meet the donor suitability requirements or is HBsAg reactive, the container shall be prominently and permanently labeled: "For autologous use only."

The instruction circular must provide adequate directions for use. Instruction circulars are provided by the product manufacturers and must include the following information:

1. The statement: "Mix before use."

2. The statement: "Use a filter in administration equipment."

3. A statement: "Do not add medications" or an explanation concerning allowable additives.

4. A list of known sensitizing substances.

5. A description of the product, its source and preparation, including the name and proportion of the anticoagulant used in collecting the whole blood from which each product is prepared.

6. Statements that the product was prepared from blood that was nonreactive when tested for hepatitis B surface antigen by an FDA-required test and nonreactive when tested for syphilis by a serologic test for syphilis (STS). (The STS test will not be required in the near future.)

7. The statement: "Warning. The risk of transmitting hepatitis is present. Careful donor selection and available laboratory tests do not eliminate the hazard."

8. The names of cryoprotective agents and other additives that may still be present in the product.

9. The names of all tests performed and results when necessary for safe and effective use.

10. The use of the product, indications, contraindications, side effects and hazards, dosage, and administration recommendations.

11. For Whole Blood units from which Cryoprecipitate has been removed, instructions not to use the unit of blood for patients requiring antihemophilic factor.

12. For Red Blood Cells, the instruction circular shall contain: (a) instruction to add a suitable plasma volume expander if Red Blood Cells are substituted when Whole Blood is required; and (b) a warning not to add lactated Ringer's injection (U.S.P.) solution to Red Blood Cell products.

13. For Platelets, the instruction circular shall contain: (a) the approximate volume of plasma the Platelets were prepared from; and (b) instructions to use as soon as possible, but not more than 4 hours after entering the container.

14. For Plasma, the instruction circular shall contain: (a) a warning against further processing of the frozen product if there is evidence of breakage or thawing; (b) instructions to thaw the frozen product at a temperature between 30 and 37°C; (c) when applicable, instructions to use the product within 6 hours after thawing; (d) instructions to administer to ABO group compatible recipients; and (e) the statement that "This product has the same hepatitis risk as Whole Blood; other plasma volume expanders without this risk are available for treating hypovolemia."

15. For Cryoprecipitate, the instruction circular shall contain: (a) the statement that "Average potency is 80 or more units of antihemophilic factor"; (b) the statement "Usually contains at least 150 mg of fibrinogen," or, alternatively, the average fibrinogen level determined by assay; (c) a warning against further processing of the product if there is evidence of breakage or thawing; (d) instructions to thaw the product for 15 minutes at a temperature of 37°C; (e) instructions to store at room temperature after thawing and use as soon as possible, but not more than 4 hours after entering or pooling and within 6 hours after thawing; (f) a statement that saline is the preferred diluent; (g) adequate instructions for pooling to ensure complete removal of all concentrated material from each container; and (h) the statement that "Good patient management requires monitoring treatment responses to Cryoprecipitate transfusions with periodic plasma factor VIII or fibrinogen assays in hemophilia A and hypofibrinogenemic recipients, respectively."

PROPER NAMES OF PRODUCTS

Proposed changes in the proper names of biologic products to more accurately identify the products and, in some cases, to shorten the name are as follows:

Proposed Name	Present Name
Albumin Human	Normal Serum Albumin (Human)
Antihemophilic Factor	Antihemophilic Factor (Human)
Cryoprecipitate	Cryoprecipitated Antihemophilic Factor (Human)

Proposed Name	Present Name
Factor IX Complex	Factor IX Complex (Human)
Fibrinolysin	Fibrinolysin (Human)
Plasma	Single Donor Plasma (Human)
Fresh-Frozen Plasma	Single Donor Plasma (Human), Fresh-Frozen
Liquid Plasma	Single Donor Plasma (Human), Liquid
Platelet-Rich Plasma	Single Donor Plasma (Human), Platelet-Rich
Plasma Protein Fraction	Plasma Protein Fraction (Human)
Platelets	Platelet Concentrate (Human)
Red Blood Cells	Red Blood Cells (Human)
Red Blood Cells Deglycerolized	Red Blood Cells (Human), Deglycerolized
Red Blood Cells Frozen	Red Blood Cells (Human), Frozen
Rh(D) Immune Globulin	$Rh_0(D)$ Immune Globulin (Human)
Whole Blood	Whole Blood (Human)
Whole Blood Cryoprecipitate Removed	Whole Blood (Human), Modified

REFERENCES

1. JUDD, WJ: *Blood Banking: Past, Present and Future. Presented by Pfizer Diagnostics.*
2. MYHRE, BA: *Quality Control in Blood Banking.* John Wiley & Sons, New York, 1974, p 213.
3. *Principles and Practice of Quality Control in the Blood Bank.* American Association of Blood Banks, Washington, DC, 1980, p x.
4. *Code of Federal Regulations, Title 21, Parts 600–799.* Food and Drug Administration, U.S. Government Printing Office, Washington, DC, 1981.
5. SOLOMON, JM: *Ortho Blood Lines* (newsletter of Ortho Diagnostics). Vol 1, No 2, 1977.
6. MYHRE, BA: *Blood Transfusion, Blood Components and Hepatitis.* U.S. Department of Health and Human Services, NIH Publication No. 80–1958, Public Health Service, 1980, p 173.
7. HOPPE, PA: *Performance criteria for blood grouping sera.* In *A Seminar on Performance Evaluation.* American Association of Blood Banks, Washington, DC, 1976, pp 1–24.
8. HOPPE, PA: *The role of the Bureau of Biologics in assuring reagent reliability.* In *Considerations in the Selection of Reagents.* American Association of Blood Banks, Washington, DC, 1979, pp 1–33.

BIBLIOGRAPHY

A Seminar on Blood Components: E Unum Pluribus. American Association of Blood Banks, Washington, DC, 1977.

A Seminar on Performance Evaluation. American Association of Blood Banks, Washington, DC, 1976.

GLENN, GC and HATHAWAY, BS: *Quality control by blind sample analysis.* Am J Clin Pathol 72:156, 1979.

Guide for Hospital Committees on Transfusions. American Medical Association, Chicago, 1976.

INHORN, SL (ed): *Quality Assurance Practices for Health Laboratories.* American Public Health Association, Washington, DC, 1978, pp 411–450.

MOORE, BPL, HUMPHREYS, P and LOVETT-MOSELEY, CA: *Serological and immunological methods.* In *Technical Manual of the Canadian Red Cross Blood Transfusion Service,* ed 7. Canadian Red Cross Society, Toronto, 1975.

MYHRE, BA: *Quality Control in Blood Banking.* John Wiley & Sons, New York, 1974.

ROBERTS, S and FRANKS, M: *Quality control for cryopreserved red blood cells: A blood banker's approach.* In *Clinical and Practical Aspects of the Use of Frozen Blood.* American Association of Blood Banks, Washington, DC, 1977.

SOLOWAY, HB: *Seven fallacies about quality control.* Medical Laboratory Observer 7:41, 1975.

Standards for Blood Banks and Transfusion Services, ed 10. American Association of Blood Banks, Washington, DC, 1981.

TASWELL, HF, et al.: *Quality control in the blood bank—a new approach.* Am J Clin Pathol 62:491, 1974.

ZUCK, TF and GERGIN, JJ: *Laboratory interface with transfusion therapy.* In *Transfusion Therapy.* American Association of Blood Banks, Washington, DC, 1974, pp 15–28.

APPENDIX

BLOOD BANK CHECKLIST

<table>
<tr><td colspan="4" align="center">DEPARTMENT OF HEALTH AND HUMAN SERVICES
BLOOD BANK INSPECTION CHECKLIST AND REPORT</td></tr>
<tr><td>1a.   NAME OF INVESTIGATOR(S)</td><td>b.   DATES OF INSPECTION</td><td colspan="2">c. TOTAL INSPECTION
TIME IN BLOOD BANK</td></tr>
<tr><td></td><td></td><td colspan="2"></td></tr>
<tr><td></td><td></td><td colspan="2"></td></tr>
<tr><td></td><td></td><td colspan="2"></td></tr>
</table>

2. REGISTRATION NO./MEDICARE NO./CLIA NO.	3. U.S. License No. & Location No.
4. a. Legal Name of Blood Bank	5. a. Address and Zip Code of Establishment being Inspected
b. DBA	b. Telephone No. ( ) —
6. Name of Medical Director	7. a. Name of Responsible Head if Licensed [600.10(a)] b. Name of Director if not Licensed [606.20(a)]

8 a. Name of Person(s) With Whom Overall Inspection Discussed.	9. Type of Operation (Check all applicable)
	     ☐ 1. Blood Bank
	     ☐ 2. Donor Center
	     ☐ 3. Transfusion Service

b. Form FDA 483 Issued?
 	
     ☐ Yes   ☐ No
	10. Type of Inspection (Check all Applicable)
	     ☐ 1. Scheduled
	     ☐ 2. Follow-up
	     ☐ 3. Prelicense
	     ☐ 4. Investigation

11. Are there corrections to be made on the Establishment Registration (Form FDA 2830)? ☐ Yes ☐ No (if "Yes," specify on reverse)	12. RESOURCE DATA a. Approximately how many units of whole blood are drawn per year? b. Approximately how many units of whole blood and red cells are received from outside sources per year? c. Approximately how many units whole blood and red blood cells are transfused per year? d. Approximately how many units of red blood cells are prepared per year?

APPLICABLE SECTIONS	YES	NO	PAGE
A. WHOLE BLOOD (Donor Suitability and Collection)			2
B. LABORATORY AND LABELING (Only establishments which collect blood and/or prepare components)			3
C. RED BLOOD CELLS			5
*D. PLASMA AND RECOVERED PLASMA			6
*E. PLATELETS			7
*F. CRYOPRECIPITATED AHF			8
G. COMPATIBILITY TESTING AND TRANSFUSION REACTIONS			9
H. STORAGE, DISTRIBUTION AND GENERAL			10
I. UNIFORM BLOOD LABELING			11
*NOTE: If Plasmapheresis is performed, also complete Form FDA 2722.			

COMMENTS OR SUMMARY:

ITEM	CFR No.	Yes	No	ITEM	CFR No.	Yes	No
A1. Is Donor Suitability determined at this Blood Bank?				A11. PILOT TUBE SAMPLES:			
A2. DONATION INTERVAL: Is it 8 weeks or greater unless a physician gives written approval?	640.3(b) 640.3(f)			a. Are laboratory tubes adequately identified?	640.4(g)(3)		
A3. DONOR HISTORY & EXAM:				b. Are they collected at time containers are filled?	640.4(g)(2)		
a. Acute and chronic disqualifying diseases	640.3(b)(4) & (5)			A12. AUTOLOGOUS COLLECTION:			
b. Endemic malaria area: Anti-malarial drugs taken?	640.3(b)(2)			a. Are autologous units collected?			
c. Viral hepatitis history?	640.3(c)(1)			b. Are records maintained of the extent of testing and final disposition?			
d. Viral hepatitis exposure: contact with afflicted person in last 6 months?	640.3(c)(2)			A13. DATING PERIOD: Are units assigned proper dating periods?	610.53		
e. Blood or blood derivatives received within 6 months?	640.3(c)(3)			A14. STORAGE: Is blood product placed at proper storage temperature after drawing?	640.4(i)		
f. Do Donor suitability areas provide for privacy?	606.40(a)(1)			A15. QUALITY CONTROL CHECKS FOR COLLECTION:			
A4. DONOR EXAM: Does donor screening include:				a. Are blood container scales standardized against container of known weight?	606.60(b)		
a. Temperature? [<37.5° C (99.6° F)]	640.3(b)(1)			b. Can blood container lot number be related to donor?	606,160(a)(2)		
b. Blood pressure? 90-180mm/50-100mm	640.3(b)(2)			A16. DONOR AND COLLECTION RECORDS:			
c. Determining acceptable hemoglobin (>12.5gm/100ml)? or equivalent hematocrit (>38%)?	640.3(b)(3)			a. Are the records maintained as required?	606.160(a)		
				b. Are the records complete as required?	606.160(b)(1)		
d. Examination of both arms for narcotic addiction scars?	640.3(b)(7)			c. Do the records include reasons for permanent or temporary deferral?	606.160(b)(1)(ii)		
A5. Was the determination of donor suitability observed?				d. Are adverse reactions, complaints, reports, and follow-up included?	606.160(b)(1)(iii)		
A6. ARM PREPARATION:				e. Do the records identify the phlebotomist?	606.160(b)(1)(vi)		
a. Was procedure observed?				f. Do the records indicate whether the bleeding was successful or unsuccessful?			
b. Was procedure performed satisfactorily?	640.4(f)			g. Indicate number of records checked.			
A7. ARM PREPARATION SUPPLIES:				A17. Was blood collection observed by investigator?			
a. Are prepackaged supplies used?							
b. If not, are supplies properly sterilized before use? i.e., for 20 minutes in saturated steam [121.5°C(251°F)]? or for 2 hours with dry heat [170°C(338°F)]?	600.11(b) 606.60(c)			A18. NOTE: Therapeutic Bleedings — see question H12.			
				ADDITIONAL QUESTION FOR LICENSED ESTABLISHMENTS			
A8. BLOOD UNIT NUMBER: Is blood unit number marked on blood container?	640.4(e)			A19. a. Is physician on premises during donor suitability determination and blood collection?	640.3(a) 640.4(a)		
A9. COLLECTION CONTAINER: Is an approved collection container used?				b. If not, is SOP manual approved by Bureau of Biologics?	640.3(a)(1) 640.4(a)(1)		
A10. COLLECTION:				c. If a physician is not on premises, is a responsible person designated as required?	640.3(a)(2) 640.4(a)(2)		
a. Is the venipuncture performed with "non-touch" technique?	640.4(f)						
b. Is blood drawn by a method that insures a correct amount?	606.100(b)(5)						
c. Is container hermetically sealed?	640.2(c)						

COMMENTS:

QUALITY CONTROL AND REGULATORY REQUIREMENTS   **313**

ITEM	CFR No.	Yes	No	ITEM	CFR No.	Yes	No
B1. Is Whole Blood collected routinely *(anytime other than under therapeutic or emergency conditions)*?				B7. SEROLOGICAL TEST FOR SYPHILIS: Are all units tested?	640.5(a)		
B2. ABO TESTING: Are red cells tested with Anti-A and with Anti-B and is serum tested with known A and known B cells?	640.5(b) 405.1317(b) (4)(i) HCFA			B8. REAGENTS:			
				a. Are only licensed antisera used for HB$_S$Ag, ABO, and Rh tests?	610.40(b) 640.5(b)(c)		
B3. Rh TESTING:				b. Do all test methods conform to manufacturer's current specifications?	606.65(e) 640.5(b)(c)		
a. Are red cells tested with Anti-D?	640.5(c) 405.1317(b) (4)(ii) HCFA			c. Are all reagents used in date?	606.65(e)		
b. Are D negatives confirmed by further testing?	640.5(c)			B9. LABORATORY RECORDS:			
B4. HB$_S$Ag TESTING:				a. Are records maintained as required?	606.160(a)(1)		
a. Is each unit of blood tested for HB$_S$Ag by a 3rd generation test?	610.40(a)			b. Are manufacturer, lot number, and expiration date of reagents recorded?	606.160 (b)(7)(v)		
b. Is test made on a sample taken at time of donation?	610.40(b)			c. Do the records include the identification of the persons responsible for labeling all products?	606.160(b) (2)(v)		
B5. HB$_S$Ag TESTING *(Performed on Premises)*:				B10. QUALITY CONTROL CHECKS:			
a. Is HB$_S$Ag testing performed in segregated area?	600.11(e)(1) 606.40(a)(7)			a. Are specificity and reactivity of reagents recorded each day of use?	606.65(c)		
b. Are the supplies and reagents used in HB$_S$Ag testing properly disposed of?	606.40(d)(1)			b. Is laboratory equipment standardized and/or calibrated as specified in the regulations?	606.60(b)		
B6. HB$_S$Ag TESTING *(Testing by Outside Laboratory)*:							
a. If HB$_S$Ag testing is not performed on premises, list laboratory performing test.							
(1) Name							
(2) Address							
(3) City (4) State (5) Zip							
b. Are written test results in the possession of the collection facility before units are issued?	610.40(b)(3)						

COMMENTS:

314   MODERN BLOOD BANKING AND TRANSFUSION PRACTICES

ITEM	CFR No.	Yes	No	ITEM	CFR No.	Yes	No
B11. LABELING OF WHOLE BLOOD AND RED BLOOD CELLS: Paste label below.				B13. AUTOMATED TESTS:			
a. Does label of unit ready for issue include all of the items listed below? ABO Rh STS HB$_S$Ag Mix Proper Name Donor No. Crossmatch Use Filter Expiration Date Name & Address Hepatitis Warning See Circular Storage Temp. Volunteer or Paid Donor Volume *("prepared from. . ." for RBC's)* "Caution: Federal Law Prohibits. . ." Quantity and Kind of Anticoagulant License No. *(if applicable)*.	640.7 610.62 610.61 606.120(b) 21 U.S.C. 353(b)(4)			a. If an automated system is used then write name and model in comments.			
				b. Is the equipment set up and labeled so that an investigator can follow how the equipment operates?	606.140(a) and (b)		
				c. Are appropriate controls tested at the beginning and end of each run to confirm channel identification and specific reactivity of every reagent used?	606.140(a) and (b)		
b. Group O classification?	640.7(e)			d. Are all reagents dated when put into use?	606.160(a)		
c. Is D^U performed on D negative?				e. If unlicensed reagents are used, has the appropriate reagent evaluation been conducted?			
d. If D^U not performed on D negative, does label so indicate?	640.5(c)			B14. a. Have there been any laboratory or labeling errors since the last inspection?	600.14		
e. Whole Blood *(Human)* Modified: 1. Proper name	640.7(g)(1)			b. Are records of laboratory and labeling errors maintained as required?	606.160(b)(7)(iii)		
2. Factor(s) removed	640.7(g)(2)						
3. Restrictions on use, if applicable.	640.7(g)(3)			c. Is BoB notified if HB$_S$Ag positive blood products are issued?	600.14		
f. Are HB$_S$Ag reactive units used in research or the manufacture of HB$_S$Ag test reagents?				B15. a. Are units from an outside source retested?			
g. If so, are units labeled to indicate reactive results and possible transmission of hepatitis?	610.40(d)			b. If yes, are records maintained?	606.160(a)(1)		
B12. Were the following tests observed *(check all applicable)*? ☐ ABO & Rh ☐ HB$_S$Ag ☐ STS ☐ Labeling							

COMMENTS:

QUALITY CONTROL AND REGULATORY REQUIREMENTS   **315**

	ITEM	CFR No.	Yes	No		ITEM	CFR No.	Yes	No
C1.	Are Red Cells prepared routinely *(anytime other than under therapeutic or emergency conditions)*?				C5.	IF DEGLYCEROLIZED RED BLOOD CELLS ARE PREPARED: a. Is the temperature of thawing apparatus monitored and recorded?	606.60(b)		
C2.	If cells are prepared in open system, is a 24 hour expiration date assigned?	610.53				b.q Is the dating period for deglycerolized Red Blood Cells ≤24 hours?	610.53		
C3.	State in comments how plasma is disposed of. *(If it is used to make Plasma or Recovered Plasma, fill in applicable sections of Part D.)*					c. Are Quality Control tests performed on deglycerolized Red Blood Cells?	640.17		
						d. Are records kept of Quality Control tests?	606.160(b)(5)		
C4.	IF FROZEN RED BLOOD CELLS ARE PREPARED: a. Is the dating period <3 years?	610.53			C6.	RED BLOOD CELL RECORDS: a. Are records maintained as required?	606.160(a)		
	b. Is a caution prominently displayed on the label, e.g., "Do Not Use Without Further Processing"?	606.120(b)(6)				b. Are records complete as required?	606.160(b)(2)(ii)		
					C7.	Was the preparation of Red Blood Cells observed by the investigator?			

COMMENTS:

MODERN BLOOD BANKING AND TRANSFUSION PRACTICES

ITEM	CFR No.	Yes	No	ITEM	CFR No.	Yes	No

OPTICAL STEPS IN PROCESSING SINGLE DONOR PLASMA	(640.30– 640.34,			D5. LABELING: *(Paste label on reverse)*
				 a. S ndard items:
				    ABO HB$_S$Ag
				    STS Donor No.
				    Proper Name Volume of Plasma
				    Use Filter Expiration Date
				    Name and Address See Circular
				    Volume and type of anticoagulant
				    "Caution: Federal law. . .",
				    License No. *(if applicable)*
				    Volunteer or Paid Donor
					640.35
					 21 U.S.C.
					 353(b)(4)		

Closed system from whole blood collection or by plasmapheresis.*							

PLASMA FRESH FROZEN:
   Collected with minimal damage to tissues.
   Separated from RBC and frozen solid within 6 hours.
   Stored at -18°C or colder for ⩽1 year.
   May have PC removed from product.
				b. Expiration date?	640.35(f)		

				c. Proper storage temperature?	640.35(i)		
				d. Instructions to thaw frozen product at 30–37°C?	640.35(k)		

PLASMA:
   Separated from the RBC within 26 days after phlebotomy *(within 40 days after phlebotomy wnen CPDA-1 solution is used as the anticoagulant).*
   Stored at -18°C or colder within 6 hours after separation.
   Dating period – 5 years.
   PC and/or CAHF may be removed from product.
				e. Warning not to use if frozen product has evidence of thawing or breaking?	640.35(j)		

				f. Instructions to use frozen product within 6 hours after thawing?	640.35(l)		
				g. Instructions to administer to ABO compatible recipients?	640.35(n)		

PLASMA PLATELET RICH:
   Collected with minimal damage to tissues.
   Separated from RBC within 4 hours after phlebotomy.
   Procedure must produce a product with at least 250,000 platelets/microliter.
   Stored at 1–6°C, or at 20–24°C with agitation, for 72 hours.
				h. When applicable, instructions to agitate SDP Plasma Platelet Rich during storage?	640.35(o)		

				D6. Was the preparation of plasma observed by the investigator?			
				RECOVERED PLASMA			

PLASMA LIQUID:
   Separated from the RBC within 26 days after phlebotomy *(within 40 days after phlebotomy when CPDA-1 solution is used as the anticoagulant).*
   Stored at 1–6°C for total of 26 days.
				Recovered Plasma is obtained from single units of expired or unexpired whole blood, outdated Plasma or as a bv-product in blood component preparation.			

				CRITICAL STEPS IN PROCESSING RECOVERED PLASMA Must be able to relate Plasma unit to donor. Each unit must be tested for HB$_S$Ag			
*If Plasma is prepared by plasmapheresis, complete all questions on Plasma in this section and additionally the applicable sections of Form FDA 2722.				D7. PREPARATION: Is Recovered Plasma prepared?			
				D8. CRITICAL STEPS: Are all the critical steps followed?			
D1. PREPARATION: Is Single Donor Plasma prepared?				D9. Is the procedure for preparing and shipping Recovered Plasma described in SOP?	606.100(b) (18)		
D2. CRITICAL STEPS: For the specific products prepared, are all of the critical steps followed?	640.34(a-d)			D10. a. Shipped under short supply?	601.22		
				b. If so, to which ilcensed manufacturer(s)? *(Specify in comments)*			
D3. FROZEN PRODUCTS: Are frozen products stored so as to detect thawing?	640.34(g)(2)			D11. Shipped for in-vitro reagent use?			
				D12. LABELING: Paste label on reverse. a. Descriptive neme, e.g,, "Recovered Human Plasma"	606.120(b)		

D4.   PLASMA RECORDS:
      a. Are records maintained as required?
	606.160(a)			b. Standard items:
				         Quantity anticoagulant(s),
				         donor or pool no. collection date
				                        HB$_S$Ag
					606.120(b)		

b. Are critical steps documented?	606.160(b) (2)(ii)			c. Storage temperature	606.120(b)		
				d. Name and address of manufacturer	606.120(b)		
COMMENTS:				e. If under short supply: "Caution! For Manufacturing Use Only"?	606.120(b)		

				f. If not under short supply:
				        1. "Caution: For Use In Manufacturing Noninjectable Products Only";
				        2. "Caution: Not for use in products subject to license under §351 of the PHS Act"?			

				D13. RECOVERED PLASMA RECORDS: a. Are records maintained as required?	606.160(a)		
				b. Are records complete as required?	606.160(b) (2)(iii)		
				D14. Was the preparation of Recovered Plasma observed by the investigator?			

QUALITY CONTROL AND REGULATORY REQUIREMENTS   **317**

ITEM	CFR No.	Yes	No		ITEM	CFR No.	Yes	No
CRITICAL STEPS IN PROCESSING	640.20– 640.25 640.27			E4.	Is corrective action taken if Q.C. results are unsatisfactory?	640.25(b)(3)		
Prepared from plasma obtained from whole blood collection, plasmapheresis*, or plateletpheresis. Uninterrupted, free flowing venipuncture. Source blood or plasma at 20–24°C until PC removed. Separated appropriately in a closed system within 4 hours of collection. Stored in 30–50 ml at 20–24°C with agitation, or in 20–30 ml at 1–6°C. 72 hour expiration date. Q.C. – 4 units, 72 hours old, each month of preparation; platelet count 5.5×10^{10}; pH6; volume as above.				E5.	RECORDS: a. Are records maintained as required?	606.160(a)		
					b. Are critical steps documented?	606.160(b)(2)(ii)		
				E6.	a. If Platelets are collected by platelet-pheresis, write name and model number of machine in comments.			
*If Platelets are prepared by plasmapheresis, complete all questions in this section and additionally the applicable sections of Form FDA 2722.					b. Is SOP followed?	606.100(b)(17)		
E1. PREPARATION: Are Platelets prepared?				E7.	LABELING: Paste platelet concentrate label below.			
E2. CRITICAL STEPS: Are all of the critical steps followed?	640.20– 640.25				a. Standard items: ABO HB_sAg STS Donor No. Proper Name Use Filter Volume Exp. Date and Hour Name and Address See Circular Kind and Volume of Anticoagulant "Caution: Federal law . . .", Volunteer or Paid Donor License No. *(if applicable)*	640.26 21 U.S.C. 353(b)(4)		
E3. MANUFACTURING RESPONSIBILITY: If Q.C. is not performed under the supervision and control of this establishment, then indicate in comments where Q.C. testing is done.	640.25(c)							
					b. Recommended storage temperature, and to continually agitate gently if at 20–24°C?	640.26(j)		
COMMENTS:					c. Use as soon as possible, but not more than 4 hours after entering the container?	640.26(k)		
				E8.	Was the preparation of Platelets observed by investigator?			

ITEM	CFR No.	Yes	No		ITEM	CFR No.	Yes	No
CRITICAL STEPS IN PROCESSING	640.50– 640.56			F5.	RECORDS: a. Are records maintained as required?	606.160(a)		
Closed system from whole blood collection or by plasmapheresis.*					b. Are critical steps documented?	606.160(b) (2)(ii)		

Starting plasma:
  at least 200 ml;
  frozen within 6 hours after blood collection;
  stored at –18°C or colder until thawed;
  thawed at 1–6°C.
Procedure produces average of no less than 80 units
  AHF per container.
Q.C. test of at least 4 units each month of
  preparation; average 80 units AHF per
  container; results available within 30
  days of preparation.
Stored at –18°C or colder for one year.
 	
*If CAHF is prepared by plasmapheresis, complete
all questions in this section and additionally the
applicable sections of Form FDA 2722.
				F6.	LABELING: Paste cryoprecipitate
					label below.
					a. Standard items:
					  ABO HB$_s$Ag
					  STS Proper Name
					  Donor No. Use Filter
					  Expiration Date Name and Address
					  See Circular
					  "Caution: Federal Law . . ."
					  License No. *(if applicable)*
					  Volunteer or Paid Donor
						640.57
						21 U.S.C.
						353(b)(4)		

					b. Average potency is 80 or more units of antihemophilic factor.	640.57(h)		
F1. PREPARATION: Is Cryoprecipitated AHF prepared?					c. Warning against further processing if evidence of breakage or thawing.	640.57(j)		
F2. CRITICAL STEPS: Are all of the critical steps followed?					d. Instructions to store at –18°C or colder?	640.57(i)		
					e. "Thaw at 30–37°C"?	640.57(k)		
F3. MANUFACTURING RESPONSIBILITY: If Q.C. is not performed under the super- vision and control of this establishment, then indicate in comments where Q.C. testing is done?	640.56(c)				f. Store at room temperature after thawing and use as soon as possible but no more than 4 hours after entering or pooling and within 6 hours after thawing.	640.57(l)		
				F7.	Was the preparation of CAHF observed?			
F4. Is corrective action taken if Q.C. results are unsatisfactory?								

COMMENTS:

QUALITY CONTROL AND REGULATORY REQUIREMENTS   319

ITEM	CFR No.	Yes	No	ITEM	CFR No.	Yes	No
COMPATIBILITY TESTING				G7. COMPATIBILITY TEST RECORDS:			
				a. Are records maintained as required?	606.160(a)(1)		
G1. RECIPIENT SAMPLE ID: Does the labeling of the recipient's blood sample insure positive ID?	606.151(a)			b. Do the records include results of compatibility tests, testing of patient samples, anti-body screening, and identification?	606.160(b)(4)(i)		
G2. REAGENTS:	606.65(e)						
a. Are reagents used according to manufacturer's directions?	610.40(b) 640.5(b)(c)			c. Do the records include results of ABO and Rh confirmatory testing?	606.160(b)(4)(ii)		
b. Are the reagents used for required tests in date?	606.65(e)			d. Do the records include date of receipt of recipient's sample?	606.160(b)(4)		
c. Are reagent performance checks done each day of use?	606.65(c)			G8. Were the following testing procedures observed by the investigator (check all applicable)?			
G3. MAJOR CROSSMATCH: Does it include the antiglobulin (Coombs) method?	606.151(c)			☐ ABO & Rh ☐ Crossmatching			
G4. ANTIBODY TESTING OF DONOR BLOOD:				**RECIPIENT REACTIONS (Transfusion Services):**			
a. Do the labels indicate that donor blood is tested for unexpected antibody?				G9. RECIPIENT REACTIONS:			
b. If not, do records show a minor crossmatch (i.e., donor's serum and recipient cells) is performed?	606.151(d)			a. Are records kept of reports of suspected transfusion reactions?	606.170(a)		
G5. EMERGENCY TRANSFUSIONS:				b. Does the blood bank have an SOP for investigating suspected transfusion reactions?	606..100(b)(9)		
a. Are procedures available for life-threatening emergencies?	606.151(e)			c. Are suspected hemolytic transfusion reactions reviewed by appropriate personnel?			
b. Are records maintained of units issued before completion of crossmatches?	606.151(e)			d. When a hemolytic transfusion reaction results from a faulty product, do the records indicate that the manufacturer or collecting facility was notified?	606.170(a)		
c. Do the records show subsequent completion of crossmatches?	606.160(b)(4)(i)						
d. Do the records include documentation of need for emergency procedures?	606.151(e)			G10. RECORD OF RECIPIENT REACTIONS:			
G6. PLASMA DERIVATIVES: If plasma derivatives are distributed by blood bank, do the records identify lot numbers and recipients?	606.160(b)(3)(i)			a. Records are maintained as required?	606.170(a)		
				b. Were reports of recipient reactions reviewed by investigator?			

COMMENTS:

ITEM	CFR No.	Yes	No
STORAGE			
H1. PHYSICAL STORAGE:			
a. Are blood products stored on premises?			
b. Are they stored separately from hazardous or contaminated items?	606.40(a)		
c. Are quarantine areas provided for storage of blood or components:			
1. prior to completion of tests?	606.40(a)(3)(4)		
2. not suitable for use?	606.40(a)(6)		
H2. STORAGE TEMPERATURES AND RECORDS:			
a. Do all observed temperatures and temperature records meet standards?	610.53 606.160(b)(3)(iii)		
b. Is there an explanation for any temperature deviation?	606.160(a)(1) 606.160(b)(3)(iii)		
c. Is temperature recorder used?			
d. If yes, is it compared against thermometer daily?	606.60(b)		
e. If yes, are the blood bank temperature recorder charts changed at proper intervals?	600.12(a) 606.160(b)(3)(iii)		
f. If yes, are the charts retained (dated and initialed)?	606.160(d)		
GENERAL OPERATIONS			
H3. PERSONNEL: Do personnel appear familiar with the current applicable regulations?	600.10(b) 606.20(b)		
H4. SOP:			
a. Is SOP maintained as required?	606.100(b)		
b. Do personnel appear familiar with it?	606.100(b)		
H5. FACILITIES: Are all facilities clean and suitable?	606.40		
H6. FATAL REACTIONS:			
a. Were there any fatal donor and/or recipient reactions in the last 24 months?			
b. Was Bureau of Biologics notified of any fatal reactions?	606.170(b)		
H7. CIRCULARS: Are current circulars available for all products prepared or used at this blood bank?	606.120(b)(8)		
H8. RECORDS:			
a. Are records retained for at least 5 years after processing?	606.160(d)		
b. Are they traceable to the donor?	606.160(c)		
DISTRIBUTION			
H9. RECORD SYSTEM: Is a record of unsuitable donors used to prevent the distribution of products collected from such individuals?	606.160(e)		
H10. INSPECTION:			
a. Are whole blood and red blood cells visually inspected at the time of issue?	640.5(e) 640.11(b)		
b. Is a record of such inspections maintained?	606.160(b)(3)(ii)		
H11. REISSUE:			
a. Is blood reissued?			
b. Does reissued blood meet all requirements as stated?	640.2(e)		

ITEM	CFR No.	Yes	No
H12. THERAPEUTIC BLEEDINGS:			
a. Is the request for a therapeutic donation by the attending physician on file?	606.160(b)(1)(iv)		
b. Are therapeutic bleedings used for transfusions?			
c. If therapeutic bleedings are used for transfusion, does label indicate disease?	640.3(d)		
d. Is disposition recorded?			
H13. EMERGENCY ISSUE: When blood is issued in an emergency:			
a. is it properly labeled?	640.7(f)		
b. are required records kept?	640.2(f)(2) 606.160(b)(3)(v)		
H14. SHIPPING:			
a. Are blood products distributed to outside facilities? If so,			
b. Are blood products shipped in such a manner as to assure maintenance of proper temperature?	600.15(a)		
c. Has the establishment periodically verified capacity of shipping containers to maintain proper temperature?	606.160(b)(5)(iv)		
H15. DESTRUCTION RECORDS:			
a. Are destruction records maintained?	606.160(b)(3)(i)		
b. Do records indicate reason for destruction?	606.160(a)		
c. Do records indicate method of destruction (If HB$_s$Ag reactive, by autoclaving or incineration.)?	606.160(a)		
d. Do the records include all components prepared from an HB$_s$Ag reactive unit?	606.160(a)		
H16. DISTRIBUTION RECORDS:			
a. Are all distribution records complete as required?	606.160(b)(3)(i) 606.165(b)		
b. Do distribution records enable a unit of Whole Blood and all of its components to be traced?	606.165(a) 606.165(b)		
PREVIOUS EXCEPTIONS			
H17. PREVIOUS EXCEPTIONS:			
a. Have deviations cited in previous inspection been corrected?			
b. If not, list continuing deviations in comments citing applicable question number.			

COMMENTS:

QUALITY CONTROL AND REGULATORY REQUIREMENTS   **321**

PART I				UNIFORM BLOOD LABELING				
ITEM	CFR	Yes	No	ITEM	CFR	Yes	No	

	ITEM	CFR	Yes	No		ITEM	CFR	Yes	No
I1.	Is uniform blood labeling being used?				I3. a.	Is approved circular of information available for each product?			
I2.	Labeling for all blood products:				b.	Is circular distributed/received with blood shipments?	Proposed 606.122		
	a. Does label of unit ready for issue include all of the items listed below in eye readable form?	Proposed 606.121 21 U.S.C. 353(b)(4)			c.	Is current AABB-ARC circular used?			
	Proper name Storage temp. Name & Address ABO Donor No. Rh Expiration date Hepatitis warning Paid or Volunteer donor Volume *(except cryo)* "Caution: Federal Law Prohibits..." See Circular "Properly identify intended recipient" Identity & volume of source material License No. *(if applicable).*				d.	If not AABB-ARC circular does circular contain all information required in uniform labeling guideline?			

COMMENTS:

CHAPTER 14

TRANSFUSION THERAPY

PAUL R. SOHMER, M.D.

In the past 2 decades, newly developed strategies for the collection and preservation of blood have made it possible to separate individual blood components from whole blood. Today, the indiscriminant use of whole blood is neither required nor justified. The blood component that is considered most likely to correct a specific deficiency is administered, just as antibiotics are administered, according to the specific and known sensitivity of an infectious agent.

The efficacy of blood component therapy is dependent on (1) an accurate assessment of the patient's needs; (2) the appropriate choice of blood product; and (3) the conscientious monitoring of transfusion effect. Since generalizations are often not applicable to a specific clinical setting, the principles of blood component therapy are best defined using a clinically derived, problem-oriented approach.

HEMORRHAGE

The hemodynamic response to acute blood loss is initiated rapidly and with great vigor. However, in the face of severe hemorrhage, the effectiveness of circulatory compensation is diminished by associated volume depletion. When blood loss exceeds the body's ability to compensate, the response to hemorrhage becomes self-defeating. The uninhibited release of catecholamines causes sustained arteriolar and venular vasoconstriction. The deleterious effects of hypovolemia are compounded by the effects of a maldistribution of blood flow, which further impedes tissue perfusion. This may result in severe pulmonary, hepatic, and renal dysfunction. In the face of severe hemorrhage and reduced blood volume, the capacity for hemodynamic compensation is eventually exhausted.

ASSESSMENT OF NEED

In 1794, Dr. Benjamin Rush[1] described the response of yellow-fever victims to "therapeutic" phlebotomy as follows: "1) It raised the pulse when depressed and quickened when it was preternaturally slow or subject to intermissions. 2) It reduced its force and frequency." Read these two statements carefully—they are contradictory! Rather than indicating a lack of clarity in verbal expression or thinking, this contradiction reflects an observation that is of great significance to the accurate assessment of patients who have suffered a loss of blood: *No two individuals will respond in exactly the same manner.* Each patient must be evaluated individually and considered relative to the specific nature of his or her underlying disorder, condition prior to injury, and ongoing response to therapy. Generalized quantitative guidelines can be seriously misleading and often have no value in the specific clinical setting.

The extent of blood loss may be estimated from the site and severity of injury. Injuries that result in significant soft tissue and skeletal damage are often associated with a significant loss of blood. Penetrating wounds of the abdomen and chest and pelvic fractures are most often associated with severe hemorrhage into body cavities; the likelihood of concealed hemorrhage in the presence of such injuries prevents an accurate assessment of blood loss.

When the extent of injury cannot be estimated from inspection (e.g., gastrointestinal bleeding), it is obviously difficult to accurately assess the volume of blood lost. A useful guide is provided by the observations made by Shenkin and associates[2] in 1944 of *normal human volunteers* who were bled 10 percent (500 ml), 20 percent (1000 ml), and nearly 25 percent (over 1000 ml) of their estimated blood volumes. Symptoms observed at rest, such as hypotension, pallor, diaphoresis, cold extremities, and loss of consciousness, occur with a significant blood loss of approximately 25 percent of the blood volume; symptoms not present at rest, but elicited by a change in position (orthostatic hypotension), suggest a blood loss of at least 20 percent of the blood volume. However, the patient who is compromised by associated renal, cerebral, pulmonary, or coronary insufficiency is less tolerant: serious symptomatology may be induced by an apparently less-than-significant loss of blood volume.

Pulse rate and blood pressure are often misleading. Neither is a reliable index of either the extent or rate of bleeding. Similarly, the hematocrit is equally unreliable. Central venous pressure (CVP) is a sensitive indicator of functional blood volume; it reflects the extent of hypovolemia and may provide the earliest indication of decompensation.

CHOICE OF PRODUCT

The principal variables of oxygen delivery are quantitatively expressed by the Fick equation:

$$VO_2 = Q \times 1.34 \times Hb \times (SaO_2 - SvO_2)$$

where VO_2 is the volume of oxygen delivered in liters per minute, Q is the blood flow in liters per minute, 1.34 is the volume of oxygen in milliliters that is bound to each gram of hemoglobin, and SaO_2 and SvO_2 are the percentage of arterial and mixed venous oxygen saturations. A small amount of oxygen that is physically dissolved in blood is not described by the equation.

Since the basic underlying pathophysiologic defect of hemorrhagic shock and hypovolemia is impaired oxygen transport, the Fick equation, which quantitatively defines oxygen delivery, can be applied as a guide to the priorities of treatment. The first priority is restoration of blood volume and flow. When commenced with a non-oxygen-carrying solution, volume resuscitation alone will improve oxygen delivery and increase oxygen consumption.[3] Indeed, since shock is rarely caused by anemia and may result from hypovolemia not associated with red cell loss, it is most appropriate to commence therapy with fluids other than blood, unless there is pre-existing cerebrovascular, or cardiopulmonary insufficiency.

Initial fluid replacement with either crystalloid (e.g., lactated Ringer's solution) or colloid (e.g., 5 percent albumin, plasma protein fraction, dextrans, hydroxyethyl starch) solutions is fundamental to the treatment of hypovolemia regardless of its cause. The choice of fluid is, as yet, a matter of great controversy. Those who favor resuscitation with colloid solutions argue that control of the colloid oncotic pressure is of paramount importance to the maintenance of intravascular fluid volume and that its preservation by infusion of colloid-containing solutions will result in long-term volume expansion, promotion of capillary perfusion, and reduction in the incidence of postresuscitation pulmonary complications.[4-9] Laboratory observations of the mechanism of fluid shift and restitution of plasma protein in response to hemorrhage,[10] however, have supported the importance of restoration of extracellular fluid losses in the treatment of hypovolemia.[10-14] Indeed, maintenance of extracellular fluid volume (and, therefore, interstitial pressure) with non-colloid-containing solutions will drive the physiologic mechanism by which colloid osmotic pressure is restored by endogenous protein.[14] Those who favor the use of crystalloid solutions have stressed the need to replenish extracellular fluid losses, the attendant increase in capillary perfusion that occurs with hemodilution caused by the infusion of low-viscosity crystalloids, and the significant reduction in cost of therapy associated with their use.[15-18] In a carefully controlled study, Lowe, Moss, and Jilek[19] observed no difference in alveolar-arterial oxygen difference, pulmonary function, or survival in patients treated with either colloid or crystalloid solutions.

Obviously, a detailed description of the properties of crystalloid and colloid solutions, the physiology attendant with their use, and an in-depth treatise of this controversy far exceeds the scope of a general text in blood banking. The author will resist the temptation to thrust upon the reader his own personal preference in this matter. Instead, the reader is referred to the publications cited above.

The second and third variables of the Fick equation describe the "functional" oxygen content of arterial blood, that is, the concentration of red cell hemoglobin that is available to carry oxygen and the ability of hemoglobin to carry, bind, and release oxygen. A significant blood loss signifies a reduction in both cardiac output (blood volume) and hemoglobin concentration. These reductions are additive in limiting the availability of oxygen. The number of circulating red cells and their hemoglobin content is crucial. Since large numbers of circulating red blood cells will be lost, restoration of the circulating red cell volume by transfusion is warranted. The British and American experience with combat casualties in North Africa nearly 40 years ago clearly demonstrated that conventional cell-free resuscitation fluids alone (e.g., 5 percent albumin, Ringer's lactate) are inadequate in the face of severe hemorrhage.[20,21] Thus, conventional wisdom dictates that restoration of the patient's oxygen-carrying capacity with transfusions of erythrocyte-containing blood products is imperative. (Significantly, the third variable of the Fick equation, the fractional unloading of oxygen, has largely been ignored.)

There is obvious logic in the use of whole blood in the treatment of massive hemorrhage. Transfusion of whole blood is the simplest way to simultaneously infuse plasma and red blood cells. However, the notion that stored whole blood is closest in composition to the fluid that has been lost and, therefore, is the component of choice, is a potentially dangerous untruth. The biochemical and metabolic properties of blood are significantly altered during in-vitro storage (see Chapter 1). Although the plasma of whole blood is no more effective than 5 percent albumin as a volume expander, it contains significant quantities of cellular debris, adenine, citrate, sodium, potassium, and ammonia, which may impose a significant metabolic burden on the bleeding patient, who typically requires large volumes of transfused blood. The removal of excess plasma may significantly reduce the metabolic burden of massive transfusion.

Whole blood is *not* essential to the treatment of hemorrhage. Indeed, restoration of the circulating hemoglobin concentration can be accomplished effectively and with reduced risk of metabolic complications with packed red cell transfusions rather than whole blood. After centrifugation, the remaining packed cell unit contains the same volume of hemoglobin in its 300-ml volume as does the 500-ml volume of whole blood. The load per unit of adenine, citrate, potassium, sodium, ammonia, plasma protein antigens, and antibodies in a packed cell unit is typically at least one third to one half of that found in a comparable (in length of storage) unit of whole blood.

The two major criticisms of the use of packed cells in this setting are derived from economic considerations and the practical problem of flow rate. Unfortunately, in many instances plasma and albumin have been used to supplement packed cell transfusions without regard to specific indications of patient need. Obviously, this adds greatly to the cost of transfusion and is an extravagance not previously associated with the routine use of whole blood. It is clear that "adequate" fluid replacement most often requires volumes that exceed "normal" blood volume. The volume in excess of "normal" should consist of fluids other than blood to allow for ease of removal after resuscitation has been accomplished. Recent experience with crystalloid solutions demonstrates that this required supplementation of blood transfusions can be accomplished effectively and inexpensively. Regardless of the fluid used to initiate resuscitation (colloid or crystalloid), the adoption of crystalloid solutions to supplement packed cell transfusions renders the economic criticism invalid, particularly in light of the distinct metabolic advantages gained by avoiding massive transfusion with whole blood.

The viscosity of blood stored as packed cells is obviously greater than that of whole blood. As viscosity is inversely related to flow, a reduction in transfusion flow rate accompanies the use of packed cells. This is easily remedied by infusing blood through a "Y" set, such that the rapid resuspension in saline, when necessary, is facilitated. With a minimum of experience this technique is easily mastered. However, the present trend to prepare packed cells at the highest hematocrit possible—so as to remove additional plasma for the procurement of fractionation products—does significantly reduce the transfusibility of blood. Beyond the clinical considerations described above, the repeated observation that post-transfusion red blood cell viability is reduced in packed cells stored at higher hematocrits in newer blood preservation systems is evidence enough that this practice should be condemned. A rational and practical compromise is to prepare packed cells to a hematocrit of approximately 0.75 ± 0.05. This level has been shown to be appropriate for maintenance of red cell viability and generally does not adversely effect flow rate, although resuspension in saline may be required.

Initiation of therapy with cell free solutions has the practical advantage of providing time for a specimen to be carried to the laboratory for the determination of the patient's ABO and $Rh_0(D)$ blood group and the selection of compatible donor blood for transfusion. Under most conditions, adequate time is available to prepare at least type-specific blood. It has been said that other than in a military context, there is no indication for uncrossmatched, group O, "universal donor" blood transfusions. However, the modern civilian trauma center faces a number of problems that are reminiscent of the military experience and often functions under virtual battlefield conditions. All admitted patients have suffered massive multisystem injuries and profound blood loss. The simultaneous admission of more than one severely injured patient is common. Time delays are incurred prior to the initiation of therapy because patients are often transported over previously unprecedented distances to facilities that are prepared to care for their needs. No matter how seasoned the staff or rigorous the treatment protocols, the initial resuscitation of critically injured patients is highly charged and always hectic. When faced with multiple admissions there is always an added sense of urgency. Obviously, the risk of clerical error is vastly increased in this setting. The trauma center and the patient population it serves are highly specialized and defined. Their support requires an aggressive and heroic approach that, until recently, was considered heretical by civilian standards and appropriate only in the context of military medicine.

The planned but limited, closely monitored, and strictly controlled utilization of uncrossmatched group-O blood transfusions may provide an important margin of safety and may facilitate the early resuscitation of simultaneously admitted patients who have suffered profound blood loss and whose treatment has been delayed by the time required for transportation to the treatment facility.[22] However, the use of uncrossmatched group-O blood is clearly not without risk. Naturally occurring anti-A and anti-B isoagglutinins in the plasma of blood drawn from group-O donors may cause acute hemolysis of the erythrocytes of A, B, and AB recipients.[23] In addition, subsequent transfusions with type-specific blood may induce an acute hemolytic transfusion reaction owing to the presence of these passively transferred antibodies.[24,25] The military experience with transfusions of uncrossmatched group-O whole blood selected for low titers of isoagglutinins has emphasized the importance of this phenomenon.[26] It has been recommended that transfusion with blood of the recipient's hereditary blood group should either not be attempted or, at the very least, be delayed for a minimum of 14 days in group-A recipients who have received 4 or more units of group-O whole blood.[24,27] Removal of the plasma and transfusion of group-O packed cells reduce the amount of antibody transferred to the recipient and the attendant risk.[22] However, if the antibody is strong, considerable activity will remain and the risk of incompatibility will persist.[28] In any event, uncrossmatched group-O blood should never be administered unless a blood sample is first drawn from the recipient to ascertain his or her hereditary blood group.

Because of the risk of Rh incompatibility and sensitization, $Rh_0(D)$-negative group-O blood is preferred for uncrossmatched blood transfusions. However, since the transfusion of $Rh_0(D)$-positive blood poses no immediate threat to the $Rh_0(D)$-negative recipient, unless the recipient has been sensitized by prior pregnancy or transfusion, it has been used in emergency situations when supplies of group-O, $Rh_0(D)$-negative blood are limited. Uncrossmatched group-O blood transfusions without regard to Rh incompatibility and sensitization have been used routinely for the resuscitation of battle casualties. For the military, the future risk of hemolytic disease of the newborn in recipient offspring has not been a consideration in selection of transfusion materials. However, when the principles of uncross-matched group-O transfusion therapy are applied to the civilian setting, where considerable numbers of female patients of child-bearing age may be involved, Rh sensitization becomes a very real and significant consideration. The transient immune paralysis associated with trauma and massive transfusion does not protect from Rh sensitization.[22] Similarly, in the civilian setting the presence of antibodies other than anti-A and anti-B in recipient plasma because of prior pregnancy or transfusion must be considered. Simply put, there is no such thing as "universal donor" blood. If this fact is understood, it becomes clear that the use of group-O blood transfusions for patients of blood groups other than group O should be limited to emergency situations that have been clearly defined by predetermined and specific criteria.

Uncontaminated hemorrhage into the chest or abdominal cavity may provide an additional source of red blood cells for transfusion. An effective intraoperative blood salvage system can provide a source of blood that is immediately available and readily accessible. Such blood is obviously type and group specific, crossmatch compatible, warm, and fresh. The choice of system is in part dictated by the setting in which intraoperative autotransfusion is contemplated. In an emergency in which the purity of the final product is of somewhat less concern since alternative sources of red blood cells for transfusion may be limited, the Sorenson Autologous Transfusion System developed by Noon[29] has proven effective.[30] In this system, pooled mediastinal, chest, or abdominal blood is aspirated with a suction tip, anticoagulated with CPD or ACD (in the usual blood-to-anticoagulant ratio of 7:1), and reinfused through two 170-micron filters. Labile clotting factors are retained and are active as well as platelets, unless a microaggregate filter is used.[31] Indeed, this system has been proved safe and effective when used for the postoperative salvage of blood in both adult and pediatric cardiac surgery patients,[32] as well as in the emergency room.[30,33]

The major disadvantage of the Sorenson system is the reinfusion of contaminants that may potentiate pathologic bleeding or organ dysfunction. Thus, an alternative system, the Haemonetics Cell Saver,[34,35] which permits the relative atraumatic collection of blood, filtration through a microfilter, and preparation and washing of red cell concentrates, is preferred for the nonemergent, elective setting. This system provides a final product that is of high hematocrit and is free of particulate matter, products of hemolysis, and other contaminants. In addition, platelet concentrates may be prepared intraoperatively using this system. The major disadvantages of this system are its cost, the requirement for a knowledgeable operator, and the time delay required for preparation of the final product (which would be of consideration in the emergency situation). As with the Sorenson Autologous Transfusion System, intraoperative autotransfusion with the Haemonetics Cell Saver is contraindicated in the presence of contamination (e.g., fecal contamination of an abdominal wound) or when tumor surgery results in dislodging of material whose metastatic dissemination may be facilitated by the reinfusion of shed blood.

TRANSFUSION EFFECT

Initial blood studies should include hematocrit, hemoglobin concentration, blood type, antibody screen and/or crossmatch, pH, blood gases, electrolytes, albumin concentration, and serum glucose concentration. Successful therapy is indicated by the maintenance of circulatory homeostasis without drug support, adequate urine output, normal central venous and pulmonary wedge pressures, a blood pressure of at least 90/60, and normal serum electrolytes, pH, and blood gases. Obviously, this is a gross simplification of the appropriate manner by which critically ill patients are monitored, but must suffice, because this is not the primary focus of this book.

ANEMIA

ASSESSMENT OF NEED

In general, chronic anemia is best treated without blood transfusion. Anemias that are expected to respond to specific therapy, such as iron deficiency and megaloblastic anemia, do not require transfusion unless significant symptoms of decompensation such as decreased exercise tolerance, tachycardia, tachypnea, and angina pectoris are present. Transfusion therapy is indicated when the patient fails to respond to hematinic therapy or when a delay in response cannot be tolerated because of the severity of symptoms. Transfusion therapy for chronic stable anemia is almost never indicated when the hemoglobin concentration is greater than 10 g per dl. Mild symptoms are often associated with hemoglobin levels of 8 to 10 g per dl; severe symptoms are often associated with levels of 5 to 8 g per dl. However, especially when the onset of anemia is gradual, a patient may adapt to severe anemia such that he or she appears well compensated despite having hemoglobin levels of 5 to 8 g per dl. This is particularly true of patients who suffer anemia in association with chronic liver or renal disease.

It is not necessary to transfuse patients to a high level of hemoglobin in preparation for surgery. The indications for preoperative and operative transfusion are based on assessment of the patient's general condition and underlying illness, the predicted and actual blood loss, the length and extent of the operative procedure, and residual pathology. In general, a preoperative hemoglobin level of 11.0 g per dl is satisfactory for procedures associated with a loss of 500 ml of blood.

The anticipation of intraoperative transfusion is, obviously, of practical importance to the blood bank. An awareness of the usual blood loss associated with specific surgical procedures (and surgical teams performing these procedures) will facilitate the management of the blood bank inventory.

With a routine review of blood utilization, specific guidelines may be established for not only blood supply, but the extent of pretransfusion testing. When blood requirements are routinely minimal, "type and screen" rather than preoperative crossmatch has been recommended.[36] Determination of the patient's ABO and Rh blood group and a screen of the patient's serum for unexpected antibodies may be adequate preoperative preparation for cholecystectomy, thyroidectomy, colostomy, abdominal and vaginal hysterectomy, ovarian wedge resection, total knee replacement, removal of hip pins, reduction mammoplasty, skin graft, and transurethral resection of the prostate.[36] If transfusion becomes necessary, a complete crossmatch can be completed within 15 to 30 minutes if low ionic strength media or other potentiators are utilized. An abbreviated crossmatch, however, may be completed in 5 minutes by performing the immediate-spin room-temperature phase only. Type-specific uncrossmatched blood also can be administered with relative safety as a last alternative. Specific guidelines should be generated by each transfusion service after consultation with surgical colleagues.

CHOICE OF PRODUCT

The danger of fluid load is significant when blood is administered to severely anemic patients. A reasonable approach is to give the maximal number of red cells in the smallest practical volume. Therefore, only packed red cells should be given for transfusion treatment of anemia. Whole blood is never indicated in this setting.

TRANSFUSION EFFECT

One 300-ml unit of packed red cells should raise the hemoglobin concentration by 1.0 g per dl or hematocrit by 3 percent in an adult of average size. If the hemoglobin yield is less than expected or if the transfusion effect is short-lived, bleeding or alloimmunization should be suspected.

The severely anemic patient should be closely monitored for signs of volume overload, such as elevated central venous pressure, jugular venous distension, and audible chest rales. Congestive heart failure may develop up to 12 hours after transfusion. The rapid administration of intravenous diuretics may reduce the risk of circulatory failure.

THROMBOCYTOPENIA

A minimal number of normal platelets is required for adequate hemostasis. The platelet has three major hemostatic functions: (1) formation of the hemostatic plug; (2) release of platelet phospholipid to enhance the conversion of prothrombin to thrombin; and (3) maintenance of capillary endothelial integrity. A definitive platelet hemostatic threshold is not known.

ASSESSMENT OF NEED

The clinical response to thrombocytopenia is highly variable. An individual may adapt such that sustained and severe thrombocytopenia is well tolerated; others will suffer spontaneous hemorrhage when the platelet count is only moderately depressed. The indications for platelet transfusion are not rigid. Each patient must be evaluated individually relative to his or her underlying disorder, the clinical setting (e.g., surgery), and factors that increase the risk of spontaneous hemorrhage, such as infection,[37] fever, and a precipitous fall in the platelet count.[38]

Although prolongation of the template bleeding time suggests that the risk of hemorrhage is increased in the face of platelet counts of less than 100,000 per cu mm,[39] spontaneous bleeding occurs only rarely when the count is greater than 20,000 per cu mm.[40] A platelet count of 20,000 per cu mm to 70,000 per cu mm, although adequate for the prevention of spontaneous bleeding, may be hazardous in surgery. However, a platelet count of 30,000 per cu mm does provide adequate hemostasis for most surgical procedures.[41,42] Higher counts may be required for longer or more technically difficult operative procedures. Owing to the high probability of spontaneous hemorrhage associated with platelet counts of less than 20,000 per cu mm, prophylactic platelet transfusions are recommended for the prevention of bleeding in patients whose bone marrow function is impaired owing to aplastic anemia, myelofibrosis, acute leukemia, or cancer chemotherapy.[43] However, in the face of risk factors such as fever or infection, prophylactic platelet transfusions may be indicated at only modest levels of thrombocytopenia. In general, bleeding associated with platelet counts of less than 50,000 per cu mm is an indication for platelet transfusion therapy. However, causes for bleeding other than thrombocytopenia must be carefully ruled out.

Patients whose bone marrow function is depressed as the result of a primary disease process such as aplastic anemia or leukemia, or as the result of an exogenous insult such as ionizing radiation or cancer chemotherapy, will often require frequent platelet transfusions. Whereas patients suffering from aplastic anemia will in all likelihood require prolonged platelet support, exogenously induced thrombocytopenia is generally transient and requires only intermittent platelet support. Obviously, the former group is at highest risk of developing alloimmunization.

The results of platelet transfusions in patients whose primary underlying disorder has resulted in peripheral platelet destruction are generally disappointing. Platelet transfusion therapy is of limited value in antibody-induced thrombocytopenias such as idiopathic thrombocytopenia purpura, since infused platelets are rapidly destroyed and cleared from the circulation. In these patients, platelet transfusions are reserved for the treatment of life-threatening hemorrhage. Although splenectomy has been safely performed with platelet counts as low as 20,000 per cu mm,[44] intraoperative platelet transfusion may be indicated after clamping of the splenic pedicle. Similarly, platelet transfusion has only a limited effect in the consumptive thrombocytopenia associated with infection and disseminated intravascular coagulation.

A 50 to 70 percent reduction in platelet count is associated with cardiopulmonary bypass because of platelet adherence to bypass equipment, platelet sequestration, and hypothermia.[45-47] Abnormalities of in-vitro platelet function, which have been described in these patients,[48-51] do not correlate with excessive bleeding after cardiac surgery. In fact, bleeding most often occurs as the result of a failure to effect mechanical hemostasis. Platelet transfusions cannot compensate for the loose ligature. Prophylactic platelet transfusions are neither required nor justified in cardiac surgery.

The massive transfusion of bank blood and cell-free solutions that are lacking in platelet content is often associated with significant thrombocytopenia. This is most often the case when the transfusion exceeds one blood volume within a short period of time. The change in platelet count and final post-transfusion platelet count correlates with the total volume infused. However, there is no direct correlation between the volumes infused and the incidence of post-transfusion bleeding. If bone marrow function is intact, most patients tolerate a simple dilutional thrombocytopenia as the platelet count is restored to a securely hemostatic level within several days of massive transfusion. Indeed, postresuscitation hemorrhage correlates far better with the severity and extent of the underlying and precipitating injury than with the total volume of fluids or blood infused. Therefore, it has been this author's practice to use the following guidelines for platelet transfusions in patients who have suffered severe multisystem trauma. Platelet concentrates are transfused if the patient demonstrates: (1) a platelet count of 50,000 per cu mm or less *in the face of active bleeding;* (2) a platelet count of 30,000 per cu mm or less with no active bleeding, but *with further surgery anticipated;* and (3) a platelet count of less than 20,000 per cu mm with no active bleeding or surgery anticipated.

CHOICE OF PRODUCT

The use of fresh whole blood for the treatment of thrombocytopenia invariably results in circulatory failure. Fortunately, modern technology has made it possible to harvest platelets from whole blood and has thus facilitated the treatment of thrombocytopenia. Basically, there are three transfusion products available for the treatment of thrombocytopenia: (1) random donor platelet concentrates, which are prepared by mechanical centrifugation from whole blood units; (2) single donor platelet packs, which are collected from one donor using a cell separator and contain the equivalent in platelets of 6 to 10 units collected by conventional whole blood donation; and (3) single donor, HLA-matched platelet packs, which are drawn from a single donor (related or unrelated) who has been determined to be HLA compatible with the potential recipient.

The random donor platelet concentrate should contain a minimum of 5.5 $\times$ 10^{10} platelets.[52] Pooled random donor platelet concentrates are well suited for the short-term requirement of patients who suffer a transient bleeding episode, such as those who have suffered traumatic injury. Although the use of single donor platelet packs at the outset of long-term transfusion support in patients with depressed marrow function is theoretically appealing, at this time it is standard practice to transfuse pooled random donor platelet concentrates unless there is evidence of alloimmunization. Single donor (not HLA-matched) platelet packs containing approximately 5 $\times$ 10^{11} platelets[53] are particularly useful in patients with hematologic disorders with thrombocytopenia secondary to drug therapy, who have not alloimmunized or do not require long-term support.

In general, HLA-matched, single donor platelet packs are reserved for the alloimmunized patient who has become refractory to random donor platelets. This fascinating but complex subject of HLA compatibility is discussed in Chapter 22.

It is generally acceptable to transfuse random donor platelets without regard to ABO compatibility. However, A and B antigens are found on donor platelets. The post-transfusion recovery of A_1 platelets is reduced when these are administered to group-O recipients.[54] The administration of platelets from a group-A donor to a group-O recipient is, therefore, best avoided. In fact, although the question of platelet transfusion and ABO compatibility is as yet unsettled, it is probably prudent to transfuse ABO-compatible platelets whenever possible. When group-compatible platelets are unavailable and large volumes of pooled random donor concentrates or single donor platelet packs are contemplated for transfusion, consideration must be given to potential sensitization or hemolysis caused by red cell contaminants or incompatible donor plasma. Rh antigens are not found on platelets, but may be of concern because of their presence on red blood cells that may contaminate platelet packs.

TRANSFUSION EFFECT

The hemostatic response to platelet transfusion is most accurately assessed by the clinical observation of cessation of bleeding or performance of the template bleeding time. The latter approach, however, is sometimes associated with scarring and may provide a nidus for infection in patients who are concomitantly granulocytopenic. The platelet count correlates well with the bleeding time.[55] In practice, then, determination of the platelet count following the infusion of viable platelets is usually an adequate monitor of transfusion effect. Although some splenic sequestration will occur, platelet recovery may be estimated from a platelet count 1 hour after transfusion. Platelet survival is estimated from a platelet count drawn at 18 to 24 hours after transfusion and daily thereafter. The platelet increment is defined as:

$$\frac{\text{post-transfusion count minus pretransfusion count}}{\text{number of units infused}} \times \text{body surface area}$$

A platelet increment of 6000 to 8000 per cu mm is most often observed in an adult of average size (1.7 sq m body surface area). Higher normal increments, such as 9000 to 10,000 per cu mm, are often observed and reported. However, the numbers reported above are consistent with the author's present experience.

The alloimmunized patient will rapidly destroy transfused platelets such that neither a 1-hour nor a 24-hour increment is observed. In most nonalloimmunized thrombocytopenic patients, the survival of transfused platelets is either normal (post-transfusion life span of 8 to 9 days[56]) or slightly reduced.[57] Of course, the recovery is reduced in patients with significant splenomegaly.[58]

HEREDITARY HEMORRHAGIC DISORDERS

Hereditary hemorrhagic disorders invariably involve the isolated deficiency of a single coagulation factor. As such, an accurate clinical and laboratory diagnosis is critical to the management of these disorders.

The two most frequently encountered and most severe disorders are associated with deficiencies of factor VIII and factor IX, hemophilia A and B. These are inherited in a sex-linked recessive fashion. Except for von Willebrand's disease, which is an autosomal dominant disorder, all coagulation factor deficiencies are autosomal recessive.

Hereditary hemorrhagic disorders are treated by replacement of the deficient factor with components and derivatives of fresh plasma. Coagulant activity is preserved by freezing plasma within 8 hours of donation.[59] Cryoprecipitate is particularly rich in factor VIII, von Willebrand's factor, and fibrinogen. Concentrates of specific coagulation factors are prepared from plasma by chemical fractionation.

HEMOPHILIA

Hemophilia is defined as severe, moderate, or mild depending on the extent of factor deficiency. Patients with less than 2 percent procoagulant activity are said to suffer from severe hemophilia most often presenting with spontaneous joint and soft tissue bleeding. Moderate hemophilia is defined by the presence of from 2 to 5 percent procoagulant activity. Although spontaneous bleeding is rare with such activity, minor trauma may lead to major bleeding. Mild hemophilia is defined by procoagulant activity within the range of 5 to 30 percent. These patients may present with severe bleeding following trauma or surgery.

ASSESSMENT OF NEED

The requirements for replacement therapy are determined by the severity of bleeding, the time elapsed from the onset of bleeding, the nature and location of the tissue area involved, and the patient's ongoing response to therapy. Replacement therapy is specifically indicated for the treatment of episodic bleeding. Some therapeutic guidelines are summarized in Table 14-1.

CHOICE OF PRODUCT

Fresh-frozen plasma contains all plasma coagulation factors. Approximately 1 unit of coagulation factor activity is present in each milliliter of plasma. The infusion of 10 to 15 ml of fresh-frozen plasma per kilogram of body weight will raise the recipient's plasma clotting activity by approximately 15 to 20 percent. The therapeutic efficacy of fresh-frozen plasma is limited by the infusion volume required to achieve appropriate factor levels. Neither surgical coverage nor medical therapy of the severe deficiency can be accomplished without causing circulatory overload.

Cryoprecipitate is rich in factor VIII. Approximately 30 to 80 percent of donor factor VIII may be recovered in cryoprecipitate. In general, 1 ml of cryoprecipitate contains approximately 5 to 10 units of factor VIII coagulant activity. Although cryoprecipitate is an effective therapeutic agent for the treatment of hemophilia A, rational therapy is made difficult by the wide variation in factor VIII content found in this product.

TABLE 14-1. Therapeutic Guidelines for Factor VIII Replacement Therapy

	Percentage Level to Control Bleeding[60,61]	Factor Dosage[60]
Spontaneous hemorrhage	15–20	10 units/kg
Deep muscle hematomata	50	20–30 units/kg
Hemarthrosis	20–60	20–30 units/kg
Retropharyngeal hemorrhage	80	40 units/kg
Retroperitoneal hemorhage	80	40–50 units/kg
Head injuries	100	40–50 units/kg
Surgery		
Preoperative	100	40–50 units/kg
Postoperative: Day 1–4	60	30 units/kg
Day 4–8	20–40	10–20 units/kg
Orthopedic surgery		
Preoperative	100	40 units/kg
Postoperative: Day 1–4	80	20 units/kg
Day 4–8	40	10 units/kg
Until ambulation	20	

Lyophilized factor VIII (AHF) concentrate is prepared from pooled plasma. When reconstituted in sterile water the concentrate is a potent and predictable therapeutic agent. This material is easily stored at 4°C and rarely causes allergic reactions. Since the concentrate contains 10 to 20 times the factor VIII content of plasma, circulatory overload is not likely, even when high activity levels are required. Dosage calculation is facilitated since the known factor activity is stated on each bottle. The use of factor VIII concentrate is associated with a significant risk of hepatitis and the passive transfer of group-A and group-B red blood cell isoagglutinins.

Concentrates of factors II, VII, IX, and X (prothrombin complex) are manufactured primarily for the treatment of hemophilia B. The two presently available products contain either 18 or 25 units of factor IX activity in each milliliter of concentrate. As with the factor VIII concentrates, prothrombin complex also carries the risk of hepatitis transmission; however, it is easily stored and administered and has a standardized and predictable dose activity.

TRANSFUSION EFFECT

The dosage may be calculated on the basis of the patient's weight, approximate plasma volume, and severity of bleeding. An estimation of the patient's residual factor activity is of vital importance. For simplicity, it has been suggested[60] that one may assume that one unit of factor VIII concentrate per kilogram body weight will raise the patient's plasma level by 2 percent, and that one unit of factor IX concentrate per kilogram of body weight will raise the patient's factor IX plasma level by 1.5 percent. The biologic half-life of factor VIII is 8 to 12 hours; the half-life of factor

IX reportedly ranges from 12 to 40 hours.[61] Therefore, to maintain a factor VIII level of greater than 30 percent, for example, it is necessary to raise the patient's plasma level to 60 percent every 12 hours.

While transfusion effect is best monitored by the specific factor assay, good intralaboratory clinical correlations suggest that the activated partial thromboplastin time will provide a fairly dependable measurement of factor recovery and survival.

Resistance to therapy may signify the development of an acquired inhibitor to factor VIII or factor IX. This occurs most often in the young patient whose plasma factor level is less than 1 percent. Acquired inhibitors are detected in 5 to 20 percent of patients with factor VIII deficiencies and 2 to 3 percent of patients with factor IX deficiencies.[60,61] The inhibitors are usually monoclonal IgG and occur most commonly during the first 50 days of therapy, but are unusual after more than 100 transfusions.

When an acquired inhibitor has been identified, it is best to withhold therapy except for the treatment of life-threatening hemorrhage. When therapy is withheld, there may be a gradual fall in antibody titer, and in many patients, the antibody will completely disappear. In most cases, however, antibody titers will rise again approximately 5 to 10 days after rechallenge. Neutralization of the inhibitor may be accomplished by the continuous infusion of high doses of factor concentrate.[62] Hemostasis may be achieved without appreciable increments in factor levels. Plasma exchange has only a temporary effect but may be of value in the treatment of life-threatening hemorrhage. Immunosuppressive therapy has been partially successful.[63]

VON WILLEBRAND'S DISEASE

ASSESSMENT OF NEED

Von Willebrand's disease is a mild to moderately severe hemorrhagic disorder that affects both sexes. Bleeding most often occurs from mucous membranes, typically as epistaxis, gastrointestinal bleeding, and menorrhagia.

Because von Willebrand's factor is required for normal platelet adhesion and formation of the platelet hemostatic plug, this disorder is most consistently characterized by prolongation of the bleeding time. The deficiency in von Willebrand factor may also be reflected by impaired ristocetin-induced platelet aggregation. The partial thromboplastin time is usually, but not always, prolonged. The plasma levels of factor VIII required for hemostasis are roughly equivalent to those required for hemophilia.[61]

CHOICE OF PRODUCT

The concentration of von Willebrand's factor in most commercial factor VIII concentrates is inadequate for replacement therapy. Therefore, fresh-frozen plasma or cryoprecipitate should be employed.

TRANSFUSION EFFECT

In von Willebrand's disease the transfusion of either fresh-frozen plasma or cryoprecipitate is followed by a prolonged and progressive rise in factor VIII levels. This effect may be due to the presence of a factor that stimulates either the release or production of factor VIII clotting activity. Because of this effect, hemostatic levels of factor activity are more easily achieved and maintained than in classic hemophilia.

A reduction in bleeding time may follow the infusion of fresh-frozen plasma or cryoprecipitate. In most cases, this reduction is short-lived. Performance of the partial thromboplastin time and factor VIII assays may be required to properly monitor therapy.

FIBRINOGEN DEFICIENCY

Fibrinogen deficiency is most commonly associated with acquired hemorrhagic disorders. Rarely, a hereditary autosomal recessive form is encountered.

ASSESSMENT OF NEED

A minimum fibrinogen level of 100 mg per dl appears to be adequate to control most bleeding. Fibrinogen levels of less than 100 mg per dl and a prolonged thrombin time indicate a need for therapy.

CHOICE OF PRODUCT

A fibrinogen concentrate made from pooled plasma is no longer available for clinical use. Cryoprecipitate is particularly rich in fibrinogen and can be used for replacement therapy. Between 28 and 50 percent of plasma fibrinogen is concentrated in a unit of cryoprecipitate. Although units of cryoprecipitate may vary widely in fibrinogen content, for ease of calculation, each bag of cryoprecipitate should be considered to contain approximately 150 mg of fibrinogen. Cryoprecipitate should be administered as ABO compatible owing to the presence of anti-A and anti-B isoagglutinins.

TRANSFUSION EFFECT

A therapeutic goal of 100 to 200 mg per dl is recommended. Since transfused fibrinogen has a biologic half-life of 96 to 120 hours, prophylactic maintenance is possible for patients who suffer frequent hemorrhagic episodes. However, fibrinogen infusion has been associated with the development of fibrinogen antibodies.[64] The author has observed that on the average, four units of cryoprecipitate given for each 10 kg body weight will raise the fibrinogen level by approximately 150 mg per dl (approximately 7.5 mg per dl per 5-ml bag).

FACTOR II DEFICIENCY

ASSESSMENT OF NEED

A deficiency of factor II may be associated with severe hemorrhage and death at an early age. Epistaxis, ecchymoses, and postoperative hemorrhage are commonly associated with this disorder. Factor II levels of 30 to 40 percent are required for hemostasis.

CHOICE OF PRODUCT

Although fresh-frozen plasma contains all coagulation factors, the post-transfusion recovery of factor II is generally so poor that levels of greater than 20 percent cannot be achieved without plasma exchange. Higher levels can be achieved with prothrombin complex, whose post-transfusion recovery is approximately 40 to 50 percent.[65]

TRANSFUSION EFFECT

Laboratory measurement of recovery is provided by the prothrombin time, partial thromboplastin time, and a specific factor assay. The transfusion half-life of factor II is approximately 72 hours.[65]

FACTOR V DEFICIENCY

ASSESSMENT OF NEED

Factor V deficiency is usually a mild bleeding disorder. Therapy may be indicated for the treatment of epistaxis, menorrhagia, hemarthroses, and postoperative bleeding. The level of factor V required for hemostasis is thought to range from 10 to 15 percent.[65]

CHOICE OF PRODUCT

Approximately 80 percent of transfused factor V activity is recovered following the infusion of fresh-frozen plasma. Factor levels that provide adequate hemostasis are readily achieved with infusion of fresh-frozen plasma.[65]

TRANSFUSION EFFECT

Laboratory measurement of recovery is provided by the prothrombin time, partial thromboplastin time, and specific factor assay. The transfusion half-life of factor V is approximately 12 hours.[65]

FACTOR VII DEFICIENCY

ASSESSMENT OF NEED

The inherited deficiency of factor VII is associated with a mild bleeding disorder characterized by epistaxis, menorrhagia, and ecchymoses. Hemarthroses and postoperative hemorrhage are uncommon. Factor VII levels of approximately 5 to 10 percent are required for hemostasis.

CHOICE OF PRODUCT

Replacement therapy for factor VII deficiency is best achieved with the transfusion of fresh-frozen plasma. Levels adequate for hemostasis are easily achieved. Because of the efficacy of fresh-frozen plasma, prothrombin complex is not required.

TRANSFUSION EFFECT

Therapy is most properly monitored by performance of the prothrombin time and a specific factor assay. The transfusion half-life of factor VII is approximately 4 to 6 hours.[65]

FACTOR X DEFICIENCY

ASSESSMENT OF NEED

Factor X deficiency may be characterized by repeated hemarthroses and severe postoperative hemorrhage. The level of factor X required for hemostasis is approximately 10 to 15 percent.[65]

CHOICE OF PRODUCT

The replacement of factor X can be effected with either fresh-frozen plasma or prothrombin complex. A dosage of 10 to 15 ml of fresh-frozen plasma per kilogram body weight should adequately replace 10 to 15 percent of factor activity.

TRANSFUSION EFFECT

Factor X recovery is monitored by the prothrombin time, the partial thromboplastin time, and the specific factor assay. The transfusion half-life of factor X is approximately 10 to 15 hours.[65]

FACTOR XI DEFICIENCY

ASSESSMENT OF NEED

Factor XI deficiency is associated with a relatively mild bleeding disorder. Bleeding does not correlate well with factor assay levels. Although guidelines are difficult to determine, levels of 25 percent are generally regarded as adequate for preparation for surgery. A deficiency of factor XI is associated with prolongation of the partial thromboplastin time.

CHOICE OF PRODUCT

Approximately 90 percent of factor XI activity is recovered after transfusion of fresh-frozen plasma. Levels of greater than 30 percent are achieved with infusion of 15 to 20 ml of fresh-frozen plasma per kilogram of body weight.

TRANSFUSION EFFECT

Replacement of factor XI is monitored by the partial thromboplastin time and the specific factor assay. The transfusion half-life of factor XI is approximately 60 to 90 hours.[65]

FACTOR XIII DEFICIENCY

ASSESSMENT OF NEED

Less than 5 percent total activity is required for hemostasis. Therefore, bleeding will occur only with total deficiency of factor XIII. In such cases, delayed wound healing and recurrent hemorrhage are typical.

CHOICE OF PRODUCT

Factor XIII deficiency is best treated with a single dose of fresh-frozen plasma.

TRANSFUSION EFFECT

The factor XIII assay provides a fairly dependable monitor of the recovery of transfused factor XIII. The transfusion half-life of factor XIII is approximately 6 to 10 days.[65]

ACQUIRED HEMORRHAGIC DISORDERS

Most acquired hemorrhagic disorders are associated with multiple coagulation factor deficiencies. These bleeding disorders may occur as the result of deficient factor synthesis, "disseminated intravascular coagulation," or fibrinolysis.

VITAMIN K DEFICIENCY AND ORAL ANTICOAGULANTS

Vitamin K is an essential cofactor for the synthesis of factors II, VII, IX, and X. Vitamin K deficiency caused by inadequate dietary intake or steatorrhea may be associated with a hemorrhagic diathesis owing to a deficiency of these factors. A "vitamin K deficiency-like" state is induced by the use of oral anticoagulants whose therapeutic effect is derived from the inhibition of vitamin K dependent factor synthesis.

ASSESSMENT OF NEED

Because multiple factors are involved, the bleeding tendency associated with vitamin K deficiency or oral anticoagulants is less predictable than that of the patient who suffers from an inherited coagulation factor deficiency. In general, this disorder is characterized by ecchymoses, epistaxis, hematuria, gastrointestinal bleeding, and postoperative hemorrhage. Intracranial hemorrhage may also occur.

Combined deficiencies of factors II, VII, IX, and X cause prolongation of the prothrombin time. The partial thromboplastin time may be normal, but is generally prolonged in severe vitamin K deficiency. A factor is depleted in accordance with its respective intravascular half-life. Factor VII, whose half-life is approximately 4 to 6 hours, disappears first and is followed by factors IX, X, and II. Therefore, the prothrombin time is most sensitive and is altered earlier than is the partial thromboplastin time.

CHOICE OF PRODUCT

The prophylactic intramuscular administration of vitamin K_1 has virtually eliminated primary hemorrhagic disease of the newborn. Adults most often require treatment with 10 mg or more of vitamin K_1. In the face of severe bleeding a more rapid response than can be obtained with vitamin K_1 is required. In this setting, the intravenous administration of 10 mg of vitamin K_3 or fresh-frozen plasma is usually effective. Also, fresh-frozen plasma is quite useful when coumadin overdosage has occurred and incomplete correction with maintenance of therapeutic anticoagulation is desired.

TRANSFUSION EFFECT

The prothrombin time is an appropriate monitor of therapy. A delay in response should be expected after the administration of vitamin K_1.

DISSEMINATED INTRAVASCULAR COAGULATION (DIC)

Characterized by an acute or chronic acceleration of coagulation factor and platelet utilization and secondary fibrinolysis, excessive intravascular coagulation results in the consumption and depletion of coagulation factors and platelets, which may lead to a hemorrhagic diathesis.

Excessive intravascular coagulation may be induced by the release of thromboplastic material into the circulation (e.g., amniotic fluid emboli, abruptio placentae, hemolytic transfusion reaction), by conditions associated with vascular endothelial damage (e.g., shock, rickettsial infection), by stasis in blood flow (e.g., giant hemangioma, shock), or as a complication of septicemia. When the underlying stimulus is removed, the syndrome of DIC is self-limiting.

ASSESSMENT OF NEED

In the presence of DIC the peripheral smear most often reveals red cell distortion and fragmentation. The platelet count is markedly reduced. Levels of 20,000 to 40,000 per cu mm are common in acute DIC. The prothrombin time, partial thromboplastin time, and thrombin time are prolonged by deficiencies of factors V, VII, VIII, and XIII, fibrinogen, and interference by fibrinogen degradation products. The protamine paracoagulation test, which is indicative of active procoagulant activity, is positive. The euglobulin lysis time is shortened. In primary fibrinolysis (see below) the protamine sulfate paracoagulation test is negative.

CHOICE OF PRODUCT

The successful management of DIC is dependent on removal of the underlying cause. All other therapy is supportive and not of fundamental importance unless the initiating process is controlled. The factor deficit and resultant bleeding correlate well with the severity of the underlying disorder, shock, and acidosis. Blood flow and tissue perfusion must be maintained. Transfusion of fresh-frozen plasma and platelet concentrates may be required to replace depleted factors. The specific replacement of fibrinogen with cryoprecipitate is frequently indicated. It has been suggested that when the underlying cause cannot be eliminated, as in a hemolytic transfusion reaction, the coagulation process may be controlled with heparin. When used, the infusion of 500 to 1000 units of heparin per hour in adults is continued until the hemorrhagic process is corrected. Replacement of coagulation factors and platelets is required after heparinization.

Primary fibrinolysis is a rare cause of pathologic bleeding. It may be induced by major trauma, electrical shock, acute hypoxia, extracorporeal circulation, or prostatic manipulation.[66-68] Epsilon-aminocaproic acid, which is administered to interfere with fibrinolysis, has been reported to be useful in the treatment of this rare disorder.[69-72] Concomitant administration of coagulation factors may be required.

TRANSFUSION EFFECT

The therapy of DIC should be monitored by performance of the most readily available and relevant laboratory tests. Performance of the prothrombin time, partial thromboplastin time, and thrombin time and measurement of the platelet count and fibrinogen level are fundamental.

LIVER DISEASE

Since the liver is intimately involved in the synthesis and catabolism of the components of coagulation, hepatocellular disease is often associated with a complex coagulation disorder. Biliary obstruction or poor bile flow will impede the assimilation of vitamin K. Parenchymal liver disease is associated with diminished synthesis of all coagulation factors except factor VIII. Hepatocellular damage is associated with impaired clearance of activated coagulation factors and plasminogen activators that potentiate the development of a hypercoagulable state and abnormal fibrinolysis. Portal hypertension and associated splenomegaly may cause a moderate thrombocytopenia. Bone marrow production of platelets is also diminished.

ASSESSMENT OF NEED

Liver disease may be associated with extensive epistaxis, ecchymoses, postoperative hemorrhage, and gastrointestinal hemorrhage. The severity of bleeding often correlates with the extent of hepatocellular damage.

Liver failure is often associated with a moderate prolongation of the prothrombin time and partial thromboplastin time. A moderate degree of thrombocytopenia is most common. A sudden prolongation of the prothrombin time and partial thromboplastin time, a fall in platelet count and fibrinogen concentration, and a sudden elevation in fibrinogen degradation products indicate the onset of acute DIC.

CHOICE OF PRODUCT

As suggested by its pathogenesis, bleeding in liver disease is unpredictable and difficult to manage. Large volumes of fresh-frozen plasma may be required. Prothrombin complex is of limited value since it supplies only factors II, VII, IX, and X. It has been reported that epsilon-aminocaproic acid is effective in this setting.[69] Cryoprecipitate and platelet transfusions may be indicated.

TRANSFUSION EFFECT

Therapy is properly monitored by performance of the prothrombin time and partial thromboplastin time and by measurement of the platelet count and fibrinogen level. Careful observation for evidence of circulatory overload and evaluation of electrolyte and nitrogen balance are critical.

REFERENCES

1. Rush, B: *An account of the bilious remitting yellow fever as it appeared in the city of Philadelphia in 1793.* Dolson, Philadelphia, 1794.

2. Shenkin, HS, et al.: *On the diagnosis of hemorrhage in man.* Am J Med Sci : 421, 1944.

3. Shoemaker, WC and Bryan-Brown, CW: *Resuscitation and the immediate care of the critically ill and injured patient.* Seminars in Drug Treatment 3:249, 1973.

4. Collins, JA, Braitberg, BS and Butcher, HR: *A direct comparison of fluid regimens in the resuscitation of rats following hemorrhage.* In Malinin, RI, et al. (Eds): *Acute Fluid Replacement in the Therapy of Shock.* Stratton Intercontinental Book Corporation, 1973, p 169.

5. Shoemaker, WC: *Comparison of the relative effectiveness of whole blood transfusions and various types of fluid therapy in resuscitation.* Crit Care Med 4:71, 1976.

6. Shoemaker, WC, Matsuda, T and State, D: *Relative pulmonary hemodynamic effectiveness of whole blood and plasma expanders in burned patients.* Surg Gynecol Obstet 144:909, 1977.

7. Boutros, AR, et al.: *Comparison of hemodynamic, pulmonary, and renal effects of use in three types of fluids after major surgical procedures on the abdominal aorta.* Crit Care Med 7:9, 1979.

8. Skillman, JJ, Parikh, BM and Tanenbaum, BJ: *Pulmonary arteriovenous admixture: Improvement with albumin and diuresis.* Am J Surg 119:440, 1970.

9. Skillman, JJ, Restall, DS and Salzman, EW: *Randomized trial of albumin vs. electrolyte solutions during aortic operations.* Surgery 78:291, 1975.

10. Shires, GT and Canizaro, PC: *Fluid resuscitation in the severely injured.* Surg Clin North Am 53:1341, 1973.

11. Carrico, CJ et al.: *Extracellular fluid replacement in hemorrhagic shock.* Surg Forum 14:10, 1963.

12. Crenshaw, CA, et al.: *Changes in extracellular fluid during acute hemorrhagic shock in man.* Surg Forum 13:6, 1962.

13. Rocchio, MA, Di Colo, V and Randall, HT: *Role of electrolyte solutions in hemorrhagic shock.* Am J Surg 125:488, 1973.

14. Gann, DS: *Endocrine control of plasma protein volume.* Surg Clin North Am 56:1135, 1976.

15. Virgilio, RW, et al.: *Crystalloid vs. colloid resuscitation: Is one better?* Surgery 85:129, 1979.

16. Lucas, CE, et al.: *Effects of albumin versus non-albumin resuscitation on plasma volume and renal excretory function.* J Trauma 18:564, 1978.

17. Moss, GS: *An argument in favor of electrolyte solutions for early resuscitation.* Surg Clin North Am 52:3, 1972.

18. Zarins, CK, et al.: *Lymph and pulmonary response to isobaric reduction in plasma oncotic pressure.* Circ Res 43:925, 1978.

19. Lowe, RJ, Moss, GS and Jilek, J: *Crystalloid versus colloid in the etiology of pulmonary failure after trauma—a randomized trial in man.* Crit Care Med 7:107, 1979.

20. The Board for the Study of the Severely Wounded: *The Physiologic Effects of Wounds.* Office of the Surgeon General, Department of the Army, Washington, DC, 1952, pp 5–9.

21. Kendrick, DB: *Blood Program in World War II.* Office of the Surgeon General, Department of the Army, Washington, DC, 1964, pp 54–59.

22. Sohmer, PR, et al.: *Universal donor blood transfusions in civilian trauma.* Presented at the Society of Critical Care Medicine, San Francisco, California, May 1979.

23. Gardner, J and Tovey, G: *Potentially dangerous group O blood.* Lancet i:1001, 1954.

24. Kendrick, DB, op cit, p 805.

25. Kiel, F: *Development of a blood program in Viet Nam.* Milit Med 131:1469, 1966.

26. Barnes, A, Jr and Allen, TE: *Transfusions subsequent to administration of universal donor blood in Vietnam.* JAMA 204:695, 1968.

27. Camp, FR and Shields, CE: *Military blood banking—identification of group O universal donor for transfusion of A, B, and AB recipients—an enigma of two decades.* Milit Med 132:426, 1967.

28. Inwood, MI and Zuliani, BA: *Anti-A hemolytic transfusion with packed O cells.* Ann Int Med 89:515, 1978.

29. Noon, G: *Intraoperative autotransfusion.* Surgery 84:719, 1978.

30. Sohmer, PR: *Hemotherapy in a major trauma center.* In Barnes, A and Umlas, J (eds): *Hemotherapy in Trauma and Surgery.* American Association of Blood Banks, Washington, DC, 1979.

31. Bell, WR: *The hematology of autotransfusion.* Surgery 84:695, 1978.

32. Schaff, H, et al.: *Autotransfusion in cardiac surgical patients after operation.* Surgery 84:713, 1978.

33. Mattox, KL, et al.: *Blood availability for the trauma patient-autotransfusion.* J Trauma 14:663, 1975.

34. Orr, M and Gilcher, R: *Autotransfusion—perioperative blood salvage in nonheparinized patients.* Crit Care Med 4:103, 1976.

35. Gilcher, RO and Orr, M: *Intraoperative blood salvage.* In Barnes, A and Umlas, J (eds): *Hemotherapy in Trauma and Surgery.* American Association of Blood Banks, Washington, DC, 1979, p. 57.

36. Henry, JB, Mintz, P and Webb, W: *Optimal blood ordering for elective surgery.* JAMA 237:451, 1977.

37. Higby, DJ, et al.: *The prophylactic treatment of thrombocytopenic patients with platelets. A double blind study.* Transfusion 14:440, 1974.

38. Sohmer, PR and Dawson, RB: *Transfusion therapy in trauma. A review of the principles and techniques practiced in the MIEMS program.* Am Surg 45:109, 1979.

39. Harker, LA and Slichter, SJ: *The bleeding time as a screening test for evaluation of platelet function.* N Engl J Med 287:155, 1972.

40. Freireich, EJ.: *Effectiveness of platelet transfusion in leukemia and aplastic anemia.* Transfusion 6:50, 1966.

41. Bergin, JJ and Zuck, TF: *Selected aspects of component therapy: Platelets.* In Dawson, RB (ed): *Transfusion Therapy.* American Association of Blood Banks, Washington, DC, 1974, p 1.

42. Bergin, JJ, Zuck, TF and Miller, RE: *Compelling splenectomy in medically compromised patients.* Ann Surg 178:761, 1973.

43. Aisner, J, Schiffer, CA and Wiernik, PJ: *Cell support.* In Spivak, J (ed): *Fundamentals of Clinical Hematology.* Harper & Row, Hagerstown, MD, 1980, p 357.

44. Ellman, C, et al.: *Platelet autoantibodies in a case of infectious mononucleosis presenting as thrombocytopenia purpura.* Am J Med 55:723, 1973.

45. Bjork, VO and Hultquist, G: *Brain damage in children with deep hypothermia for open heart surgery.* Thorax 15:284, 1960.

46. de Leval, MR, et al.: *Blood platelets and extracorporeal circulation.* J Thorac Cardiovasc Surg 69:144, 1975.

47. Dutton, RC, et al.: *Platelet aggregate emboli produced in patients during cardio-pulmonary bypass with membrane and bubble oxygenators and blood filters.* J Thorac Cardiovasc Surg 67:258, 1974.

48. Bachman, E, et al.: *The hemostatic mechanism after open heart surgery.* J Thorac Cardiovasc Surg 70:76, 1975.

49. Bick, RL: *Alterations of hemostasis associated with cardiopulmonary bypass: Pathophysiology, prevention, diagnosis, and management.* Semin Thromb Hemostas 3:59, 1976.

50. McKenzie, FN, et al.: *Blood platelet behavior during and after open heart surgery.* Br Med J 2:795, 1969.

51. Moriau, M, et al.: *Hemostasis disorders in open-heart surgery with extracorporeal circulation.* Vox Sang 32:41, 1977.

52. *Standards for Blood Banking and Transfusion Services,* ed 10. American Association of Blood Banks, Washington, DC, 1981.

53. Widmann, FK (ed): *Technical Manual,* ed 8. American Association of Blood Banks, Washington, DC, 1981.

54. Aster, R: *Effect of anticoagulant and ABO incompatibility on recovery of transfused human platelets.* Blood 26:732, 1965.

55. Harker, LA and Slichter, SJ: *The bleeding time as a screening test for evaluation of platelet function.* New Engl J Med 287:155, 1972.

56. Najean, Y, et al.: *Survival of radiochromium-labelled platelets in thrombocytopenia.* Blood 22:718, 1963.

57. Platelet Transfusion Subcommittee of the Acute Leukemia Task Force: *Platelet transfusion procedures.* Cancer Chemotherapy Reports, Part 3, 1:1, 1968.

58. Aster, RH and Jandl, JH: *Platelet sequestration in man. II. Immunologic and clinical studies.* J Clin Invest 43:856, 1964.

59. Sohmer, PR, Scott, RL and Smith, DJ: *Effect of delayed refrigeration on plasma components in whole blood stored in CPDA-2.* Transfusion (in press).

60. Hilgartner, MW: *The management of hemophilia.* In Morrison, F (ed): *Hemophilia.* American Association of Blood Banks, Washington, DC, 1978, p 17.

61. Biggs, R: *Plasma concentrations of factor VIII and factor IX and treatment of patients who do not have antibody directed against these factors.* In Biggs, R (ed): *The Treatment of Hemophilia A and B and Von Willebrand's Disease.* Blackwell Scientific Publications, Oxford, 1978, p 110.

62. Kessler, CM and Bell, WR: *Coagulation factors.* In Spivak, J (ed): *Fundamentals of Clinical Hematology.* Harper & Row, Hagerstown, MD, 1980, p 319.

63. Kasper, CK, et al.: *Proceedings: A more uniform measurement of factor VIII inhibitors.* Throm Diath Haemorrh 34:612, 1975.

64. De Vries, A and Cohen, I: *Hemorhagic and blood coagulation disturbing action of snake venoms.* In Poller, L (ed): *Recent Advances in Blood Coagulation.* Churchill, London, 1969, p 277.

65. Macfarlane, RG: *Blood coagulation and haemostasis.* In Biggs, R (ed): *The Treatment of Haemophilia A and B and Von Willebrand's Disease.* Blackwell Scientific Publications, Oxford, 1978, p 1.

66. Silver, D and Daniel, TM: *Diagnosis and management of non-mechanical bleeding.* In Berk JL, et al. (eds): *Handbook of Critical Care Medicine.* Little, Brown & Co., Boston, 1976, p 373.

67. Andersson, L and Nilsson, IM: *Effect of E-amino-n-caproic acid (EACA) on fibrinolysis and bleeding conditions in prostatic disease.* Acta Chir Scand 121:291, 1961.

68. Douglas, AS, et al.: *The haemostatic defect following extracorporeal circulation.* Br J Surg 53:455, 1966.

69. Marengo-Rowe, AJ: *The management of multiple coagulation factor deficiencies.* In Dawson, RB (ed): *Hemostasis for Blood Bankers.* American Association of Blood Banks, Washington, DC, 1977, p 59.

70. Gans, H and Krivit, W.: *Problems in hemostasis during and after open heart surgery. III. Epsilon aminocaproic acid as an inhibitor of plasminogen activity.* Ann Surg 155:268, 1962.

71. McNicol, GP, et al.: *Use of epsilon aminocaproic acid in management of postoperative hematuria.* J Urol 86:829, 1961.

72. Sack, E, et al.: *Reduction of prostatectomy bleeding by epsilon aminocaproic acid.* N Engl J Med 266:541, 1962.

CHAPTER 15

APHERESIS

BRIAN E. RITCHEY, R.N.

I. CYTAPHERESIS

II. PLASMA EXCHANGE

III. PHARMACOLOGY

IV. TYPES OF APHERESIS EQUIPMENT

Blood, a subject of fascination since the dawn of history, continues to mystify man. Early medical practitioners must have wondered at the separation of blood as it clotted in ceremonial bowls, leaving the retracted clot and serum. To this day, medical science capitalizes on this phenomenon when performing tests in chemistry, microbiology, or in the blood bank. Early workers, seeking to satisfy their curiosity, sought techniques to further understand this wonderful "life force" called blood. Various methods were used to study "corpuscles" as blood cells were known. Gradually, tiny pieces of the puzzle began to fall into place. In the 1830s, "albumin" was defined, and other "proteins" were identified in the plasma.[1] Nearly 100 years passed, though, until the rate of discovery accelerated. Sodium citrate used as an anticoagulant was a landmark event of the late 19th century that allowed more sophisticated manipulation of the elements of the blood.

Pioneering work by Landsteiner in the early 1900s opened a new era in modern medicine by revealing the possibilities of blood transfusion.[2,3] The military organizations of the world saw the possibilities that transfusion of blood products held for treatment of injured soldiers and "blood banking" became a reality. Since O.H. Robertson's work in World War I[2] with the first blood bank, new and exciting possibilities continue to arise. With the advent of the nuclear age, two separate events further increased application of transfusion concepts: (1) radioisotopes became available for diagnostic and research techniques, and (2) following the bombing of Hiroshima and Nagasaki in 1945, interest in treatment of leukemia and aplastic anemia was stimulated.[2,4] These diseases led to interest in platelet and leukocyte transfusions. Terasaki's work with the human leukocyte antigen system (HLA) further enhanced the interest in the availability of leukocyte and platelet transfusion.[5,6]

While manual, multiple blood bag techniques are still used to harvest plasma, leukocytes, and platelets, these techniques are time consuming and inefficient. Automated equipment developed by International Business Machines in the early 1960s opened the way for "single donor" platelet products for transfusion and research and later for leukocyte concentrate transfusion.[7] In the last 20 years, very sophisticated apheresis equipment has been made available. This new equipment has moved blood banking into the forefront of modern medicine, particularly in the treatment of cancers. *Apheresis,* a Greek word meaning to "separate" or "take out of," became the name used for the technology of separating blood into components with subsequent manipulation of some or all of its components. The original automated apheresis equipment involved very basic concepts using a centrifuge and peristaltic pumps to move the blood components. While space-age advances have changed the form of this equipment, the basic principle remains the same: anticoagulated blood centrifuged in a test tube will separate into red blood cells (RBCs), white blood cells (WBCs), platelets, and plasma (Fig. 15-1). By placing a pipette at the appropriate level in the test tube one can aspirate any of these components. Apheresis technology applies the same concept, but utilizes an "in-vitro-in-vivo" technique. Blood is removed from an individual, usually with a large bore needle, anticoagulated, and transported directly to the centrifuge bowl, where it is separated into specific com-

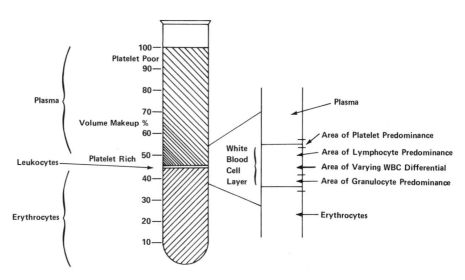

FIGURE 15-1. Sedimented blood sample. (Courtesy of IBM)

MODERN BLOOD BANKING AND TRANSFUSION PRACTICES

ponents. Once the blood has been separated, any component can be withdrawn and then used for transfusion, treatment of disease, or research (Fig. 15-2). The remaining portions of the blood are remixed and returned to the donor. Depending on the intent of the individual procedures (of which there are many), the instruments must be adjusted appropriately. The general conditions are (1) centrifuge speed and diameter, (2) length of dwell time of the blood in the centrifuge, and (3) the type of solutions added, such as anticoagulants or sedimenting agents. By manipulating these variables, the operator can harvest plasma, platelets, or cells in large quantities for commercial or therapeutic purposes.

Apheresis can be divided into two broad categories, cytapheresis and plasmapheresis. Cytapheresis is the withdrawal of one or more cellular constituents; plasma and the remaining cellular elements are returned to the patient or donor. Plasmapheresis is the removal of plasma; cellular constituents are returned to the donor/patient. This procedure is generally performed on patients who manifest one of many plasma abnormalities. The patient's own plasma is collected and discarded and the lost fluid volume is replaced with normal plasma; the process is known as plasma exchange. Plasmapheresis is also performed on healthy donors whose plasma contains some commercially desirable substance such as antibodies against the $Rh_0(D)$ blood group antigen or against hepatitis B. The collected plasma is then employed in the manufacture of Rh immune globulin or hepatitis B immune globulin.

CYTAPHERESIS

LEUKAPHERESIS

Collection of granulocytes for transfusion to leukemic or aplastic anemia patients is one major application of apheresis technology. Since the treatment goal for a leu-

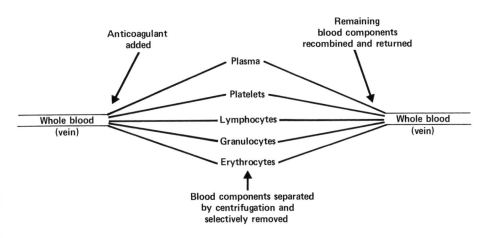

FIGURE 15-2. Principles of apheresis.

kemic patient is to eradicate the malignant cell population, chemotherapy is used to force the bone marrow into remission, that is, to halt leukemic cell production. The chemotherapeutic agents used today are rather specific in their action and agents act directly on bone marrow. This results in prolonged aplasia not only of leukemic cells but also of RBCs, platelets, and nonleukemic nucleated cells.[8] Historically, this was associated with death caused by bleeding (thrombocytopenia) or by overwhelming infection (granulocytopenia). While RBCs may be readily available to correct anemia and platelets may be available from random sources to correct thrombocytopenia, WBCs (specifically granulocytes) may be needed to aid antibiotics in fighting infection. The generally accepted guidelines for beginning WBC support are (1) the presence of infection, (2) no response to antibiotics for 48 hours, and (3) profound granulocytopenia, <500 per cu mm.*[9-12] When these conditions are present, granulocyte support can be obtained from hospital-based apheresis centers, regional blood banks, or commercial apheresis centers.

WBC donors usually meet the whole blood donor criteria of the American Association of Blood Banks (AABB). Some centers request that donors take steroid medication prior to the donation in order to stimulate granulocyte production.[12,13] This increases harvests of WBCs significantly. Granulocyte donors are usually ABO compatible with the recipient because of the inevitable RBC contamination found in granulocyte concentrates.[11] While there are currently numerous types of apheresis machines available, collection procedures are similar. Since granulocytes do not separate well from RBCs, a sedimenting agent such as hydroxyethyl starch (HES) may be added.[14,15] HES causes the RBCs to form rouleaux and releases the WBCs from suspension (some European centers use dextrans, which cause similar actions). Once a suitable donor has been selected, whole blood is drawn from one arm and anticoagulated, usually with a citrate product. The blood enters the centrifuge, where it is separated into components. Granulocytes are harvested via various mechanisms and the RBCs, lymphocytes, platelets, and plasma are recombined and returned to the donor, usually into the opposing arm.[7] With this technique, granulocytes can be harvested over several consecutive days with little demonstrable toxicity to the donor (Table 15-1).[10] The centrifugal force that is required for WBC collection is different from that used for platelet collection, and some instruments are provided with adjustable collection parameters. Some equipment is not adjustable and relies on operator experience to begin and end cell withdrawal. Since granulocytes separate adjacent to RBCs in the centrifuge bowl, some RBC contamination is inevitable. AABB criteria call for granulocyte concentrates to be prepared in such a way as to contain 1.0×10^{10} granulocytes per concentrate.[16,17] Granulocyte yields have been reported as high as 4 to 5×10^{10}, but no standard "dose" has been stipulated.[15,18]

While few side effects are common, donors may experience citrate toxicity from the anticoagulant or hemodilution from repeated administration of HES, which acts as a volume expander.[17] HES is excreted slowly by the kidneys and evidence indicates that some starch may persist for several months following one

---

*Recommendations for initiation of support vary widely.

MODERN BLOOD BANKING AND TRANSFUSION PRACTICES

TABLE 15-1. Apheresis Side Effects*

1. Numbness, tingling, cramps, chills, convulsions—Citrate toxicity
2. Hyperventilation—Anxiety
3. Shock, fainting—Hypovolemia, Anxiety
4. Bruising—Improper needle position/fragile vein condition
5. Headache, edema, hives, shock—Hydroxyethyl starch
6. Air embolism—Administration of air by venous return

*Side effects may be expressed in many ways, such as localized pain, abdominal discomfort, or feelings of fullness. Each complaint must be investigated and donors should be free to express anxiety, pain, or general misgiving.

500-ml administration.[16] Since granulocytes are produced at a very rapid rate, cells are replaced quickly with no apparent harm to the donor. Occasional allergic responses to HES have been reported. Citrate toxicity is not uncommon, especially when the ionized calcium levels of donors are below normal.[17] Recommendations for transfusion of granulocytes are similar to RBC transfusion protocols. Febrile reactions to granulocyte transfusions are relatively common and respond to administration of diphenhydramine hydrochloride (Benadryl) or acetaminophen (Tylenol).[11,19] Febrile reactions are not a reason for discontinuance of the transfusion. Granulocyte concentrates are administered over a 2-hour period via standard blood administration sets. Micropore filters should *not* be used.[19] Granulocyte products should be infused as soon as possible after the end of collection.

Mononuclear WBCs also can be harvested by apheresis techniques. Since monocytes and lymphocytes separate cleanly from RBCs, sedimenting agents are not necessary.[20] These cells are used for research purposes since lymphocyte transfusions are not currently in clinical use. It has been suggested that lymphocyte concentrates may be effective against viral infection but would likely result in graft versus host (GVH) disease if not irradiated. However, irradiated lymphocytes do not function properly.

Some attempts had been made to collect stem cells for use in bone marrow transplantation, but circulating stem cell levels were too low to provide sufficient quantities for transplantation.[21] Recently, however, Abboud and associates[32] modified the approach to stem cell collection. They showed that a single plateletpheresis procedure stimulated the release of large numbers of non-lymphoid hematopoietic stem cells into the peripheral circulation. A subsequent leukapheresis, performed 48 to 72 hours after the plateletpheresis, yielded a leukocyte concentrate that was rich in these stem cells. Specifically, they were able to harvest large numbers of granulocyte-monocyte colony forming units (CFU-C) and erythrocyte burst forming units (BFU-E). Increases were not noted in any lymphoid cells. This study concluded that transfusions of these stem cell-rich preparations might one day be used to facilitate remission induction in aplastic patients.

PLATELETPHERESIS

Platelet transfusion therapy has been used for many years. Platelets are generally harvested from routine whole blood units, resulting in one "unit" of platelets (5.5×10^{10} platelets).[16,22] For surgical or trauma patients, random pooled platelet products generally function very well. However, when leukemic or aplastic anemia patients have received multiple blood product transfusions, they may become "refractory" or immune to platelet transfusion. This is recognized when there is no increment in post-transfusion platelet count.

Following the development of the refractory state in multiply transfused patients, such patients are at severe risk of death from hemorrhage caused by thrombocytopenia. While little is known about development of the refractory state, it appears that stimulation of the immunologic system by repeated administration of foreign proteins is the culprit.[6,8,23] The body recognizes antigens on platelets as foreign and mounts an immune response against them, resulting in alloimmunization. At this time, the only treatment for this condition is the administration of platelets from a histocompatible donor,[8] also referred to as a "tissue-typed" or human leukocyte antigen (HLA) identical donor.[24] If HLA-typing of the patient can be accomplished, HLA identical donors can be located by local blood centers that have HLA "catalogues." Platelets from such a compatible donor can be transfused with favorable results. Since the recipient's immune system does not recognize the platelets as being foreign, the thrombocytes circulate and function normally. If tissue-typing of the patient cannot be accomplished (not enough circulating WBCs), parents or siblings can be used with some degree of success.[5,24] However, age, physical condition, and geographic availability of the donor often limit the success of this approach.

Platelets are collected in much the same manner as are WBCs.[22] A harder (faster) centrifuge spin may be used since platelets are one thirteenth the size of RBCs. An anticoagulant is added to the whole blood as it is drawn from the donor's arm. Sedimenting agents are not necessary.[20] Platelet yields depend on (1) initial donor platelet count and (2) length of collection. Six to ten units (5.0×10^{11}) of platelets can usually be harvested in about 90 minutes, depending on the type of equipment used.[17] Side effects to the donor are usually limited to citrate toxicity. Repeated platelet collections may result in depletion in platelet stores and should be done only after checking platelet counts on subsequent donations. Since platelet concentrations generally lack RBC contamination, they can be administered rapidly, if necessary, and need not be ABO compatible. Occasional febrile reactions may occur in the recipient since the concentrates may contain significant WBC contamination.

NEOCYTAPHERESIS

Patients with thalassemia major require continuous red cell transfusion therapy in order to survive. This is a result of the underlying mechanism of the disease. Homozygous inheritance of a genetic defect results in the inability of the patient to manufacture β-globin chains, which are essential for the production of normal adult hemoglobin. Consequently, insufficient hemoglobin is produced and severe anemia presents very early in life. Unless treated, the survival time of these patients is very short—only a few years.

Transfusion therapy became the therapy of choice in 1964 and has permitted these patients to live years longer than they otherwise might have. The treatment, however, produces its own characteristic pathology: siderosis. The human body has no mechanism for the rapid excretion of iron. Since chronic transfusion provides large numbers of red blood cells that eventually become senescent, iron overload occurs. This iron may accumulate in tissues such as liver, heart, and endocrine glands. If iron accumulation were to continue unabated, the majority of β-thalassemia patients would succumb to associated complications, especially heart failure. In the past, iron overload was minimized through the use of iron chelating agents, which enhanced the urinary excretion of iron, thus reducing the body's iron load.

A new form of treatment was studied by Propper and colleagues[33] in order to further diminish iron overload in thalassemia patients. This treatment utilized a form of apheresis and has been named "neocytapheresis." The basis of the procedure involves the withdrawal of donor "neocytes," that is, young red blood cells or reticulocytes.

Based on the observation that young erythrocytes are less dense than adult erythrocytes, the investigators found that neocytes could be collected in sufficient quantities to provide needed blood transfusions for their patients. Their study concluded that neocytes provided two advantages over traditional blood transfusions: the interval of time between transfusions could be prolonged and iron accumulation was further reduced.

THERAPEUTIC APPLICATIONS

Although the primary purpose of cytapheresis is to collect blood components for transfusion, it also has certain therapeutic applications.

Plateletpheresis may be used for direct patient therapy. It has been shown that in patients with excessively elevated platelet counts, hemostatic effectiveness is compromised. This has been verified in many patients with idiopathic thrombocythemia and polycythemia vera. Sequential plateletpheresis was shown to substantially reduce the platelet count; hemostatic efficiency was then restored.

A therapeutic modification of leukapheresis has been utilized in treating patients with chronic leukemia. When the leukocyte count of these patients is grossly elevated, they may suffer the effects of vascular sludging and stasis of blood flow. Reduction of the vascular cellular load would alleviate this leukostasis. This procedure is not used routinely as yet and is still considered a research modality.

Patients with polycythemia vera are routinely treated by therapeutic phlebotomy. Units of whole blood are sequentially withdrawn until a desired hematocrit has been reached. Reducing the patient's red cell content thus alleviates the adverse effects of vascular sludging. The technique of apheresis could be utilized for this type of therapy. The advantage would be that the patient would only need to sit through one apheresis procedure, rather than donate two to four units of whole blood over a period of several weeks. The main disadvantage, however, is the exorbitant cost of apheresis. Because of this, the conventional therapy is still the therapy of choice in this disease.

Finally, patients in sickle cell anemia crisis have been treated successfully by red cell exchange; sickled cells are removed and replaced with normal, viable red cells.

The techniques used for therapeutic cytapheresis are similar to those previously described.

PLASMA EXCHANGE

Plasma constitutes approximately 60 percent of blood volume and plays an essential role in regulation of physiologic processes. Control of temperature and osmotic pressure, circulation of blood cells, and transport of enzymes, hormones, coagulation factors, and tissue nutrients are some of plasma's functional tasks. Albumin and blood fibrin were analyzed in the late 1830s, but definitive work with proteins was delayed almost 100 years until newer equipment, techniques, and assays were developed.[1] Only recently has understanding of individual proteins advanced with the advent of protein sequencers, analyzers, and high pressure liquid chromatography (HPLC). One-dimensional and two-dimensional electrophoresis has revealed additional information.

It is essential to note that when one manipulates the blood, as in apheresis, fluid balance, clotting mechanisms, and basic immunologic functions can be dangerously altered. Of primary interest are the immunoglobulins A, D, E, G, and M and plasma albumin. In many diseases the immune system, for unknown reasons, becomes faulty and an "autoimmune" condition develops. The results of this condition can be painful, debilitating, and possibly fatal. These autoimmune conditions can attack many different tissues producing a variety of results. Treatment for these immune system dysfunctions are varied and generally follow the principle "treat the symptoms." Steroids and chemotherapeutic agents have been used with less than ideal response. Falling short of successful treatment with these modalities, therapeutic plasma exchange has led, with some degree of success, to treatment of several disease entities. The term "plasma exchange" refers to the separation of plasma from the cellular components and subsequent replacement of that plasma in the patient with various substitutes.[25] Characteristically it is the IgA, IgG, or IgM that constitutes the offending antibody; however, when manipulating the plasma it is difficult to remove specific immune globulins.[1] Instead we are forced to discard all the plasma which includes coagulation factors, nutrients, medications, albumin, and so on. The choice of replacement or exchange solutions is very important. When crystalloid substitutes (saline, lactated Ringer's solution, or other such fluids) are used, severe cardiovascular hypotension may result owing to osmotic pressure changes. The volume of exchange will, in part, determine the solution to be used. For example, if only 1 or 2 liters of plasma will be removed, saline may function adequately. A one volume exchange for a 70-kg adult is considered to be 4 liters of plasma. If 4-liter exchanges are performed, it is recommended that some colloid solution such

356

as 5 percent albumin be used. If larger volumes of exchanges (10 liters) are performed, then other components must be used, including fresh-frozen plasma (FFP). Coagulation, blood chemistry, and cardiovascular status must be very carefully monitored, especially in larger volume exchanges.[26]

IgM is found predominantly in interstitial tissue. To remove significant amounts the exchange can be done slowly to enhance the movement of IgM from a higher gradient (interstitial tissue) to a lower gradient (circulation). The specific disease may also dictate what replacement solution is used. Thrombotic thrombocytopenic purpura (TTP), for example, appears to respond to the use of FFP, although some workers report success with other solutions.[27] A summary of determining factors in plasma exchange, then, is as follows: (1) component to be removed, (2) rate of exchange, (3) volume of exchange, and (4) exchange replacement solution.

Definitive statements regarding plasma exchange as a therapeutic tool are difficult to make. Many disease entities have been reported to be successfully treated with therapeutic plasma exchange, including such diverse maladies as Raynaud's disease, cutaneous vasculitis, hypertension, and asthma.[25] Clearly, plasma exchange is not successful in all these diseases. The "powerful placebo" effect must be suspected in some reports. Several diseases have been accepted rather widely as being amenable to treatment with plasma exchange. Goodpasture's syndrome and glomerulonephritis, systemic lupus erythematosus, renal allograft rejection, and thrombotic thrombocytopenic purpura are only a few of those reported.[25,27-31]

Apheresis technology also has been applied for collection of plasma to be used for production of blood bank reagents. Individuals with rare antibodies or multiparous females who have had antigenic stimulus from multiple antigens may be candidates for donation of plasma. Hyperimmune globulins also have been manufactured from plasma obtained from apheresis procedures. Strict limitations are placed on the amount of plasma collected and frequency of donation.

PHARMACOLOGY

Manipulation of blood and blood components depends on alteration of the normal clotting system. Citrate products are used to provide adequate anticoagulation. Citrate has been used as a whole blood anticoagulant since the inception of the earliest blood banks. Acid citrate dextrose (ACD) is used for most apheresis. While side effects are relatively frequent, they are generally mild and easily managed. ACD binds ionized calcium[16] and thus interferes with function of the clotting cascade. Ionized calcium levels below normal or rapid administration of citrate may result in perioral paresthesia, chills, or convulsions. ACD is available in different strengths from manufacturers or can be prepared by a pharmacist. In procedures in which HES is used, trisodium citrate is added to make a "double duty" solution that both enhances red cell sedimentation (rouleaux) and provides for anticoagulation. Side effects are similar to those of ACD but may also include side effects observed during the administration of HES. Blood volume expansion from HES may result in headache or hemodilution.[16]

Steroids such as prednisone, dexamethasone, or hydrocortisone are used by many apheresis centers to stimulate granulocyte yields in leukapheresis donors. Stimulation of moderate leukocytosis by way of steroid administration, when used in conjunction with HES, may double granulocyte harvests.[16] Dosages may vary from center to center. Steroids should not be administered to individuals with a history of diabetes, ulcers, or hypertension.

Heparin, another anticoagulant, is used in some apheresis applications, alone or as an adjunct to ACD. Drug effects are longer lasting than with citrate and may result in dangerous prolongation of coagulation times. Heparin should not be administered to females during menses or to patients with clotting disorders. Protamine sulfate, a heparin antidote, is sometimes used to negate heparin's anticoagulation effect, but must be given slowly. Side effects are flushing, diaphoresis, or hypotension.

TYPES OF APHERESIS EQUIPMENT

Cell separation equipment is available from several manufacturers (Fenwal, Haemonetics, IBM). Instruments are available in a wide range of purchase prices. While each specific instrument, may have features or accessories available, there are three basic types of equipment: (1) Continuous flow centrifugation (CFC) which results in simultaneous extraction and return of blood from and to the donor, (2) Intermittent flow centrifugation (IFC) which entails removal of an aliquot of blood with delayed return of blood to the donor, (3) Filtration leukapheresis which relies on adherence of granulocytes to nylon fibers with subsequent elution of the cells from the fibers.

Specific procedures and techniques vary from instrument to instrument and manufacturers' recommendations should be consulted.

Numerous applications have been found for apheresis equipment. It should be noted by both experienced practitioners and newcomers to the field that apheresis has limitations. While some claims have been made regarding the use of granulocytes as therapeutic agents in sepsis and the use of plasma exchange for rheumatoid arthritis and other diseases, it is *not* universally successful. The technique of apheresis has changed and is changing rapidly. New claims of successful treatments are being made daily; old claims are being discarded. This equipment can be dangerously misused by inexperienced operators. Careful, scientific, controlled studies must be made with each disease or application before claims of success can be made.

REFERENCES

1. PUTNAM, FW: *The Plasma Proteins (I)*. Academic Press, New York, 1975, p 6.
2. WINTROBE, MM: *Blood, Pure and Eloquent*. McGraw-Hill, New York, 1980, p 691.
3. LANDSTEINER, K: *Obituary notices of Fellows of the Royal Society*. 5:295, 1947.
4. CONGDON, CC: *Bone marrow transplantation*. Science 171:1123, 1971.
5. WIECKOWICZ, M: *Single donor platelet transfusions*. Transfusion 16:195, 1976.
6. GOLDSTEIN, IM, et al.: *Leukocyte transfusions*. Transfusion 2:19, 1971.

7.   HESTER, JP, et al.: *Principles of blood separation and component extraction in a disposable continuous-flow single stage channel.* Blood 54:254, 1979.

8.   LOKICH, JJ: *Managing chemotherapy-induced bone marrow suppression in cancer.* Hosp Pract 2:61, 1976.

9.   FORTUNY, IE, et al.: *Granulocyte transfusion: A controlled study in patients with acute nonlymphocytic leukemia.* Transfusion 15:548, 1975.

10. VOGLER, WR: *A controlled study of the efficacy of granulocyte transfusions in patients with neutropenia.* Am J Med 63:548, 1977.

11. BURNETT, D AND HIGBY, DJ: *Granulocyte transfusions: Current status.* Blood 55:2, 1980.

12. FORD, JM and CULLEN, MH: *Prophylactic granulocyte transfusions.* Exp Hematol (Suppl) 5:65, 1977.

13. WINTON, EF AND VOGLER, WR: *Development of a practical oral dexamethasone premedication schedule leading to improved granulocyte yields with the continuous-flow centrifugal blood cell separator.* Blood 52:249, 1978.

14. SUSSMAN, LN, et al.: *Harvesting of granulocytes using a hydroxyethyl starch solution.* Transfusion 15:461, 1975.

15. HUESTIS, DW, et al.: *Use of hydroxyethyl starch to improve granulocyte collection in the Latham blood processor.* Transfusion 15:559, 1975.

16. WIDMANN, FK (ed): *Technical Manual*, ed 8. American Association of Blood Banks, Washington, DC, 1981.

17. BERKMAN, EM and NUSBACHER, J (eds): *Fundamentals of a Pheresis Program.* American Association of Blood Banks, Washington, DC, 1979, p 53.

18. STRAUSS, RG: *Therapeutic neutrophil transfusions.* Am J Med 65:1001, 1978.

19. INMAN, M: *Leukapheresis, Transfusion, and Observed Reactions. Vein to Vein: A Seminar for Phlebotomists and Transfusionists.* American Association of Blood Banks, Washington, DC, 1976.

20. AISNER, J: *A standardized technique for efficient platelet and leukocyte collection using the Model 30 blood processor.* Transfusion 16:437, 1976.

21. WEINER, RS, et al.: *Semi continuous flow centrifugation for the pheresis of immunocompetent cells and stem cells.* Blood 49:391, 1977.

22. KISKER, CT, et al.: *Combined platelet leukapheresis: A technique for preparing separate platelet and granulocyte-platelet units from single donors.* Transfusion 19:173, 1979.

23. YANKEE, RA, et al.: *Selection of unrelated compatible platelet donors by lymphocyte HL-A matching.* N Engl J Med 288:760, 1973.

24. DUQUESNOY, RJ, et al.: *ABO compatibility and platelet transfusions of alloimmunized thrombocytopenic patients.* Blood 54:595, 1979.

25. LOCKWOOD, CM: *Plasma exchange: An overview.* Plasma Therapy. 1:1, 1979.

26. CARRERA, CJ: *Procedural Guidelines for Large Volume Plasma Exchange, and Therapeutic Cytapheresis Using IBM Blood Cell Separator.* University of California Press, San Francisco, 1979.

27. OKUNO, T and KOSOVA, L: *Plasmapheresis for thrombotic thrombocytopenic purpura (TTP).* Transfusion 19:342, 1979.

28. WALLACE, D, et al.: *A therapeutic role for pheresis in the management of rheumatoid arthritis.* Proceedings of Haemonetics Research Institute Advanced Component Seminar, Boston, Massachusetts, 1979.

29. JONES, JV, et al.: *A therapeutic role for plasmapheresis in the management of acute systemic lupus erythematosus.* Proceedings of Haemonetics Research Institute Advanced Component Seminar, Boston, Massachusetts, 1976.

30. LOCKWOOD, CM and PETERS, DK: *The role of plasma exchange and immunosuppression in the treatment of Goodpasture's syndrome and glomerulonephritis.* Plasma Therapy 1:19, 1971.

31. CARDELLA, CJ, et al.: *Renal allograft rejection and intensive plasma exchange.* Proceedings of the Haemonetics Research Institute Advanced Component Seminar, Boston, Massachusetts, 1979.

32. ABBOUD, CN, et al.: *Quantification of erythroid and granulocytic precursor cells in plateletpheresis residues.* Transfusion 20:9, 1980.

33. PROPPER, RD, BUTTON, LN, and NATHAN, DG: *New approaches to the transfusion managment of thalassemia.* Blood 55:55, 1980.

CHAPTER **16**

THE HAZARDS
OF TRANSFUSION

FRANCES K. WIDMANN, M.D.

Blood transfusion often causes unexpected adverse effects. Since blood is an enormously complex biologic product, and the patient who receives the transfusion is an enormously complex biologic organism, the occurrence of adverse reactions is hardly surprising. We should perhaps be surprised that no more than 5 to 6 percent of recipients manifest recognizable adverse effects to transfused blood and components.[1]

Hemolytic transfusion reaction (HTR) is the adverse effect most widely feared because an antibody-mediated hemolysis of transfused red cells can rapidly produce severe symptoms and sometimes death. The possibility of this type of reaction reminds both clinical and laboratory personnel to establish and adhere to rigorous standards of sample and patient identification, and to employ meticulous technique. The blood bank worker should also be aware that other problems that occur more commonly also require continuing attention to observation, investigation, and prevention.

The law requires that transfusion-related deaths be reported to the Office of Biologics of the Food and Drug Administration.[2] Between mid-1976 and the end of 1979, there were 110 fatalities reported; an estimated 37 million units were transfused during this period,[3] giving a reported fatality rate of 0.00023 percent. Of these 110 fatalities, hemolytic reactions accounted for 63 and post-transfusion hepatitis for 33. A variety of problems caused the remaining 14.

It is instructive to examine the causes for the 63 HTRs. A crossmatch that failed to detect antibody caused only 4; 3 were delayed reactions caused by anamnestic appearance of previously undetectable antibody. Laboratory errors in blood typing resulted in 4. In 5 cases, giving uncrossmatched blood during an emergency resulted in administering incompatible blood. The remaining 47 deaths resulted from ABO incompatibility. Either the patient (31), the blood sample (7), or the laboratory records (9) were misidentified through human carelessness. The miscellaneous causes included anaphylaxis (4), respiratory distress syndrome (4), gram-negative endotoxemia (2), disseminated intravascular coagulation (2), graft-vs-host reaction (1) and overheating the donor blood (1).

No doubt other transfusion-related deaths occurred but were not reported because the causes of death were complex and association with transfusion was not clearcut. The dramatic fact remains, however, that most hemolytic transfusion reactions result from human carelessness. ABO mix-ups kill patients. Subtle deficiencies of laboratory technique do not cause ABO mix-ups; carelessness and failure to follow established routines do.

The list of transfusion-related problems is far longer than the list of fatal events. Although a few are potentially life-threatening, the vast majority of adverse effects cause relatively minor discomfort or morbidity. Tables 16-1 to 16-4 classify the types, the relative frequency of adverse effects, and the clinical significance of adverse effects that may follow transfusion of blood or components.

PROBLEMS WITH NONIMMUNOLOGIC CAUSES

Blood bankers tend to think primarily in immunologic terms. Certainly the largest number of transfusion problems arise from immune-mediated mechanisms, but

TABLE 16-1. Hemolysis Associated with Transfusion

Nonimmunologic mechanisms
    Physical damage to transfused cells
        Overheating
        Incompatible fluid
        Excessive pressure during infusion
    Physical damage to recipient's cells
        Infusion of hypotonic solutions
        Entrance of irrigating fluids to blood stream
    Microbial agent damage to donor's or recipient's cells
        Gram-negative bacteria in blood or platelets
        Clostridial sepsis pre-existing in recipient
        Malaria
    Destruction of patient's abnormal cells
        G-6-PD deficiency
        Paroxysmal nocturnal hemoglobinuria
        Sickle cell disease in crisis

Antibody-mediated mechanisms
    Immediate intravascular hemolysis
        Usually ABO mix-up
        Complement-activating antibody
        Destruction of transfused cells
    Immediate extravascular hemolysis
        Attachment of antibody (usually complement-activating IgG) to cells
        Rapid destruction of coated cells in reticuloendothelial system
    Delayed hemolysis
        Nearly always extravascular
        Attachment of rapidly developing IgG antibody to donor cells
    Effect of donor's antibody on recipient's cells
        Nearly always group O plasma, with high-titered anti-A or anti-B
        Development of positive direct antiglobulin test in recipient
        Possible gradual occurrence of extravascular hemolysis

some problems result from nonimmunologic causes. The commonest nonimmunologic complication is disease transmission. Physical mishaps may cause red cell destruction, and other problems that may follow transfusion can have many causes.

HEMOLYSIS

If a transfusion recipient exhibits free hemoglobin in his plasma, marked hemoglobinuria, or shortened red cell survival, immediate investigation should focus on antibody-mediated cell destruction. If this initial testing for antibody-mediated destruction proves negative, however, pursuit of other possibilities should follow. The first hypothesis to test is that the donor cells were damaged before or during infusion. This occurs if the cells were exposed to extremes of heat or cold; if they were infused under excessive pressure through a too-small needle; or if there was contact with incompatible intravenous solutions.

    Investigating nonimmunologic hemolysis requires detailed inquiry into the circumstances of the transfusion. Visual examination of the blood remaining in the bag

TABLE 16-2. Nonhemolytic Adverse Effects of Transfusion

Allergic reactions
   Urticaria/hives
   Anaphylaxis
Febrile reactions
   Possible chills
Volume overload
   Acute systemic hypertension
   Pulmonary edema
Disease transmission
   Non-A non-B hepatitis
   Hepatitis B
   Malaria
   Cytomegalovirus
Immunization to blood-borne antigens
   Red cell antigens
   HLA antigens, stimulated by white cells or platelets
   Granulocyte antigens
   Platelet antigens
   IgA: class-specific or allotypic
Noncardiac pulmonary events
   Leukoagglutinin reactions
   Complement-induced granulocyte aggregation
   Adult respiratory distress syndrome
Hemostatic effects
   Dilutional thrombocytopenia after massive transfusion
   Citrate toxicity, with massive transfusion and depressed liver function
Hypothermia
   Occurs with massive transfusion, in patients with impaired thermal control
Graft-vs-host disease
   Only in immunologically compromised recipients
Transfusional hemosiderosis
   After years of transfusion to patients with chronic severe hemolysis

or the blood in the administration tubing may reveal red cell damage if hemolysis is evident. If blood warming devices were used, these should be tested for malfunction. American Association of Blood Banks (AABB) standards[4] forbid the use of microwave blood warmers or other devices that heat the entire unit of blood, but these may still be used in some settings. In-line blood warmers, the only kind permitted by the AABB, may malfunction, and this should be evaluated if circumstances warrant. Infusion solutions that may damage red cells if mixed with blood in infusion tubing include 5 percent dextrose in water, 5 percent dextrose in one fourth normal saline and lactated Ringer's solution, and other calcium-containing solutions.[5]

    Sometimes post-transfusion hemolysis involves the recipient's cells. If hypotonic solutions enter the blood stream, circulating red cells experience osmotic rupture. This can occur in irrigation accidents, or if the wrong bottle is hung for intravenous infusion. Severe sepsis may destroy circulating cells, especially in massive clostridial infection. Some patients have red cells that are intrinsically abnormal, susceptible to hemolysis induced by transfusion or by the illness that necessitated the

TABLE 16-3. Relative Frequency of Adverse Effects

Very common: Follows 1% or more of transfusions
    Febrile reactions
    Allergic reactions
    Non-A non-B hepatitis
    Immunization to red cell, white cell, platelet, or protein antigens
Somewhat common
    Circulatory overload
    Dilutional thrombocytopenia
    Delayed hemolytic reaction
    Hepatitis B (becoming less common)
Rare
    Intravascular hemolysis (ABO)
    Extravascular hemolysis (other blood groups)
    CMV transmission
    Malaria transmission
    Hypothermia
    Physical damage to transfused cells
    Transfusional hemosiderosis
Very rare
    Anaphylactic reactions
    Noncardiac pulmonary reactions
    Graft-vs-host disease
    Bacterial contamination
    Citrate toxicity

transfusion. Patients with paroxysmal nocturnal hemoglobinuria (PNH) experience massive hemolysis following transfusion of blood products that contain substantial amounts of plasma. Red cells deficient in glucose-6-phosphate dehydrogenase may hemolyze in conditions of stress and metabolic derangement. A hyperhemolytic episode in sickle cell disease may provoke or accompany the need for transfusion. A patient with malaria could experience a hemolytic episode temporally related to transfusion. Drug-induced hemolysis may complicate the clinical condition of a patient receiving blood. Laboratory tests for these conditions should not be routine in evaluating post-transfusion hemolysis, but they may be useful if hemolysis cannot otherwise be explained.

Hemoglobinemia may be unrelated to transfusion, but if the temporal sequence is suggestive or the clinical circumstances ambiguous, transfusion reaction may be suspected. Extracorporeal oxygenators often damage enough circulating cells to cause visible hemoglobinemia. (At plasma hemoglobin levels of 25 mg per dl, pink discoloration is apparent to the unaided eye.) Valvular or arterial prostheses may cause chronic low-grade hemolysis, while acute hemolysis is a manifestation of thrombotic thrombocytopenic purpura and hemolytic-uremic syndrome. Patients with hematomas in soft tissue or body cavities may have elevated serum levels of hemoglobin or bilirubin irrespective of damage to circulating red cells. Thermal burns may cause hemolysis and hemodynamic alterations that are easily confused with transfusion reaction.

TABLE 16-4. Relative Significance of Adverse Effects

Serious, potentially life-threatening
    Intravascular hemolysis (ABO)
    Extravascular hemolysis, if severe
    Circulatory overload, if severe
    Hepatitis B
    Anaphylactic reactions
    Bacterial contamination
    Noncardiac pulmonary reactions
    Graft-vs-host disease
    Malaria
Serious but rarely life-threatening
    Extravascular hemolysis (most)
    Delayed hemolytic reactions, if severe
    Coagulation problems
    Transfusional hemosiderosis (except in thalassemia major)
    Non-A non-B hepatitis
    CMV transmission in infants
Rarely cause major clinical problems
    Febrile reactions
    Allergic reactions
    Delayed hemolytic reactions (most)
    Immunization to blood-borne antigens (except immunization to high-incidence red
      cell antigens and development of refractory state to platelet transfusion)
    Cytomegalovirus transmission in adults

CARDIORESPIRATORY EVENTS

Blood transfusion causes chemical, physical, and hemodynamic alteration of the patient's circulation. Volume overload is, unfortunately, a fairly common complication of transfusing whole blood. Specific incidence figures are difficult to obtain, because the resulting respiratory difficulties can usually be corrected by medical means or, at worst, by phlebotomy, so that this adverse effect is seldom reported. Patients with severe anemia or impaired cardiac function are especially at risk; red blood cells, not whole blood, should be used to raise their oxygen-carrying capacity.

Respiratory complications unrelated to volume overload occur infrequently and are difficult to diagnose, treat, or prevent. Interaction between leukoagglutinins and white blood cells has been implicated in some cases of impaired respiratory function with radiologic evidence of pulmonary infiltration. The interaction of complement with white cells has been implicated[6] as a cause of adult respiratory distress syndrome, which can accompany or follow blood transfusion and may be fatal. Laboratory evaluation of this complex series of events is very difficult.

Some workers implicate infusion of microaggregates as a cause of adult respiratory distress syndrome in massively transfused patients. The physiologic effect of these small (20 to 120 μ) aggregates of fibrin and cellular debris is controversial; clinical studies of microaggregate filters have given conflicting results. So many clinical variables affect the outcome of massive transfusion that controlled studies of microaggregate filtration are difficult to perform. Complicating the physiologic picture is evidence that microaggregates may reoccur after blood has passed through the special small-pore filters.[7]

HEMATOLOGIC EVENTS

Massive transfusion sometimes affects circulating levels of platelets or coagulation proteins. Large-volume transfusion, by itself, rarely causes significant dilution of coagulation proteins, but the patient with disseminated intravascular coagulation may have massive hemorrhage, requiring large-volume replacement at the same time that levels of coagulation proteins decline. Low platelet counts are a somewhat more frequent consequence when transfusion volume equals two or more times the patient's original blood volume, but even here observations and opinions differ. Dilutional thrombocytopenia is by no means universal, despite transfusion of 20 or more units of blood, and platelet replacement should not be administered according to a set formula. The platelet count should be monitored during and after massive transfusion, and platelet concentrates should be available if there is a significant drop.

Citrate toxicity is an extremely rare cause of disordered hemostasis since unmetabolized citrate accumulates dangerously only if there is profound hepatic dysfunction or hypothermia, or if blood is administered at rates at or above 100 ml per minute.

Whole-body chilling from rapid transfusion of cold blood may occur when a large volume rapidly enters the circulation, or when the patient has poor thermal homeostasis, such as in anesthetized patients and very small children. With transfusion volumes below 3000 ml, and at infusion rates slower than 100 ml per minute, adult patients very rarely experience hypothermia.[8] Except for patients with astronomic titers of cold agglutinins, it is rarely necessary to warm blood transfused at moderate rates. At rapid infusion rates, the transfused red cells have less time to warm before encountering circulating cold antibodies. Blood or red blood cells hung as a gravity drip usually warm to room temperature in the time it takes to complete infusion.[9]

TRANSMISSION OF ORGANISMS

Blood can transmit infectious organisms as a result either of pre-existing disease in the donor or of bacterial growth in the stored unit. With disposable phlebotomy equipment and aseptic venipuncture technique, bacteria rarely enter a unit as it is being drawn. Earlier requirements for periodically culturing stored blood reflected conditions when needles, tubing, and bottles had to be cleaned for repeated re-use and the seal of the empty blood container had to be punctured by the phlebotomist. At present, barring a leak in the plastic equipment or faulty sterilization by the manufacturer, the only way for bacteria to enter the unit is if incompletely cleansed skin fragments enter the container with the flowing blood. Gram-negative organisms, notably Citrobacter freundii, some Escherichia coli, and some species of pseudomonas, can grow at refrigerator temperatures. Gram-negative endotoxemia may follow transfusion of blood that contains significant numbers of organisms. Some such units can be seen to have clots, excessive hemolysis, or purple or brown discoloration, but there may be no abnormalities of appearance to signal the presence of bacterial growth.

Components carry a somewhat higher risk of bacterial contamination or growth than does whole blood. With integral transfer bags and tubing, the process of component preparation itself rarely constitutes a hazard, but the conditions of storage and administration can be a problem. Platelet concentrates stored at room temperature may support bacterial multiplication, although studies on the incidence of bacterial contamination of platelet concentrates have given conflicting results. Cryoprecipitate and frozen plasma, thawed at 37°C and subjected to considerable manipulation, may also allow bacterial multiplication. In thawing frozen products, it is extremely important to avoid contact between the outlet ports of the blood container and the water in the warming bath, which may harbor pseudomonas or other water-borne organisms. Pooling platelet concentrates or cryoprecipitates provides ample potential for bacterial contamination. Components should not be entered for pooling until the time of administration, and the pooled material should not be left unduly long at room temperature before or during administration.

Symptoms usually develop quite rapidly after transfusion of contaminated blood. Hypotension, fever, disseminated intravascular coagulation and renal failure unrelated to antibody-mediated hemolysis should arouse suspicion of bacterial septicemia, and all the blood bags and infusion equipment should be promptly examined. Gram stains are rarely positive but culturing the residual material and equipment should reveal the nature of the problem.

Syphilis is virtually never transmitted by transfusion. The one reported case occurred in a 28-year-old man who received several freshly drawn units among the numerous transfusions from donors with negative serologic tests (STS).[10] Spirochetes do not survive refrigerator storage for 3 days. Theoretically, fresh blood could transmit the organisms, but spirochetemia cannot be detected by laboratory means other than animal inoculation. By the time an infected individual develops a positive STS, the phase of spirochetemia has passed. Routine performance of an STS on donor blood provides no protection to recipients and is difficult to justify on the grounds of public health screening. A patient can acquire a positive STS from transfused blood; this will persist for 4 to 10 days if the donor's antibody titer is 1:64 or greater.[11]

Malaria has been transmitted by transfusion of red cells from infected individuals; components that contain no intact red cells will not contain infective parasites. Transfusion-associated malaria is rare; only three cases were reported in the U.S. in 1978. Careful history taking and stringent adherence to donor standards should avoid this preventable hazard of transfusion.

Infection with cytomegalovirus (CMV) can be transmitted by blood from donors with prior CMV infection, even though the donors are in good health and have anti-CMV antibodies.[12] This rarely causes problems with adult recipients, but newborn infants may acquire clinically significant CMV-associated symptoms. It has been suggested that newborn infants should be given blood only from donors who lack anti-CMV.

Such other parasites as trypanosomes (Chagas' disease, sleeping sickness), toxoplasma, leishmania (kala-azar), and babesia (Nantucket fever) will survive in stored blood and can potentially cause disease, but are so rare in U.S. transfusion practice that there is no justification for routine preventive measures other than taking a careful donor history.

Hepatitis is far and away the commonest and the most dangerous disease transmitted by blood transfusion. All blood and components and some bulk-processed blood products can transmit hepatitis viruses. The most severe clinical disease results from hepatitis B infection, which has markedly declined in frequency with the advent of sensitive tests for hepatitis B markers in donors. Careful prospective studies of transfusion recipients reveal, however, that most post-transfusion hepatitis is due to one or several other viruses collectively designated non-A, non-B hepatitis. A complete discussion of hepatitis testing, prevention, and treatment is found in Chapter 17.

FEBRILE AND ALLERGIC REACTIONS

Immunologic mechanisms lie behind most adverse effects of transfusion, from the common to the rare, from the trivial to the fatal. The adverse effects most often reported to the blood bank are febrile reactions and urticarial reactions. The frequency with which these reactions are reported is directly proportional to the care with which transfusion recipients are observed. In a transfusion service with high-quality serologic testing and careful clinical surveillance and reporting, as many as 6 percent of recipients, representing 1.5 percent of units transfused, had transfusion-related clinical consequences.[1] The patient with an isolated hive or a transient temperature rise need not occasion alarm or require therapeutic intervention. Careful observation and reporting are important because serious adverse effects, if they occur, will be noted promptly and treated with minimal delay. A high level of reported reactions does not signify a careless laboratory; it indicates careful clinical observation.

URTICARIAL REACTIONS

Urticarial reactions (hives and itching) occur frequently and have little significance except to the patient, who may be uncomfortable. Histamine-mediated skin symptoms of this sort are thought to follow an immunologic reaction between some soluble material in the transfused unit and an antibody in the patient's circulation. Antibodies to serum proteins, especially to IgA subclasses, are often considered the culprit, but experimental evidence for this is limited. Many patients who experience urticarial reactions have antibodies against IgA allotypes, but similar antibodies exist in recipients who do not have reactions, and some patients with these reactions do not have demonstrable antibodies.[13,14]

Urticarial reactions tend to recur in susceptible patients and are more frequent in those who have had multiple transfusion. It would, in theory, be possible to test these patients' sera against a panel of IgA-coated cells and test all the donor units for IgA allotype, but this is neither practical nor likely to be clinically useful. Urticarial reactions can usually be reversed by administering antihistamines and can often be prevented by giving antihistamines before transfusion. The patient who suffers frequent or severe reactions should receive packed red blood cells or washed red cells rather than whole blood to minimize the volume of transfused plasma.

Hives or other skin manifestations sometimes occur with febrile nonhemolytic reactions (see below), but they do not accompany hemolytic transfusion reactions[15] and can be considered annoying but not dangerous. Transfusion need not be stopped if hives are observed, because hives are not prodromal of more severe hemolytic events. These reactions should be observed as part of good patient surveillance and reported on the patient's chart and to the blood bank as part of good record-keeping, but further action by the laboratory is not necessary.

ANAPHYLACTIC REACTIONS

Anaphylactic reactions, which may assume life-threatening proportions, are quite different from relatively trivial histamine-mediated urticarial reactions to poorly defined antigens. Probably the result of massive histamine release, these reactions begin with sudden onset of flushing and hypertension, followed by hypotension, widespread edema, respiratory distress, and, sometimes, nausea, vomiting, and diarrhea. Smooth muscle constriction and increased vascular permeability account for most of these observed effects. Triggering histamine release appears to be a reaction between IgA in the transfused product and a class-specific anti-IgA in the patient's circulation. A few milliliters of blood, red cells, or plasma contain enough IgA to initiate the reaction.

Patients susceptible to such reactions seem to be those congenitally deficient in the entire IgA class. Immunoglobulin A exists in several allotypes, and individuals whose IgA molecules are of one allotype may develop antibodies against other allotypes. Such antibodies, with limited specificity, are the type suggestively implicated in the urticarial reactions described above; their clinical impact is relatively modest. Some persons, however, have no IgA in their plasma and can form antibodies against molecules of the entire IgA class. IgA-deficient patients rarely have clinical signs of immunodeficiency and thus are usually unaware that the condition exists.

An IgA-deficient patient exposed by transfusion to IgA may develop powerfully reactive class-specific antibodies. Most of the relatively few patients in whom anaphylactic reactions have been reported had had previous immunizing exposure to transfusion products before the transfusion that elicited the reaction. Because IgA deficiency is relatively common (f $\leq$ 1:1000), there must be many IgA-deficient patients who have received more than one transfusion and have not developed antibodies. The frequency of immunization cannot be determined, so the factors that affect the likelihood of immunization cannot be characterized.

If anaphylactic syndrome does develop during transfusion, the transfusion must be stopped immediately, and therapy instituted to combat hypotension, laryngeal edema, and bronchiolar constriction. Investigation should be deferred until the clinical condition has been stabilized. Investigation should include the usual search for evidence of red cell incompatibility but should also include determination of immunoglobulin levels in pretransfusion serum. If preliminary radial immunodiffusion testing reveals deficiency of IgA, the specimen should be referred to a laboratory that can quantify immunoglobulins and antibodies to immunoglobulins.

Not every IgA-deficient patient with anti-IgA experiences life-threatening anaphylaxis. Symptoms may be considerably less severe the first time they occur, but it is important to avoid stimulating their recurrence. An IgA-deficient patient who has once had anaphylactic manifestations should not be transfused with IgA-containing material. For red cell transfusion, deglycerolized frozen cells are the best product; washed cells are also effective. Platelet concentrates or other components that unavoidably contain plasma should be prepared from donors who are, themselves, IgA-deficient. The American National Red Cross and the Immunohematology Reference Laboratory program of the American Association of Blood Banks can provide such components or the names of suitable donors. Susceptible patients should carry a wallet card or medallion warning against the hazards of unmodified transfusion.

FEBRILE REACTIONS

Comparable in frequency to urticarial reactions are febrile nonhemolytic reactions to transfusion. These reactions are defined as temperature rise of $1°C$ or $2°F$ occurring during or within an hour or so after transfusion, in a patient with no other reason for acute temperature elevation. Chills and subjective malaise may accompany the fever but other signs or symptoms rarely occur. Febrile reactions have been attributed to reaction between granulocyte antigens and antibody (usually the recipient's antibody, but sometimes an antibody in transfused plasma), causing release of lysosomal enzymes. The transfused granulocytes need not be viable; febrile reactions can follow transfusion of stored blood.

Transfusion services do not ordinarily look for white cell antibodies in the serum of every patient with febrile reactions. When large scale studies have been performed, the incidence of positive results has varied with the method used. Anti-leukocyte antibodies may have a range of specificities, including but not confined to the well-defined antigens of the HLA system and the known granulocyte systems. Leukoagglutination testing correlates better with the incidence of febrile reactions than does cytotoxicity testing. Approximately 65 to 70 percent of febrile reactors have broadly reactive leukoagglutinating antibodies, and another 10 percent can be shown to have antibodies to specific granulocyte antigens.[16] Pregnancies and prior transfusions predispose to development of such antibodies, and it is usually the multitransfused patient who experiences febrile reactions.

Clinical symptoms do not fully correlate with the presence of antibodies. In the more extreme setting of granulocyte transfusions, 16 percent of recipients in one series had febrile reactions, sometimes accompanied by systemic symptoms. Agglutination and cytotoxicity tests were negative in nearly all the reactors, while 13 of 14 transfusions to patients with one or both tests positive were uneventful.[17]

Mild febrile reactions can effectively be treated with antipyretics. Febrile reactions are often recurrent, although for any given patient experiencing a febrile reaction, the odds are only one in eight that fever will follow a subsequent transfusion.[18,19] A patient who repeatedly experiences febrile reactions should receive components that are as free as possible from intact or disintegrating white cells. Leukocyte-poor red cells can be prepared by centrifugation and washing of blood stored in liquid state up to 10 days,[20] by double centrifugation of freshly drawn blood,[21] or by passing freshly drawn heparinized blood through a nylon filter. Deglycerolized frozen red cells or washed cells are leukocyte-poor but expensive. A simple and inexpensive means of administering leukocyte-poor blood is to transfuse standard red cell units through a microaggregate filter.[22]

HEMOLYTIC REACTIONS

Antibody-mediated red cell destruction, that is, hemolysis, is the most feared hazard of blood transfusion. It is difficult to estimate how often hemolytic transfusion reactions occur. As with febrile or allergic reactions, reported frequency increases with the diligence with which these reactions are investigated. Some hemolytic reactions cause prompt, dramatic symptoms and can hardly fail to be noticed. Others occur more subtly and may escape detection, especially delayed reactions in which red cell destruction begins 2 to 10 days after transfusion.

The incidence of hemolytic reactions has declined dramatically as pretransfusion serologic testing has become more sensitive and more sophisticated. When pretransfusion testing consisted only of ABO matching and immediate-spin major and minor crossmatch, approximately 1 in every 500 transfusions resulted in hemolysis.[23] As the range of known antibodies has expanded and antiglobulin testing has become nearly universal, this incidence has fallen to 1 in 6000 to 7000, according to one extremely careful series of observations.[15] Where surveillance is less intense, observed incidence tends to be much less.

Biologic variability is so complex and wonderful that it is difficult to generalize about the effects of antibodies on red cells. Major side incompatibility, the presence of antibody in the patient's serum directed against antigens present on donor cells, is likely to be dangerous or fatal. Most blood bank procedures are directed toward preventing transfusion of incompatible cells, and in general these procedures are extremely effective. Most experienced blood bankers, however, have "war stories" about patients who inadvertently received ABO-incompatible blood and displayed only trivial clinical effects. Conversely, severe hemolysis may follow transfusion of seemingly compatible blood, or transfusion to recipients with very weakly reactive antibodies of obscure or unlikely specificity. The following discussion of antibodies and red cells summarizes observations on which general agreement exists, but to which many exceptions can be cited.

MECHANISMS OF HEMOLYSIS

Antibodies damage red cells in one of two ways: by initiating attachment of complement to the cell membrane, with subsequent sequential activation of complement components; or by remaining attached as immunoglobulin on the surface of circulating cells, thereby rendering them susceptible to accelerated destruction in the reticuloendothelial system. In neither case is the cell damaged directly by the attachment of antibody molecule to cell surface antigen. If complement activation continues through activation of C8 and C9, these complement proteins pierce the red cell membrane, and the red cell lyses in the blood stream. This process is described as intravascular destruction. Sometimes the complement sequence goes no farther than attachment of C4 or C3; in such cases, the presence of complement proteins on the red cell surface has the same effect as the presence of antibodies on the cell surface. These coated cells are susceptible to phagocytic attack in the reticuloendothelial system, resulting in extravascular hemolysis.

Intravascular hemolysis occurs only when the responsible antibody is one that activates complement. Hemolytic activity can often be demonstrated in vitro. Anti-A and anti-B are the major offenders, often causing extraordinarily rapid destruction of transfused incompatible cells. Other antibodies lytic in vitro, such as the Lewis antibodies and anti-PP_1P^k, tend to cause less rapid and less exclusively intravascular destruction. Antibodies that bind complement but, despite all techniques to increase sensitivity, do not cause in-vitro hemolysis, tend to cause extravascular destruction occurring largely in the liver. Antibodies that do not bind complement cause extravascular destruction occurring primarily in the spleen.

With intravascular rupture of red cells, hemoglobin enters the plasma. Haptoglobin, a normal plasma protein, can bind small amounts of hemoglobin, but quantities of hemoglobin greater than 100 mg per dl remain free in the plasma. As blood flows through the kidney, plasma hemoglobin crosses the glomerular filter into renal tubules, where tubular epithelial cells reabsorb a substantial quantity. Unbound hemoglobin is visible to the naked eye as faint pink discoloration of plasma at levels of 25 mg hemoglobin per dl plasma; overt hemoglobinuria rarely occurs at plasma hemoglobin levels below 150 mg per dl. Plasma hemoglobin is rapidly converted to bilirubin and other pigments. Each gram of hemoglobin yields about 40 mg of bilirubin, which is excreted through the bile in a matter of hours unless there is hepatic dysfunction, biliary obstruction, or massive bilirubinemia.

Extravascular red cell destruction sometimes causes hemoglobinemia, but this is usually less intense than the discoloration that accompanies intravascular hemolysis. Antibody- or complement-coated cells undergo progressive damage and membrane loss as they encounter the macrophages of the reticuloendothelial system. Some cells escape immediate destruction by the phagocyte and re-enter the circulation as damaged or spherocytic cells. As these subsequently undergo intravascular rupture, their hemoglobin enters the plasma.

Although hemoglobinemia and hemoglobinuria are the most conspicuous results of cell incompatibility, the mere presence of circulating hemoglobin has little deleterious effect. Indeed, stroma-free hemoglobin solutions have been moderately effective as volume expanders in experimental hemorrhagic hypovolemia.[24] The clinical problems resulting from incompatible transfusion seem to be consequences of massive antigen-antibody reactions and the damage inflicted on the red cells.

Severe intravascular hemolytic reactions elicit a syndrome characterized by cardiovascular instability, autonomic dysfunction, smooth muscle spasm, and disturbances of hemostasis; these may progress to irreversible shock or, as a later phenomenon, renal failure. Reactions of this sort result almost exclusively from ABO catastrophes. Carelessness and failure to follow established routines are the only cause for these events; ABO catastrophes do not result from insufficient serologic sophistication. Serious consequences may follow the action of other antibodies, but the sequence of events is more limited and less rapid; death, if it occurs, almost always results from complications involving pre-existing medical problems exacerbated by the effects of the transfusion reaction.

The occurrence of a large-scale antigen-antibody reaction initiates a complex sequence of inter-related and mutually enhancing events involving the complement system, the coagulation system, the kinin system, and the autonomic nervous system. Complement activation releases intermediary products (C3a and C5a) into the circulation. These protein fragments exert direct effects on vascular permeability and on smooth muscle contraction. Damage to red cells releases thromboplastic activity that initiates the coagulation sequence, causing disseminated intravascular coagulation (DIC) and reinforcing complement activation. Antigen-antibody complexes can affect Hageman factor, which initiates not only the early steps of the coagulation cascade but also the interactions that generate bradykinin. Bradykinin causes arterioles to dilate and the systemic blood pressure to fall; it also increases capillary permeability so that venous return to the heart declines, as does systemic blood pressure. Hypotension stimulates the sympathetic nervous system to discharge catecholamines, which cause vasoconstriction of vascular beds high in alpha-adrenergic receptors, notably the renal and splanchnic vasculature. Massive discharge of the autonomic nervous system may also produce nausea, vomiting, diarrhea, and incontinence of urine or feces. Histamine and substances with similar action are probably responsible for the bronchospasm and vasospasm experienced subjectively as chest pain, lumbar pain and difficulty in breathing.

Hemostatic dysfunction, hypotension, and renal damage, either singly or in combination, cause the most sinister clinical consequences. Treatment should aim at breaking the vicious circle of mutual enhancement. Disseminated intravascular coagulation may further damage the kidney through widespread formation of microthrombi and stimulation of platelets to release the vasoactive agents histamine and serotonin. A hemolytic transfusion reaction should be treated essentially in the same manner as any form of shock, that is, aggressive fluid therapy and drugs as needed or indicated. Maintaining adequate renal blood flow and adequate systemic blood pressure are the most important immediate goals. Prompt support of blood pressure prevents or reverses the tissue effects of impaired perfusion, especially in the renal cortex. Mannitol, an osmotic diuretic, was for many years the cornerstone of treatment, but intravenous furosemide (Lasix) is now preferred by most clinicians. Lasix not only acts as a diuretic, but also improves renal blood flow by vasodilatation. Dopamine, which increases cardiac output as well as dilating renal vessels, has also proved useful (in low doses).[25] Attempting to elevate the blood pressure with vasoconstrictors like epinephrine dangerously reduces renal blood flow. Some workers[26] advocate treating hemolytic reactions with heparin to prevent or reverse disseminated intravascular coagulation, but this agent and the entire field of treating DIC remain controversial.

Extravascular red cell destruction may be very rapid. If there is active splenic destruction or if complement-coated cells are cleared by the liver, the half-life may be as short as 2 minutes. Cells not coated with complement are destroyed more effectively by the spleen than by the liver, with a usual half-life of hours rather than minutes. Clinical severity of transfusion reactions owing to antibodies other than anti-A or anti-B can be very variable. The speed of red cell destruction sometimes parallels the intensity of clinical symptoms, if the antibody is one with high biologic activity, but it is often difficult to correlate clinical effects with red cell hemolysis. Antibodies in the Rh, Kidd, Kell, and Duffy systems have caused reactions ranging in severity from fatal to virtually unnoticeable; there are no good explanations for this individual variability.

In the early days of transfusion, many Rh-negative patients received Rh-positive blood and developed anti-D. When pretransfusion testing was rather crude, Rh-negative patients sometimes received a second Rh-positive transfusion and suffered a hemolytic reaction. Anti-D is now an uncommon cause of hemolytic reactions because, on the few occasions that Rh-positive blood is given to Rh-negative recipients, there is very careful pretransfusion investigation.

Antibodies with virtually any specificity can cause hemolysis if they are active at body temperature. Many antibodies that develop without known antigenic stimulus ("naturally occurring") react only at low temperatures. Thus, hemolytic reactions caused by anti-P_1, anti-M, anti-N, and anti-I are very rare, although the antibodies are fairly common. Most Lewis antibodies react best at temperatures below 30°C, but occasional examples have wider thermal amplitude. Although occasional hemolytic reactions caused by anti-Le^a or anti-Le^{a+b} have been reported, Lewis antibodies rarely cause hemolysis because Lewis antigens are not intrinsic to the red cell membrane and tend to elute from the red cell during storage and after transfusion to a Lewis-negative recipient.

The frequency with which specific antibodies cause hemolytic transfusion reactions does not entirely parallel the frequency with which they occur in the general population. Anti-D continues to be frequent in older patients and in women who were pregnant before the institution of effective Rh immunoprophylaxis. Nonetheless, anti-D rarely figures prominently in recent lists of antibodies causing transfusion reactions. Anti-K and anti-Fy^a are high on the lists both for overall incidence and for causing reactions. Kidd antibodies, on the other hand, cause more transfusion reactions than their absolute incidence might suggest. Anti-Jk^a and anti-Jk^b exhibit capricious serologic reactivity and are often difficult to identify in weakly reactive form or in a serum that contains other antibodies.

CLINICAL CONSIDERATIONS

Transfusion reactions tend to occur in settings of hasty or massive transfusion. The likelihood of ABO mishaps increases when clinician or blood bank or both are operating at crisis level; the operating room, the recovery room, and the intensive care units are the prime sites for mistaking identification.[27] Problems other than misidentifying recipient or donor unit are also more frequent when there is insufficient time to test the patient's blood before transfusion. Early symptoms of transfusion reaction are often masked by the circumstances surrounding massive transfusion. The anaesthetized patient cannot report subjective events, and blood pressure and temperature control are often aberrant under anaesthesia. Hypotension caused by transfusion accident is difficult to distinguish from the hypovolemic shock for which transfusion is given.

Fever, with or without chills, is probably the commonest presenting event, usually coinciding with the occurrence of the antigen-antibody event.[15] In immediate reactions, a temperature rise of 1°C or more accompanies administration of the unit, while in delayed reactions, the temperature rise occurs several days after transfusion. Hypotension is the other common event that heralds hemolysis. Chest pain, dyspnea, flushing, and nausea occur rather irregularly, as does the onset of the hemorrhagic diathesis that characterizes DIC.

Changes in temperature and blood pressure are easily detected. Because the severity of clinical effects varies directly with the volume of incompatible blood transfused, it is important to monitor the vital signs of all transfusion recipients. The patient undergoing anaesthesia or emergency treatment for a medical, surgical, or traumatic catastrophe will necessarily be under continuous surveillance. When transfusions are given in elective circumstances, the need for careful observation may be overlooked. The transfusionist should take and record the patient's vital signs before starting the transfusion. Blood should be started slowly, no more than 15 to 25 ml in the first 15 minutes, so that incipient symptoms can be observed before a large volume is infused. At the end of 15 minutes, the patient's condition should be noted; the rate of infusion can be increased if all is going well. Before starting the transfusion, the transfusionist should note whether any conditions exist that might complicate the diagnosis of transfusion reaction, such as spiking fevers, recurrent dyspnea, a tendency to vasomotor instability, and so on. The responsive patient should be told what symptoms should prompt him to call for clinical attention; some member of the clinical team should observe the patient and record vital signs every 30 minutes.

At completion of the transfusion, the transfusionist should note the time and the patient's general condition. Surveillance should continue for at least the subsequent hour, with a record of the patient's condition and vital signs at 30 to 60 minutes after the transfusion. If subsequent units are to follow the initial transfusion, the post-transfusion vital signs for the first unit become the pretransfusion observation for the later unit. A permanent record must exist, either in the patient's chart or in the blood bank, of the identification and volume of each unit transfused. The empty blood bag need not be returned to the blood bank because the blood bank keeps a sample from each transfused unit for at least 7 days after transfusion. Returning blood bags creates problems of filing and storage and exposes personnel to potentially dangerous contact with unsealed containers and dripping administration sets.

DELAYED HEMOLYTIC REACTIONS

Transfusion complications may occur well after infusion is completed. In addition to disease transmission, the commonest late-developing adverse effect is delayed hemolysis, that is, antibody-mediated destruction of transfused red cells occurring 2 or more days after transfusion. Clinical manifestations vary enormously in severity, ranging from the existence of a positive direct antiglobulin test in an asymptomatic patient through oliguria or renal shutdown (in fewer than 10 percent of cases)[28] to DIC (very rare). Delayed hemolytic reactions, by themselves, are rarely if ever fatal, but the resulting fever, anemia, and renal complications may aggravate the patient's other clinical problems.

Delayed hemolysis occurs when the transfused cells possess an antigen to which the recipient has, at some time in the past, already been immunized. The level of immunization may be so low that no circulating antibody exists to be detected by pretransfusion testing, or there may be antibody present but at a concentration below the sensitivity threshold of the tests routinely performed. Sometimes the antibody exists as a weakly reactive component in a serum that contains other antibodies, and its presence is overlooked.

The patient has always had some prior immunizing exposure to human red cells, either by pregnancies or transfusions or both. The antigens on the recently transfused cells constitute a secondary immunizing stimulus, which provokes rapid anamnestic production of IgG antibody in these already-immunized individuals. As the concentration of circulating antibody increases, the transfused red cells come under attack, usually within 2 to 8 days after the transfusion, but occasionally as long as 14 days later.

Because the antibody is largely IgG, which rarely causes direct intravascular cell destruction, the pathologic events in delayed reactions are those of extravascular hemolysis. In patients who develop clinical symptoms, the commonest presenting event is fever, developing several days after transfusion. Unexplained fever should provoke the suspicion of delayed hemolysis in any transfusion recipient. Hemoglobinuria occurs much less commonly, and oliguria or renal shutdown is rarer still. Often delayed hemolysis is discovered only because the patient's hemoglobin level drops from the previously achieved post-transfusion level. Hemoglobin levels may decline after transfusion because of overt or occult bleeding, but the suspicion of delayed hemolysis should exist whenever the hemoglobin value exhibits a defined drop 2 to 10 days after transfusion. A common mode of discovery is to observe a positive direct antiglobulin test on a sample drawn for subsequent crossmatching. Many delayed reactions cause so few signs or symptoms that only the chance performance of a direct antiglobulin test reveals that there are antibody-coated cells in the patient's circulation.

The antibodies that most often cause delayed hemolytic reactions are those of the Kidd system (Jk^a and Jk^b), anti-E, anti-C, and anti-Fy^a. Kidd antibodies are notoriously evanescent in their appearance, difficult to detect with routine serologic procedures, and likely to be a weakly reactive component in a serum with other, stronger antibodies. Anti-E and anti-C are especially likely to be troublesome when they exist in a serum that contains other antibodies in the Rh system. The patient with delayed hemolysis caused by anamnestic antibody production may be immunized only to a single antigen, but mixtures of antibodies are frequently found.[29]

The most conclusive diagnostic finding in delayed hemolytic reactions is a positive direct antiglobulin test. Ideally, the eluate should contain identifiable antibody that reacts with a cell sample from the transfused units. Often, however, the antiglobulin results are positive only weakly or transiently, and it is not possible to prepare a diagnostic eluate. The serum may contain no free antibody at all when antibody attachment and hemolysis first occur, but within several days circulating antibody concentration usually reaches a level that readily allows serologic identification. Demonstrating the existence of hemolysis by measuring haptoglobin, hemoglobin, or bilirubin in serum and hemoglobin, hemosiderin, or urobilinogen in urine may be confirmatory but is not consistently helpful. Often these tests are ordered later than the time at which maximally abnormal findings existed.

INVESTIGATION OF THE HEMOLYTIC REACTION

CLINICAL CONSIDERATIONS

When a transfusion reaction is reported, the first goal of investigation is to ascertain what kind of reaction has occurred. The nursing service procedure manual should contain explicit instructions for handling suspected transfusion reactions. The following points should be included: stop the transfusion; keep the intravenous line open; draw a blood sample as soon as possible; send the post-reaction specimen, the blood container, the attached administration set, and a written description of the observed clinical events to the blood bank. The procedure manual should also state when postreaction urine specimens should be collected and examined. Many blood bank directors include, in the clinical procedures manual, a qualification that the transfusion need not be discontinued if a patient experiences only hives or urticaria, especially if previous transfusions have elicited similar allergic manifestations.

If ABO incompatibility has occurred, clinical treatment should begin immediately, even before laboratory findings are available. Since most ABO catastrophes occur when blood intended for one patient is given to another, clinical personnel should check the identification tag on the blood with the patient's wrist band as soon as symptoms become apparent. Identification errors are not always detected immediately but if the patient manifests a sudden drop in blood pressure, rise in temperature, or onset of arm, chest, or lumbar pain, the clinician may choose to assume that there is intravascular hemolysis and administer immediate therapy.

Treatment aims at maintaining adequate systemic arterial blood pressure and tissue perfusion and preventing renal damage. Diuretics and antihypotensive agents, if indicated, should be administered promptly; if the patient's problems are not due to a hemolytic reaction, this therapy will not, ordinarily, have caused the patient any harm. The clinician usually administers antipyretics for febrile reactions or antihistamines for allergic reactions before the laboratory has completed its investigation.

IMMEDIATE LABORATORY PROCEDURES

When the report and the specimens from a suspected transfusion reaction come to the laboratory, several tests must be done immediately. The identifying information on the blood bag, the compatibility label, the transfusion request, and the labora-tory sign-out log should be checked. The postreaction blood sample should be cen-trifuged and the color of the serum observed. Pink, red, or brown discoloration in the post-transfusion serum indicates the presence of free hemoglobin or its deriva-tives. Subtle color changes may be perceived more readily by comparing the pre-transfusion and post-transfusion serum side by side. Hemolysis in the pretransfusion sample caused by storage may be observed and should not mislead the technologist. The cells of the post-transfusion sample must be examined for the presence of cell-bound antibody, so a direct antiglobulin test should be performed immediately.

Negative results on these three procedures—checking identification, looking for free serum hemoglobin, and looking for antibody attached to circulating cells—are usually sufficient to rule out the occurrence of a hemolytic transfusion reaction. One or more positive findings signal the necessity for immediate and detailed further investigation. It is not necessary to pursue further investigations if the screening tests are negative, unless the patient's clinical condition strongly sug-gests that the preliminary results are misleading.

If the identification check reveals discrepancies, more than one patient may be at risk. If John Jones has received blood intended for Richard Smith, it is essential to check on Richard Smith to see if he has received or is about to receive the unit in-tended for Jones. Less obvious identification mix-ups may come to light as serologic tests continue. Investigating a hemolytic episode requires repeat ABO and Rh testing on the pretransfusion specimen and comparison with findings on the postreaction specimen. If these are not identical, the indication is that one (possibly both) of the specimens was misidentified. Usually it turns out that the tube used for pretransfu-sion testing, while labeled for the intended recipient, contains someone else's blood. If this is the case, it is essential to check when the specimen was received in the blood bank, who drew the specimen, and when and where it was drawn and labeled. If another one or several specimens were drawn at the same time by the same person, there is a strong likelihood that at least one of the other specimens was also mislabeled, and these specimens should be found and examined. If feasible, it is desirable to draw a new, confirmatory specimen from each of the patients potentially implicated in a labeling mix-up. Labeling errors occur when the phlebotomist fails to check the label on the tube against the patient's wrist band before leaving the bedside. Prelabeling a handful of tubes before beginning phlebotomy or applying labels at the nursing station to previously filled tubes is the usual explanation.

Examining the postreaction specimen for free hemoglobin in the serum and for a positive direct antiglobulin test is usually adequate to indicate the presence or absence of hemolysis. Intravascular hemolysis of as little as 25 ml of blood will release sufficient hemoglobin to impart visible discoloration to the serum or plasma. Extravascular hemolysis less often produces hemoglobinemia, but the serum may contain free hemoglobin if large numbers of cells undergo rapid damage in the reticuloendothelial system.

Hemoglobin molecules pass surprisingly readily through the glomerular filter, and hemoglobinuria frequently follows either intravascular or extravascular hemol-ysis. If hemolysis is not suspected until several hours after the transfusion, the serum may no longer contain hemoglobin, but hemoglobinuria can often be detected. The significant observation is hemoglobin in the supernatant urine, not the presence of red cells in the sediment. Testing for hemoglobin in uncentrifuged urine or in the sediment may be misleading since hematuria (the presence of red cells in the urine) may have a number of causes unrelated to transfusion. The appropriate examination is to centrifuge a fresh urine sample and test for hemoglobin in the supernatant. If the specimen is not examined promptly, red cells present may hemolyze and cause the spurious presence of hemoglobin outside of the sediment.

The direct antiglobulin test may be positive only transiently after a reaction if the antibody-coated red cells are rapidly destroyed. Only the transfused cells are attacked by antibody, giving a mixed-field pattern to the positive test because the antiglobulin serum does not agglutinate the patient's own cells.

MORE DETAILED TESTING

Additional tests should be done on the patient's pretransfusion and post-transfusion samples and on the unit of transfused blood if the screening tests suggest that hemolysis exists. The ABO and Rh group and the antibody screening test should be repeated on the pretransfusion sample and on a sample from the donor unit at the same time that the postreaction specimen is examined for ABO, Rh, and the presence of unexpected antibody. Errors in identification or labeling become apparent at this point. Errors in serologic technique rarely cause discrepant findings, but sometimes a missed unexpected antibody or overlooked variant A, B, or D reactivity may be detected. If the postreaction specimen has been drawn more than 18 hours after the transfusion, anamnestic antibody production could cause a positive result in the later sample, with the pretransfusion results being genuinely negative.

Crossmatching should be repeated, testing both the pretransfusion and the post-transfusion serum against cells taken from a segment attached to the donor unit. If incompatibility is noted in both, this suggests that the pretransfusion crossmatch was incorrectly interpreted, or that the test was done with incorrectly identified specimens. If the pretransfusion specimen gives compatible results but the post-transfusion serum is incompatible, the usual cause is anamnestic antibody production. This is unlikely to occur in less than 12 to 18 hours after transfusion, but is a frequent finding when delayed adverse effects are noted. If there is a discrepancy with a specimen drawn shortly after transfusion, it could be that the pretransfusion specimen was incorrectly identified, but the problem could also be anamnestic antibody response to an earlier transfusion. Very rarely, the serum may contain transfused antibody from a donor unit that contained a strong antibody. Checking the patient's transfusion history is an essential part of the detailed investigation of reported reactions.

If antibody is found in the patient's specimens or the donor unit, it should be identified. If the donor unit contains antibody, the recipient's cells should be tested for the presence of the corresponding antigen. If either or both of the patient's specimens contain antibody, it is desirable to check for the corresponding antigen in all donor units given during the current transfusion episode. The unit thought to be implicated in a reaction could be an innocent bystander to hemolysis involving blood given hours or days earlier.

If hemoglobinemia or hemoglobinuria indicates hemolysis, but serologic tests fail to reveal any antibody, nonimmunologic causes of hemolysis should be sought. Residual blood in the bag and the administration set should be examined for hemolysis, and the circumstances of the transfusion should be investigated. Even if the residual donor cells are intact, there could have been damage to cells as they entered the patient's circulation through a malfunctioning blood warmer or under excessive external pressure. Thermal damage to the unit, bacterial contamination, or admixture with unsuitable intravenuous solutions becomes apparent on examining the residual blood. Occasionally, distilled water or other solutions have entered the circulation and damaged red cells if the patient was undergoing irrigation procedures or other instrumentation involving fluids of various sorts.

Hemolysis may involve the patient's own cells if they are intrinsically abnormal. Glucose-6-phosphate dehydrogenase deficiency is fairly common in black males, and affected patients may experience hemolysis in settings of infection, drug administration, acidosis, or other medical conditions in which transfusion might be given. Hemolytic crisis in sickle cell disease is another event that may occur at the same time as transfusion. Patients with paroxysmal nocturnal hemoglobinuria (PNH) have red cells that are abnormally sensitive to complement-mediated hemolysis, and transfusion of whole blood, plasma, or red blood cells may precipitate striking hemolysis.

If initial serologic investigations are negative, it may be necessary to intensify the search for antibody and red cell destruction. The patient whose clinical condition strongly suggests hemolysis should remain under careful observation. In a patient who is not bleeding, serial drops in hematocrit and hemoglobin strongly suggest continuing red cell destruction. The antibody screening test should be repeated several times in the week or two after transfusion because exposure to incompatible cells may stimulate antibody production. If the initial antibody was weak, the immediate postreaction specimen may have no serum antibody activity because all the free antibody attached to the transfused cells. The direct antiglobulin test could be negative if there was prompt sequestration and destruction of the antibody-coated cells. Within several days, however, the antibody should achieve clearly detectable levels in the serum.

It is often desirable to use serologic techniques additional to those in routine use. Enhanced sensitivity can often be achieved by using low ionic strength solutions, if these are not routinely used; by enzyme treating reagent or donor cells or both; by increasing the volume of serum relative to the concentration of cells; or by employing enhancing media, automated techniques, radioisotope techniques, or other specialized methods.

Whatever tests and procedures are used in investigating a reported reaction, it is essential to keep complete records of all results and interpretations. An important safeguard against the development of transfusion reactions is routine scrutiny of the patient's transfusion history whenever blood is ordered. The blood bank must have available for immediate examination records on all patients in the preceding 5 years who have had significant unexpected antibodies or problems in ABO typing.[30] It should be standard practice to check the problem patient file whenever a crossmatch request is received.

THE HAZARDS OF TRANSFUSION   **381**

There is no perfect pretransfusion test, and it is impossible to guarantee normal cell survival after every transfusion. Stringent adherence to routines for identification and for serologic testing will reduce to a minimum the incidence of untoward reactions. If adverse effects do occur, careful investigation and meticulous documentation are the best safeguards of the patient and of the laboratory's reputation.

REFERENCES

1. Mollison, PL: *Blood Transfusion in Clinical Medicine*, ed 6. Blackwell Scientific Publications, Oxford, 1979, p 617.
2. *Code of Federal Regulations, Title 21, Part 606. 170(b)*. U.S. Government Printing Office, Washington, DC, 1980.
3. Tullis, JL: *The impact of advances in blood transfusion*. In Hubbell, RC (ed): *Advances in Blood Transfusion*. American Blood Commission, Arlington, Virginia, 1979, p 40.
4. Oberman, HA (ed): *Standards for Blood Banks and Transfusion Services*, ed 10. American Association of Blood Banks, Washington, DC, 1981, J2.100.
5. Ryden, SE: *Compatibility of blood with intravenous solutions*. In *From Vein to Vein. A Seminar for Phlebotomists and Transfusionists*. American Association of Blood Banks, Washington, DC, 1976, pp 33–36.
6. Jacob, HS, et al.: *Complement-induced granulocyte aggregation. An unsuspected mechanism of disease*. N Eng J Med 302:789, 1980.
7. Eiser, WG and Eckert, G: *Current problems and results in testing microaggregate filters*. Vox Sang 37:310, 1979.
8. Snyder, EL: *Non-infectious and non-immunologic complications of blood transfusion*. Conn Med 43:206, 1979.
9. Polesky, HF and Manske, WJ: *Rate of temperature change in whole blood and red cells in a controlled environment* (abstr). Transfusion 18:385, 1978.
10. Chambers, RW, Foley, HT and Schmidt, PJ: *Transmission of syphilis by fresh blood components*. Transfusion 9:32, 1969.
11. Walker, RH: *The disposition of STS reactive blood in a transfusion service*. Transfusion 5:452, 1965.
12. Yeager, AS, et al.: *Prevention of transfusion-acquired cytomegalovirus infections in newborn infants*. J Pediatr 98:281, 1981.
13. Koistinen, J and Leikola, J: *Weak anti-IgA antibodies with limited specificity and nonhemolytic transfusion reactions*. Vox Sang 32:77, 1977.
14. Rivat, L, et al.: *Comparative frequencies of anti-IgA antibodies among patients with anaphylactic transfusion reactions and among normal blood donors*. Clin Immunol Immunopathol 7:340, 1977.
15. Pineda, AA, Brzica, SM and Taswell, HF: *Hemolytic transfusion reaction. Recent experience in a large blood bank*. Mayo Clin Proc 53:378, 1978.
16. McCullough, J, et al.: *Microcapillary agglutination for the detection of leukocyte antibodies: Evaluation of the method and clinical significance in transfusion reactions*. Transfusion 14:425, 1974.
17. McCullough, J, et al.: *The role of histocompatibility testing in granulocyte transfusion*. In Greenwalt, TJ and Jamieson, GA (eds.): *The Granulocyte: Function and Clinical Utilization*. Alan R Liss, New York, 1977, pp 321–327.
18. Mollison, PL, op cit, p 572.
19. Kevy, SV, et al.: *Febrile, non-hemolytic transfusion reactions and the limited role of leukoagglutinins in their etiology*. Transfusion 2:7, 1962.
20. Meryman, H, Bross, J and Lebovitz, R: *The preparation of leukocyte-poor red blood cells: A comparative study*. Transfusion 20:285, 1980.

21. Miller, WV, Wilson, MJ and Kalb, HJ: *Simple methods for production of HL-A antigen poor red blood cells.* Transfusion 13:189, 1973.

22. Wenz, B, et al.: *Leukocyte-poor red blood cells prepared by microaggregate blood filtration (MABF)* (abstr). Transfusion 19:645, 1979.

23. Kilduffe, RA and DeBakey, M: *The Blood Bank and the Technique and Therapeutics of Transfusions.* CV Mosby, St. Louis, 1942, p 483.

24. Rabiner, SF, et al.: *Further studies with stroma-free hemoglobin solution.* Ann Surg 171:615, 1970.

25. Ruiz, CE, Weil, MH and Carlson, RW: *Treatment of circulatory shock with dopamine; Studies on survival.* JAMA 242:165, 1979.

26. Goldfinger, D: *Adverse reactions to blood transfusion.* In Mayer, K (ed): *Guidelines to Transfusion Practices.* American Association of Blood Banks, Washington, DC, 1980, pp 137–154.

27. Schmidt, PJ: *Transfusion mortality: With special reference to surgical and intensive care facilities.* J Fl Med Assoc 67:151, 1980.

28. Pineda, AA, Taswell, HF and Brzica, SM, Jr: *Delayed hemolytic transfusion reaction. An immunologic hazard of blood transfusion.* Transfusion 18:1, 1978.

29. Mollison, PL, op cit, p 579.

30. Oberman, HA, op cit, M2.100.

CHAPTER **17**

HEPATITIS

HERBERT F. POLESKY, M.D.

The most common complication of transfusion is hepatitis.[1] Two groups of viruses, hepatitis B (HBV) and non-A, non-B (NANB) can be transmitted to and may cause problems in up to 10 percent of the recipients of blood and components. It is difficult to ascertain the exact incidence of this complication because a large proportion of affected recipients are asymptomatic and will not be recognized unless prospective studies of liver function are carried out. Hepatitis may also be the major cause of mortality associated with transfusion. The true incidence is unknown since the patient often is transfused in a tertiary care facility located in a different area than where he resides. Furthermore, the delay in onset of symptoms of hepatitis after transfusion and features of the patient's disease often make it difficult to distinguish between transfusion-associated hepatitis and complications of the primary illness.

NOMENCLATURE AND CHARACTERISTICS OF AGENTS

HEPATITIS B VIRUS (HBV)

Though no one has grown the agent causing hepatitis B in tissue culture, it has been isolated from serum, body fluids, and the liver of patients with acute hepatitis. Using ultracentrifugation and electron microscopy, the virus appears to be a 27-nm core particle that is surrounded by a coat protein (Fig. 17-1). The total virion—core and surrounding coat—is 42 nm across and is called the Dane particle.[2] There are several antigens associated with the coat protein and the core particle. These antigens and their corresponding antibodies occur at different stages of clinical hepatitis and can be used to establish the diagnosis, to screen for potentially infectious donors, and to make decisions about prophylactic therapy in cases of accidental exposure (Fig. 17-2).

The first marker to appear in the serum of an individual infected with HBV is hepatitis B surface antigen (HBsAg).[3] This is the coat protein, which is produced by the liver in large amounts even though very few viral particles are present. HBsAg has also been called Australia antigen (Au antigen), SH antigen, and HAA (hepatitis-associated antigen). There are several antigenic characteristics of HBsAg that are determined by the subtype of the virus infecting the individual.[4] All subtypes share some antigenic determinants but also have some unique properties. The subtypes occur with different frequencies in certain geographic areas and can be useful in studying the epidemiology of a hepatitis B outbreak (Table 17-1).

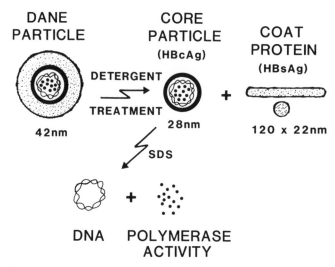

FIGURE 17-1. Diagram of the intact HBV virion (Dane particle) and its component parts as seen by electron microscopy. The coat protein (HBsAg) particles can be isolated from serum. The Dane particles are rare in serum but can be recovered from the liver.

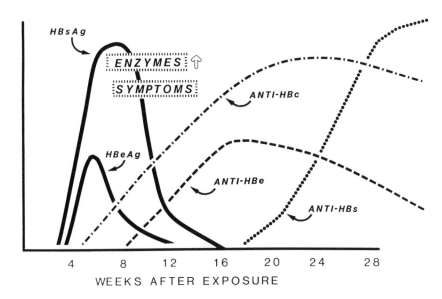

HBsAg

ENZYMES ↑

SYMPTOMS

ANTI-HBc

HBeAg

ANTI-HBe

ANTI-HBs

4	8	1 2	1 6	2 0	2 4	2 8

WEEKS AFTER EXPOSURE

FIGURE 17-2. Markers in acute HBV infection. The sequential appearances of antigens and antibodies occur at different times in each case. Shown is a typical pattern for an acute case that manifests recovery and development of immunity.

TABLE 17-1. HBsAg Subtypes by Geographic Areas[4]

	Percentage Positive in Representative Samples			
	ad	ay	w	r
Americas	85	15	95	5
Europe (Central)	75	25	99	1
Africa (Central)	10	90	100	–
Middle East	5	95	100	–
Far East	90	10	40	60

The second marker to appear is antibody to the hepatitis B core antigen, anti-HBc. Some reports have suggested that an IgM anti-HBc may be detectable before HBsAg. Cores isolated from Dane particles treated with detergent contain DNA and DNA polymerase activity. Under appropriate conditions this material produces DNA that has both double and single stranded segments.[5] Using special histologic techniques, such as immunoperoxidase or fluorescent labeled antibody, core particles can be found in the nuclei of infected hepatocytes.[6]

The hepatitis Be antigen (HBeAg) is another marker that appears during acute infection. This antigen is usually detectable only when HBsAg is also present in serum. HBeAg has at least three subtypes and probably is composed of portions of both surface and core material.[7] The presence of HBeAg has been associated with infectivity and vertical transmission (transplacental).[8]

Antibodies to HBsAg (anti-HBs) and HBeAg (anti-HBe) develop during convalescence and recovery from HBV infection. The development of anti-HBe in a case of acute hepatitis is the first serologic evidence of resolution of the disease. Antibodies are also produced in response to active immunization (e.g., anti-HBs after injection of heat-treated purified HBsAg). They may also be detected in the serum after transfusion of plasma from a donor who has antibody.

HEPATITIS A VIRUS (HAV)

The virus causing hepatitis A or infectious hepatitis is a 27-nm RNA virus, which has been isolated from the stool of acutely ill patients.[9] This picornavirus localizes primarily in the cytoplasm of the liver. It does not produce a coat protein like HBV and is not detectable in serum. HAV has not been grown in tissue culture. However, both chimpanzees and marmosets (small monkeys found in tropical forests of the Americas) have been infected with HAV isolated from human stool. Antibodies to HAV, anti-HAV, appear in the plasma at the onset of clinically apparent disease (Fig. 17-3). The initial antibody is an IgM (anti-HAV-IgM), which is subsequently replaced by an IgG antibody that will persist for years.

NON-A, NON-B VIRUSES

The availability of reliable test systems for the serologic markers of HBV and HAV made it possible to establish that the majority of cases of transfusion-associated hepatitis (TAH) are caused by other viral agents.[10] Careful studies also rule out other agents, such as the Epstein-Barr virus (EBV) and the cytomegalovirus (CMV). Thus, by exclusion, cases not caused by HBV, HAV, bacteria, chemicals (drugs and alco-

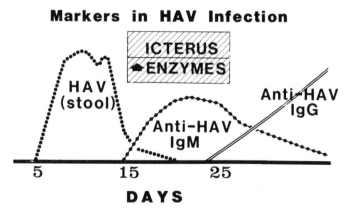

FIGURE 17-3. Markers in acute HAV infection. The typical pattern of HAV infection includes early shedding of virus in the stool, appearance of IgM anti-HAV with the onset of symptoms, and development of IgG anti-HAV and immunity on recovery.

hol), and so on have been classified as non-A, non-B. The agent or agents causing these infections are transmissible from man to man and man to chimpanzee.[11] Several candidate viruses have been seen by the electron microscope and a variety of test systems for antibody and antigen have been described. None of the candidate viruses or test systems have been universally accepted as markers of non-A, non-B infection.

CLINICAL FEATURES

The incidence of HBV infection varies from one geographic area to another and certain "high-risk" groups have been identified. Among these are health care workers, homosexuals, military recruits, patients on chronic renal dialysis, and individuals from areas in which the virus is endemic (Table 17-2). HBV infection varies from an inapparent or unrecognized course to a rapidly fatal, fulminant course. The majority of cases are probably asymptomatic or are thought to be a mild "flu" syndrome. Thus, many individuals with no history of hepatitis have serologic evidence of prior exposure to HBV and HAV (Table 17-3).

In individuals exposed by an accidental needle puncture or transfusion, the usual symptoms of weakness, fatigue, nausea, and jaundice may not appear for 10 to 16 weeks after exposure. In some individuals a prodrome of joint pain and/or rash or urticaria may occur several weeks before the illness is recognized as hepatitis. Table 17-4 summarizes the features of hepatitis in a blood bank technologist who was accidentally exposed through a cut on his finger while crossmatching. In this

TABLE 17-2. Hepatitis Markers in High-Incidence Groups

Marker	Percentage Positive		
	Southeast Asian Immigrants (483)*	Male Homosexuals (1077)	Renal Dialysis Patients (163)
Anti-HAV			
IgG	90.2	35.6	–
IgM	1.0	–	–
HBsAg	20.3†	4.5	71.7‡
Anti-HBs and Anti-HBc	46.8	50.4	–
Anti-HBs	2.9	–	–
Anti-HBc	1.4	5.1	–
HAV and/or HBV	94.6	67.9	–

*Number tested
†50% HBeAg positive, 50% anti-HBe positive, and 100% anti-HBc positive
‡71.8% HBeAg positive and 100% anti-HBc positive

TABLE 17-3. Viral Hepatitis Markers in Blood Donors With and Without a History of Prior Exposure

	Percentage Positive for One or Several Markers				
	HBsAg	Anti-HBc	Anti-HBc/HBs	Anti-HBc/HBs/HAV	Anti-HAV
Random donors (529)*	0	0.2	4.0	3.5	19.1
Health care personnel (donors) (569)	0	0.002	4.3	0.005	7.7
Donors rejected for hepatitis history (203)	0	0	5.1	1.0	27.6

*Number tested

TABLE 17-4. Clinical and Serologic Features of Acute Hepatitis in a Blood Bank Technologist

Weeks After Exposure	Clinical and Serologic Features
4	Complained of joint pain Liver function tests normal, started on steroids for arthritis
8	Nausea, jaundice developed HBsAg positive, HBeAg positive, anti-HBc positive, SGOT 690 IU, Bili 3.0 mg/dl, steroid treatment discontinued
10	Symptoms subside with restricted activity HBsAg positive, HBeAg positive, anti-HBc positive
12	Disease resolved HBsAg positive, HBeAg negative, anti-HBc positive, anti-HBe positive SGOT 85 IU, Bili 0.9 mg/dl
14	Recovered, resumed normal activity HBsAg negative, anti-HBc positive, anti-HBe positive SGOT 15 IU, Bili 0.4 mg/dl
16	HBsAg negative, anti-HBc positive, anti-HBe positive, anti-HBs negative
20	HBsAg negative, anti-HBc positive, anti-HBe positive, anti-HBs positive

case, HBV infection was not recognized until the onset of mild jaundice. The diagnosis was then confirmed by serologic testing.

The acute phase is also of variable length but usually lasts only a few weeks. Most persons who develop acute hepatitis completely recover and develop immunity. About 3 percent do not show an immunologic response to the virus and may become chronic carriers or develop chronic active or chronic persistent hepatitis. The reason that some people become chronic carriers is unknown; however, it is probably associated with their immunologic status at the time of exposure.

Acquisition of HBV infection can occur in several ways, including transfusion, needle puncture, accidental ingestion, and transplacental (vertical) exposure. In cases of accidental exposure to HBV, passive immunization with hepatitis B immune globulin (HBIG) may prevent the disease or prolong the incubation period (up to 9 to 12 months).[12,13] Some protection is also afforded by normal immune serum globulin (ISG). Studies of active immunization with heat-treated purified HBsAg suggest this will be very useful in reducing the incidence in high-risk populations.[14]

The licensing of a vaccine for prevention of HBV infection was announced by the FDA in 1981. Prepared from formalin-treated, purified HBsAg obtained from chronic carriers, this material has been shown to produce an antibody (anti-HBs) response in 96 percent of vaccinated individuals after two injections given one month apart.[14] In a high-risk population (male homosexuals) the incidence of HBV infection (both clinical and subclinical) was significantly less in the vaccinated group (1.4 to 3.4 percent) compared with the control group (18 to 27 percent). Side effects from the vaccine were minimal; however, it is likely that because of cost and limited supplies, only individuals at high risk for HBV infection will be considered for vaccination. Those individuals who already are immune (i.e., have anti-HBs and anti-HBc or only anti-HBs) will not require this treatment. It is possible that the vaccine may also be effective in preventing infection even if it is administered after an exposure to HBV. Although this product is available, it is not intended for use in transfusion practice since most cases of transfusion-associated hepatitis are caused by non-A, non-B viruses.

The clinical signs and symptoms of HAV infection are almost identical to those seen in acute HBV disease. Usually HAV has an incubation period of 20 to 45 days. Contaminated food or water and exposure to stool material from an infected individual are the common modes of transmission. Often HAV occurs as an epidemic. Although this disease used to occur primarily in pediatric patients, improved sanitation has resulted in a shift in the incidence to older age groups. Normal ISG contains antibody to HAV and is often used to treat individuals exposed in point source outbreaks, family members, and travelers to endemic areas.

The majority of patients with non-A, non-B hepatitis have minimal clinical manifestations. In prospective studies of transfused patients, about two thirds of cases of non-A, non-B hepatitis are only recognized by slight elevations of alanine aminotransferase (ALT).[10] The incubation period of non-A, non-B varies from 5 days to several months; however, most cases occur about 8 weeks after exposure. Though clinical signs and symptoms are usually mild, persistent ALT elevation or chronic active hepatitis may develop as a complication of non-A, non-B hepatitis. ISG may provide protection in cases of accidental exposure, but is probably not effective in preventing transfusion-associated cases.

TESTING FOR HEPATITIS MARKERS

Prior to the discovery of Australia antigen (Au) in 1964 by Blumberg and coworkers,[15] the etiology of a hepatitis case was based on clinical features. The recognition that this immunoprecipitin found in the serum of an Australian aborigine was a marker of HBV infection led to the development of numerous specific test systems for HBsAg. These test systems have been classified by the Office of Biologics of the FDA as first, second, and third generation based on their ability to detect dilutions of HBsAg (Table 17-5).[16] Though third generation tests may detect as little as 10^{-9} g per ml of HBsAg, less than 10^{-11} g per ml will cause infection in an experimental animal.[17]

The tests for markers of hepatitis viruses depend on detection of specific antigens or antibodies. Blumberg and coworkers used an Ouchterlony double diffusion system to identify Au. In this agar gel diffusion method (AGD), serum containing a known antibody (or antigen) is placed in a central well cut in an agarose plate. Peripheral wells are filled with unknown serum samples. After incubation to allow the reactants to reach equilibrium by passive diffusion, the plates are examined for precipitin lines. These tests, though very specific, are insensitive and relatively slow.

Counterimmunoelectrophoresis (CEP) tests for HBsAg were introduced in 1970. These tests depend on migration of antigen and antibody in opposite directions during electrophoresis in agarose.[18] Because the electrical field focuses the direction of movement of the reactants, these systems are more sensitive and much faster than AGD. The end point in the test is an immunoprecipitin line. In doing CEP careful attention must be paid to pH and purity of the agarose.

The third generation tests for HBsAg depend on use of an indicator system to enhance sensitivity. The most commonly used test, radioimmunoassay (RIA), depends on ^{125}I as the indicator. The commercially available RIA kits for HBsAg detection are sandwich type, direct assays. The test sample is added to a solid phase (bead or other type surface) coated with purified anti-BHs. After incubation and washing, radiolabeled (^{125}I) anti-HBs is added. If HBsAg was present in the test serum, an antibody-antigen-antibody sandwich will be formed. After incubation the sample is washed to remove unbound label. The solid phase is then placed in a gamma counter and the counts per minute (cpm) of each sample are monitored. The counts on the unknown are compared with a mean value obtained from a group of negative controls. A cutoff value (or ratio) between positive and negative samples is calculated by multiplying the mean value of the negative control cpm by a predetermined factor. The amount of HBsAg present in a positive sample is roughly proportional to the ratio of the unknown to the negative control mean. Table 17-6 summarizes the principles of the various test systems and calculations required to determine the level of radioactivity that separates reactive from nonreactive samples.

TABLE 17-5. Relative Sensitivity of HBsAg Test Methods[17]

Test System	Grams HBsAg per Milliliter Detectable
First generation	10^{-3}
Second generation	10^{-6}
Third generation	10^{-9}
Required to infect chimps	10^{-12}

TABLE 17-6. RIA Tests for Viral Hepatitis Markers: Principles and Calculations

Principle	Method			Calculation	Test For
DIRECT Sandwich — Antibody-coated solid phase	Unknown	+ ^{125}I labeled antibody	→ ↑cpm	A	HBsAg HBeAg
Antigen-coated solid phase	Unknown	+ ^{125}I labeled antigen	→ ↑cpm	A	Anti-HBs
Double Sandwich — Anti-IgM-coated solid phase	Unknown (specific Aby-IgM class)	+ Antigen + ^{125}I labeled antibody	→ ↑cpm	B	IgM Anti-HAV
INDIRECT — Antigen-coated solid phase	Unknown + ^{125}I labeled antibody	+ ^{125}I labeled antibody	→ ↓cpm	C	Anti-HBc Anti-HAV
Competitive — Antibody-coated solid phase	Unknown + antigen	+ ^{125}I labeled antibody	→ ↓cpm	C	Anti-HBe

Method of calculating negative cutoff:
A. Factor (e.g., 2.1) × mean negative control cpm*
B. Mean negative control cpm + 0.1 (mean positive control cpm)
C. $\dfrac{\text{Mean negative control cpm} + \text{mean positive control cpm}}{2}$

*Mean cpm = Gross cpm − background cpm

Another method, the enzyme-linked immunoassay (ELIA), is based on the same sandwich principle as the RIA test, but an enzyme label rather than a radiolabel is used as the indicator. In this test, after incubation and washing to remove unbound label, a chromogenic substrate is added. Degradation of the substrate by bound enzyme produces a color change and an optical density increase that is proportional to the HBsAg concentration in the unknown sample (Fig. 17-4).

The sensitivity and specificity of these tests is influenced by several factors, including the time and temperature of incubation, reagent variability, and the condition of the sample. Lot-to-lot variation and storage time affect the sensitivity of the reagent. These changes can be monitored by the inclusion of a low-level (borderline) positive control with each batch of unknown samples.

The sensitivity of some tests for HBsAg can be improved by lowering the negative cutoff level recommended by the reagent manufacturer.[19] Attempts to increase the sensitivity of the methods may result in a slight decrease in the specificity of the test.

Most methods give occasional false-positive results. On many samples these reactions are not reproducible on retesting. However, in cases in which a questionable result is repeatable, neutralization or inhibition with anti-HBs or testing the sample for the presence of other HBV markers is a method that can be used to establish HBsAg specificity.

Two third generation test systems, reverse passive hemagglutination (RPHA) and reverse passive latex agglutination (RPLA), depend on subjective observation of antibody-coated, stabilized red cells or latex particles. In RPHA the settling pattern of the cells is observed. If the unknown contains HBsAg, matting of the cells occurs be-

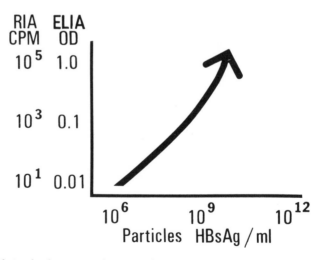

FIGURE 17-4. Relationship between end point reading in RIA and ELIA and relative quantity of HBsAg in an unknown sample. These values are only approximations since there is no standard HBsAg preparation. An occasional strongly reactive sample will appear to give increased reactivity on dilution.

cause the antigen cross links with antibody on the indicator cells. In the absence of HBsAg a discrete button occurs. In RPLA one sees a smooth suspension (negative) or a rough suspension (positive) of particles. Though these tests require minimal equipment and are rapid, they have a higher incidence of false positives and are not as sensitive as other third generation tests (Table 17-7).

Test systems for antibodies to HBV markers include both direct (sandwich) and indirect (competitive) methods (see Table 17-6). In the former, antigen-coated beads and labeled antigen are used to form the sandwich with the antibody in the unknown. In the latter, the antibody in the unknown competes with labeled antibody for antigen-binding sites on a solid phase. The tests for antibody have good specificity and sensitivity.

Several serologic techniques have been described to identify anti-HAV, including complement fixation, immune adherence, hemagglutination, and radioimmunoassay. Only RIA will be discussed since tests employing the other methods are not commercially available. The RIA test for anti-HAV (HAVAB, Abbott Laboratories) uses a solid phase (bead) that is coated with an anti-HAV-HAV complex. This is incubated with a mixture of patient's serum and ^{125}I-labeled anti-HAV. Anti-HAV in the patient's serum competes with the known labeled antibody for the available binding sites, resulting in a decrease in cpm (see Table 17-6). A 50 percent or greater reduction in the counts when compared with the negative control count per minute indicates that the unknown contains anti-HAV.

The use of staphylococcal protein A (Newman DC or Cowen strain) to adsorb IgG from diluted serum prior to testing for anti-HAV is one of several methods available to identify IgM antibody. Other methods, including column chromatography and labeled anti-IgM, have been used. In the RIA test for detecting IgM anti-HAV (HAVAB-M, Abbott Laboratories), patient's serum is incubated with an anti-IgM-coated solid phase. Purified HAV particles are added to the bound IgM fraction of the patient's serum. These will bind to IgM having anti-HAV specificity. After incubation and washing to remove unbound protein, ^{125}I-labeled anti-HAV is added. An increase in the counts per minute of the test when compared with the negative control indicates the presence of IgM-anti-HAV in the unknown sample (see Table 17-6).

TABLE 17-7. Sensitivity and Specificity of Third Generation Tests for HBsAg*

Test Method	Number of Laboratories Reporting	Participants Reporting Correct Answer (%)	
		HBsAg Positive Samples	HBsAg Negative Samples
RIA	530	95.9	99.3
ELIA	27	83.3	98.1
RPHA	101	68.2	99.5
LATEX	20	44.8	100

*Based on AABB-CAP Viral Hepatitis Marker Survey

PREVENTION OF TRANSFUSION-ASSOCIATED HEPATITIS

The prevention of TAH depends on several factors in addition to testing for HBsAg. Careful selection of donors is an important step in assuring safe blood. Donors from high-risk categories and those who might have recent exposure to HBV or non-A, non-B agents can be detected by an appropriate history. The motivation for giving blood (e.g., cash, a 2-day pass) can affect the reliability of the history.

Testing for HBsAg by specific and sensitive methods has eliminated much of the risk of HBV infection from transfusion. Testing for other markers such as anti-HBc will have little effect on prevention and add considerable cost to donor screening. Test methods for carriers of non-A, non-B depend on nonspecific evaluation of liver function.[20] Though several reports suggest that elevated ALT levels in donors correlate with increased risk of non-A, non-B transmission, the overall significance and cost effectiveness of this type of screening is not established.

Another facet of TAH prevention is surveillance of recipients. Careful reporting of TAH may identify some donors who have a higher risk than others. Several methods of followup on recipients have been suggested, including review of hepatitis admissions and discharges for prior transfusion, review of patients with abnormal liver function tests, and postcard followup to the physicians of any patient transfused in the past 3 months.[21] When cases are found they must be reported to the donor center so that high-risk individuals can be identified and eliminated from the donor pool.

The most effective way of preventing TAH is education of clinicians about the risks of blood and components. The fact that these risks are greater with certain derivatives (e.g., coagulation concentrates prepared from large donor pools) and increase with each unit administered should be emphasized so as to reduce unnecessary transfusions.

REFERENCES

1. POLESKY, HF: *Serologic tests in viral hepatitis.* In Homburger, HA and Batsakis, JG (EDS): *Clinical Laboratory Annual,* vol. 1. Appleton-Century-Crofts, New York, 1982.

2. DANE, DS, CAMERON, CH and BRIGGS, M: *Virus-like particles in serum of patients with Australia-antigen-associated hepatitis.* Lancet i:694, 1970.

3. KRUGMAN, S, et al.: *Viral hepatitis, type B. Studies on natural history and prevention re-examined.* N Engl J Med 300:101, 1979.

4. COUROUCÉ, AM, et al. (EDS): *HBs antigen subtypes. Proceedings of the International Workshop on HBs Antigen Subtypes, Paris, 1975.* Bibl Haematol (Monograph 42), 1976.

5. ROBINSON, WS: *Hepatitis B Dane particle DNA structure and the mechanism of the endogenous DNA polymerase reaction.* In Vyas, G, Cohen, S and Schmid, R (EDS): *Viral Hepatitis.* Franklin Institute Press, Philadelphia, 1978, p 139.

6. LAMOTHE, F, LAURENCINE-PICHÉ, J and COTÉ, J: *Detection of surface and core antigens of hepatitis B virus in the liver of 164 human subjects. A study by immunoperoxidase and orcein staining.* Gastroenterology 71:102, 1976.

7. Trepo, C, et al.: *Heterogeneity and significance of HBeAg: Characterization of a third specificity (e₃).* In Vyas, G, Cohen, S and Schmid, R (EDS): *Viral Hepatitis.* Franklin Institute Press, Philadelphia, 1978, p 203.

8. Stevens, CE, et al.: *HBeAg and anti-HBe detection by radioimmunoassay: Correlation with vertical transmission of hepatitis B virus in Taiwan.* J Med Virol 3:237, 1979.

9. Feinstone, SM, et al.: *Characterization of HAV.* In Vyas, G, Cohen, S and Schmid, R (EDS): *Viral Hepatitis.* Franklin Institute Press, Philadelphia, 1978, p 41.

10. Alter, HJ, et al.: *Non-A/non-B hepatitis: A review and interim report of an ongoing prospective study.* In Vyas, G, Cohen, S and Schmid, R (EDS): *Viral Hepatitis.* Franklin Institute Press, Philadelphia, 1978, p 359.

11. Tabor, E, et al.: *Experimental transmission and passage of human non-A/non-B hepatitis in chimpanzees.* In Vyas, G, Cohen, S and Schmid, R (EDS): *Viral Hepatitis.* Franklin Institute Press, Philadelphia, 1978, p 419.

12. Grady, GF and Lee, VA: *Hepatitis B immune globulin—prevention of hepatitis from accidental exposure among medical personnel.* N Engl J Med 293:1067, 1975.

13. Hoofnagle, JH, et al.: *Passive-active immunity from hepatitis B immune globulin. Reanalysis of a Veterans Administration cooperative study of needle-stick hepatitis. The Veterans Administration Cooperative Study Group.* Ann Int Med 91:813, 1979.

14. Szmuness, W, et al.: *Hepatitis B vaccine: Demonstration of efficacy in a controlled clinical trial in a high-risk population in the United States.* N Engl J Med 303:833, 1980.

15. Blumberg, BS, Alter, HJ and Visnich, S: *A "new" antigen in leukemia sera.* JAMA 191:541, 1965.

16. *Code of Federal Regulations, Title 21, Part 610:40.* 1980, p 47.

17. Gerety, RJ, et al.: *Tests for HBV-associated antigens and antibodies.* In Vyas, G, Cohen, S and Schmid, R (EDS): *Viral Hepatitis.* Franklin Institute Press, Philadelphia, 1978, p 121.

18. Ashcavai, M and Peters, RL: *Manual for Hepatitis B Antigen Testing.* WB Saunders, Philadelphia, 1973.

19. Polesky, HF and Hanson MR: *Results of HBsAg testing of AABB-CAP survey samples.* Am J Clin Pathol 68:210, 1977.

20. Aach, RD, et al.: *Transfusion-transmitted viruses: Interim analysis of hepatitis among transfused and nontransfused patients.* In Vyas, G, Cohen, S and Schmid, R (EDS): *Viral Hepatitis.* Franklin Institute Press, Philadelphia, 1978, p 383.

21. Polesky, HF and Hanson M: *Transfusion Associated Hepatitis.* American Society of Clinical Pathology, Chicago, ASCP Check Sample IH-109, 1980.

CHAPTER **18**

HEMOLYTIC DISEASE OF THE NEWBORN

SANDRA ALM BUCK, MT(ASCP)SBB

Hemolytic disease of the newborn (HDN) is a unique isoimmune disease. It is characterized by red cell destruction during fetal life and is caused by a feto-maternal blood group incompatibility.

The greatest risk of HDN occurs in offspring from an Rh-negative mother and an Rh-positive father. The mother can develop an antibody (anti-D) that is directed against the Rh_0 (D) antigen on the infant's red cells. This antigen is inherited from the father. In about 1 out of every 10 pregnancies a mother is Rh negative and the infant is Rh positive. HDN can also result from incompatibilities caused by many other red cell antibodies, although this occurrence is much less frequent. HDN caused by Rh incompatibility (Rh-HDN) is responsible for most of the cases of moderate and severe disease and essentially all instances of HDN mortality. For this reason the etiology, diagnosis, clinical findings, and treatment of HDN covered in this chapter will be from studies primarily done on Rh-HDN. These findings are also applicable to most other antibodies that may cause HDN, with the exception of ABO antibodies.

Feto-maternal incompatibility occurring within the ABO system also may cause HDN (ABO-HDN). While ABO incompatibility is very common, one out of every five pregnancies, the symptoms associated with ABO-HDN are most often mild or subclinical. Almost every aspect of ABO-HDN differs from HDN caused by other antibodies and shall be discussed separately.

Numerous advances have been made in the diagnosis and management of HDN and have greatly decreased infant morbidity and mortality. The greatest of these advances has been made in disease prevention. Although there is no cure for HDN, a method of antibody immunosuppression was developed to prevent Rh immunization in the mother and has been widely available since 1968. Passive antibody in the form of Rh immune globulin (RhIG) is given to Rh-negative women after delivery of an Rh-positive infant to prevent immunization to the Rh antigen and the resulting production of anti-D. Although only effective against immunization to the Rh antigen, treatment with RhIG has greatly reduced the overall incidence and severity of HDN.

Blood bank technology provides information necessary for the diagnosis and clinical management of HDN. Technologists need to identify the specific feto-maternal incompatibility, provide the safest possible blood for transfusion therapy, and identify the candidate for RhIG immunosuppression. They must also be knowledgeable in the etiology, diagnosis, and clinical manifestations of HDN.

ETIOLOGY

Hemolytic disease of the newborn has been described throughout medical history. Although the disease appeared to be inherited, it was noted that first-born infants were rarely affected, and the true etiology remained elusive. In 1939 Levine and Stetson[1] correlated the presence of an irregular antibody in the serum of a woman to the stillbirth of her infant and a transfusion reaction that occurred when she received blood from her husband. The suggestion was later made that red cells from the fetus can sensitize the mother to produce antibody that is directed against a red cell antigen that the fetus inherited from the father.[2] In 1940 Landsteiner and Wiener[3] discovered the Rh antigen and demonstrated its presence in 83 percent of the population, and the relationship between Rh negative women and Rh incompatibility causing HDN was established.

A number of conditions must be met for HDN to occur:

1. The woman must be exposed, either through pregnancy or transfusion, to a red cell antigen that she lacks;

2. The antigenic exposure must result in immunization and production of antibody;

3. The antibody must have the ability to cross the placenta and be of sufficient concentration to cause red cell destruction; and

4. The infant must possess the antigen corresponding to the maternal antibody.

Immunization of a mother through pregnancy is depicted in Color Plate 16.

During the first pregnancy no incompatibility exists and the first infant is unaffected. At birth red cells from the fetus enter the maternal circulation as the placenta separates from the uterus. These red cells may be recognized as antigenic and stimulate the maternal immune system to produce specific antibody. Once the mother has produced an antibody, all subsequent offspring who inherit the corresponding antigen from the father will be affected. During the next pregnancy with an incompatible fetus, maternal antibody crosses the placenta and reacts with the antigen on the fetal red cells.

The antigen-antibody complex on the red cell causes increased red cell destruction in the fetus, which continues throughout the pregnancy. Maternal antibody levels in the fetus are maximal at birth and the hemolytic process continues in the newborn until the antibody is eliminated.

Many variables affect the immunization of a woman through pregnancy. Theoretically a woman may become immunized any time an infant is positive for a red cell antigen that she lacks. This occurs in essentially all pregnancies considering the number of known red cell antigens. Fortunately, immunization occurs in very few women. Factors that affect immunization of a woman through pregnancy include the exposure to antigen, the immune response of the woman, and the type and strength of antibody produced.

EXPOSURE TO ANTIGEN

The incidence of immunization to red cells is related to the volume of the red cell exposure. In Rh-negative individuals who receive one unit of Rh-positive blood, approximately 50 percent will become immunized. Rh-negative women who deliver Rh-positive infants will become immunized approximately 10 percent of the time (when untreated with RhIG). The volume of antigenic exposure is the greatest factor responsible for this difference in immunization rates.

The most common exposure to red cells in a woman is through pregnancy. Fetal red cells enter the maternal circulation in about half of all deliveries with an average volume of less than 1.0 ml, although it is not uncommon for larger volumes to challenge the maternal immune system. It has been demonstrated that in difficult deliveries the volume of feto-maternal bleeding may be greater.

Exposure to fetal red cells also occurs during pregnancy. The placenta does not allow free passage of red cells; however, red cells can enter the maternal circulation throughout pregnancy. The volume of early feto-maternal bleeding is usually insufficient to cause maternal immunization. When early immunization does occur, it often results in low levels of antibody, which may be undetectable.

Early feto-maternal bleeding is very significant in an already sensitized woman. Volumes of fetal red cells that are insufficient to cause primary immunization can induce an anamnestic response and rapid production of antibody in a previously immunized woman.

Immunization by red cells is associated more with some blood group antigens than others. The incidence of immunization to the D antigen is the greatest. For this reason it has been emphasized that Rh-negative individuals only receive Rh-negative blood. Other antigens in the Rh system, such as C(rh′), E(rh″), and c(hr′), are also strong antigens. While the Kell (K) antigen is quite immunogenic, the frequency of the gene in the population is low, and it is therefore not a prevalent cause of HDN.

Immunization through pregnancy is almost exclusively associated with the D antigen. When other irregular antibodies are detected in the serum of a pregnant woman, they are usually the result of exposure to antigen by transfusion rather than by pregnancy.

The number of antigen sites on a red cell influences the number of antibody molecules that will be attached. Large amounts of antibody attached to a red cell facilitate the removal and destruction of that cell. In the Rh system the red cell genotype also affects the number of D sites per cell. A red cell that is genotypically $R_2 R_2$ (DcE/DcE) contains more antigenic sites than one that is $R_1 R_1$ (DCe/DCe). As would be expected in the presence of maternal anti-D, $R_2 r$ (DcE/dce) infants are more severely affected by HDN than $R_1 r$ (DCe/dce) infants.[4]

An incompatible fetus is always heterozygous for the antigen corresponding to the maternal antibody. This reduces the immunogenicity of many blood group antigens on the fetal red cell by reducing the number of antigen sites per cell. A red cell that is heterozygous for an antigen may also be less susceptible to red cell destruction by corresponding antibody.

PRODUCTION OF ANTIBODY

The ability of individuals to produce antibody following antigenic exposure varies considerably. In deliberate immunization studies it has been noted that certain individuals fail to produce antibody after repeated antigenic exposure. These individuals are termed "nonresponders" and constitute approximately 30 percent of the general population.[5] Other individuals produce multiple antibodies quite readily and may be termed "hyper-responders."

An individual may respond to antigenic stimulation in various ways. Following exposure to red cell antigens most people do not respond at all. Those who do respond may produce very weak or very potent antibody.

Primary sensitization occurs when an individual is exposed to a foreign antigen for the first time and antibody is produced. Detectable levels of antibody occur within 6 to 8 weeks of initial stimulation. Occasionally a second antigenic exposure is necessary for antibody to be serologically detectable.

An antibody that has been produced may persist for many years or, in time, may decrease and no longer be detectable. Once an individual has been immunized, reintroduction of antigen to the immune system will cause an anamnestic response.

CLASSIFICATION AND SPECIFICITY OF ANTIBODY

The classification and specificity of the maternal antibody are important factors that determine the severity of HDN in the infant. For maternal antibody to cause HDN it must cross the placenta, react with the fetal red cell antigen, and initiate the destruction of these cells.

Of the three main classes of immunoglobulins produced—IgM, IgG, and IgA—only IgG antibodies are able to traverse the placenta and cause HDN. IgM antibodies cannot cross the placenta and therefore are not implicated in this disease. The placental passage of antibody is accomplished by an active transport mechanism determined by the Fc portion of the IgG molecule.

The passage of gamma globulins to the fetus provides antibody protection against disease in the first weeks of neonatal life. The fetus does not make substantial antibody; essentially all antibody in the fetus is maternally derived. The concentration of IgG antibody in the fetus may be similar to or greater than the concentration in the mother.

Four subclasses of IgG antibody (IgG1, IgG2, IgG3, and IgG4) are defined and vary in their abilities to traverse the placenta, bind complement, and initiate red cell destruction by binding to macrophage receptors. IgG1 and IgG3 subclasses possess properties that are associated with greater red cell destruction and are potentially more harmful to the fetus.

HDN has been associated with almost all IgG red cell antibodies and may be classified by specificity into three categories: (1) Rh-HDN, (2) ABO-HDN, and (3) HDN caused by all other antibody specificities. Rh-HDN and ABO-HDN represent over 95 percent of all HDN, and the other antibodies constitute less than 5 percent. While the incidence of ABO-HDN is now greater than the incidence of Rh-HDN, the clinical importance of the latter disease is much greater.

"Other" antibodies that are the most common cause of HDN are anti-c (hr'), anti-E (rh"), and anti-K (Kell).[5] Frequently anti-G is detected as a component of anti-D. These antibodies have been associated with moderate and severe forms of HDN. An extensive list by Sabo[6] gives reference to over 70 different antibodies reported to cause HDN, including those directed against high-frequency, low-frequency, and private antigens.

Autoantibody that causes autoimmune hemolytic anemia in a pregnant woman may cause HDN in the fetus. The limited number of cases in the literature suggest that the infants at greatest risk are those born to mothers with severe hemolysis and very low hemoglobin levels. The hemolysis increases as pregnancy progresses and it has been suggested that women with autoimmune hemolytic anemia be closely monitored for the duration of their pregnancy.[7]

Antibodies such as anti-Le^a, anti-Le^b, anti-P$_1$, anti-M, and anti-N are usually IgM and do not cause HDN. Rarely, one of these antibodies, such as anti-M, will be IgG and may cause HDN. Anti-Le^a and anti-Le^b may never be associated with HDN because the antigen is not developed on fetal red cells.

ABO GROUP

ABO incompatibility occurs when a mother has an antibody directed against the infant's A or B red cells. Investigators have noted that severe HDN occurs more frequently in ABO-compatible infants than in ABO-incompatible infants. Ironically ABO incompatibility can cause mild ABO-HDN and may also protect against Rh immunization. This type of protection may occur when an unsensitized Rh-negative mother is also ABO incompatible with an Rh-positive infant. The fetal red cells presumably are prevented from stimulating the mother to the Rh antigen because these cells are rapidly hemolyzed by ABO antibody when they enter the maternal circulation. Exactly why this happens is unknown and ABO protection is not predictable.

EFFECTS OF RED CELL DESTRUCTION

Maternal antibody can cross the placenta and be present in the fetus during the second trimester. Since most red cell antigens are quite well developed at this time, red cell destruction may then begin. The hemolytic process generally increases toward the end of pregnancy and hemolysis rarely causes fetal death before 20 weeks gestation.[5]

Maternal antibody attached to antigen sites on the fetal red cell is recognized by macrophages in the reticuloendothelial system of the fetus. The red cells are altered, removed, or hemolyzed, resulting in a shortened life span. Red cell hemolysis in the infant can cause anemia and bilirubinemia and can indirectly lead to enlargement of the liver and spleen.

ANEMIA

The disease findings of HDN range from subclinical red cell destruction to profound anemia that may cause stillbirth and neonatal death. Anemia can stimulate the erythropoietic system of the fetus to release erythroblasts into the circulation. The term *erythroblastosis fetalis* has been commonly used to describe this feature of HDN. Severe anemia may lead to heart failure and generalized edema, called *hydrops fetalis.* Anemia poses the greatest risk to the fetus and the newborn in the first 24 hours of life, while hyperbilirubinemia is the greatest concern thereafter.

BILIRUBINEMIA

Hemoglobin is released as a product of red cell degradation. It is broken down into bilirubin and removed by the liver. Bilirubin in the form of indirect or unconjugated bilirubin is of greatest concern in infants. In the fetus bilirubin traverses the placenta and is excreted by the mother. In the neonate, however, the ability to conjugate and remove bilirubin is not well developed. High levels of unconjugated bilirubin in the brain result in *kernicterus,* causing irreversible brain damage. The risks associated with hyperbilirubinemia are also related to the maturity of the infant, with premature infants at higher risk than full-term infants.

LATE ANEMIA

Frequently HDN presents as a mild clinical disease. Neonates with HDN can have normal cord blood hemoglobins and low bilirubin levels that slowly rise and peak at around the third day of life. This is typical of ABO-HDN. Exchange transfusion may not be indicated in the first week; however, late anemia occasionally develops. The newborn who has been treated by exchange transfusion may still have circulating maternal antibody capable of destroying fetal red cells as they are released from the bone marrow. This also may cause late anemia. These infants may require transfusion therapy at 3 to 5 weeks after birth to correct the anemia.

DIAGNOSIS AND TREATMENT

When an antibody is detected in the serum of a pregnant woman, it is often difficult to predict the occurrence of fetal red cell destruction. Paternal antigen typing, maternal antibody titrations, and obstetric history provide information that may be significant in predicting the outcome to the fetus.

General conclusions can be made from studying the pattern of disease in successive siblings in a family affected with HDN. The infant from the first pregnancy in which an antibody is detected does not usually have severe disease. A subsequent infant may have a similar disease process or may be more severely affected. Once a severely affected infant is born, the chance of stillbirth in subsequent pregnancies is quite high.

When evaluating the significance of an antibody detected during pregnancy, it may be important to determine if the father possesses the corresponding red cell antigen. When the father is negative for the antigen, HDN cannot occur. Should the father be positive for the antigen, it is advantageous to determine if he is homozygous or heterozygous for the gene. In a homozygous father, all offspring will be affected. If it can be shown that he is heterozygous for the gene, statistically 50 percent of the offspring will be antigen negative and unaffected.

This information is also considered in the decision to perform an amniocentesis on the mother that directly monitors the degree of red cell destruction in the fetus.

AMNIOCENTESIS

Amniocentesis is the single most important procedure used to assess the severity of HDN in utero. A needle is inserted through the maternal abdominal wall and the interuterine wall, and into the fetal amniotic sac. An aliquot of amniotic fluid is withdrawn for bilirubin analysis. The optical density of the amniotic fluid is measured at 450 nm. The difference between the measured optical density and a baseline value is determined and the final value is plotted on a Liley graph[8] as seen in Figures 18-1 and 18-2. Three zones are associated with the severity of the disease. Levels corresponding to zone one indicate that the infant is unaffected or not in danger. Infants whose levels correlate with zone two should be closely monitored and retested. Levels corresponding to zone three indicate that the fetus is endangered. The fluid is also analyzed for fetal lung maturity and a decision can then be made regarding early delivery. When the infant is under 34 weeks gestation or immature for gestational age, an intrauterine transfusion (IUT) may be indicated to treat the life-threatening anemia.

INTRAUTERINE TRANSFUSION

Intrauterine transfusion (IUT) is a method of transfusing the fetus directly through its abdominal wall. Successful treatment of the anemia is dependent upon the ability of the fetus to absorb red cells through its peritoneum. The risk to the fetus associated with intrauterine transfusion is high and the procedure is performed only to treat severe prenatal HDN.

SPECTRAL ABSORPTION CURVE
AMNIOTIC FLUID

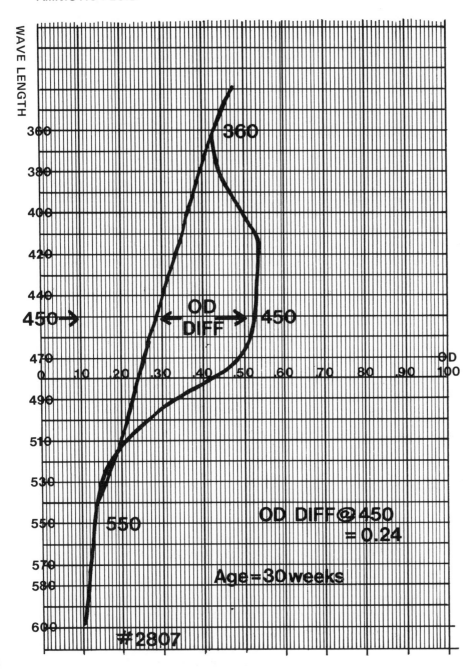

FIGURE 18-1. Spectral scan of bilirubin in amniotic fluid.

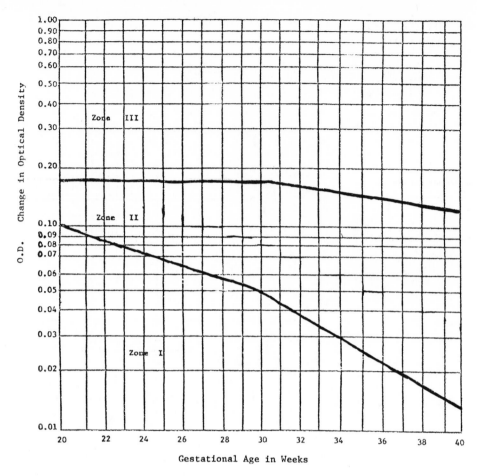

FIGURE 18-2. Liley graph. (Modified from Liley.[8])

EXCHANGE TRANSFUSION

Exchange transfusion is used in the treatment of both the anemia and hyperbilirubinemia. Small amounts of blood are continuously removed from the neonate and replaced with donor blood compatible with the maternal antibody until a one or two blood volume exchange is achieved. Performing the procedure in this manner is necessary to maintain blood volume and to prevent circulatory overload. Exchange transfusion removes bilirubin and circulating maternal antibody in the infant's plasma in addition to replacing antibody coated red cells with compatible donor cells.

The efficiency of a two volume exchange transfusion is approximately 80- to 90-percent removal of red cells and 25- to 35-percent removal of bilirubin.[5,20] The inefficient removal of bilirubin is due to extravascular bilirubin, which is not removed by the procedure and is released into the plasma following exchange transfusion. It is, therefore, more effective to perform exchange transfusion before the red cells are destroyed and high levels of bilirubin produced.

The criteria considered in the decision to perform an exchange transfusion include the degree of anemia, the bilirubin level, the rate of the rise of bilirubin, and the maturity of the infant. The average normal hemoglobin level of a newborn is 14 to 20 g per dl. Mild anemia is present in infants with cord blood hemoglobins of 13 g per dl, while below 8 g per dl the anemia is considered severe. The hemoglobin level from a cord blood specimen is a more reliable indicator of red cell destruction than a heel-prick specimen. Often a specimen taken from the infant following delivery will have a considerably higher hemoglobin level owing to infusion of blood from the placenta.

The management of hyperbilirubinemia in the neonate is based on the prevention of kernicterus, which may occur at bilirubin levels of 20 mg per dl in a full-term infant and at lower levels in a premature infant. Generally a bilirubin increase greater than 0.5 mg per dl per hour or a rise to 10 mg per dl in the first 24 hours is an indication for treatment by exchange transfusion. In a 3- or 4-day-old full-term infant, the liver may already be able to conjugate sufficient levels of bilirubin and thus may tolerate much higher levels. The premature infant is treated at much lower levels.

PHOTOTHERAPY

Phototherapy is the exposure of an infant to light, which slowly decomposes bilirubin into a nontoxic substance. It is used to treat low levels of bilirubin not associated with a rapid hemolytic process. This is commonly seen in ABO-HDN. Phototherapy is also used in conjunction with exchange transfusion.

SEROLOGIC INVESTIGATION

PRENATAL ANTIBODY DETECTION

The protocol for monitoring pregnant women must include: (1) ABO grouping, (2) D and D^u typing, and (3) an antibody screening procedure. These tests should be performed at 2 to 3 months and again at 7 to 8 months of pregnancy. Early detection of antibodies is important for monitoring a potentially affected infant.

When an antibody is detected during pregnancy, the specificity and class of the antibody must be determined and its ability to cause HDN assessed. The potential clinical significance of the antibody must be noted and reported to the obstetrician. In addition, the patient's transfusion and obstetric histories may be of value whenever an irregular antibody is detected that indicates that the fetus may be at risk. As an example, passive anti-D may be detected in prenatal studies that is acquired by the antenatal or postpartum treatment of Rh-negative women with Rh immune globulin (RhIG). RhIG antibody is readily demonstrable for 2 to 3 months, but occasionally may persist longer. The obstetric history of the patient will be necessary to distinguish RhIG from maternal antibody formed following immunization.

When prenatal antibody screening procedures detect the presence of multiple antibodies, it is necessary to determine which of these antibodies is capable of causing HDN. When multiple IgG antibodies are present, blood that is negative for the antigens may be difficult to obtain. A unit of blood suitable for transfusion to the mother and infant should be procured and be readily available during the last 2 months of pregnancy. It may be necessary in the presence of high-incidence antibodies to draw and freeze blood from the mother for use at delivery.

Antibodies to low-incidence or "family" antigens may go undetected by routine prenatal screening procedures. The newborn, if affected, will have an unexplained positive direct antiglobulin test (DAT). The antibody can then be detected if the maternal serum or an eluate prepared from the infant's red cells is tested for compatibility against the father's red cells or sometimes those of another sibling.

ANTIBODY TITRATION

An antibody titration is a technique in which serum is serially diluted and tested against appropriate red cells to determine the highest dilution in which a specific antibody demonstrates reactivity. The result is expressed as the reciprocal of the titration end point or as a titer score.

In HDN caused by anti-D, maternal antibody titers above 32 have been associated with infants who are more severely affected and require treatment more often than lower maternal antibody titers. Exceptions are not uncommon. Mothers with a low-titer antibody occasionally have infants who are severely affected, while those with a high titer may not.

The first prenatal titer that is performed is an estimate of maternal antibody concentration. Subsequent titers performed throughout pregnancy offer more valuable information in estimating the potential severity of HDN in utero. If an antibody shows a rapid rise in titer during pregnancy, this may indicate that the infant is affected. Only a difference of greater than two dilutions or a score change of more than 10 should be considered a significant change in titer.

Antibody titers may lead to further diagnostic procedures and must be carefully controlled to eliminate as many variables as possible. The first specimen for titration should be frozen and run in parallel with later specimens. The technique must be performed exactly the same way each time and only titers that measure IgG antibody are relevant. The blood bank should develop meaningful interpretive values for antibody titrations, as these values may vary between laboratories. Red cells used for each titration should be of the same genotype, approximately the same age, and the same concentration. Even though titration results may not always correlate with the severity of red cell destruction in the infant, if carefully controlled, they may be valuable in the prenatal diagnosis of HDN.

NEONATAL STUDIES

ABO grouping, Rh typing, and DATs should be performed on cord blood specimens from infants in question. Some unique problems exist in working with cord bloods.

ABO GROUPING

Wharton's jelly is an occasional contaminant in cord blood specimens that causes red cell clumping and may result in false-positive test results. This can usually be alleviated by washing the cells in saline three to five times. Hyaluronidase may also be added to reverse the agglutination.

The A and B antigens are not fully developed in newborns and occasionally very weak reactions will occur with anti-A or anti-B commercial grouping sera. The grouping of the infant may have to be delayed until the antigen is better developed on the red cell, perhaps until the infant is 6 months of age. Since the neonate does not have its own natural isoagglutinins, reverse grouping cannot be done to confirm the ABO group.

Rh TYPING

When an infant's red cells have a strongly positive DAT, typing for red cell antigens causes certain problems. Some anti-D typing sera contain up to 30 percent albumin. Red cells coated with antibody may agglutinate in such a high-protein medium and cause a false-positive D typing. The negative control tube will usually detect false agglutination of this type, as it should also show agglutination.

To avoid the problems associated with high-protein reagents, all red cells with a positive DAT should be tested using saline reagents. These are prepared from human IgM antibody or from chemically modified IgG antibody. Saline reagent anti-D, however, may fail to agglutinate red cells in which all the D sites are blocked by maternal anti-D, resulting in a false-negative Rh typing. An eluate prepared from red cells will demonstrate anti-D. Cells from which antibody has been eluted may be used for repeat Rh typing.

DIRECT ANTIGLOBULIN TEST

The DAT is the single most important serologic test in the diagnosis of HDN after birth. A positive DAT indicates that antibody is coating the infant's red cells in vivo. The DAT correlates well with the presence of HDN; however, the strength of the test does not correlate well with the severity of the disease.

Hemolytic disease of the newborn by definition indicates that red cell destruction is occurring. Antibody may be detected on the red cells of infants when there are no indications of clinical disease. When this happens, as determined by a positive DAT test or by the elution of antibody from the red cells, it is referred to as subclinical HDN. This is very typical of ABO-HDN.

ELUATES

When a newborn has a positive DAT, an eluate prepared from the red cells should be done and the antibody identified to conclusively prove that the HDN is caused by a particular antibody. The antibody specificity of an eluate should be determined by standard techniques that detect IgG antibody. When the infant is ABO incompatible with the mother, the eluate should also be tested against the appropriate A or B adult cells.

SELECTION OF BLOOD
EXCHANGE TRANSFUSION

Blood for exchange transfusion must be negative for any red cell antigen to which the mother has corresponding antibody. It must also be ABO and Rh compatible with the infant's blood group.

Rh-positive blood may be given to any Rh-positive infant whenever the mother does not have anti-D.

The selection of the ABO group for exchange transfusion is shown in Table 18-1. Whenever the infant or the mother is group O the red cells for exchange transfusion must always be group O. When group O blood is selected for exchange transfusion of a group A or B infant, all the plasma must be removed and replaced with compatible donor plasma. If it is necessary to crossmatch blood prior to delivery for immediate transfusion, it is convenient to use group O, Rh-negative red cells reconstituted with group AB plasma. When possible it is desirable to use the infant's ABO and Rh group.

Individuals who are heterozygous for the gene that codes for hemoglobin S (sickle cell trait or hemoglobin AS) may donate blood that is acceptable for most transfusion purposes. However, exchange transfusion may be performed under con-

TABLE 18-1.   ABO Group of Red Cells for Exchange Transfusion

Infant	Mother	Donor Red Cells
Group O	O, A, or B	O
Group A	O, B	O
	A, AB	A or O
Group B	O, A	O
	B, AB	B or O
Group AB	A	A or O
	B	B or O
	AB	AB, A, B, or O

ditions of decreased oxygen tension, which may cause the cells to sickle. Consequently all blood to be used for exchange transfusion must be tested and found negative for hemoglobin S.[9]

Transfusion of blood carries a risk of transmitting cytomegalovirus (CMV), which can result in CMV infection, particularly in infants. Some evidence suggests that donors with CMV antibodies pose a greater risk of transmitting CMV than those without.[10]

INTRAUTERINE TRANSFUSION

For intrauterine transfusion, group O, D-negative red cells compatible with the mother are used and should be as fresh as possible. Viable lymphocytes present in the donor blood are capable of causing graft-versus-host disease in the fetus. For this reason, it is recommended that blood for intrauterine transfusion be irradiated or as free of lymphocytes as possible.

ANTICOAGULANT

The anticoagulant selected for exchange transfusion may be CPD, CPDA-1, or heparin. The selection may depend upon the resources of the blood bank.

Blood drawn in CPD or CPDA-1 less than 5 days old has acceptable pH, 2,3-DPG, and potassium levels. The citrate in CPD and CPDA-1 binds to ionized calcium, which may produce low ionized calcium levels deleterious to some infants. Blood drawn in heparin is the most physiologic in pH and electrolytes and does not contain citrate. Heparinized blood, however, should be transfused within 24 hours and, therefore, is not often available.

Frozen red cells are readily available to many transfusion facilities and are often preferred because they are free of isoagglutinins and leukocytes. Exchange transfusion with frozen red cells depletes an infant of platelets and coagulation factors and requires pH monitoring of the infant. Frozen red cells may be reconstituted with fresh-frozen plasma or 5 percent albumin solution. Rare blood from the mother may be stored as frozen blood, then thawed and deglycerolized at delivery, enabling rare blood types to be readily available.

Although many institutions advocate blood up to 5 days old for exchange transfusion, fresher blood is always advantageous. Mollison[5] notes that red cell loss caused by the normal lesion of storage in a unit of older blood may result in unacceptable bilirubin levels, particularly when exchange transfusion is performed for hyperbilirubinemia.

COMPATIBILITY TESTING

Red cells selected for transfusion of the neonate must always be compatible with the mother since the infant has circulating maternal antibody. The specimen to be used for compatibility testing may depend upon the circumstances and the urgency of the request for exchange transfusion blood. The preference of specimen for compatibility testing is: (1) mother's serum, (2) an eluate prepared from the infant's red cells, and (3) infant's serum. The mother's serum should be used for compatibility testing whenever possible. The strength of the antibody in the infant's serum is unreliable and this specimen should only be used when the mother's serum is not available and time does not allow for the preparation of an eluate.

When the mother's specimen is not available, it must be assumed that an ABO incompatibility may exist and group O red cells should be selected for exchange transfusion. The infant's serum should be used for compatibility testing for subsequent transfusion, when the infant may have had time to develop an irregular antibody.

In the presence of multiple antibodies in which a maternal IgM antibody interferes with compatibility testing, a crossmatch technique that only detects IgG antibody is appropriate in finding compatible blood.

Exchange transfusion with reconstituted red cells utilizes one unit of donor plasma, which is equal to the total plasma volume in an infant. Compatibility testing of the donor plasma with the donor red cells has been recommended as a precaution against potential incompatibility between donors.[11]

It is also notable that even incompatible blood has been successfully used for urgent exchange transfusion when compatible blood could not be obtained.

ABO-HDN

ABO incompatibility occurs whenever the mother has an antibody directed against the infant's ABO red cell antigens. Although this event happens in about one out of every five pregnancies, fewer than 10 percent of these infants will require treatment.

ABO feto-maternal incompatibility had been noted prior to the discovery of the Rh factor, although reports were conflicting. The association between Rh incompatibility and HDN around 1940 stimulated new interest in ABO incompatibility. It is not surprising that earlier investigators were confused. The symptoms of HDN do not correlate well with the incidence of ABO incompatibility. As seen in Table 18-2, the serologic and clinical findings associated with ABO-HDN differ substantially from Rh-HDN and HDN caused by other antibodies.

ETIOLOGY

The natural presence of IgG antibody in ABO-HDN is one characteristic that differentiates it from all other types of HDN. In addition, many individuals make "naturally occurring" IgG antibody. The term "naturally occurring" is used because the antibody develops in the absence of any known red cell stimulus. These antibodies are the result of early environmental stimulus and occur more frequently in group O individuals. Anti-A,B is produced only in group O individuals and is described as an antibody that crossreacts with both group A and group B red cells; it is most responsible for HDN caused by ABO incompatibility.

As would be expected, ABO-HDN is a disease that is virtually limited to infants of group O mothers. Most cases of HDN occur in group A infants in the white

TABLE 18-2. Comparison of Rh-HDN and ABO-HDN

	Rh-HDN	ABO-HDN
Type of antibody:	Immune IgG	"Naturally occurring" IgG
In presence of antibody:	All affected	90% are subclinical or untreated
Prenatal evaluation:	Assess antibody titers and obstetric history	No prenatal evaluation
Obstetric history:	First unaffected, disease is more severe in subsequent offspring, stillbirth common	First may be affected, disease is not predictable, no stillbirth
Anemia:	Moderate to severe	Absent or mild
Bilirubinemia:	Rapid rise	Peak at 1–3 days
DAT:	Positive	Weakly positive or negative
Blood picture:	No microspherocytes	Microspherocytes
Prevention:	RhIG	None

population. In the black population group B infants are more often affected, while the overall incidence of HDN is several times greater.

The relatively mild clinical course of ABO-HDN is more related to the antigenic development of the fetal red cell than to properties of maternal antibody. A group-A infant of a group-O mother may be unaffected by maternal antibody that is incompatible with group-A donor blood.

The A and B antigens are not fully developed until the first year of life. This is well demonstrated by the A antigen. Group A_1 infant red cells are serologically more similar to A_2 adult red cells, and A_2 infant red cells are much weaker.[12] Indeed, A_2 infants and premature infants do not suffer from ABO-HDN.[13]

The hematologic findings in ABO-HDN differ from those in Rh-HDN, as seen in Table 18-2. Microspherocytes in a peripheral blood smear are indicative of ABO-HDN and not seen in Rh-HDN. Many infants suffering from ABO-HDN also have increased red cell fragility. These factors may be taken into consideration when a diagnosis of ABO-HDN is difficult to confirm.

ABO SEROLOGY

In ABO-HDN there is minimal red cell destruction in utero and no prenatal protocol has been established for identifying women whose infants may be affected.

Many investigators have attempted to predict or diagnose ABO-HDN by serologic studies with maternal and infant blood. Techniques using maternal serum only should be indicative of the presence and strength of IgG antibody. This can be accomplished by using anti-IgG-specific antihuman globulin reagent, treating the serum with 2-mercaptoethanol or dithiothreitol, or neutralizing the antibody with

HEMOLYTIC DISEASE OF THE NEWBORN

415

soluble A and B substance. The serum then may be titered, tested for hemolysins, or reacted with the infant's red cells. These tests are laborious and at best will demonstrate the presence of IgG maternal antibody, but they will not correlate well with the degree of fetal red cell destruction.

The infant's serum often contains circulating maternal antibody, which is IgG. Tests performed on this specimen also do not correlate well with indicators of red cell destruction.

DIRECT ANTIGLOBULIN TEST

Numerous conflicting papers have been published concerning the validity of the DAT in diagnosing infants with ABO-HDN. While some authors report that the DAT is rarely positive, others state that it is frequently positive.[14] These papers are difficult to compare. Among many variables are the definitions of ABO-HDN, the techniques employed, and the reagents utilized. Generally higher percentages of positive DATs will be obtained if the tests are read microscopically using fresh cord blood specimens.

ABO-HDN is known to occur in infants whose red cells have a negative DAT. Several theories have been proposed to explain this. (1) A weak interaction between the antigen and antibody may cause the antibody to be eluted off the red cell during the washing phase of the testing process. (2) The antibody molecules may not be present in sufficient numbers on the red cell antigens to facilitate a reaction with antihuman globulin serum. (3) The red cells with sufficient antibody attached may hemolyze intravascularly. (4) The population of fetal red cells may vary in their antigenic development according to their age, the younger fetal red cells being more developed and possessing more antigen sites than older red cells. The younger red cells may consequently be destroyed while older fetal red cells may not react with maternal antibody.

While the DAT is not consistently positive in ABO-incompatible infants, it has been shown to be positive in the majority of infants requiring treatment.[15] Accordingly, it remains a good indicator of clinically significant ABO-HDN.

In ABO-incompatible infants displaying no clinical evidence of HDN, the DAT may also be positive, which indicates that these infants have subclinical disease or compensated anemia, or that the antibody coating the red cells does not readily destroy them.

While the secretor status of the infant does not seem to be a significant factor in the severity of HDN, ABO antigens are widely dispersed in fetal tissue, thus absorbing some of the maternal antibody. All these factors probably contribute to the mild hemolytic process typical of ABO-HDN.

ELUATE

In ABO-HDN an eluate prepared from the infant's red cells will usually demonstrate the presence of maternal antibody. This may occur in the absence of clinical disease even when the DAT is negative. The antibody is readily eluted from infant red cells using heat, freeze-thaw, ether, or other eluate techniques. An eluate may be tested against group O screening cells in addition to A or B cells to rule out the existence of an irregular antibody. The strength of an eluate when titered against appropriate adult cells may correlate with the degree of jaundice in the infant.[16]

There is no single serologic test that is diagnostic for ABO-HDN. When an eluate demonstrates the presence of incompatible maternal antibody, the diagnosis of ABO-HDN is straightforward. However, when the DAT and an eluate are negative in an ABO-incompatible infant who is jaundiced, the clinician may be faced with a diagnostic problem. It is often quite difficult to distinguish between jaundice associated with ABO-HDN and that of "unexplained origin" or physiologic jaundice. Physiologic jaundice is quite common in neonates and is characterized by a slow increase in bilirubin levels, which disappear at about 1 week of age. It is nonimmunologic and may occur in normal, full-term and preterm infants.

CONSEQUENCES AND TREATMENT

ABO-HDN is typically much milder than Rh-HDN but represents the greatest cause of neonatal jaundice.[16] Typically, red cell destruction begins late in fetal life and anemia is not present at birth. The bilirubin level rises slowly, peaks at 1 to 3 days, and is followed by delayed anemia. The most serious consequences of HDN—stillbirth, hydrops fetalis, and kernicterus—are extremely rare in ABO-HDN.

Infants suffering from ABO-HDN are treated for anemia and hyperbilirubinemia when indicated, although few require treatment. Phototherapy is frequently used to control slowly rising bilirubin levels.

HDN caused by ABO incompatibility, in the past, has been overshadowed by the more severe disease caused by Rh incompatibility. As the incidence of Rh-HDN has declined, ABO-HDN has become the prevalent cause of hemolytic disease of the newborn.

PREVENTION WITH Rh IMMUNE GLOBULIN

PRINCIPLE

Rh immune globulin (RhIG) is concentrated and purified human anti-D gamma globulin. RhIG acts as an immunosuppressant and is given to *nonimmunized* Rh-negative mothers who have given birth to Rh-positive infants to suppress the development of anti-D. RhIG became widely available in 1968 and is 98- to 99-percent effective as a prophylactic treatment against Rh immunization.

Rh-negative mothers are treated with RhIG following pregnancy with an Rh-positive infant. The prophylactic mechanism is depicted in Color Plate 17. In untreated mothers fetal red cells are eventually removed from the maternal circulation, primarily in the spleen. The fetal red cells are immunogenic and sensitize the mother to produce anti-D. HDN can then occur in a subsequent Rh-positive fetus.

In mothers treated with RhIG, sensitization to the Rh antigen is prevented. RhIG is given within 72 hours of delivery while the fetal red cells are still in circulation. It attaches to the Rh antigen on the red cell and these antibody-coated red cells are systematically removed from the maternal circulation. The red cells are no longer immunogenic and do not sensitize the mother. The exact mechanism in which immunization is blocked is unknown. RhIG may be detectable in maternal serum for 2 to 3 months. Since maternal anti-D is not produced, a subsequent Rh-positive infant is unaffected with Rh-HDN. The mother must be treated in this manner following every exposure to Rh-positive red cells.

POSTPARTUM INDICATIONS

In Rh-negative mothers the standard method of treatment consists of an intramuscular injection of 300 μg of RhIG within 72 hours of delivering an Rh-positive infant. A 300-μg dose is accepted as sufficient for prophylactic treatment against 15 ml of fetal red cells (30 ml of whole blood). The following standard criteria are used for administering RhIG: (1) the mother must be Rh negative, D^u negative, (2) the mother must not be immunized to the D antigen, and (3) the infant must be Rh positive, or D^u positive, or assumed Rh positive in the case of abortion.

Rh-negative women who have developed antibodies other than anti-D should be considered RhIG candidates if all the above criteria are met. Women who give birth to Rh-negative infants or who already have produced anti-D should not be RhIG candidates. As previously mentioned, anti-D at delivery may occasionally be present from antenatal treatment with RhIG. Under such conditions RhIG should again be administered to ensure proper levels of passive antibody. Women whose red cells type as D^u positive should not receive RhIG; however, the D^u type should be firmly established and must be distinguished from a positive D^u test caused by large numbers of fetal cells in the mother's circulation (see below). RhIG has also been successfully administered to women with low levels of anti-D to prevent the development of a high-titer antibody.[22]

Prior to the administration of RhIG, a D^u test on a postpartum maternal specimen should be read microscopically to detect a large volume of feto-maternal bleeding. This is a simple screening procedure, which should detect feto-maternal bleeding greater than 35 ml.[5] When a D^u test is positive on a postpartum specimen, further investigation is necessary.

DETECTION OF FETO-MATERNAL BLEEDING

When a large volume of feto-maternal bleeding is suspected, the presence of fetal red cells in the maternal circulation should be demonstrated. Techniques for demonstrating these cells include the ELISA technique, mixed agglutination, rosette formation, fluorescent antibody techniques, and the acid-elution technique, which is the most commonly employed method. The Kleihauer-Betke technique of acid elution is based on the resistance of fetal hemoglobin to elution in an acid media. A maternal blood slide preparation is fixed in alcohol, treated with acid buffer, and stained. The fetal red cells appear intact on a field of maternal hemolyzed "ghost" cells. The fetal cells are counted and an estimate of their percentage is made. It is then decided, calculating 20 μg RhIG per 1.0 ml fetal red cells, how many vials of RhIG should be given to adequately protect the mother. Since the technique is not exact, the estimate of fetal red cells should be doubled when calculating the dosage of RhIG to be injected.

The termination of pregnancy at any time may cause feto-maternal bleeding. Thus, all unsensitized Rh-negative women who have spontaneous or induced abortions also should receive RhIG; lower doses of RhIG are recommended for this purpose. A 50-μg dose is recommended up to 12 weeks gestation and a 100-μg dose at 12 to 20 weeks.[17]

FAILURE OF TREATMENT

Treatment with RhIG is said to fail when a previously unsensitized Rh-negative mother produces anti-D following pregnancy in which treatment was received within 72 hours of the birth of an Rh-positive fetus. Postpartum prophylactic treatment with RhIG currently has an overall 1- to 2-percent failure rate. Failures are attributed to several factors. The dose of RhIG given may be insufficient for a large volume of feto-maternal bleeding. A pregnancy may terminate unknowingly, causing a woman to be untreated or the treatment to be delayed. The most probable cause, however, is feto-maternal bleeding that occurs during pregnancy. Shortly after termination of pregnancy, antibody appears in the serum of about 1 percent of RhIG-treated mothers. An additional 1 percent without detectable antibody has been stimulated, as evidenced by rapid antibody production following a subsequent exposure to antigen. This antigenic exposure usually occurs early in a second pregnancy.

ANTENATAL PROGRAM

Bowman and Pollock[18] have shown that the failure rate can be significantly reduced by treating Rh-negative women with 300 μg of RhIG at 28 weeks of pregnancy in addition to postpartum treatment. Low doses of RhIG have no apparent deleterious effects on an Rh-positive fetus.[19] Unfortunately, the antenatal program greatly increases the demand for RhIG. All Rh-negative RhIG candidates in an antenatal program receive the standard dose of RhIG twice so that less than 2 percent are prevented from becoming immunized. While this program reduces the incidence of immunization in the mother, additional factors should be considered. It appears that women who receive RhIG and become immunized have infants with milder Rh-HDN than infants from untreated immunized women.[21] Also the severity of HDN decreases as the average family size has been reduced in the last 2 decades. The incidence of infant morbidity and mortality reduction from mothers who would benefit from an antenatal program is under debate.

OTHER APPLICATIONS

The fact that RhIG may be given during pregnancy has important implications for treating women undergoing amniocentesis and other procedures known to cause risk of feto-maternal bleeding, and Rh-negative women undergoing such procedures should receive RhIG.

Frequently Rh-negative patients develop anti-D following the inadvertent administration of Rh-positive red cells and following the infusion of whole blood components such as platelet concentrates. RhIG may be given to any Rh-negative individual, but it is particularly important for the treatment of females of child-bearing age and under. In the United States the incidence of Rh-HDN has been reduced by almost 80 percent following the widespread use of RhIG.[23] A further reduction is anticipated in the near future.

Prophylactic treatment is not available to prevent the formation of other antibodies that occasionally cause HDN. Although the same mechanism most probably would apply, the incidence and severity of HDN caused by other antibodies do not appear to warrant such a program.

REFERENCES

1. LEVINE, P and STETSON, RE: *An unusual case of intra-group agglutination.* JAMA 113:126, 1939.
2. LEVINE, P: *Erythroblastosis fetalis and other manifestations of isoimmunization.* Symposium on Erythroblastosis Fetalis, Second American Congress on Obstetrics and Gynecology, St. Louis, 1942.
3. LANDSTEINER, K and WIENER, AS: *An agglutinable factor in human blood recognized by immune sera for Rhesus blood.* Proc Soc Exp Biol Med 43:223, 1940.
4. MURRAY, S, KNOX, E and WALKER, W: *Hemolytic disease and the rhesus genotypes.* Vox Sang 10:257, 1965.
5. MOLLISON, P: *Blood Transfusion in Clinical Medicine,* ed 6. Blackwell Scientific Publications, Oxford, 1979.
6. SABO, BH: *Evaluation of the neonatal direct antiglobulin test: Notes on low-frequency antigens in hemolytic disease of the newborn.* In BELL, CA (ED): *A Seminar on Perinatal Blood Banking.* American Association of Blood Banks, Washington, DC, 1978, pp 31–54.
7. PETZ, LD and GARRATTY, G: *Acquired Immune Hemolytic Anemias.* Churchill Livingstone, New York, 1980, pp 321–327.
8. LILEY, AW: *Liquor amnii analysis in management of pregnancy complicated by rhesus sensitization.* Am J Obstet Gynecol 82:1359, 1961.
9. MURPHY, RJC, MALHOTRA, C and SWEET, AY: *Death following an exchange transfusion with hemoglobin SC blood.* J Pediatr 96:110, 1980.
10. YEAGER, AS, et al.: *Prevention of transfusion-acquired cytomegalovirus infections in newborn infants.* J Pediatr 98:281, 1981.
11. KEVY, SV: *Pediatric transfusion therapy.* In DAWSON, RB (ed): *Transfusion Therapy.* American Association of Blood Banks, Washington, DC, 1974.
12. GRUNDBACKER, FJ: *The etiology of ABO hemolytic disease of the newborn.* Transfusion 20:5, 1980.
13. SCHELLONG, G (ed): Proceedings of the 10th Congress International Society of Blood Transfusion. Karger (Basel), Stockholm, 1964 (German with English abstract, 1965).
14. GOLD, ER and BUTLER, NR: *ABO Hemolytic Disease of the Newborn.* John Wright & Sons, Ltd., London, 1972, pp 46–62.
15. DESHARDINS, L, et al.: *The spectrum of ABO hemolytic disease of the newborn infant.* J Pediatr 95:447, 1979.
16. DUFOUR, DR and MONOGHAN, WP: *ABO hemolytic disease of the newborn. A retrospective analysis of 254 cases.* Am J Clin Pathol 73:369, 1980.
17. *McMaster Conference on Prevention of Rh Immunization.* Vox Sang 36:50, 1979.

18. BOWMAN, JM and POLLOCK, JM: *Antenatal prophylaxis of Rh immunization: 28 weeks gestation service program.* Can Med Assoc J 118:627, 1978.

19. BOWMAN, JM, et al.: *Rh iso-immunization during pregnancy: Antenatal prophylaxis.* Can Med Assoc J 118:623, 1978.

20. QUEENAN, JT: *Modern Management of the Rh Problem,* ed 2. Harper & Row, New York, 1977.

21. TOVEY, LAD and TAVERNER, JM: *A case for the antenatal administration of anti-D immunoglobulin to primigravidae.* Lancet i:878, 1981.

22. TOVEY, LAD and SCOTT, JF: *Suppression of early Rhesus sensitization by passive anti-D immunoglobulin.* Vox Sang 39:149, 1980.

23. POLLACK, W, GORMAN, JG and FREDA, VJ: *Rh immune suppression: Past, present, and future.* In FRIGOLETTA, FD, JEWETT, JF and KONUGERS, AA (EDS): *Rh Hemolytic Disease. New Strategy for Eradication.* GK Hall and Co, Boston, 1982, p 9–70.

CHAPTER 19

RED BLOOD CELL AUTOANTIBODIES

SUSAN STEANE, M.S., MT(ASCP)SBB

In the preceding chapters red cell *alloantibodies* have been described. The individual who made the antibody, either as a response to RBC sensitization (e.g., anti-D and anti-Fy^a) or as a result of non-RBC sensitization (e.g., anti-A, anti-B, and anti-P$_1$), lacked the antigen. Therefore, the serum did not react with the cells of the antibody-maker; the autologous control was negative. This chapter will address those antibodies that are directed against the individual's own red cells, *autoantibodies*. Most autoantibodies react with high-incidence antigens; they will agglutinate, lyse, or sensitize RBCs of most random donors in addition to autologous cells.

It is currently believed that production of antibodies against "self" occurs because there is a failure of the mechanism regulating immune response. Briefly, under normal circumstances immunoglobulins are made by B lymphocytes. Other lymphocytes, T cells, modulate the activity of antibody-producing cells. Helper T cells, one population of T lymphocytes, help immunocompetent B cells make antibody against some foreign antigens. Another population of T lymphocytes, suppressor T cells, has the opposite effect on B cell activity; they prevent excessive proliferation of B cells and overproduction of antibodies. Suppressor T cells are thought to act through a feedback mechanism. An increasing concentration of antibody activates these T cells and suppresses further antibody production.[1]

Autoantibody production may be prevented through a similar mechanism. Suppressor T cells induce tolerance to "self" antigens by inhibiting B-cell activity. Conversely, loss of suppressor T-cell function could result in autoantibody production. Support for this concept comes from studies in animal models[2] and in patients taking alphamethyldopa.[3] The cause of dysfunction of the regulatory system is not understood, but microbial agents and drugs have been suggested.[4] The reader is referred to Chapter 3 for more discussion of the immune response.

Autoantibodies are important for two reasons. First, they can cause red cell destruction. Second, when an individual's cells are coated with antibody and his serum contains antibody reactive with most random donor cells, it may be difficult to interpret routine cell grouping, antibody detection and identification, and compatibility tests correctly. The effect of autoantibodies on routine tests and techniques to resolve the problems are discussed below. It is important to realize that serologic and clinical problems can be found separately or together.

The presence of autoantibodies in a patient's serum or on his cells may be indicative of autoimmune hemolytic anemia (AIHA), but additional information is needed before one draws this conclusion. One must establish that RBCs are being destroyed and that the destruction is immune-mediated. Individuals who are experiencing immune red cell destruction may or may not be anemic (decreased hemoglobin and hematocrit) depending upon whether red cell production has increased to compensate for the loss, but they will have increased reticulocyte counts and unconjugated bilirubin levels and decreased haptoglobin levels. If red cell destruction is predominantly intravascular, hemoglobinemia and hemoglobinuria may occur. There are other causes of hemolysis (e.g., hereditary spherocytosis and hemoglobinopathies); therefore, AIHA must be confirmed by additional serologic tests. Diagnostic tests include (1) the direct antiglobulin test (DAT) using polyspecific and monospecific reagents, and (2) characterization of autoantibody in the serum and eluate. Based on these results and the clinical evaluation of the patient, AIHA can be diagnosed and classified as cold reactive or warm reactive. The expected laboratory findings for each type are discussed below. Petz and Garratty[5] devote a chapter in their book, *Acquired Immune Hemolytic Anemias,* to the diagnosis of the hemolytic anemias. The reader is referred to this text for a complete discussion.

There are individuals who have autoantibodies in their sera and on their red cells but who display no evidence of decreased RBC survival. For example, as many as 8 percent of hospitalized patients have a positive DAT.[6,7] Most have only complement on their cells but some have IgG. The differences between individuals who are affected (i.e., have AIHA) and those who are unaffected by autoantibodies are not clearly understood. Among the possibly significant factors are

1. Thermal amplitude of antibody reactivity[8]
2. IgG subclass of the antibody[9]
3. Amount of antibody bound to red cells[10]

4. Ability of the antibody to fix complement in vivo[10]
5. Activity of the individual's macrophages[5]

The opposite situation also occurs; there are patients with immune hemolytic anemia in whom autoantibodies cannot be demonstrated by routine techniques. Some patients have more IgG on their RBCs than is normal but less than the amount detected by the antiglobulin technique.[11] In other cases the patient's cells are sensitized with IgA molecules.[12,13] Since polyspecific antiglobulin reagents must contain only anti-IgG and anti-C3d,[14] anti-IgA is not consistently present and IgA-sensitized cells may not give a positive test. Finally, prior to the current requirements for polyspecific antiglobulin reagents, many commercial reagents did not agglutinate cells coated with complement components.[15] Therefore, a negative DAT was not an unusual finding in patients with cold agglutinin hemolytic anemia. The reader is cautioned to note the date of a publication in which AIHA associated with a negative DAT is reported.

As stated earlier, autoantibodies can be divided into two main groups, those that react best in the cold (4°C) and those that react best at a warmer temperature (37°C). Characterization of autoantibodies is important because treatment of the patient and resolution of the serologic difficulties differ according to the optimal temperature of reactivity. The clinical and laboratory aspects of cold reactive and warm reactive autoantibodies are discussed separately.

COLD REACTIVE AUTOANTIBODIES

BENIGN COLD AUTOAGGLUTININS

The most commonly encountered autoantibody is a benign cold agglutinin that is demonstrable in the serum of most individuals when testing is done at 4°C. It is usually not noticed because routine tests are never done at this temperature. The typical cold autoagglutinin has a relatively low titer; at 4°C it is less than 64. Occasionally, the antibody has increased thermal amplitude and will agglutinate cells at room temperature (20 to 24°C). However, even in this situation one obtains the strongest reactions at 4°C. Most cold agglutinins react best with enzyme-treated cells; therefore, one is more likely to detect them if, for example, ficin-treated cells are tested at room temperature. Cold autoantibodies are of the IgM class and can activate complement in vitro; therefore reactions may be seen in the antiglobulin phase. The reactions shown in Table 19-1 can be seen when these agglutinins are present.

LABORATORY TESTS AFFECTED BY COLD AUTOAGGLUTININS

Because cold autoagglutinins have the serologic characteristics described above, they sometimes interfere with routine cell and serum tests. The degree to which they cause problems depends on how strongly the antibody reacts at room temperature, that is, the concentration and thermal amplitude of the antibody. Although the au-

TABLE 19-1. Serologic Reactions of a Typical Cold Autoagglutinin

	Screening Cells		Autologous Cells
	I	II	
4°C	4+	4+	4+
RT*	+	+	+
37°C	0	0	0
AGT†	+w	+w	+w

*RT = Room temperature reactions, 20–24°C.
†AGT = Antiglobulin test using polyspecific reagent.

toantibody found in the serum of most people does not routinely interfere with testing, it is one of the more common causes of problems. Therefore, one should be familiar with the recognition and methods of resolution of problems associated with these antibodies.

ABO GROUPING

If an individual's RBCs are heavily coated with cold autoagglutinins, they may spontaneously agglutinate. Consequently one can obtain false-positive reactions with anti-A and anti-B reagents. In most cases valid testing can be done using cells washed once or twice with normal saline. The autoantibody elutes during washing. For example, group O cells coated with a cold agglutinin might give the following reactions before and after washing:

	Anti-A	Anti-B
Serum suspended RBCs	+	+
Saline washed, suspended RBCs	0	0

If more potent agglutinins are present, one may have to incubate the cells in saline at 37°C and use warm (37°C) saline for washing.[16] In the very rare situation in which 37°C saline washing is not effective, thiol reagents (e.g., dithiothreitol) can be used to disperse the autoagglutination.[17] (See Procedures A and B in Appendix of this chapter.)

Since ABO serum grouping is done at room temperature, cold autoagglutinins reactive at this temperature can cause discrepancies between cell and serum results. In the following example, the results indicate that the cells are group AB. Therefore, one does not expect the serum to agglutinate A_1 and B cells. Although a number of explanations are possible, an interfering cold autoagglutinin is a likely cause; when autologous cells are agglutinated, as shown, it is the probable cause.

	Anti-A	Anti-B	
RBCs	4+	4+	

	A₁ cells	B cells	Autologous cells
Serum	+	+	+

Such a discrepancy is easily resolved if the cold reactive autoantibody is removed by an autoabsorption technique and the tests with A$_1$ and B cells are repeated with autoabsorbed serum.

	A₁ cells	B cells	Autologous cells
Autoabsorbed serum	0	0	

Rh GROUPING

As with ABO cell grouping, one can find false-positive reactions when one tests RBCs coated with cold autoagglutinins with anti-D reagents. In this case one is alerted to a false-positive reaction when the cells agglutinate in the Rh control diluent. Usually, valid Rh grouping can be performed on washed cells. As mentioned above, thiol reagents can be used when elution with warm saline washes does not resolve the problem.

Since cold autoagglutinins can activate the complement cascade, components of complement may be attached to RBCs. Therefore one can find false-positive reactions in the D^u test when polyspecific antiglobulin reagents are used. The control will also be positive. As shown in the following example, one can use monospecific anti-IgG reagents for D^u testing. The problem of in-vitro complement activation can also be avoided if the RBCs are collected into EDTA or some other suitable anticoagulant.

	Anti-D	Rh control	
Immediate spin	0	0	
Antiglobulin phase (polyspecific reagent)	+	+	Detects complement components
Antiglobulin phase (anti-IgG reagent)	0	0	Does not detect complement
Red cells collected in EDTA	0	0	Complement not bound

Similar problems can be encountered in other cell phenotyping tests (e.g., K, Fy^a) if the antiglobulin test is used.

DIRECT ANTIGLOBULIN TEST

When a properly collected specimen is used, the DAT on cells from patients with benign cold autoagglutinins is negative. However, one frequently obtains a positive result if a clotted specimen is used because complement can be activated in vitro. If monospecific reagents are used, these cells are agglutinated by anti-C3 but not by anti-IgG. As discussed in the preceding section, one can obtain false-positive antigen typings when clotted specimens and polyspecific reagents are used. Sometimes cold autoagglutinins are sufficiently potent to cause autoagglutination at room temperature and a false-positive DAT, even though the RBCs have been washed several times. In this situation one can use cells washed with 37°C saline or treated with a thiol reagent.

ANTIBODY DETECTION AND IDENTIFICATION

The frequency with which cold autoagglutinins interfere with detection and identification of red cell alloantibodies depends to a large extent on the routine procedures one uses for these tests. As shown in Table 19-1, cold agglutinins react best at 4°C, but they are not detected because testing is never done at this phase. Room-temperature reactive autoantibodies may not be found because many laboratories no longer use this technique. Antibodies reactive only at this phase are clinically insignificant.[18] Benign cold autoantibodies do not react at 37°C; therefore, the antiglobulin test is the phase in which cold agglutinins are most likely to interfere. They bind to the cells at lower temperatures when the serum and cells are mixed or during centrifugation following 37°C incubation and activate complement. The antibody elutes during the 37°C incubation or the washing phase, but complement remains attached. If the antiglobulin serum contains anti-C3 activity, the cells will be agglutinated. When enzyme-treated cells are used, reactions in all phases may be stronger.

Many antibodies capable of causing accelerated cell destruction are detected by the antiglobulin test; therefore, reactions observed in this phase may be clinically significant and should be investigated. The reactions may be caused by a cold reactive autoantibody alone, or AGT reactive alloantibodies may be present in addition to, but masked by, an autoantibody.

To detect significant alloantibodies in a serum but not cold reactive autoantibodies, most technologists use a prewarmed technique or perform tests with autoabsorbed serum.[16] By prewarming the serum and cells prior to mixing, avoiding room temperature centrifugation after 37°C incubation, and washing the cells with 37°C saline, one can prevent the reaction between autoantibody and antigen and prevent complement activation. Alloantibodies reactive at 37°C, however, can bind to the cells and activate complement. (See Procedure C in Appendix of this chapter.) An example of the results of testing a serum that contains a cold autoagglutinin and a weakly reactive anti-Fy[a] by a standard technique and by the prewarmed technique is shown in Table 19-2. This is the simplest technique and is successful in most cases, but if very potent autoagglutinins are present, it may be difficult to keep the serum and cells at a high enough temperature through every phase of testing to avoid antigen-antibody interaction and complement activation.

TABLE 19-2. Reactions Observed with a Serum Containing Anti-Fy^a and a Cold Autoagglutinin

Reagent RBCs	Standard AGT Technique	Prewarmed AGT Technique
Fy(a+)	+	+
Fy(a−)	+w	0
Fy(a+)	+	+
Fy(a−)	+	0
Fy(a−)	+w	0
Fy(a−)	+w	0
Fy(a+)	+	+
Fy(a+)	+	+

When potent autoantibodies are present or if one wishes to identify a room temperature reactive antibody, autoabsorbed serum should be used. One incubates an aliquot of the patient's cells with an equal volume of the patient's serum at 4°C. Autoantibody is removed; alloantibody remains in the serum. It may be necessary to repeat the absorption several times if the autoantibody is particularly strong. Since enzymes enhance the reactivity of most cold agglutinins, most technologists enzyme-treat the patient's cells prior to absorption. (See Procedure D in Appendix of this chapter.) When a patient has been recently transfused, one must interpret results obtained with autoabsorbed serum with caution. Circulating donor RBCs may absorb additional alloantibody. Most technologists prefer to use the prewarmed technique in this situation. In some cases, however, it may be impossible to interpret test results unless some autoantibody has been removed.

If monospecific anti-IgG reagents are used for the antiglobulin test, one can avoid the problem caused by most cold autoagglutinins. However, one can miss very rare clinically significant alloantibodies that are detected only because they bind complement. (See Chapter 12 for a discussion of the importance of anti-C3 activity for detecting alloantibodies.) Use of anti-IgG reagents is an attractive alternative when prewarming is not effective and there is not enough time to absorb the serum.

COMPATIBILITY TESTING

The difficulties encountered in antibody detection and identification tests are also found in compatibility tests because the most commonly encountered antibody (auto-anti-I) is directed against an antigen that is found on the RBCs of most random donors as well as on most reagent red cells. Compatibility tests, like antibody detection and identification tests, can be done with prewarmed or autoabsorbed serum or anti-IgG reagents.

Two of the other common cold agglutinins, anti-IH and anti-H, distinguish between reagent red cells and random donor cells. As discussed in the following section on specificity, anti-IH and anti-H show a distinct preference for group O cells; they react least well with group A$_1$ and A$_1$B cells. Anti-IH and anti-H are most often found in the serum of group A_1 and A_1B persons; therefore, the units of blood most likely selected for compatibility testing are those that will give the weakest, if any reactivity. On the other hand, group O reagent RBCs give the best reactions.

SPECIFICITY OF COLD AUTOAGGLUTININS

ANTI-I, ANTI-i

Most cold reactive autoantibodies have anti-I specificity. The I antigen is fully expressed on the RBCs of essentially all adults, whereas it is only weakly expressed on cord RBCs. As infants mature, the amount of I antigen on their cells increases until adult levels are reached at about 18 months. Very rare adults lack I antigen; they are called i adults.

The reactivities of several examples of anti-I are given in Table 19-3. As shown, I specificity may be apparent when a serum is simply tested with adult and cord RBCs. Serum 1, for example, reacts with adult and not with cord cells. Serum 2 reacts with both adult and cord RBCs, but the preference for adult cells is still obvious. In many cases, one may have to test dilutions of a serum to determine specificity. Serum 3 is an example of such an anti-I. Allo-anti-I is frequently present in the serum of i adults.

Anti-i is a relatively uncommon autoantibody. As shown in Table 19-4, this antibody reacts in an antithetical manner to anti-I. Cord cells and i adult cells have the most i antigen; random adult cells, the least.

TABLE 19-3. Reactions of Serums Containing Anti-I with Adult and Cord Cells

	Serum Dilution	RBCs	
		Adult	Cord
Serum 1	neat	3+	0
Serum 2	neat	4+	2+
	1:2	4+	+
	1:4	3+	0
	1:8	2+	0
Serum 3	neat	4+	3+
	1:2	4+	2+
	1:4	4+	+
	1:8	3+	0
	1:16	2+	0
	1:32	+^{s}	0
	1:64	+	0

TABLE 19-4. Serologic Reactions of Cold Autoantibodies*

RBC Phenotype	Anti-I	Anti-i	Anti-H	Anti-IH
O I_{adult}	4+[†]	+	4+	4+
$A_1 I_{adult}$	4+	+	+	+
$A_2 I_{adult}$	4+	+	2+	2+
O i_{cord}	2+	3+	4+	+
O i_{adult}	+	4+	4+	0
$A_1 i_{adult}$	+	4+	+	0
$A_2 i_{adult}$	+	4+	2+	0
$O_h I_{adult}$	4+	+	0	0

*Serums are ABO-compatible with RBCs.
[†]Relative strengths of reactivity are given.

ANTI-H, ANTI-IH

Cold agglutinins found in the serum of group A_1 and A_1B individuals (and sometimes group B) may have anti-H specificity. This antibody distinguishes between cells of various ABO groups. Group O cells and group A_2 cells react best because they have the most H substance. Group A_1 and A_1B cells have the least H antigen, so they react weakly. The pattern of reactivity one sees with anti-H is also shown in Table 19-4. See Chapter 5 for a discussion of H substance.

It is very important not to confuse cold reactive anti-H with the anti-H found in the serum of O_h individuals who are H negative. Cold reactive anti-H is an autoantibody even though the cells of the antibody-maker (A_1 or A_1B) may give considerably weaker reactions. Bombay (O_h) anti-H is a potent alloantibody, reacts at 37°C and at lower temperatures, and is capable of causing rapid cell destruction.

Anti-IH, another of the usually harmless cold autoagglutinins, is also found in the serum of group A_1 and A_1B persons. This antibody agglutinates only those RBCs that have both I and H antigens. As with anti-H, group O and A_2 cells react best. The difference between these two antibodies is that group O i_{cord} cells and group O i_{adult} cells react as strongly as group O I_{adult} cells with anti-H, but not with anti-IH (see Table 19-4).

OTHER COLD REACTIVE AUTOANTIBODIES

A number of other less commonly encountered cold agglutinins have been described (e.g., anti-Pr, anti-Gd, anti-Sd^x). The reader is referred to the review by Marsh[19] for additional information. Most workers agree that specificity of cold reactive autoantibodies is primarily of academic interest and not clinically important.

PATHOLOGIC COLD AUTOAGGLUTININS

COLD AGGLUTININ DISEASE

In most cases cold autoagglutinins do not cause RBC destruction, but in some patients they can cause hemolytic anemia that varies in severity from mild to life-threatening intravascular lysis. Cold reactive immune hemolytic anemia may be a chronic, idiopathic condition or an acute, transient disease that is usually associated with *Mycoplasma pneumoniae* pneumonia (occasionally with infectious mononucleosis). Cell destruction occurs when antibody binds to RBCs, usually in the peripheral circulation where the temperature is lower, and complement is activated. Hemolysis increases if the patient is exposed to the cold. Patients with the chronic form of the disease are advised to avoid cold weather. They frequently require no other treatment.[5]

LABORATORY FINDINGS

Since complement is activated, patients may have hemoglobinemia and hemoglobinuria. Most have bilirubinemia relative to the degree of cell destruction. The reticulocyte count is also increased. The most striking finding is that autoagglutination occurs as blood samples cool to room temperature. Autoagglutination may make it difficult to determine the patient's hemoglobin and hematocrit on a Coulter counter or to prepare a satisfactory peripheral blood smear.

Since individuals can have potent cold autoagglutinins that are benign, one must characterize the antibody before concluding that an anemic patient has cold agglutinin disease. The following tests are useful in differentiating harmless and harmful antibodies: (1) DAT using polyspecific and monospecific reagents; (2) determination of thermal amplitude of antibody using saline-suspended and albumin-suspended RBCs; and (3) titration of serum.

Table 19-5 summarizes results one usually obtains when samples from patients with pathologic and benign cold agglutinins are tested. Specific instructions for sample collection and test procedures are described by Petz and Garratty.[5] These authors find that one can make a diagnosis of cold reactive immune hemolytic anemia if the patient's cells are coated with C3d but not with IgG, if the antibody reacts at 30°C with albumin-suspended cells, and if the patient's clinical condition is consistent with the diagnosis. The titer gives valuable information but is not definitive. It is interesting to determine specificity, but it is not clinically important. Both pathologic and benign antibodies usually have anti-I specificity.

SELECTION OF BLOOD FOR TRANSFUSION

Most patients with cold agglutinin disease do not require transfusion, but when they do it is sometimes very difficult to select blood. As previously described, potent cold agglutinins interfere with most routine tests. Perhaps the most difficult problem is to detect and identify alloantibodies. Procedures to manage these problems have been

TABLE 19-5. Serologic Results Observed with Benign and Pathologic Cold Autoagglutinins

	Benign		Pathologic	
Direct antiglobulin test				
Polyspecific	0		+	
Anti-IgG	NT		0	
Anti-C3d	NT		+	
Titer				
4°C	<64		>1000	
Thermal amplitude	Saline Suspended RBCs	Albumin Suspended RBCs	Saline Suspended RBCs	Albumin Suspended RBCs
4°C	+	+	+[s]	+[s]
20°C	0–+	0–+	+[s]	+[s]
30°C	0	0	0–+	+
37°C	0	0	0–+	0–+

described earlier in this chapter. It is important that one gives blood compatible with clinically significant alloantibodies. Most patients are transfused with blood positive for the autoantibody. Units of i_{adult} RBCs are extremely rare and should be reserved for patients with allo-anti-I.

PAROXYSMAL COLD HEMOGLOBINURIA

Paroxysmal cold hemoglobinuria (PCH) is the rarest form of autoimmune hemolytic anemia (AIHA). The mechanism of cell destruction is similar to that in cold agglutinin disease, but there are notable differences. Both antibodies bind at lower temperatures, then activate complement as the temperature increases. However, the PCH antibody is IgG rather than IgM. It can agglutinate cells at 4°C, but the titer is usually low (<64). Unlike most pathologic cold reactive autoantibodies, the PCH antibody does not interfere with most routine cell and serum tests. In PCH the DAT is weakly positive, and the cells are coated only with complement components even though the antibody is IgG. The IgG antibody elutes at warmer temperatures and during washing. The antibody usually has anti-P specificity. (See Chapter 8 for a description of the P blood group antigens.)

The unique characteristic of the PCH autoantibody is that it is a *biphasic* antibody. It binds to RBCs during a 4°C incubation, and when the mixture is moved to 37°C, it lyses the cells. This is the basis for the Donath-Landsteiner test, the diagnostic test for PCH[16] (see Procedure E in Appendix of this chapter).

Paroxysmal nocturnal hemoglobinuria (PNH) is often confused with PCH because of the similarity of the names and acronyms. Red cell destruction in PNH is complement-mediated, but the mechanism is not clearly understood. An autoantibody has not been implicated; a membrane defect is thought to be involved. The only reason for including these comments is to alert the reader to a common error.

WARM REACTIVE AUTOANTIBODIES

Autoantibodies that react best at 37°C are not found as often as the almost ubiquitous cold auto-anti-I. However, many more of the autoimmune hemolytic anemias are of the warm reactive type (70 percent) than the cold reactive type (16 percent).[5] Warm reactive AIHA may be idiopathic (i.e., not associated with another disease), secondary to another disease such as systemic lupus erythematosus (SLE), or drug-induced (see Chapter 20). As with the cold reactive autoantibodies, there are individuals who have apparently harmless warm reactive autoantibodies (some of the possible explanations for why some of these antibodies cause cell destruction and others do not are given on pages 424 to 425). The harmless autoantibodies are serologically indistinguishable from the harmful ones. There are no diagnostic tests that can be performed. When a warm reactive autoantibody is encountered, it should be characterized as such and reported to the patient's physician. The antibody may alert the physician to an underlying autoimmune disease.

SEROLOGIC CHARACTERISTICS

Warm reactive autoantibodies are typically IgG immunoglobulins that react best by the antiglobulin technique. As a rule, they do not agglutinate saline suspended RBCs after 37°C incubation. However, if one adds albumin or another agglutination potentiator to the reaction mixture, one may observe agglutination in this phase. They may activate complement, and they are usually enhanced by enzyme techniques. Most of these autoantibodies react with a high-incidence antigen and have specificity within the Rh blood group system, but there are reports of antibodies associated with most of the other blood group systems. Identification of autoantibodies is discussed in the following section. The reactions in Table 19-6 are typical.

TABLE 19-6. Serologic Reactions of Typical Warm Reactive Autoantibodies

	Screening Cells		Autologous Cells
	I	II	
RT	0	0	0
37°C*	0	0	0
AGT	2+	2+	4+

*Agglutination is frequently observed if the RBCs are suspended in albumin or LISS or if they are enzyme-treated.

LABORATORY TESTS AFFECTED BY WARM REACTIVE AUTOANTIBODIES

Warm reactive autoantibodies can interfere with most routine blood bank tests and they may be more of a problem than cold autoagglutinins. Many cold autoagglutinin problems can be avoided if one simply performs the tests at 37°C. In this case, both significant alloantibodies and autoantibody react best at 37°C. Therefore one may have to use more complicated procedures to resolve any problems.

ABO GROUPING

Since warm reactive autoantibodies are not direct agglutinins, ABO grouping is usually not affected. Even though the patient's cells may be heavily coated with antibody, they do not spontaneously agglutinate when reagent anti-A and anti-B sera are added. Similarly, warm autoantibodies in the serum do not agglutinate saline suspended A_1 and B cells.

Rh GROUPING

False-positive Rh grouping tests can be a problem when the patient's cells are coated with 37°C reactive autoantibodies. Agglutination potentiators are added to the most commonly used Rh grouping reagents (slide and modified tube) so that D-positive cells, once coated with anti-D, will agglutinate. Potentiators are beneficial because they allow one to perform an immediate spin Rh grouping test. The disadvantage of adding potentiators is that cells coated with any antibody may be agglutinated, including D-negative cells coated with autoantibody. For this reason a control test, consisting of cells and Rh diluent, must be performed in parallel with the Rh test. The results of Rh grouping tests are valid only when the control is negative.

Similar problems occasionally occur when cells are coated with cold reactive autoantibodies, but the problem is usually easily resolved by washing the cells several times with saline. Warm reactive autoantibodies do not elute during saline washing, so another approach must be taken. Most of the time saline reactive anti-D sera (IgM and IgG chemically modified) will give valid tests. (See Chapter 6 on Rh blood groups.) In an extreme situation, autoantibody can be eluted from the cells with chloroquine prior to testing.[20]

If one wishes to test for the weak expression of the D antigen, D^u, one must use chloroquine-eluted RBCs, because prior to elution the cells are coated with IgG. Monospecific antiglobulin sera are no help in this situation. An absorption technique is an alternative method. This test is based on the fact that antigen-positive cells will remove antibody from a serum even though they are coated with antibody of another specificity; antigen-negative cells will not.[21] It is not necessary to go to such great lengths to determine if such a patient is D^u positive. One would select D-negative blood for transfusion. However, the same methods (chloroquine elution and absorption) may be valuable to determine if the patient is antigen-positive or antigen-negative if one suspects that the patient has an antibody in his serum. For example, one may wish to determine if a patient is Fy(a+) or Fy(a−) if anti-Fy^a is in his serum.

DIRECT ANTIGLOBULIN TEST

A positive DAT is characteristically associated with warm reactive autoantibodies. The RBCs may be coated with IgG, IgG and complement, or complement.[5] In rare cases of warm-reactive AIHA, the DAT may be negative[11] or only IgA[12] may be present.

ANTIBODY DETECTION AND IDENTIFICATION

The serum of a patient with warm reactive antibodies may contain only autoantibody or it may contain a mixture of autoantibodies and alloantibodies. In some cases all the autoantibody has been absorbed by the patient's cells in vivo and is not demonstrable in the serum.

When warm reactive autoantibodies are present in the serum or on the patient's cells one should (1) establish that the antibody on the patient's cells is an *auto*antibody, (2) do limited testing to determine the specificity of the autoantibody, and (3) detect and identify any clinically significant alloantibody.

EVALUATION OF AUTOANTIBODY

Positive DATs caused by RBC alloantibodies or by drug-induced antibodies can occasionally be confused with those caused by warm reactive autoantibodies because in some cases they have serologic features in common, for example, IgG on the RBCs and antibody not demonstrable in the serum. It is important that one distinguish between the possibilities because one selects blood and treats the patient accordingly. To make the distinction one must first have the patient's medical history, including transfusion history, diagnosis, and medications. When a patient has been recently transfused, one must consider that alloantibodies are coating the RBCs. In most cases, by examining the DAT microscopically for mixed field agglutination and by determining specificity of the antibody in the eluate, one can establish alloantibodies as the cause (see Chapter 16 for a discussion of delayed transfusion reactions). Since warm reactive autoantibodies are frequently associated with certain diseases, such as SLE, and with medications, such as Aldomet, the patient's diagnosis and drug history are informative. As discussed below, the specificity of the antibody may be helpful in differentiating between autoantibody and alloantibody.

To identify the specificity of a warm reactive autoantibody, one must test an eluate prepared from the patient's RBCs and the serum against a panel of reagent red cells. (See Procedure F in Appendix of this chapter for instructions for preparing an ether eluate.) If the patient has not been transfused, one can assume that any antibody activity in the eluate is autoantibody. Serum may contain alloantibody in addition to autoantibody.

The reactions of an autoantibody may be different in the serum and eluate. Such an example is shown in Table 19-7. When the serum is tested, an antibody of limited or simple specificity can be identified, anti-e. The ether eluate, however, reacts with all cells; it has broader or complex specificity. Some workers suggest that these results indicate that there are two autoantibodies present. Others suggest that there is a single antibody present that reacts with all cells but shows a preference for e-positive cells.[22] When the antibody is present in lower concentration, as in the serum, the preference can be seen. When the relatively ineffective heat elution technique is used, anti-e-like specificity may be demonstrable in the eluate (see Table 19-7). The difference between ether and heat elution results may also reflect a difference in antibody concentration in the eluate.

Many warm reactive autoantibodies have Rh-like specificity similar to those shown in Table 19-8. Occasionally they have simple specificity such as anti-e, but more often they have complex specificity; they react with all RBCs of normal Rh phenotype (e.g., cde/cde, CDe/cDE). To categorize them as anti-nl, anti-pdl, or anti-dl one must use very rare RBCs, for example, partially deleted ($-D-/-D-$) and fully deleted (Rh_{null}).[23]

There are numerous reports of autoantibodies with specificity other than Rh. Among the other specificities are auto-anti-U, -Wr[b], -En[a], and -Kp[b]. The reader is referred to Chapter 7 of Petz and Garratty[5] for a detailed discussion of autoantibody specificity.

Most workers agree that it is not necessary to do extensive studies to identify autoantibodies, but they do recommend limited testing. By testing a commercial red cell panel one can identify an antibody of simple specificity. Specificity is useful in evaluating whether the antibody is autoantibody or alloantibody. For example, if anti-Fy[a] is found in the eluate, it is probably an alloantibody, since auto-anti-Fy[a] has not been described. On the other hand an antibody reactive with all cells is probably an autoantibody. However, there are numerous exceptions to these interpretations. The need to consider the medical history in making the interpretation cannot be

TABLE 19-7. Serologic Reactions of Serum and Eluates Containing Warm Reactive Autoantibodies

RBC Phenotype	AGT Reactions		
	Serum	Ether Eluate	Heat Eluate
e positive	+	4+	3+
e positive	+	4+	3+
e positive	+	4+	3+
e negative	0	4+	+
e negative	0	4+	+
e positive	+	4+	3+
e positive	+	4+	3+
e positive	+	4+	3+

TABLE 19-8. Serologic Reactivity of Warm Reactive Autoantibodies with RBCs of Selected Rh Phenotypes[23]

	RBC Phenotype		
	Normal	Partially Deleted	Fully Deleted
	cde/cde, etc.	-D-/-D-, etc.	Rh_{null}
anti-nl	+	0	0
anti-pdl	+	+	0
anti-dl	+	+	+

over-emphasized. Specificity is also helpful in selecting blood for transfusion. Some workers prefer to transfuse RBCs that are compatible with autoantibody when, for example, the specificity is e-like.

DETECTION AND IDENTIFICATION OF ALLOANTIBODIES

All workers agree that detection and identification of alloantibodies are of primary concern when one must transfuse a patient with warm reactive autoantibodies. When autoantibody is cell-bound and not free in the serum, one can use standard methods. However, when autoantibody is free in the serum, it will probably mask any alloantibodies present. In this situation one can use several techniques:

1. Test cells that are compatible with the autoantibody
2. Absorption of autoantibody with autologous cells
3. Absorption of autoantibody with cells from selected donors
4. Dilution of the patient's serum

When the autoantibody has simple specificity, one can test a panel of negative cells that are positive for selected antigens. For example, when auto-anti-e is present, the best way to detect other antibodies is to test e-negative cells that are positive for K, Fy^a, Jk^a, and so on.

When autoantibodies have broader specificity, one must use an absorption technique, preferably autoabsorption. In this procedure one removes autoantibody by incubating serum and autologous cells at 37°C and leaves alloantibody in the serum. To improve antibody-uptake one can elute some of the antibody bound in vivo and then treat the RBCs with a proteolytic enzyme. If there is a high concentration of autoantibody in the serum, one may have to use several aliquots of cells (see Procedure G in Appendix of this chapter). Table 19-9 gives an example of antibody detection tests using unabsorbed, once-absorbed, and twice-absorbed serum. In this example one absorption did not remove all the autoantibody, but two absorptions were effective. No alloantibodies are present.

TABLE 19-9. Antibody Detection Tests Using Unabsorbed and Auto-absorbed Serum

Reagent Red Cells	Unabsorbed 37°C	AGT	Once-Absorbed 37°C	AGT	Twice-Absorbed 37°C	AGT
I	+	3+	0	$+^s$	0	0
II	+	3+	0	$+^s$	0	0

There are several problems with autoabsorptions. First, if the patient has been transfused, donor RBCs might remove more alloantibody during the procedure. Alloantibody absorption by donor RBCs does occur in vivo, but even more antibody might be removed when the cells are eluted and enzyme-treated. Therefore, one must interpret the results with "autoabsorbed" serum carefully. Second, if the patient is severely anemic, there may not be enough autologous cells to remove all the autoantibody. Third, whenever an absorption is done, with autologous cells or with cells of selected phenotypes, the serum is diluted to some degree. Some saline is present in "packed" RBCs. A very weakly reactive alloantibody might be missed if multiple absorptions are done.

When the patient has been recently transfused or is severely anemic, one can use cells of selected phenotypes. They should lack antigens for the more commonly encountered alloantibodies that are clinically significant (e.g., anti-K, anti-E, anti-Fy^a). As shown in Table 19-10, if one absorbs the patient's serum with cells from donors A, B, and C and then tests the absorbed sera, one can detect many important alloantibodies. It is not possible to detect all alloantibodies by this technique. For example, anti-k, an alloantibody to a high-incidence antigen, will be removed by cells from donors A, B, and C. For this reason autoabsorption is always preferable, but when indicated this procedure is invaluable.

The fourth procedure suggested, testing dilutions of the serum, will detect alloantibodies if they are present in higher concentration that the autoantibody. In the example shown in Table 19-11, all cells react with undiluted serum, but at a 1:10 dilution only the K+ cells react. These results suggest that the autoantibody is present in lower concentration than anti-K. In a critical situation this procedure may be helpful because it is not as time-consuming as absorption techniques. However, it is not always as reliable.

SELECTION OF BLOOD

Many patients with warm reactive AIHA never require transfusion; they can be managed by steroid therapy and splenectomy. Occasionally, however, the anemia is so severe that transfusion can not be avoided.[5] Other patients who pose similar laboratory problems are those with nonhemolytic warm reactive autoantibodies who require blood for a surgical procedure. In these cases compatibility of the donor's

TABLE 19-10. Differential Absorption Technique for Detecting Allo-antibodies in the Serum of a Patient with Warm Reactive Autoantibodies

Donor	RBC Phenotype	Antibody Remaining in Absorbed Serum
A	R_1R_1, Ss, Fy(a−b+), Jk(a+b−), kk	c, E, Fy^a, Jk^b, K
B	R_2R_2, ss, Fy(a+b+), Jk(a−b+), kk	C, e, S, Jk^a, K
C	rr, SS, Fy(a+b−), Jk(a+b+), kk	C, D, E, s, Fy^b, K

TABLE 19-11. Dilution Technique for Identifying Allo-anti-K in the Presence of Warm Reactive Autoantibody

RBC Phenotype	Undiluted Serum AGT	1:10 Dilution of Serum AGT
K+	2+	+
K−	2+	0
K−	2+	0
K−	2+	0
K−	2+	0
K+	2+	+

RBCs with any alloantibodies is the main concern. Of secondary importance is compatibility with the autoantibody, and this is only important when the antibody has limited specificity. Compatible units should be selected using techniques described in the preceding section.

REFERENCES

1. BANACERRAF, B and UNANUE, ER: *Textbook of Immunology.* Williams & Wilkins, Baltimore, 1979.
2. BARTHOLD, DR, KYSELA, S and STEINBERG, AD: *Decline in suppressor T cell function with age in female NZB mice.* J Immunol 112:9, 1974.
3. KIRTLAND, HH, HORWITZ, DA, and MOHLER, DN: *Inhibition of suppressor T cell function by methyldopa: A proposed cause of autoimmune hemolytic anemia.* N Engl J Med 302:825, 1980.
4. VAN LOGHEM, JJ: *Concepts on the origin of autoimmune diseases: The possible role of viral infection in the etiology of idiopathic autoimmune diseases.* Semin Haematol 9:17, 1965.
5. PETZ, LD and GARRATTY, G: *Acquired Immune Hemolytic Anemias.* Churchill Livingstone, New York, 1980.
6. WORLLEDGE, SM: *The interpretation of a positive direct antiglobulin test.* Br J Haematol 39:157, 1978.
7. JUDD, WJ, et al.: *The evaluation of a positive direct antiglobulin test in pretransfusion testing.* Transfusion 20:17, 1980.
8. GARRATTY, G, PETZ, LD and HOOPS, JK: *The correlation of cold agglutinin titrations in saline and albumin with haemolytic anaemia.* Br J Haematol 35:587, 1977.

9.   ENGELFRIET, CP, et al.: *Autoimmune hemolytic anemias. I. Serological studies with pure anti-immunoglobulin reagents.* Clin Exp Immunol 3:605, 1968.

10. ROSSE, WF: *Quantitative immunology of immune hemolytic anemia. II. The relationship of cell-bound antibody to hemolysis and the effect of treatment.* J Clin Invest 50:734, 1971.

11. GILLILAND, BC, BAXTER, E and EVANS, RS: *Red cell antibodies in acquired hemolytic anemia with negative antiglobulin serum tests.* N Engl J Med 285:252, 1971.

12. STRATTON, F, et al.: *Acquired hemolytic anemia associated with IgA anti-e.* Transfusion 12:197, 1972.

13. STURGEON, P, et al.: *Autoimmune hemolytic anemia associated exclusively with IgA of Rh specificity.* Transfusion 19:324, 1979.

14. HOPPE, PAH: *The role of the Bureau of Biologics in assuring reagent reliability.* In *Considerations in the Selection of Reagents.* American Association of Blood Banks, Washington, DC, 1979, pp 1–33.

15. GARRATTY, G and PETZ, LD: *An evaluation of commercial antiglobulin sera with particular reference to their anticomplement properties.* Transfusion 11:79, 1971.

16. WIDMANN, FK (ed): *Technical Manual.* American Association of Blood Banks, Washington, DC, 1981.

17. REID, ME: *Autoagglutination dispersal utilizing sulfhydryl compounds.* Transfusion 18:353, 1978.

18. ISSITT, PD: *Antibodies reactive at 30 Centigrade, room temperature and below.* In BUTCH, S (ed): *Clinically Significant and Insignificant Antibodies.* American Association of Blood Banks, Washington, DC, 1979, pp 13–28.

19. MARSH, WL: *Aspects of cold-reactive autoantibodies.* In BELL, CA (ed): *A Seminar on Laboratory Management of Hemolysis.* American Association of Blood Banks, Washington, DC, 1979, pp 79–103.

20. EDWARDS, JM, MOULDS, JJ and JUDD, WJ: *Chloroquine dissociation of antigen-antibody complexes: A new technique for typing red blood cells with a positive direct antiglobulin test.* Transfusion 22:59, 1982.

21. BEATTIE, KM: *Laboratory evaluation and management of antibody specificities in warm autoimmune hemolytic anemia.* In BELL, CA (ed): *A Seminar of Laboratory Management of Hemolysis.* American Association of Blood Banks, Washington, DC, 1979, pp 105–134.

22. LALEZARI, P and BERRENS, JA: *Specificity and crossreactivity of cell-bound antibodies.* In MOHN, JF et al. (ed): *Human Blood Groups.* S Karger, Basel, 1977, pp 44–55.

23. WEINER, W and VOS, GH: *Serology of acquired hemolytic anemias.* Blood 22:606, 1963.

APPENDIX

PROCEDURES

A. 37°C Elution-Wash to Remove Cold Reactive Autoagglutinins

1. Incubate approximately 1 ml of a 25 percent saline suspension of RBCs at 37°C for 15 minutes.
2. Fill the tube with saline prewarmed to 37 to 40°C.
3. Centrifuge and decant supernatant saline.
4. Add enough warm saline to make a 25 percent RBC suspension. Incubate at 37°C.
5. Repeat several times until antibody-coated RBCs no longer spontaneously agglutinate.
   (a) Add 1 drop of a 2 to 5 percent saline suspension of RBCs to each of two tubes.
   (b) To one tube add 2 drops of normal saline; to the other tube add 2 drops of inert serum, 6 percent albumin or Rh diluent.
   (c) Centrifuge; resuspend the cell buttons and observe for agglutination. If the cells do not autoagglutinate, they can be used for cell grouping tests. If they agglutinate, one needs to perform additional 37°C washes or to treat the cells with 0.01 M dithiothreitol (see below).

B. Dithiothreitol (DTT) Dispersal of Autoagglutination Caused by Cold Reactive Autoantibodies[17]

1. Prepare 0.01 M DTT in phosphate buffered saline, pH 7.3.
2. Add 1 volume of 0.01 M DTT to 1 volume of a washed 50 percent RBC suspension.
3. Mix and incubate at 37°C for 15 minutes. Mix several times during the incubation.
4. Wash the DTT-treated RBCs several times with normal saline. Resuspend to 2 to 5 percent.
5. Test the DTT-treated RBCs for autoagglutination in saline and in protein diluents.
   (a) Add 1 drop of treated cells to two tubes. One contains 2 drops of saline; the other, 2 drops of 6 percent albumin, Rh diluent, or inert serum.
   (b) Mix and centrifuge. Resuspend and observe for agglutination.
   (c) RBCs can be used for blood grouping tests and DAT if there is not autoagglutination.
   (d) DTT treatment can be repeated if initial treatment is not successful.

Comments: When RBCs are very heavily coated with cold reactive autoantibodies, they may spontaneously agglutinate and cause false-positive ABO and Rh grouping tests and DAT. When valid tests cannot be done using 37°C eluted-washed RBCs, one can treat the cells with a thiol reagent such as DTT. Thiol reagents abolish or decrease the agglutinating activity of IgM molecules. In this application the IgM molecules are bound to the RBCs surface. DTT-treated cells give reliable blood grouping and direct antiglobulin tests when controls are negative.

C. Prewarmed Technique for Testing Serum Containing Cold Autoagglutinins[16]

1. Add 2 drops of serum to each tube and incubate at 37°C for 5 to 10 minutes.
2. In separate tubes incubate cell suspensions (in saline or LISS) at 37° for 5 to 10 minutes.
3. Transfer 1 drop of prewarmed cell suspension to a tube containing prewarmed serum.
4. Incubate mixture at 37°C for 15 to 30 minutes.
5. DO NOT REMOVE TUBES. Fill the tubes with warm saline (37°C), then remove tubes from incubator and centrifuge. Repeat the washing procedure two to three more times with warm saline.
6. To a dry cell button add 1 to 2 drops of antiglobulin reagent. Centrifuge, resuspend, and record results.

Comments: Most problems encountered in compatibility tests and antibody detection and identification tests that are caused by cold autoagglutinins can be resolved if one uses this procedure. By preventing the reaction between the cold agglutinin and RBCs at room temperature (during centrifugation, and so on), one prevents complement activation. Most antibodies that react at 37°C will be detected in the antiglobulin phase.

D. Autoabsorption Technique to Remove Cold Reactive Autoantibody[16]

1. Wash the autologous RBCs several times with 37°C saline to remove some cold reactive autoantibody and other serum proteins.
2. To 1 volume of washed, packed RBCs add 1 volume of 1 percent ficin. Incubate 15 to 30 minutes at 37°C.
   NOTE: A solution of any proteolytic enzyme is satisfactory. This step is not essential, but antibody uptake is greatly enhanced. One may have to do fewer absorptions to remove most of the antibody.
3. Wash the ficin-treated cells six times with large volumes of saline to remove enzyme.
4. Centrifuge the treated cells 10 minutes at 3500 rpm. Remove and discard supernatant saline.
5. To 1 volume of cells add 1 volume of serum. Mix by inverting several times.
6. Incubate at 4°C for 30 minutes. Mix several times.
7. Centrifuge 3 to 5 minutes at 3500 rpm and collect the autoabsorbed serum.
8. Test the autoabsorbed serum using the desired techniques.

Comments: In some cases a single absorption will not remove a sufficient amount of antibody. Add the once-absorbed serum to a second aliquot of ficin-treated autologous cells and repeat the 4°C incubation. Most workers prepare several volumes of ficin-treated RBCs initially so that additional absorptions require little extra time.

E. Donath-Landsteiner Test[16]

1. Collect the specimen and keep it at 37°C while it clots. Separate the serum from the clot and use as soon as possible.
2. Add 1 ml serum to each of two tubes.
3. Add 0.1 ml 50 percent suspension of random group O RBCs to each tube. Mix well.
4. Incubate one tube at 4°C (in an ice bath) and the other tube at 37°C for 30 minutes.
5. After incubation, gently mix the contents of the cold tube and transfer it to 37°C for 30 minutes. Mix the contents of the warm tube and leave it at 37°C for 30 minutes.
6. Invert the two tubes to mix the serum and cells; centrifuge for 60 seconds at 3500 rpm.
7. Observe for hemolysis.

Comments: The test is positive for PCH when the cells incubated at 4°C then at 37°C are lysed and the cells incubated at 37°C are not lysed.

F. Ether Elution Technique[16]

1. Wash 1 volume of packed RBCs at least six times with large volumes of saline to remove all antibodies not bound to the RBCs. Save an aliquot of the last wash to test in parallel with the eluate.
2. Add 1 volume of saline (or 6 percent albumin) and 2 volumes of ether to 1 volume of packed washed RBCs.
3. Stopper and shake vigorously for 1 minute. Remove the stopper periodically to allow ether vapor to escape.
4. Heat unstoppered at 56°C for 15 to 30 minutes.
5. After centrifugation for 10 minutes at 3500 rpm, there will be three layers. The clear top layer is the ether; the middle layer is RBC debris; the eluate is heavily hemoglobin-stained and is at the bottom.
6. Remove the ether with a Pasteur pipette and discard.
7. Using a Pasteur pipette penetrate the RBC debris layer and collect the eluate from the bottom. Transfer the eluate to a properly labeled tube. Recentrifuge to remove debris if necessary.
8. Incubate the eluate for 5 to 10 minutes at 37°C to allow evaporation of residual ether.
9. Test the eluate by the antiglobulin technique. The supernatant saline from the last wash should be tested in parallel and should be negative. When testing an eluate, one wants to detect antibody eluted from the RBCs and not antibody free in the serum.

G. Autoabsorption Technique to Remove Warm Reactive Autoantibodies[16]

1. Wash an aliquot of autologous RBCs six times with large volumes of saline.
2. To 1 volume of packed, washed cells add 1 volume of saline. Mix by inverting several times.

3. Shake the mixture for 3 to 5 minutes in a 56°C waterbath. Centrifuge immediately and remove supernatant eluate.

   NOTE: This eluate can be tested but will not contain as much antibody as eluates prepared by other methods. The purpose of this step is to free antigen sites to improve removal of autoantibody.

4. Add 1 volume of 1 percent ficin (or a solution of another proteolytic ezyme) and mix.

   NOTE: Enzyme treatment improves removal of autoantibody.

5. Incubate mixture for 15 minutes at 37°C.

6. Wash the enzyme-treated RBCs several times with large volumes of saline.

7. Add 1 volume of serum to 1 volume of tightly packed enzyme-treated autologous cells and mix by inverting several times.

8. Incubate the mixture at 37°C for 15 to 30 minutes.

9. Centrifuge and harvest supernatant autoabsorbed serum.

   NOTE: One may have to use several aliquots of RBCs to remove the warm reactive autoantibody. Transfer the once-absorbed serum to a second aliquot of cells, and so on.

Comment: The same procedure can be used if one is using RBCs from donors of selected phenotypes. Steps 1 through 3 are not necessary, however, since donor RBCs are not antibody-coated.

CHAPTER **20**

DRUG-INDUCED RED BLOOD CELL SENSITIZATION AND DESTRUCTION

SUSAN STEANE, M.S., MT(ASCP)SBB

I. IMMUNE COMPLEX MECHANISM

II. DRUG ADSORPTION MECHANISM

III. MEMBRANE MODIFICATION

IV. AUTOANTIBODY FORMATION

V. SUMMARY

Drugs can cause a variety of side effects, including immune destruction of erythrocytes (RBCs) and other blood cells. Hemolytic anemia, thrombocytopenia, and agranulocytosis can occur separately, but in some patients more than one cell line can be affected. The cells may be coated with antibody, antibody and complement, or complement alone. The discussion in this chapter is limited to RBC problems, but many of the same principles could be applied to platelets and leukocytes.

Drug-mediated problems may come to the attention of a blood bank technologist in one of two ways:

1. A request for diagnostic testing on a patient with hemolytic anemia
2. Unexpected results in routine testing, for example, a positive autologous

control in the antiglobulin phase of antibody screening or compatibility testing or a positive direct antiglobulin test (DAT)

Drugs should be suspected as a possible cause for immune hemolytic anemia or positive DATs when there is no other explanation for the serologic and hematologic findings and if the patient has a history of taking the drug. Other explanations should be considered first, because, with the exception of Aldomet-induced problems, drug-induced positive DATs or hemolytic anemias are relatively rare. Petz and Garratty[1] review four different mechanisms by which drugs can induce problems: immune complex, drug adsorption, membrane modification, and autoantibody formation. Each mechanism has characteristic serologic and clinical features. Specific drugs are commonly associated with one particular mechanism but may work by another.[2-4]

IMMUNE COMPLEX MECHANISM

The largest variety of drugs causing immune-mediated problems work by the immune complex mechanism. Drugs operating through this mechanism are thought to combine with plasma proteins to form immunogens.[5] Antibody (IgG or IgM) subsequently produced recognizes determinants on the drug. If the patient ingests the same drug (or a drug bearing the same haptenic group) following immunization, the formation of a drug-anti-drug complex may occur. Following antigen-antibody interaction the complement cascade may be activated. RBCs are thought to be involved in this process only as innocent bystanders. The soluble drug-anti-drug complex nonspecifically adsorbs to the cell surface. Complement, when activated, sensitizes the cell with complement components and may cause lysis (Fig. 20-1). Drugs associated with the immune complex mechanism include phenacetin, quinine, rifampin and stibophen. For a more complete list the reader should consult *Acquired Immune Hemolytic Anemias* by Petz and Garratty.[1] These authors point out that, in

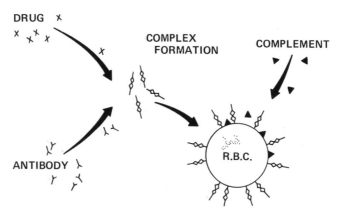

FIGURE 20-1. Immune complex mechanism. (From Petz and Garratty,[1] with permission.)

spite of the large number of drugs involved, the incidence of drug-related immune complex-mediated problems is very low.

Since complement activation is involved in the immune complex, clinically affected patients frequently present with acute intravascular hemolysis.[6] When other causes for hemoglobinemia and hemoglobinuria have been excluded (e.g., ABO hemolytic transfusion reactions or cold reactive autoimmune hemolytic anemia), one should consider a drug-anti-drug reaction. When obtaining the drug history it is important to realize that this group of patients needs to take only small doses of the drug to be affected. The patient rapidly improves once the drug is withdrawn.

The DAT on the patient's cells will usually be positive. If monospecific reagents are used, agglutination usually occurs with anticomplement but not anti-IgG (Table 20-1). Tests with anti-IgG are negative, even when the antibody in question is of the IgG class, because the drug-anti-drug complex is thought to elute from the red cells during the three or four washes prior to the antiglobulin test. Other routine blood bank tests are negative: the antibody is directed against a drug, not a red cell antigen; therefore, the antibody screen and compatibility tests are negative in all phases unless unrelated red cell alloantibodies also happen to be present. An eluate

TABLE 20-1. Serologic Reactions Observed with Drug-Induced Positive DATs

| Mechanism | Direct Antiglobulin Test | | | Serum | Eluate |
	Poly-specific	Anti-IgG	Anti-C3		
Immune complex	+	0*	+	Routine antibody screens are negative	
				Antibody demonstrable if serum, complement, drug incubated with RBCs	Antibody not demonstrable even in presence of drug
Drug adsorption	+	+	0*	Routine antibody screens are negative	
				High-titered antibody demonstrable if serum tested with drug-coated RBCs	Antibody demonstrable using drug-coated RBCs
Membrane modification	+	+	+	Routine antibody screens are negative; nonimmunologic mechanism.	
Autoantibody formation	+	+	∪*	Autoantibody reactive with normal RBCs may or may not be present	Eluate reactive with normal RBCs

*May occasionally be positive.

tested against reagent red cells is also negative even if some IgG is on the cells. A summary of typical serologic results is given in Table 20-1.

To confirm that a drug-anti-drug reaction acting through this mechanism is responsible for a positive DAT one must demonstrate the antibody in the patient's serum. One must incubate the patient's serum, a solution of the drug in question, and group compatible red cells. Complement activation is the usual indicator of an antigen-antibody reaction; therefore, one should observe for hemolysis after incubation and use reagents containing anti-C3 activity for the antiglobulin test. The patient's serum should be fresh or an aliquot of fresh normal donor serum can be added as a source of complement. A general procedure suggested by Garratty[7] for demonstrating antibodies reacting by the immune complex mechanism is given in Appendix A of this chapter.

For the test results to be interpreted correctly, adequate controls must be performed. The patient's serum must not react with the cells when saline or the diluent used to dissolve the drug is substituted for the drug solution, and the drug solution must not nonspecifically hemolyze a suspension of cells. Examples of typical reactions with the patient's serum and controls are given in Table 20-2.

An eluate prepared from the patient's red cells is usually nonreactive even if the drug and a source of complement are added. Very little antibody, if any, remains on the cells following washing.

In most blood banks confirmatory testing is done only when the patient has hematologic complications and not when the patient simply has a history of taking the drug and a positive DAT. Some of the drugs known to cause immune complex mediated problems are in frequent use, and there are a large number of patients with a positive DAT who do not have hemolytic anemia.[8,9] Therefore, a great deal of time could be spent investigating a serologic problem that has no clinical significance.

DRUG ADSORPTION MECHANISM

Unlike drugs acting through the immune complex mechanism, drugs operating through the drug adsorption mechanism bind firmly to proteins, including the proteins of the red cell membrane (Fig. 20-2). Presumably because of their ability to bind to proteins, these drugs are better immunogens. For example, antibodies to penicillin, the drug most commonly associated with this mechanism, are found in the majority of hospital patients.[10] Even with the relatively high incidence of antipenicillin antibodies and the ability of the drug to bind to the red cell membrane, penicillin-induced positive DATs are not common.[11] The low incidence is probably due to the fact that the patient must be receiving massive doses (10 million units daily) of penicillin for the cells to be coated adequately, and most antipenicillin antibodies are IgM, not IgG, and are not detected by the antiglobulin test.[7] The penicillin antibody responsible for a positive DAT is IgG. Complement activation usually does not occur.

The laboratory results are consistent with this description of the mechanism (see Table 20-1). Cells from patients with a positive DAT are usually coated with

TABLE 20-2. Interpretation of Tests to Confirm Presence of Antidrug Antibody Acting by Immune Complex Mechanism

	Patient's Serum	Fresh Serum (Complement)	Drug	RBCs	Results*	Interpretation
Tests:	✓	✓	✓	✓	Positive	Antidrug antibody present if controls working
	✓	✓	✓	✓	Negative	Antidrug antibody not present; drug not present in proper concentration, etc.
Controls: Patient's serum	✓	0†	0	✓	Negative	No alloantibody vs these RBC antigens present
Fresh serum	0	✓	✓	✓	Negative	No alloantibody vs RBC or drug present in serum of random donor (complement)
Drug solution	0	0	✓	✓	Negative	Drug solution does not cause RBCs to agglutinate or lyse

*Based on presence of hemolysis, agglutination.
†0 = Phosphate-buffered saline substituted in reaction mixture.

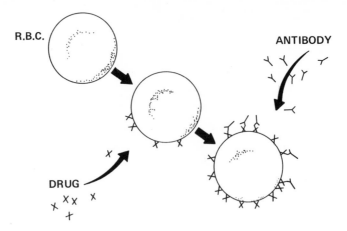

FIGURE 20-2. Drug adsorption mechanism. (From Petz and Garratty,[1] with permission.)

IgG alone. However, sometimes both IgG and complement are present on the cells. The patient's serum and eluate are nonreactive with reagent red cells and random donor cells. Therefore, antibody screens are negative and crossmatches are compatible in all phases. However, if the serum and eluate are tested with penicillin-coated cells, agglutination does occur in the antiglobulin phase. The procedure for preparing and testing penicillin-coated cells to confirm penicillin-antipenicillin activity as the cause for a positive DAT is given in Appendix B of this chapter.[7] Since many patients have antipenicillin, Garratty emphasizes that the serum antibody must be high-titered and the eluate must be positive before findings are definitive. Interpretation of confirmatory tests to demonstrate anti-penicillin antibodies is outlined in Table 20-3.

Only a small percentage of those patients who develop a penicillin-induced positive DAT exhibit hematologic complications. The clinical features of such a hemolytic episode differ from immune complex-mediated problems in several ways. Since the complement cascade is usually not activated, cell destruction is predominantly extravascular rather than intravascular. Therefore, the anemia develops more slowly and is not life-threatening unless the cause for anemia is not recognized and penicillin therapy continues. Penicillin-induced hemolysis occurs only when the patient has received a massive dose of the drug (greater than 10 million units of intravenous penicillin every day for a week). This requirement for a large dose is in contrast to the fact that only a small dose can induce immune complex-mediated hemolysis. The patient improves once penicillin is withdrawn, but hemolysis continues at a decreasing rate until cells heavily coated with penicillin are removed. The DAT may remain positive for several weeks. Mixed field agglutination will be seen in the DAT because some cells will be penicillin-coated, others will not.

Other drugs can cause a positive DAT and hemolytic anemia by this mechanism. Among these are cephalothin (Keflin) and quinidine.[1] Distinguishing between Keflin-induced problems and penicillin-induced problems is technically difficult

TABLE 20-3. Interpretation of Screening Tests for Presence of Antidrug Antibodies Acting by Drug Adsorption Mechanism

	Patient's Serum/Eluate	Drug-Coated RBCs	Uncoated RBCs*	Results†	Interpretation
Test:	✓	✓	—	Positive	Antidrug antibody present if controls working; antibody in serum usually high-titered
	✓	✓	—	Negative	Antidrug antibody not present
Controls: Patient's serum	✓	—	✓	Negative	No alloantibody vs these RBC antigens present in serum or eluate
Drug-coated RBCs	0‡	✓	—	Negative	Drug-coated RBCs do not spontaneously agglutinate or lyse

*Same RBCs as those coated with drug.
†Based on presence of agglutination (or hemolysis with serum).
‡0 = Phosphate-buffered saline substituted in reaction mixture.

because these drugs have antigenic determinants in common and antipenicillin is frequently present in serum. Antipenicillin will react with Keflin-treated cells; anti-Keflin, with penicillin-coated cells. Garratty[7] suggests that comparing the strength of reactivity (titer, score) of the serum or eluate with penicillin-coated and Keflin-coated cells may be of value.

There are additional difficulties involved with using Keflin-treated cells. As discussed in the next section, Keflin-treated cells may nonspecifically adsorb protein and give a positive indirect antiglobulin test with a serum that contains no anti-Keflin antibodies. One can avoid this problem by using a dilution of serum (1 in 20, for example). Eluates, since they contain little serum protein, do not cause this type of false-positive result.

MEMBRANE MODIFICATION

The cephalosporins, in addition to operating through the drug adsorption mechanism, are able to modify red cells so that plasma proteins (e.g., IgG, IgM, IgA and complement) can bind to the membrane (Fig. 20-3).[12] Consequently RBCs from patients receiving cephalosporins (Keflin, for example) may exhibit a positive DAT with polyspecific and monospecific reagents. The uptake of immunoglobulins or complement components is not the result of an antigen-antibody reaction, so this mechanism is nonimmunologic. Since antibody is not involved, tests with the patient's serum and eluate are negative (see Table 20-1). Several cases of cephalosporin-associated hemolytic anemia have been reported, but destruction seems to have been mediated through the drug adsorption mechanism rather than membrane modification.[13-16]

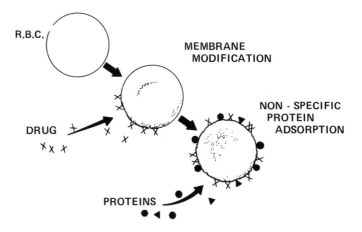

FIGURE 20-3. Membrane modification mechanism. (From Petz and Garratty,[1] with permission.)

AUTOANTIBODY FORMATION

Unlike the drugs acting through the immune complex or drug adsorption mechanisms that induce production of *allo*antibodies against a determinant on a drug, methyldopa (Aldomet) induces the production of *auto*antibodies that recognize RBC antigens.[17,18] The antibodies produced are serologically indistinguishable from those seen in patients with warm reactive autoimmune hemolytic anemia (see Chapter 19). Aldomet-induced positive DATs are frequently encountered. Approximately 10 to 20 percent of patients receiving this antihypertensive drug develop a positive DAT. However, very few (0.5 to 1 percent) of this group of patients subsequently develop immune hemolytic anemia.[1] Other drugs that also cause autoantibody production are L-dopa and mefenamic acid.[1]

Several mechanisms by which Aldomet causes the production of autoantibodies have been proposed,[18-20] but the most attractive suggestion is that of Kirtland, Horwitz, and Mohler.[21] They have shown that methyldopa alters the function of T suppressor cells and suggest that this upset in the immune system would allow production of antibody against "self."

The serologic features of this type of drug-induced problem are very different from those previously described. As shown in Table 20-1, the antibody in the eluate *will* react with normal red cells in the absence of the drug. Antibody of similar specificity and reactivity may be found in the serum. Patient's RBCs are coated with IgG, rarely with complement components.

Because the serology of Aldomet-induced positive DAT/hemolytic anemia is identical to that of warm reactive autoimmune hemolytic anemia, one cannot establish in the laboratory that Aldomet is the cause of the problem. However, if the patient is receiving the drug, one should be highly suspicious. If Aldomet is withdrawn, autoantibody production will eventually stop, but it may be several months before the DAT is negative. For some unexplained reason, withdrawal of the drug has more rapid clinical benefits; improvement is usually seen within 10 days despite the presence of the antibody on the cells or in the serum.[1]

SUMMARY

By understanding the mechanisms by which drugs can cause a positive DAT or immune hemolytic anemia, one can quickly decide which laboratory tests are most likely to be informative. Before any special testing is done, one should

1. Obtain the patient's medical history, including transfusions, medications and diagnosis.
2. Perform a DAT using RBCs collected in EDTA. Test the cells with a polyspecific antiglobulin reagent and monospecific reagents (anti-IgG and anti-C3).
3. Screen the patient's serum for RBC alloantibodies.
4. Prepare and test an eluate for RBC alloantibodies if IgG is on the cells.

After evaluating this information, one can decide if drugs are a possible cause of the problem and which of the mechanisms is involved. Then, when other causes (e.g., transfusion reactions) have been excluded and if the clinical situation warrants additional testing, drug-coated cells or solutions of the drug can be prepared for confirmatory tests.

REFERENCES

1. PETZ, LD and GARRATTY, G: *Acquired Immune Hemolytic Anemias.* Churchill Livingstone, New York, 1980.
2. KERR, RO, et al.: *Two mechanisms of erythrocyte destruction in penicillin-induced hemolytic anemia.* N Engl J Med 298:1322, 1972.
3. RIES, CA, et al.: *Penicillin-induced immune hemolytic anemia.* JAMA 233:432, 1975.
4. FREEDMAN, J and LIM, FC: *An immunohematologic complication of isoniazid.* Vox Sang 35:126, 1978.
5. SHULMAN, NR: *Mechanism of blood cell destruction in individuals sensitized to foreign antigens.* Trans Assoc Am Physicians 76:72, 1963.
6. WORLLEDGE, SM: *Immune drug-induced haemolytic anemias.* Semin Haematol 6:181, 1969.
7. GARRATTY, G: *Laboratory Investigation of Drug-Induced Immune Hemolytic Anemia and/or Positive Direct Antiglobulin Tests.* American Association of Blood Banks, Washington, DC, 1979.
8. WORLLEDGE, SM: *The interpretation of a positive direct antiglobulin test.* Br J Haematol 39:157, 1978.
9. LAU, P, HAESLER, WE and WURZEL, HA: *Positive direct antiglobulin reaction in a patient population.* Am J Clin Pathol 65:368, 1976.
10. LEVINE, BB, FELLNER, MJ and LEVYTSKA V: *Benzylpenicilloyl specific serum antibodies to penicillin in man.* J Immunol 96:707, 1966.
11. JUDD, WJ, et al.: *The evaluation of a positive direct antiglobulin test in pretransfusion testing.* Transfusion 20:17, 1980.
12. SPATH, P, GARRATTY, G and PETZ, LD: *Studies on the immune response to penicillin and cephalothin in humans. II. Immunohematologic reactions to cephalothin administration.* J Immunol 107:860, 1971.
13. KAPLAN, K, REISBURG, B and WEINSTEINS, L: *Cephaloridine studies of therapeutic activity and untoward effects.* Arch Intern Med 121:17, 1968.
14. GRALNICK, HR, McGINNISS, MH and ELTON, W: *Hemolytic anemia associated with cephalothin.* JAMA 217:1193, 1971.
15. FORBES, CD, CRAIG, JA and MITCHELL, R: *Acute intravascular hemolysis associated with cephalexin therapy.* Postgrad Med J 48:186, 1972.
16. JEANNET, M, et al.: *Cephalothin-induced immune hemolytic anemia.* Acta Haematol 55:109, 1976.
17. CARSTAIRS, KC, et al.: *Incidence of a positive direct Coombs' test in patients on α-methyldopa.* Lancet ii:133, 1966.
18. WORLLEDGE, SM, CARSTAIRS, KC and DACIE, JV: *Autoimmune hemolytic anemia associated with methyldopa therapy.* Lancet ii:135, 1966.
19. GOTTLIEB, AJ and WURZEL, HA: *Protein-quinone interaction: In vivo induction of indirect antiglobulin reactions with methyldopa.* Blood 43:85, 1974.
20. DAMESHEK, W: *Alpha-methyldopa red cell antibody: Cross reaction or forbidden clone.* N Engl J Med 276:1382, 1967.
21. KIRTLAND, HH, HORWITZ, DA and MOHLER, DN: *Inhibition of suppressor T cell function by methyldopa: A proposed cause of autoimmune hemolytic anemia.* N Engl J Med 302:825, 1980.
22. HENDRY, EG: *Osmolarity of human serum and of chemical solutions of importance.* Clin Chem 7:156, 1961.

APPENDIX

PROCEDURES

A. Test to Demonstrate Antibody Reacting by Immune Complex Mechanism[7]

1. Prepare a 1 mg per ml solution of the drug in phosphate-buffered saline, pH 7.35. See Procedure A(1) below for preparation of phosphate-buffered saline.
2. Centrifuge and remove the supernatant drug solution. Discard undissolved material.
3. Measure pH of solution; adjust to approximately 7 if not between 5 and 8.
4. Set up tube containing 2 volumes of patient's serum, complement (fresh normal serum), and drug solution. For controls substitute phosphate-buffered saline (see Table 20-2).
5. Add 1 volume of a 5 percent saline suspension of RBCs to each tube. Mix.
6. Incubate for 1 to 2 hours at 37°C.
7. Centrifuge. Observe for hemolysis and agglutination.
8. After four washes with saline add antiglobulin serum (containing anti-C3). Centrifuge and examine for agglutination.

Results: If the tube containing the patient's serum, complement, and drug solution hemolyzes, agglutinates, or coats the RBCs *and* the control tubes are negative, the test suggests that an antibody against the drug is present. If no hemolysis or agglutination is observed, it is possible that the drug did not dissolve and the manufacturer should be consulted if additional testing is necessary. The test is not valid if any of the control tubes are positive (see Table 20-2).

A(1). Preparation of Phosphate-Buffered Saline[22]

Solution A: 0.126 M Na_2HPO_4
    Dissolve 8.94 g Na_2HPO_4 in 500 ml distilled (or deionized) water.
Solution B: 0.16 M NaH_2PO_4
    Dissolve 11.04 g $NaH_2PO_4 \cdot H_2O$ in 500 ml distilled (or deionized) water.
Phosphate buffer, pH 7.35
    Mix 85 ml solution A with 15 ml solution B. Measure pH. Adjust to 7.35 by adding small aliquots of acidic (solution B) or basic (solution A) phosphate solutions.
Phosphate-buffered saline
    Mix 100 ml phosphate buffer, pH 7.35, with 900 ml normal saline.

B. Test to Demonstrate Antipenicillin Antibody in Patient's Serum or Eluate[7]

Penicillin-Coated RBCs
1. Add 1×10^6 units of penicillin G to 15 ml 0.1 M barbital buffer, pH 9.6 to 9.8. Mix well. See Procedure B(1) for preparation of barbital buffer.
    NOTE: Normal saline may be substituted for barbital buffer, but the buffer is the preferred solvent.

2. Add 1 ml washed packed RBCs to the penicillin solution (15 ml). Fresh group O RBCs are suggested.

NOTE: Reserve an aliquot of the RBCs to use as a control.

3. Incubate the RBC-penicillin mixture for 1 hour at room temperature. Mix several times during the incubation.
4. Wash the coated cells four times with saline.
5. Prepare 5 percent saline suspensions of penicillin-coated and uncoated RBCs for testing.

Screening Test to Detect Antipenicillin Antibodies in Serum and Eluate

1. Add 2 drops of serum and eluate to two tubes. To each tube add 1 drop of a 5 percent suspension of *penicillin-coated* RBCs.
2. Add 1 drop of a 5 percent suspension of *uncoated* RBCs to two tubes containing 2 drops of serum and eluate.
3. To another tube add 2 drops of saline to 1 drop of penicillin-coated cells.
4. Incubate all tubes at 37°C for 30 to 60 minutes.
5. Centrifuge and observe for hemolysis and agglutination.
6. Perform the antiglobulin test; examine for agglutination.

Results: Positive tests in the tubes containing penicillin-coated cells indicate the presence of antipenicillin if the control tests are negative. If the patient's serum and eluate react with the uncoated cells, an antibody against a RBC antigen is present and the tests are not valid. Similarly, if the penicillin-coated cells lyse or agglutinate in the absence of serum and eluate, the test is invalid (see Table 20-3). It is important to remember that IgM antipenicillin antibodies are frequently present in serum. To establish antipenicillin as the cause for a positive DAT, the eluate must contain the antibody. In samples from patients with penicillin-induced hemolytic anemia, one can demonstrate the antibody in the eluate and in the serum (titer above 1000 by the antiglobulin test).

B(1). Preparation of Barbital Buffer[7]

1. Add 2.06 g sodium barbital to 100 ml distilled (or deionized) water. Mix well.
2. Adjust the pH to 9.6 to 9.8 by adding 0.1N HCl.

CHAPTER **21**

POLYAGGLUTINATION

HELENA M. GLIDDEN, MT(ASCP)SBB

I. CATEGORIES OF POLYAGGLUTINABLE CELLS

II. IMPORTANCE IN THE LABORATORY

III. LABORATORY RECOGNITION

The terms "polyagglutination" and "polyagglutinable cells" were designated to describe abnormal or altered red blood cells that are agglutinated by virtually all normal adult human sera. It is thought that latent receptors on the red blood cell membrane become exposed or activated, notably by the action of microbial (bacterial/viral) enzymes. These exposed antigens are then available for agglutination by the corresponding IgM antibody found in the sera of most adults.

Polyagglutinability was first described in 1925 by Hübener and was also demonstrated in 1930 by Thomsen and Friedenreich.[1] Polyagglutinability thus became known as the Hübener-Thomsen-Friedenreich, or T, phenomenon. Much later, in 1957, Moreau and coworkers[2] showed that another type of polyagglutinability existed, which they called Tn. In 1959 Cameron and colleagues[3] described yet another polyagglutinable state, acquired B. Almost a decade later, Cazal and associates[4] studied a family in which the first example of Cad was found, which subsequently was shown to have an association with the super strong Sd^a antigen.[5] In 1972 Bird and Wingham reported the first example of Tk polyagglutination,[6] and they also discovered Th in 1978.[7] VA (Vienna) was identified by Graninger and coworkers[8] in

1976 and NOR, another distinct polyagglutinable condition, was described by Harris and associates in 1980.[9]

The polyagglutinable condition can be induced in vivo or in vitro. A septicemic patient infected with an organism such as Bacteroides fragilis could have altered red blood cells as a result of circulating bacterial enzymes exposing previously hidden receptors. A grossly contaminated blood specimen (e.g., by Clostridium perfringens, Streptococcus pneumoniae, or Vibrio cholerae) can also display this phenomenon, since these organisms produce an enzyme, neuraminidase, that cleaves sialic acid from the red cell membrane and exposes the crypt receptors.

The degree of polyagglutinability can vary from case to case. For example, the cells may have many exposed determinants and will demonstrate potent polyagglutinability. Alternatively, if just a few sites are exposed, only strongly reactive serum antibodies will be capable of causing agglutination of these weakly polyagglutinable cells.

When an individual's red cells become polyagglutinable by some of these mechanisms, notably T, Th, and Tk, they are said to be "activated." Thus, T-polyagglutinable cells are referred to as T-activated cells.

CATEGORIES OF POLYAGGLUTINABLE CELLS

Polyagglutinable cells have been differentiated into a number of categories: T, Tn, Tk, Th, VA, Cad, NOR, and acquired B. These categories depend primarily upon the cell's behavior in serologic testing and certain other characteristics, for example, sialic acid levels, duration of the polyagglutinable state in vivo, effect of enzyme treatment, and notably their origin. In brief, the causes of polyagglutinability are (1) the alteration of the red blood cell membrane by bacterial or viral enzymes that act to expose latent receptors (e.g., T, Tk, or Th receptor sites);[10-13] (2) an abnormality of the red blood cell membrane that is not as yet completely understood but is thought to be related to a transferase deficiency that gives rise to incomplete biosynthesis of antigen structures, thus resulting in a polyagglutinable state (e.g., Tn);[14-16] (3) an inherited condition (e.g., Cad[4] and NOR[9]); and (4) conversion of N-acetylgalactosamine (blood type A substance) to galactose (blood type B substance) by a bacterial deacetylase (e.g., acquired B).[17,18] Polyagglutination seen with acquired B may be the result of the same bacterial enzyme modification of the red blood cell membrane as is seen in Tk activation.[19-21]

Polyagglutinable states differ in how long they persist in vivo. Transient acquired types are the most common, as seen in T, Tk, or acquired B polyagglutination. Once the causative agent (e.g., bacteria) is no longer present, the red cells lose their polyagglutinability and become normal again. Tn and VA are persistent, whereas Cad and NOR have been described as permanent conditions.

Cases involving more than one type of polyagglutinability have been described. Concomitant T-activation and Tk-activation alone and in association with acquired B antigens have been reported[22,23] as has coexistent Tk and VA polyagglutinability.[24]

IMPORTANCE IN THE LABORATORY

Polyagglutinable red cells can interfere with serologic tests and must be recognized and handled appropriately. How are polyagglutinable cells detected in the laboratory? Usually they are first noticed when the most fundamental test in the blood bank is performed, the ABO blood typing. Polyagglutinable cells, capable of being agglutinated by most adult sera, will react with ABO typing reagents, which may contain anti-T, anti-Tn, and so on. This causes a forward and reverse typing discrepancy. Since forward typing reactions are normally strongly positive owing to the availability of potent anti-A, anti-B, and anti-A,B sera, an unusual appearance (e.g., mixed field agglutination, which is specifically characteristic of Tn-activation)[25] or slightly weakened reactivity with these reagents would arouse suspicion and would require further investigation (Table 21-1). Some blood typing reagents may not contain as much anti-T, anti-Tk, anti-Tn, and so on as others, and thus cells that are barely polyagglutinable might not even be detected. Since polyagglutinable cells usually react optimally upon immediate centrifugation or after room temperature incubation with the corresponding IgM agglutinin, it is not surprising that polyagglutination is first detected in the ABO typing.

An ABO discrepancy could be due to causes other than polyagglutinability. Alternatively, polyagglutination may mimic other phenomena, for example, a weak subgroup of A, a chimera, or a strongly reactive cold autoagglutinin. If polyagglutinability is suspected, however, obtaining a fresh specimen and repeating the ABO testing would rule out polyagglutinability caused by in-vitro bacterial contamination. Also, use of reagents from which polyagglutinable antibodies (e.g., anti-T) have been absorbed should result in an accurate ABO typing if either in-vivo or in-vitro polyagglutinability is involved. If the discrepancy is not resolved, phenomena other than polyagglutination must be considered.

Since Rh typing reagents and antihuman sera can contain anti-T, anti-Tn, and so on, a person's Rh type and direct antiglobulin test result may be similarly af-

TABLE 21-1. ABO Discrepancy Caused by Polyagglutination

	Forward Typing				Reverse Typing			
	Reagents				Cells			
	Anti-A	Anti-A$_1$ Lectin	Anti-B	Anti-A,B	A$_1$	A$_2$	B	Interpretation
Normal cells	0		0	0	++++	++++	++++	Type O
Polyagglutinable cells (Tn)	++ mf	+++	0	+++ mf	++++	++++	++++	? Further work needed

mf = mixed field

fected, that is, false-positive results could occur. Besides causing difficulties in ABO and Rh typing, and in obtaining accurate direct antiglobulin test results, polyagglutinable cells can cause problems in crossmatching. If a patient's serum is crossmatched with a donor cell sample that is polyagglutinable, there will be an incompatibility. Resolution of the incompatibility is necessary to ensure patient safety.

Recognition of polyagglutinability by the laboratory may provide useful information to the patient's physician. Since many polyagglutinable conditions are of microbial origin or are the result of enzyme activity exposing crypt antigens on the red blood cell membrane, a polyagglutinable condition in a patient would be of interest to the physician. Also polyagglutination, specifically the Tn type, has been reported as being associated with disease states, such as myelocytic leukemia, other myeloproliferative disorders, and pancytopenia.[26,27] In addition, VA polyagglutination has been associated with hemolytic anemia,[8] and a case of T-activation with concomitant hemolytic anemia has been reported.[28,29] Acquired B has most often been seen in association with lower intestinal obstruction, infection, or malignancy.[30]

Detecting that a patient has a polyagglutinable condition may have an impact upon transfusion therapy. If a patient's cells are markedly polyagglutinable, they are at risk of agglutinating with the anti-T, anti-Tn, and so on of infused plasma products or whole blood. This could cause decreased red cell survival or overt hemolysis.[28,29,31,32] For this reason, the physician may choose to avoid transfusion until the patient's cells are no longer polyagglutinable. Should the patient require red cells only, washed packed cells would be the transfusion product of choice since the plasma containing antibodies directed at the receptors of polyagglutinable red cells would be removed during the washing procedure.

LABORATORY RECOGNITION

It is important to recognize that a sample submitted to the laboratory is polyagglutinable. The condition can manifest itself as an ABO typing, Rh typing, or crossmatch problem. Resolution is necessary. Distinguishing between polyagglutinable and normal cells can be achieved by noting the following characteristics and testing procedures (Table 21-2).

1. Polyagglutinable cell samples are most often detected when performing ABO testing because a discrepancy is noted between forward and reverse typing. Normal cells generally react strongly with ABO typing reagents, and any reactivity less than that is suspect. Polyagglutinable cells may demonstrate mixed field agglutination with ABO typing reagents (see Table 21-1). Once other causes for the ABO discrepancy have been ruled out and polyagglutination is suspected, reagents lacking anti-T, anti-Tn, and so on should be used to obtain an accurate ABO type.

2. Polyagglutinable cells will react with ABO compatible, fresh adult sera but not with sera from newborns whose anti-T, anti-Tn, and so on have not as yet developed. Optimal reactivity occurs after immediate centrifugation or after standard room temperature incubation. Normal cells will not agglutinate with either adult or cord sera.

TABLE 21-2. Normal Versus Polyagglutinable Cells

	Screening Methods				Agglutination After Papain Treatment	Duration
	Fresh Adult Sera	Cord Sera	Polybrene	*Glycine Soja*		
Normal						
Group O	0	0	+	0	usually enhanced	—
T	+	0	0	+	no effect	transient
Tn	+	0	0/+mf	+	decreased	persistent
Tk	+	0	+	0	enhanced	transient
Cad	sometimes +	0	+	0/+w	enhanced	permanent
Acquired B	+	0				transient
VA	+w	0	+	0	no effect	persistent
Th			+	0	decreased	
NOR	+	0	+	0	enhanced	permanent

0 = no reactivity
+ = reactivity/aggregation
+w = weak reactivity/aggregation
+mf = mixed field reactivity
transient = cells revert to normal state after primary condition is resolved
persistent = essentially permanent, but rare cases have been reported in which the cells returned to normal
permanent = cells remain permanently altered and polyagglutinable

3. The serum from a polyagglutinable sample will not usually react with the person's own polyagglutinable cells. For example, if a person's cells become T-activated, the serum will lack detectable levels of anti-T for the duration of the polyagglutinable state but will still contain anti-Tk, anti-Tn, and so on. Thus, the autologous control will be negative.

4. Some forms of polyagglutinable cells have lower membrane sialic acid levels than most normal cells. In the presence of Polybrene (polylysine or protamine sulfate produces the same effect), normal cells aggregate because of their normal levels of sialic acid. Polybrene, which has a net positive charge, may act by neutralizing the negative charge of the red cell sialic acid, thereby allowing the cells to aggregate or form rouleaux. This effect is not achieved when cells have reduced sialic acid levels. Perhaps the excess positive charge of the reagent then functions to keep the cells apart. Polyagglutinable cells, then, will not aggregate in Polybrene, since their sialic acid levels are reduced.[32,33] (See Reagent Preparation A in Appendix of this chapter.)

Another reagent useful for detecting cells with lowered sialic acid levels is a plant lectin, *Glycine soja* (soybean). Those cells deficient in sialic acid (e.g., polyagglutinable cells) will react strongly with the soybean extract, whereas normal cells will not. (See Reagent Preparation B in Appendix of this chapter.)

5. Enzyme (papain) treatment is useful in distinguishing between normal cells and some forms of polyagglutination. Generally, agglutination of normal cells is enhanced following enzyme treatment. This is also true of NOR, Tk, and Cad cells.

TABLE 21-3. Differentiation of Polyagglutinable Cells Using Lectins

	Arachis Hypogaea	Dolichos Biflorus	Salvia Sclarea	Salvia Horminum	Bandeiraea Simplicifolia (BS II)	Vicia Graminea (N_{VG} Receptor)
Normal						
Group O	0	0	0	0	0	—
T	+	0	0	0	0	Enhanced
Tn	0	+	+	+	0	Depressed
Tk	+	0	0	0	+	No effect
Cad	0	+	0	+	0	
Acquired B	0				+	
VA	0	0	0		0	
Th	+		0	0	0	
NOR	0	0	0	0	0	

T-activated and VA-activated cells show no change in their ability to be agglutinated by normal adult sera and typing reagents once these cells have been enzyme treated. Tn-activated and Th-activated cells, however, will demonstrate decreased agglutinability following enzyme treatment.[34] Since enzyme treated Tn-activated and Th-activated cells will no longer agglutinate with sera containing the corresponding polyagglutinins that are found in ABO typing reagents, these cells can successfully be used in obtaining an accurate ABO forward typing, thus resolving an ABO forward and reverse typing discrepancy that occurred because of Tn or Th polyagglutination.

Identification of polyagglutinable states and further differentiation can be achieved by using a variety of plant lectins. Development of appropriate plant lectins that can be used in serologic testing for the identification of polyagglutinable states had been pioneered chiefly through the research of G. W. G. Bird.[25,35-37] The results of his work have provided the blood banker with the knowledge that a new assortment of reagents can be used that react specifically with different types of polyagglutinable cells. Plant lectins are stable and are now available commercially or are relatively easy to prepare in most cases.[38]

The most widely used lectins for differentiation of polyagglutinable states are *Arachis hypogaea* (peanut extract—see Reagent Preparation C in Appendix of this chapter),[39] *Dolichos biflorus* (A_1 activity), *Salvia sclarea, Salvia horminum*,[36,37,40] *Bandeiraea simplicifolia* (BS II lectin), and *Vicia graminea* (N activity). *Arachis hypogaea* reacts specifically with T, Tk, and Th cells and not with the other types of polyagglutinable cells. *Dolichos biflorus*, which is A_1 specific, is useful in distinguishing Tn and Cad from other polyagglutinable states. If Tn or Cad is suspected, lectins prepared from Salvia seeds can be used to differentiate between the two. Both Tn and Cad cells will react with *Salvia horminum*, but only Tn cells will react with *Salvia sclarea* (Clary seeds).[35-37,40] Acquired B and Tk polyagglutinable cells will agglutinate with the BS II component of the lectin prepared from *Bandeiraea simplicifolia* seeds.[19,41] *Vicia graminea* lectin is usually used as a typing reagent for detection of the N antigen on red blood cells. It can also be used in helping to differentiate between different polyagglutinable states[42] (Table 21-3).

REFERENCES

1. FRIEDENREICH, V: *Production of a Specific Receptor Quality in Red Cell Corpuscles by Bacterial Activity. The Thomsen Hemagglutination Phenomenon.* Levin and Munskgaard, Copenhagen, 1930.

2. MOREAU, R, et al.: *Anémie hémolytique acquise avec polyagglutinabilité des hematies par un nouveau facteur présent dans le sérum humain normal, anti-Tn.* Bull Soc Méd Hopetaux (Paris) 73:569, 1957.

3. CAMERON, C, et al.: *Acquisition of a B-like antigen by red blood cells.* Br Med J ii:29, 1959.

4. CAZAL, P, et al.: *Polyagglutinabilité héréditaire dominante: Antigène privé (Cad) correspondant à un anticorps public et à une lectine de* Dolichos biflorus. Rev Fr Transfus 11:209, 1968.

5. SANGER, R, et al.: *Plant agglutinin for another human blood-group.* Lancet i:1130, 1971.

6. BIRD, GWG and WINGHAM, J: *Tk: A new form of red cell polyagglutination.* Br J Haematol 23:759, 1972.

7. BIRD, GWG, et al.: *Th, a "new" form of erythrocyte polyagglutination.* Lancet ii:1215, 1978.

8. GRANINGER, W, et al.: *"VA," a new type of erythrocyte polyagglutination characterized by depressed H receptors and associated with hemolytic anemia.* Vox Sang 32:195, 1977.

9. HARRIS, PA, et al.: *An inherited RBC characteristic, NOR, resulting in erythrocyte polyagglutination.* Abstract, AABB annual meeting, 1979.

10. BIRD, GWG, et al.: *Tk polyagglutination in* Bacteroides fragilis *septicaemia.* Lancet i:286, 1975.

11. INGLIS, G, et al.: *Erythrocyte polyagglutination showing properties of both T and Tk probably induced by* Bacteroides fragilis *infection.* Vox Sang 28:314, 1975.

12. INGLIS, G, et al.: *Effect of* Bacteroides fragilis *on the human erythrocyte membrane: Pathogenesis of Tk polyagglutination.* J Clin Pathol 28:964, 1975.

13. INGLIS, G, et al.: *Tk polyagglutination associated with reduced A and H activity.* Vox Sang 35:370, 1978.

14. CARTRON, JP, et al.: *Selective deficiency of 3-β-D-galactosyltransferase (T-transferase) in Tn-polyagglutinable erythrocytes.* Lancet i:855, 1978.

15. STURGEON, P, et al.: *Permanent mixed-field polyagglutinability PMFP. I. Serological observations.* Vox Sang 25:481, 1973.

16. STURGEON, P, LUNER, SJ and McQUISTON, DT: *Permanent mixed field polyagglutinability PMFP. II. Hematological, biophysical and biochemical observations.* Vox Sang 25:498, 1973.

17. GERBAL, A, MASLET, C and SALMON, C: *Immunological aspects of the acquired B antigen.* Vox Sang 28:398, 1975.

18. SPRINGER, GF and ANSELL, NJ: *Acquisition of a blood group B-like antigen by human A and O erythrocytes.* Fed Proc Am Soc Exp Biol 19:70, 1960.

19. JUDD, WJ and BECK, ML: *The demonstration of Tk receptors on "acquired-B" red cells* (abstr). Transfusion 16:527, 1976.

20. MARSH, WL, JENKINS, WJ and WALTHER, WW: *Pseudo B: An acquired group antigen.* Br Med J ii:63, 1959.

21. MARSH, WL: *The pseudo B antigen. A study of its development.* Vox Sang 5:387, 1960.

22. JUDD, WJ, et al.: *Concomitant T- and Tk-activation associated with acquired-B antigens.* Transfusion 19:293, 1979.

23. PERKASH, A, CARLSON, A and ELLISOR, S: *Polyagglutination due to combined T and Tk activation.* Transfusion 20:301, 1980.

24. BECK, ML, et al.: *Coexistent Tk and VA polyagglutinability.* Transfusion 18:680, 1978.

25. BIRD, GWG, SHINTON, NK and WINGHAM, J: *Persistent mixed-field agglutination.* Br J Haematol 21:443, 1971.

26. BIRD, GWG, et al: *Erythrocyte membrane modification in malignant disease of myeloid and lym-*

phoreticular tissues. 1. Tn-Polyagglutination in acute myelocytic leukemia. Br J Haematol 33:289, 1976.

27. NESS, PM, GARRATTY, G and MOREL, PA: *Tn Polyagglutination preceding acute leukemia.* Blood 54:30, 1979.

28. GRAY, JM, BECK, ML and OBERMAN, HA: *Clostridial-induced type I polyagglutinability with associated intravascular hemolysis.* Vox Sang 22:379, 1972.

29. MOORES, P, PUDIFIN, D and PATEL, PL: *Severe hemolytic anemia in an adult associated with anti-T.* Transfusion 15:329, 1975.

30. BECK, ML, WALKER, RH and OBERMAN, HA: *A typical polyagglutination associated with acquired B antigen.* Transfusion 11:296, 1971.

31. RICKARD, KA, ROBINSON, RJ and WORLLEDGE, SM: *Acute acquired hemolytic anaemia associated with polyagglutination.* Arch Dis Child 44:102, 1969.

32. VAN LOGHEM JR, JJ, VAN DER HART, M and LAND, E: *Polyagglutinability of red cells as a cause of severe haemolytic transfusion reaction.* Vox Sang 5:125, 1955.

33. GREENWALT, TJ and STEANE, EA: *Quantitative haemagglutination. VI. Relationship of sialic acid content of red cells and aggregation by Polybrene®, protamine and poly-L-lysine.* Br J Haematol 25:227, 1973.

34. VAN DER HART, M, et al.: *A second example of red cell polyagglutinability caused by the Tn antigen.* Vox Sang 6:358, 1961.

35. BIRD, GWG and WINGHAM, J: *Seed agglutinin for rapid identification of Tn-polyagglutination.* Lancet i:677, 1973.

36. BIRD, GWG and WINGHAM, J: *Hemagglutinins from Salvia.* Vox Sang, 26:163, 1974.

37. BIRD, GWG and WINGHAM, J: *More Salvia agglutinins.* Vox Sang 30:217, 1976.

38. JUDD, WJ: *The use of purified lectins in immunohematology.* Transfusion 19:768, 1979.

39. BIRD, GWG: *Anti-T in peanuts.* Vox Sang 9:748, 1964.

40. MOORE, BPL and MARSH, S: *Identification of strong Sd (a+) and Sd (a+ +) red cells by hemagglutinins from Salvia horminum.* Transfusion 15:132, 1975.

41. JUDD, WJ, et al.: *BS II lectin. A second haemagglutinin isolated from Bandeiraea simplicifolia seeds with affinity for type III polyagglutinable red cells.* Vox Sang 33:246, 1977.

42. BIRD, GWG and WINGHAM, J: *The M, N and N_{VG} receptors of Tn erythrocytes.* Vox Sang 26:171, 1974.

APPENDIX

REAGENT PREPARATION

These procedures are for the preparation and use of Polybrene, *Glycine soja*, and *Arachis hypogaea* lectins and the in-vitro induction of T-activation, which are used by the Blood Group Reference Section, American Red Cross Blood Services, Bethesda, MD.

A. Polybrene (Hexadimethrine Bromide)

Stock Solution: 4 g Polybrene* per 100 ml saline (0.4 g per 10 ml). Store in plastic.

Daily Use: Dilute the stock 1:40 in normal saline. (Use positive and negative controls to determine optimal reactivity.)

Test: Mix 1 drop Polybrene plus 1 drop 4 percent cell suspension. Stand at room temperature for 15 minutes and observe for aggregation (DO NOT CENTRIFUGE) *or* gently shake mixture until aggregates appear.

Interpretation: Normal cells = aggregation. Cells with lowered sialic acid = negative.

B. Glycine Soja Lectin (Soybean)

Stock Solution: Grind 25 g soybean seeds.† Add 150 ml saline. Stir for 2 hours. Centrifuge for 20 minutes at 2700 rpm. Remove and filter supernatant. (Discard residue.) Determine dilution for optimal, specific reactivity using known T-activated (see Reagent Preparation D) and normal cells as controls. Store diluted solution frozen in aliquots.

Daily Use and Test: Mix 2 drops aliquot plus 1 drop 4 percent cell suspension. Centrifuge immediately and observe for agglutination.

Interpretation: Normal cells = negative. Cells with lowered sialic acid = positive (T, Tn).

C. Arachis Hypogaea Lectin (Peanuts)

Stock Solution: Grind 1 part raw peanuts‡ in 4 volumes saline. Let stand at 4°C overnight. Centrifuge for 20 minutes at 2700 rpm. Determine dilution§ for optimal, specific reactivity using T-activated and normal cells as controls. Store diluted solution frozen in aliquots.

---

*Polybrene can be ordered from Aldrich Chemical Co., Milwaukee, Wisconsin.
†Soybean seeds can be obtained from a health food store. *Glycine soja* solution is available commercially ready to use.
‡Raw peanuts can be obtained from grocery or health food stores.
§Alternatives to dilution to obtain a specific reagent:
  1. Extract the fat from peanuts by grinding the peanuts on absorbent paper (e.g., filter paper).
  2. Precipitate the fat by freezing, thawing, and refreezing peanut solution and then salvaging the supernatant.

Daily Use and Test: Mix 2 drops of lectin plus 1 drop 4 percent cell suspension. Centrifuge immediately and observe for agglutination.

Interpretation: Normal cells = negative. Polyagglutinable cells = positive (T, Tk, Th).

D. T-Activation In Vitro Using Neuraminidase

To prepare T-Activated Red Cells:
1. To 1 volume of group O washed packed red cells to be T-activated, add 1 volume of neuraminidase.‡
2. Mix and incubate at 37°C for 1 hour.
3. Wash cells thoroughly (4×) in normal saline.
4. Store in Alsever's solution at 4°C. (Stores well for at least 2 weeks.)

To Test for Proper Treatment:
1. Add 1 drop of a 4 percent cell suspension of T-activated cells to:
   (a) 2 drops *Arachis hypogaea* or *Glycine soja* lectin. Centrifuge immediately and observe for agglutination.
   (b) 1 drop Polybrene. Look for aggregation. (Do not centrifuge.)
   (c) 2 drops 22 or 30 percent bovine albumin. Centrifuge immediately and observe for agglutination.
2. Interpretation: *Arachis hypogaea* = positive; *Glycine soja* = positive; Polybrene = no aggregation; Bovine albumin = negative.

REFERENCES FOR REAGENT PREPARATION AND OTHER METHODS OF USE

Polybrene

Polyagglutination, A Technical Workshop. American Association of Blood Banks, Washington, DC, 1980, p 17.

Serological and Immunological Methods, ed 8. Canadian Red Cross Blood Transfusion Service, 1980, pp 63–64.

Glycine soja

Serological and Immunological Methods, ed 8. Canadian Red Cross Blood Transfusion Service, 1980, p 186.

Arachis hypogaea and T-activated cells

HOWARD, D: *Expression of T-antigen on polyagglutinable erythrocytes, anti-T lectin, anti-T absorbed human serum and purified anti-T antibody.* Vox Sang 37:107, 1979.

Polyagglutination, A Technical Workshop, American Association of Blood Banks, Washington, DC, 1980, pp 14–15.

Serological and Immunological Methods, ed 8. Canadian Red Cross Blood Transfusion Service, 1980, pp 184–185.

---

*Neuraminidase (*Vibrio cholerae* filtrate) can be ordered from Grand Island Biological Company, Grand Island, NY, 14072.

CHAPTER **22**

THE HLA SYSTEM

WILLIAM V. MILLER, M.D.

Evidence for human leukocyte blood groups was first advanced in 1954 by Dausset,[1] who observed that patients whose sera contained leukoagglutinins had received a larger number of blood transfusions than other patients. He also observed that these agglutinins were not autoantibodies, as had been thought previously, but, rather, alloantibodies produced by the infusion of cells bearing alloantigens not present in the recipient.

By 1958 several investigators had provided strong support for this assumption. Dausset[2] observed that the sera from seven polytransfused patients agglutinated leukocytes from about 60 percent of the French population, but not the leukocytes of seven patients. He termed the leukocyte alloantigen MAC, now known as HLA-A2; and family studies showed that leukocyte antigens were genetically determined. At about the same time, Payne[3] showed that the sera of patients with febrile nonhemolytic transfusion reactions often contained leukoagglutinins.

Van Rood and van Leeuwen[4] developed a computer analysis program to study these serologic complexities and discovered several diallelic leukocyte antigen systems, including 4A and 4B (now called Bw4 and Bw6). They also found that leukocyte antigens were present on most human tissues, the erythrocyte being the most notable exception. Because the leukoagglutination technique is complex and insensitive, the discovery in 1964 of the more sensitive microlymphocytotoxicity test by Terasaki and McClelland [5,6] was of special importance. In various modifications, it has maintained its major role in HLA typing until the present time.

Following the discovery of the first leukocyte antigens and a suitable test system, the number of defined serologic specificities increased rapidly. By 1967 they were clearly shown to belong to the same genetic system, and the term HL-A (Human Leukocyte Antigen—the hyphen has since been deleted) was approved by the World Health Organization's Committee on Nomenclature.[7] Previously, it had been suggested that the HLA system was composed of two closely linked loci with genes controlling two segregant series of antigens.[8] That model was substantiated by the discovery of a family showing crossover between the two loci and by analysis of family inheritance patterns specifically in twins and triplets. In 1970 the existence of a third serologically defined segregant series was established, and its value to the HLA system and organ transplantation was clearly established.[9]

Other research disclosed that the lymphocytes from two different individuals would undergo blast transformation and divide when mixed and cultured in vitro. This is known as the mixed lymphocyte reaction (MLR).[10,11] In 1967 Bach and Amos[12] discovered that the MLR test gave negative results when leukocytes from a pair of HLA identical siblings were mixed together, indicating that there was a separate locus controlling MLR within the HLA complex. In 1973 it became possible to type for MLR determinants by means of MLR homozygous cells, and the polymorphism at that portion of the HLA complex coding for the MLR determinants, now called the D locus, became clear.[13] In 1974 investigators found serologically demonstrable gene products closely related to the D locus, and by 1977 it was clear that these D-related (DR) antigens were present on B lymphocytes and monocytes and that they had very high association with HLA-D locus gene products.[14,34,35]

INTERSPECIES COMPARISONS

All mammalian and avian species studied have a defined major histocompatibility complex (MHC) analogous to the human HLA complex. These genetic factors were first discovered because of their ability to serve as transplantation antigens, since allograft survival between in-bred strains of mice was significantly prolonged if the strains were genetically matched for the MHC antigens. MHC antigens in all species show marked polymorphism, that is, many alternative alleles at a given locus. Initially, the only observed function of the MHC gene products was an ability to serve as transplantation antigens, but, since allograft exchanges are an artificial model that could not provide evolutionary pressures to generate the diversity of gene products found at the MHC, most investigators believe that other functions must also exist.

In the late 1960s McDevitt and his colleagues[15] observed that the immune responsiveness of normal in-bred animal strains to specific antigens was, in part, determined by genetic factors coded within the MHC. These immune response, or Ir, genes were found to be contained in the general region of the MHC, the I region. Ir genes in humans very likely exist, although this is not conclusively demonstrated, and preliminary evidence indicates that the genes at the DR locus may be analogous to the Ir genes of mice. It seems likely that some of the observed HLA associations of certain diseases may be related to genetic control of the immune response, since there is clear evidence of these associations in mice and other species.

NOMENCLATURE

The genetic region on the human C6 chromosome that encompasses this group of interrelated genetic information is called HLA. The gene loci belonging to the HLA system are designated by one or more letters following the HLA, that is, HLA-A, HLA-B, HLA-C, HLA-D, and HLA-DR. Each locus contains many individual alleles, and the corresponding allele specificities are designated by numbers following the actual locus symbol (e.g., HLA-A1, HLA-B5, and so on). Provisionally identified specificities carry the initial letter w (for workshop) inserted between the locus letter and the allele specificity number. For example, HLA-Bw44 indicates that the Bw44 specificity is not fully agreed upon by the World Health Organization's Committee on HLA Nomenclature.

Table 22-1 lists many of the current established HLA specificities and their approximate antigen frequencies in white Americans. Note that specificities within the A and the B locus are not numbered consecutively, as are those within the C, D, and DR locus. This is because many of the A and B specificities were established prior to the discovery of the latter loci, and, to avoid renumbering, the existing numbers for A and B locus were used. Also, note that there is no 4 or 6 within the A or the B locus, since these numbers were reserved for the leukocyte antigen systems under active investigation at the time the nomenclature was established. It is now clear that the antigens originally called 4 and 6 are now properly termed Bw4 and Bw6 and

TABLE 22-1. Current HLA Specificities and Their Approximate Frequencies

HLA-A	GF*	HLA-B	GF	HLA-B	GF	HLA-C	GF	HLA-D	GF	HLA-DR	GF
HLA-A1	.148	HLA-B5	.079	HLA-Bw45(12)	.009	HLA-Cw1	.039	HLA-Dw1	.069	HLA-DR1	.083
HLA-A2	.257	HLA-B7	.088	HLA-Bw46	.001	HLA-Cw2	.050	HLA-Dw2	.075	HLA-DR2	.133
HLA-A3	.116	HLA-B8	.084	HLA-Bw47	.004	HLA-Cw3	.106	HLA-Dw3	.882	HLA-DR3	.111
HLA-A9	.112	HLA-B12	.122	HLA-Bw48	.005	HLA-Cw4	.121	HLA-Dw4	.053	HLA-DR4	.114
HLA-A10	.061	HLA-B13	.027	HLA-Bw49(w21)	.023	HLA-Cw5	.062	HLA-Dw5	.056	HLA-DR5	.104
HLA-A11	.062	HLA-B14	.037	HLA-Bw50(w21)	.012	HLA-Cw6	.091	HLA-Dw6	.103	HLA-DRw6	.025
HLA-Aw19	.154	HLA-B15	.057	HLA-Bw51(5)	.062	HLA-Cw7	.031	HLA-Dw7	.103	HLA-DR7	.126
HLA-Aw23(9)†	.024	HLA-Bw16	.051	HLA-Bw52(5)	.017	HLA-Cw8	.026	HLA-Dw8	.031	HLA-DRw8	.037
HLA-Aw24(9)	.088	HLA-B17	.046	HLA-Bw53	.078			HLA-Dw9	.014	HLA-DRw9	?
HLA-A25(10)	.020	HLA-B18	.050	HLA-Bw54(w22)	.000			HLA-Dw10	.026	HLA-DRw10	?
HLA-A26(10)	.041	HLA-Bw21	.035	HLA-Bw55(w22)	.024			HLA-Dw11	?		
HLA-A28	.044	HLA-Bw22	.030	HLA-Bw56(w22)	.006			HLA-Dw12	.048		
HLA-A29	.041	HLA-B27	.038	HLA-Bw57(17)	.034						
HLA-Aw30	.026	HLA-Bw35	.093	HLA-Bw58(17)	.012						
HLA-Aw31	.028	HLA-B37	.015	HLA-Bw59	.003						
HLA-Aw32	.042	HLA-Bw38(w16)	.032	HLA-Bw60(40)	.040						
HLA-Aw33	.017	HLA-Bw39(w16)	.019	HLA-Bw61(40)	.016						
HLA-Aw34	.005	HLA-B40	.056	HLA-Bw62(15)	.050						
HLA-Aw36	.003	HLA-Bw41	.015	HLA-Bw63(15)	.007						
HLA-Aw43	.040	HLA-Bw42	.003	HLA-Bw4	.664‡						
		HLA-Bw44(12)	.113	HLA-Bw6	.823‡						
		Continues—									

*Gene frequencies are for Caucasian populations and are calculated as $G = 1 - \sqrt{1 - f}$ (G = gene frequency, f = observed antigen frequency). To convert to antigen frequency: $f = 2G - G^2$.

†Numbers in parentheses denote splits of previous, broader specificities.

‡These represent antigen or phenotype frequencies and are not gene frequencies.

(Modified from *Nomenclature for factors of the HLA system 1980. Tissue Antigens* 16:115, 1980, © 1980 Munksgaard International Publishers Ltd., Copenhagen, Denmark.)

that the Bw4 and Bw6 antigenic determinants reside in the same polypeptide chain as the other HLA-B locus determinants. It may be that Bw4 and Bw6 are alleles that code for a precursor substance upon which the later HLA-B alleles operate to form the final gene products of the HLA-B segregant series.[16,36]

HLA ANTIGENS AND ANTIBODIES

It is necessary to evaluate the HLA antigen composition in prospective donor-recipient pairs prior to organ transplantation and in candidates for long-term platelet therapy refractory to platelets from random donors. The evaluation of recipient serum for antibodies to donor leukocytes is important prior to transplantation and transfusion since evidence indicates that presensitization to HLA antigens may cause rapid rejection of transplanted tissues or poor survival of platelets following transfusion. HLA antigen testing is also used in anthropologic studies, disease correlation, and paternity testing.

As indicated above, the HLA antigens are the product of closely linked genes within the MHC at a locus on the autosomal chromosome 6, the HLA region.[17] The HLA region codes for cell surface antigens, which are defined by serologic technique (serologically defined, or SD, antigens) as well as by sophisticated techniques that identify inherited cell surface markers recognized only by response in the mixed lymphocyte reaction (lymphocyte defined, or LD, antigens). A current concept of the HLA region is depicted in Figure 22-1.

Those familiar with the complexities of the Rh blood group system will have little difficulty understanding the present concept of the HLA system. If one recalls the classic Fisher-Race model of the genetics of the Rh system, comparison with the HLA system is straightforward. Just as in the Fisher-Race model, in which closely linked genetic material codes for C, D, and E, one allele at the A locus codes for one HLA-A antigen, another, closely linked, codes for one HLA-B antigen, another one HLA-C, and so on. In the Rh system we often speak of the relationship between the alleles in a kind of shorthand, for example, R_1, R_2, and r. R_1 represents C, D, and e on the same chromosome. There is no equivalent shorthand notation in the HLA system, but it is important to think of this coupled relationship of A, B, C, D, and DR series alleles. Since each adult has two C6 chromosomes and each chromosome has an A, B, C, D, and DR locus, it follows that the products of 10 different genes may be expressed phenotypically on the cell surface. In practice, 10 antigens are not always detected, in part because of the lack of more precise technology and antiserum, in part because of homozygosity at any given locus, and in part because of the possibility of the deletion of genetic information at a portion of the locus.

The five genes on the same chromosome are called a *haplotype* and, except for the rare instance of crossing over, are always found to segregate together. For example, in the haplotype shown in Figure 22-2, HLA-A1, Cw1, B8, and so on will segregate independently and pass to the germ cells together. Note that the paternal and maternal haplotypes segregate independently so that the ratio of possible haplotypes is fixed. There is a one-in-four chance of two haplotypes segregating in the same

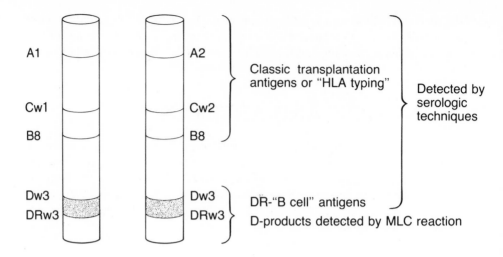

Phenotype: A1, 2, B8, Cw1, 2, Dw3, DRw3

Genotype: A1, 2, B8, 8, Cw1, 2, Dw3, 3, DRw3, 3

Haplotypes: A1, B8, Cw1, Dw3, DRw3/A2, B8, Cw2, Dw3, DRw3

FIGURE 22-1. Schematic representation of the HLA loci on the short arm of chromosome 6. (From Miller, WV and Rodey, G: *HLA Without Tears*. American Society of Clinical Pathologists, Chicago, 1981, with permission.)

way, that is, there is a one-in-four probability that two siblings will have identical HLA haplotypes. There is a one-in-two probability that two siblings will share at least one HLA haplotype and a one-in-four probability that no haplotype will be shared between two siblings. An important corollary is that a parent and child can share only one haplotype, that is, the child must have gotten one haplotype from each parent, making an identical match between child and parent unlikely. It should also be apparent that uncles, grandparents, and cousins are very unlikely to share identical haplotypes with any given child. These are important factors when looking for a well-matched organ tissue or blood transfusion.

The HLA phenotype, then, represents the notation of the surface markers detected in histocompatibility testing of a single individual. The HLA genotype represents a precise determination of the antigens represented on the two C6 chromosomes as determined by family studies, and the term haplotype refers to the antigenic makeup of a single C6 chromosome.

ANTIGENS

The HLA antigens are glycoproteins in nature and the allelic antigenic determinants rest in the polypeptide portion of the molecule, not in its carbohydrate side chains.

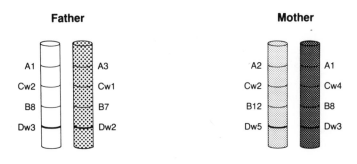

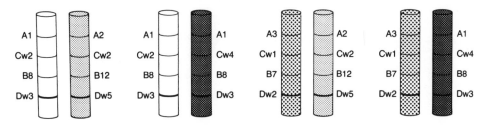

FIGURE 22-2. HLA alleles on the same chromosome are called a haplotype. Haplotypes segregate together during meiosis; only four haplotypes may result from a mating. (From Miller, WV and Rodey, G: *HLA Without Tears.* American Society of Clinical Pathologists, Chicago, 1981, with permission.)

The molecule is composed of two chains: one heavy, bearing the antigenic determinant, and one light (Fig. 22-3).[18]

Special biochemical techniques have shown that two different antigens belonging to the same series (e.g., HLA-A1 and A2), as well as antigens belonging to two different series (e.g., A1 and B8), are present on distinct and separate molecules in a cell membrane.[19,37]

Beta-2 microglobulin is a recently discovered protein of unknown function. It is present in small amounts in serum and present as a cell surface component of the HLA antigen. Beta-2 microglobulin is believed to be the light chain of the HLA molecule and has some structural similarities to the light chain in immunoglobulin.[20]

HLA-A, HLA-B, and HLA-C antigens are thought to be present on all nucleated cells, including both T and B cells, but the D and DR markers have much more restricted tissue distribution. They are found only on macrophages, B lymphocytes, endothelial cells, and spermatozoa. The structure of the D and DR molecules is less well defined, but apparently they are composed of two noncovalently linked polypeptides. Like the -A, -B, and -C antigens, they are highly polymorphic. The D alleles are T-cell activating determinants, and those B-cell antigens inducing antibody formation are DR alleles.

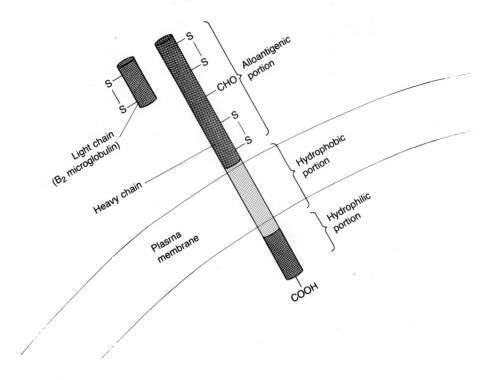

FIGURE 22-3. The HLA molecule consists of a heavy chain bearing the antigenic determinants and a light chain. (From Miller, WV and Rodey, G: *HLA Without Tears*. American Society of Clinical Pathologists, Chicago, 1981, with permission.)

ANTIBODIES

Most HLA antibodies are of the IgG class, with either lambda or kappa light chains. Since detection depends on cytotoxicity, interaction with complement is required.[21] It is likely that there are many HLA antibodies that do not bind complement and, therefore, escape detection in conventional testing systems. These antibodies might be found by agglutination or antiglobulin techniques.

Cytotoxic HLA antibodies vary in the strength and breadth of their activity. Those recognizing a large number of positives within a given population are called "long" antibodies, and those recognizing only a portion of the same positives are called "short." It was in this way that HLA-A9 was "split" into two subsets, Aw23 and Aw24, and that many other antigens have been split into more refined gene products. Long antisera will define a large class of individuals as positive, while short antisera have the ability to differentiate individuals previously thought to be the same, complicating the problems of finding a clinical match.

An additional problem in dealing with HLA antibodies is the problem of cross-reactivity. Antibodies are said to be crossreactive when they react not only with their intended specificity but with other specificities as well. For example, an anti-

HLA-A LOCUS CROSS–REACTIVITY

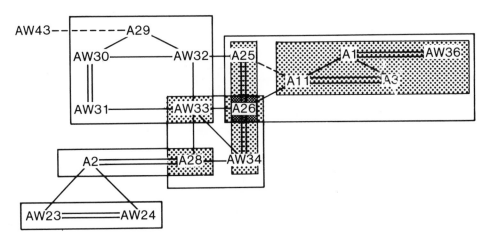

FIGURE 22-4. HLA-A locus cross-reactivities. Strong associations are shown by the double bars. (From Miller, WV and Rodey, G: *HLA Without Tears.* American Society of Clinical Pathologists, Chicago, 1981, with permission.)

body defining Bw35 may crossreact with B5 and B15. Examples of common serologic cross-reactivities are shown in Figures 22-4 and 22-5. It is apparent that one must exercise great caution when evaluating a new antibody, since it may be long or short, crossreactive or not.

A final problem is one familiar to most red cell workers. When an individual forms one HLA antibody, others are often formed as well. For example, a strong anti-HLA-A2 may be contaminated by additional antibodies of other specificities. These antibodies may be quite weak and react only with selected cells that are positive for the antigen.

LINKAGE DISEQUILIBRIUM

One other phenomenon must be described because of its importance in the HLA system. In the Rh system, the blood groups C, D, and e are found together more often than one would expect on the basis of their individual gene frequencies. The same thing is commonly found within the HLA system, and one often finds a number of genes associated in a haplotype more often than would be expected on the basis of chance alone. This linkage disequilibrium, as it is called, suggests that some selective process results in the common association of HLA-A1 and HLA-B8, of HLA-2 and HLA-B12, and others (Table 22-2). Disequilibrium between the B and D series alleles may account for some of the problems in correlating the results of serotyping with allograft survival, since matching for B series alleles would, by disequilibrium, often result in matching for D series alleles as well. Similarly, typing for associated B series alleles might result in inferential typing for associated D alleles in certain disease

HLA-B LOCUS CROSS–REACTIVITY

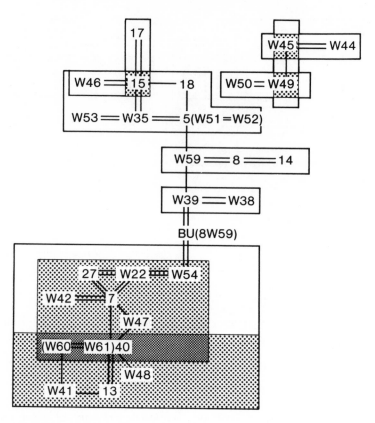

FIGURE 22-5. HLA-B locus cross-reactivity patterns. (From Miller, WV and Rodey, G: *HLA Without Tears.* American Society of Clinical Pathologists, Chicago, 1981, with permission.)

TABLE 22-2. Some of the HLA Alleles Associated by Linkage Disequilibrium

| | Haplotype | | Frequency Percentage | |
A	B	D	Observed	Expected*
A1	B8		9.8	2.1
A3	B7		5.4	2.1
	B8	D3	8.6	1.4
	B7	D2	3.9	1.8

*The expected haplotype frequencies were calculated under the assumption of no association. (From Miller, WV and Rodey, G: *HLA Without Tears.* American Society of Clinical Pathologists, Chicago, 1981, with permission.)

states. This situation has already been reported with gluten enteropathy in which there was initial association between HLA-B8 and the disease, but then a much higher association between HLA-Dw3 and the disease was subsequently demonstrated.

CROSSING OVER

Final mention should be made of another event that occasionally complicates HLA typing interpretation. During meiosis, exchange of material between the paired chromosomes occurs. The farther apart two loci are on a given chromosome the more likely are these genetic exchanges. Indeed, the frequency of these crossover events, as they are called, allows us to precisely map the genes on the chromosomes to determine their location and their distance from one another.

TECHNIQUES OF HISTOCOMPATIBILITY TESTING

The techniques employed in histocompatibility testing are basically similar to those used for erythrocyte compatibility testing, that is, known sera are used to type test cells, recipient serum is evaluated for the presence of unexpected antibodies to HLA antigens, and crossmatching of donor and recipient is customarily employed.

Preformed antibodies to tissue antigens of both donor and recipient may cause significant complications of transplantation or transfusion. Preformed antibody in donor plasma to recipient leukocytes has been associated with severe pulmonary infiltrates and respiratory distress following transfusion. Preformed recipient lymphocytotoxic or leukoagglutinating antibodies to donor antigens have been associated with accelerated graft rejection, with febrile nonhemolytic transfusion reactions, and with poor response to platelet or granulocyte transfusion.

Crossmatching in the histocompatibility system may involve examination for both serologically defined compatibility and lymphocyte-defined compatibility. Serologic crossmatching is performed by a leukoagglutination technique or by cytotoxicity, either conventional or enhanced by a variety of techniques. Lymphocyte defined compatibility is assessed by the mixed lymphocyte reaction or one of its modifications.

HLA ANTIGEN DETECTION

The agglutination methods used initially to define the HLA complex have given way to a standardized, precise microlymphocytotoxicity test.[22] Cytotoxicity methods require only 1 to 3 μl of serum, are sensitive and reproducible, and do not require exceptional skill or expensive equipment.

Heparinized blood is used, since many other anticoagulants inhibit the complement binding necessary for the test. As little as 2 ml of fresh heparinized blood is centrifuged and the buffy coat aspirated. A purified lymphocyte suspension is prepared, most commonly by centrifugation on a Ficoll-Hypaque gradient. Residual agglutinated red cells and granulocytes are packed in the bottom of the gradient, and platelets remain in the supernatant. The concentrated lymphocytes from the gradient's interface are further purified by washing to complete the cell preparation for conventional A, B, and C testing. If, however, lymphocytes for DR typing are required, further preparation is necessary. DR typing requires purified B lymphocytes with relatively few T lymphocytes present. The mixed lymphocyte suspension is incubated with neuraminidase-treated sheep erythrocytes, which react with the T lymphocytes to form large rosettes. The rosettes are removed by differential centrifugation, leaving a purified B-cell concentrate suitable for testing with DR typing sera.

Antiserum test trays are prepared by dispensing 1 μl of serum into each well and covering it with 5 μl of mineral oil to prevent evaporation. The antiserum trays are usually frozen until just prior to use.

The lymphocyte suspension is mixed and about 1 μl of cell suspension added to each well. The trays are incubated for 30 minutes at room temperature, then 5 μl of rabbit complement are added to the cell serum mixture. The complement and the cell-serum mixture are then incubated for an additional 60 minutes for the cytotoxicity reaction to occur.

Cytotoxicity is indicated by staining with special dyes, most commonly eosin: dead cells are unable to exclude the eosin; live cells exclude it normally. The reaction is fixed with formalin and each well is read in an inverted phase-contrast microscope. The strength of the reaction is coded numerically: the number 8 is used for a strong positive with essentially all cells killed; the number 1 is used for a negative reaction in which viability is the same as in the controls. By scoring the reaction of each known serum with test cells, a phenotype can be assigned.

A, B, C, and DR typings are essentially identical with the exception of the cell preparation. A, B, and C typing is performed on a mixed cell suspension, but DR typing requires a purified B lymphocyte suspension.

HLA-D TYPING

Because allografted tissue is rejected by a lymphocyte-mediated immune response, as well as by an antibody response, tests have been developed that use a biologic response of lymphocytes to foreign antigens as a measure of histocompatibility. The mixed lymphocyte reaction (MLR) test is especially important since it provides an in-vitro model in which lymphocytes can be used both as responders to foreign antigens and as stimulators carrying those antigens. For example, lymphocytes of the recipient are mixed with lymphocytes of the donor, the donor lymphocytes having been previously treated with mitomycin C to prevent mitotic activity. The response of the recipient cells to these treated donor cells in the mixed lymphocyte reaction is measured by the incorporation of radioactive thymidine into the responding cells during cell division. If the responding cells have been stimulated, large amounts of labeled thymidine are incorporated into the newly synthesized DNA. This incorporation can be quantitated in a liquid scintillation counting device. Appropriate controls and duplicate samples must be tested, which means that the procedure is not only time consuming, but also expensive. The MLR reaction recognizes the antigenic differences on stimulator cells; therefore, it follows that cells that bear the same antigens as the responding cell will cause no stimulation. This would indicate that the stimulator and the responder cells are the same HLA-D type.

In order to type for HLA-D antigens, stimulator cells from individuals known to be homozygous for HLA-D series antigens are used. Initially, these homozygous D typing cells were obtained from HLA identical children of first-cousin marriages. More recently, similar cells have been found, although infrequently, in the general population. Cells of both types are called homozygous typing cells.

In order to type, homozygous typing cells of each known phenotype are set up in MLR as stimulators against the test cells. Lack of response in MLR indicates that the test cell bears the same antigen as the homozygous typing cells.

When the DR system was discovered it was hoped that one could perform D typing serologically, which would allow detection of the HLA-D phenotype by a much simpler test than the difficult MLR. Unfortunately, DR antigens are just that—D related—but not D identical.

HLA ANTIBODY DETECTION TECHNIQUES

Demonstration and identification of HLA antibodies are similar to that of unexpected red cell antibodies, that is, the unknown serum is tested against a panel of cells whose phenotype is established. Unlike erythrocytes, however, cells from a large panel of donors must be selected if antibodies to even fairly common specificities are to be demonstrated. A panel of at least 15 to 25 carefully selected cells is required for initial screening, and a panel of at least 40 to 60 cells is required for accurate antibody identification. Because the cells can be preserved for only a short period of time, laboratories that do not have a high volume of typing must rely on a "walking panel" or frozen lymphocytes for subsequent testing. Freezing lymphocytes in trays has the advantage of rapid preparation, enabling serum to be screened in just a few hours.

The test serum is evaluated in a straightforward microlymphocytotoxicity test identical to that used for antigen detection. If antibodies to the DR system are to be identified, then purified B lymphocyte suspensions of known phenotype must be used.

OTHER TECHNIQUES

The leukoagglutination test, which provided the data for the initial description of the HLA system, is still in widespread use.[23] A mixed suspension of lymphocytes, granulocytes, and platelets is incubated with the test serum at 37°C. Direct agglutination of the suspension can be observed under a phase microscope, but, unfortunately, the test is insensitive and relatively nonspecific. Although HLA antigens can be detected by this system, under some circumstances granulocyte-specific antigens may also be detected and false negatives are extremely common. The test seems most valuable in pretransfusion testing for granulocyte transfusion. It is rarely employed prior to transplantation, and its value prior to platelet transfusion is uncertain.

Attempts to enhance the microlymphocytotoxicity test led to the addition of antiglobulin serum to the reaction. Antiglobulin serum produces a substantial increase in sensitivity and is commonly employed for crossmatching prior to allografts. It has not been used widely for HLA typing, perhaps because adequate typing sera that do not require antiglobulin conversion are available.

The improved sensitivity of the antiglobulin technique caused it to be coupled with fluorescent or enzyme labels to permit semiquantitative or quantitative reading of the result. These immunofluorescent or enzyme-linked immunospecific assays (ELISA) can be used for crossmatching prior to platelet and granulocyte transfusion and transplantation or for detection of platelet-specific and granulocyte-specific antibodies.[24]

CLINICAL SIGNIFICANCE OF THE HLA SYSTEM

Blood transfusion is a common cause of alloimmunization to HLA antigens since conventional transfusions are rich in platelets, granulocytes, and lymphocytes. Leukocyte-poor and frozen, washed erythrocytes contain few cells bearing HLA antigens and are, therefore, unlikely to produce alloimmunization or a transfusion reaction in patients previously alloimmunized. These products are usually used in patients who experience severe and recurrent febrile nonhemolytic reactions to transfusion, but their cost and availability do not warrant routine use to prevent alloimmunization.

TESTING FOR PLATELET TRANSFUSION

Combined chemotherapy programs have led to a dramatic increase in platelet transfusions in the past decade. Patients may be exposed to hundreds of different donors with as many HLA phenotypes, so that alloimmunization has become common—often limiting continuing chemotherapy. Yankee, Grumet, and Rogentine[25] found that HLA-matched platelets could sometimes restore satisfactory increments in such transfusions, and, based on their findings, blood collection agencies set up files of HLA-typed donors. Initially, it was felt that the pool necessary for effective transfusion services would necessarily be very large because the chance of finding a perfectly matched donor for a given patient would be quite small. Duquesnoy, Filip, and Aster[26] found that it might not be necessary to match perfectly for all HLA antigens, since it was often possible to substitute a crossreactive antigen. For example, an HLA-A1, B8; A11, B17 recipient might receive platelets from an A1, B8; A3, B17 donor, since A3 and A11 have been shown to be crossreactive. By substituting crossreactive antigens, a much smaller group of willing donors could serve a given group of patients. It has become clear, however, that even a close HLA matching cannot assure good platelet responses in all alloimmunized recipients. HLA-C antigens, untyped until very recently, might be responsible for some of these discrepancies, but non-HLA antigen systems seem to be even more likely candidates. Thus, it seems necessary to develop crossmatch techniques that will prevent platelet incompatibility in the face of HLA identity. A variety of techniques have been proposed, but at the time of this writing no single system has emerged.

GRANULOCYTE TRANSFUSION THERAPY

There are conflicting data on the importance of histocompatibility testing for granulocyte testing. In patients who are alloimmunized, as shown by leukoagglutination or granulocyte cytotoxicity assays, histocompatible granulocytes may prevent severe febrile reactions, although there are many false-negative and false-positive results. At this time, most would probably agree that a leukoagglutination assay is of value in granulocyte transfusion therapy and should be performed prior to transfusion. Lymphocytotoxicity seems to be of limited value in predicting either febrile reactions or transfusion response. HLA typing is probably of value in the alloimmunized recipient but of questionable value in the patient with no evidence of preformed antibodies to granulocytes.

Just as there are platelet-specific antigens detected by special techniques, so are there granulocyte-specific antigens not demonstrated by lymphocytotoxicity. They are occasionally responsible for febrile transfusion reactions and poor responses to granulocyte therapy, but have more often been implicated in neonatal granulocytopenia in which maternal antibodies to granulocytes cross the placenta to destroy the fetal granulocytes.[27]

HISTOCOMPATIBILITY TESTING FOR BONE MARROW TRANSPLANTATION

Bone marrow transplantation is used to treat patients with severe aplastic anemia, immunodeficiency disease, and various forms of leukemia. Rejection of the transplanted marrow and graft-versus-host disease are two of the major complications associated with bone marrow transplantation and histocompatibility plays a major role in both. Rejection of the marrow is unlikely if the patient is HLA identical for A, B, C, D, and DR determinants as measured by serotyping and the MLR. ABO compatibility is also important, since ABO-incompatible marrow transplants are often rejected in an accelerated fashion.[28] Even with perfectly matched donors, graft-versus-host disease poses a serious threat to bone marrow transplants. MLR tests using the donor as responder are essential and must be negative before a marrow transplant can be entertained.

HISTOCOMPATIBILITY TESTING FOR RENAL ALLOGRAFTING

Although initial studies question the value of histocompatibility testing for kidney transplant procedures, recent data strongly support the value of HLA serotyping.[29,30] The best correlations are for those donors well matched for HLA-B and DR alleles. The DR alleles seem especially important, since they provide recognition signals in the cellular immune response, and HLA-B alleles are in high linkage disequilibrium with DR alleles. Careful matching of HLA-B and DR alleles can provide a many-fold increase in the chances of kidney graft survival. HLA and ABO matching are important, but a crossmatch using the most recent serum sample from the intended recipient must be performed also. The crossmatch is usually enhanced with antiglobulin serum, and, if a previous recipient antibody screen had been positive, then that sample is crossmatched with a proposed donor as well.

It is clear that prior blood transfusion will produce a higher incidence of alloimmunization, and it might be supposed that blood transfusion should be avoided or at least that HLA antigens should be removed from donor blood. To the contrary, evidence strongly suggests that prior blood transfusion actually improves the chances of graft survival significantly over those grafts in untransfused patients[31,32].

HLA TESTING IN DISPUTED PATERNITY

While HLA polymorphism is the nightmare of transplant surgeons, it is the dream of population geneticists. It has provided the genetic tool to study population migrations and ethnic divergence not previously available. Not surprisingly, this valuable procedure has come to the attention of lawyers and courts as a more precise means of resolving cases of disputed paternity. By employing HLA-A and HLA-B locus typing, alone, the exclusion rate of falsely accused fathers is as high as 90 percent; in combination with common red cell antigen typing, exclusion rates as high as 95 percent are achieved. An example of an exclusion follows:

Mother's phenotype	A1, Aw19; B5, B17
Child's phenotype	A1, Aw32; B15, B17
Child's maternal haplotype	A1, B17
Obligatory paternal haplotype	Aw32, B15
Excluded putative father's phenotype	A1, Aw24; B8, Bw35
Excluded putative father's possible haplotypes	A1, B8/Aw24, Bw35, or A1, Bw35/Aw24, B8

In this case, the putative father is excluded because his phenotype could not have produced the obligatory haplotype.

An example of nonexclusion is illustrated as follows:

Mother's phenotype	A1, A3; B7, Bw35
Child's phenotype	A1, A11; B7, B27
Child's maternal haplotype	A1, B7
Child's obligatory paternal haplotype	A11, B27
Putative father's phenotype	A2, A11; B7, B27
Putative father's possible haplotypes	A2, B7/A11, B27, or A2, B27/A11, B7

In this case, the father cannot be excluded because he could have produced a required haplotype (A11, B27). Since A11, B27 is a relatively rare haplotype, the probability that that child and the putative father shared it by chance alone is relatively low—less than 1 percent.

In summary, in disputed paternities that cannot be resolved by simple ABO testing, HLA-A and HLA-B locus testing permits absolute exclusion of up to 90 percent of falsely accused males and can statistically include true fathers with the probability of greater than 90 percent in most cases.

HLA AND DISEASE ASSOCIATION

To date, more than 30 diseases have been described in which significant HLA antigen frequency deviations occur relative to comparably matched control groups.[33] The number of HLA antigens showing significant association with disease is somewhat restricted relative to the total number of specificities. HLA-B27 increases are found in a variety of rheumatologic disorders; HLA-B27 and Dw3 are increased in many diseases with autoimmune features. Of the more than 75 HLA specificities, only about 20 are associated with diseases, and of the 20 all but 4 are HLA-B, HLA-D, or HLA-DR specificities. Associated diseases tend to share some general features: weak, familial propensity; chronicity; disease onset in adulthood; suspected environmental ideologies; and immunologic aberrations, such as autoimmunity, often occur.

There are possible explanations to account for these associations, but the exact causes are unclear. There is no question that genetic factors coded within or near the HLA complex confer susceptibility to the development of a variety of diseases. The mechanisms by which this occurs are still unsolved, but it seems likely that this susceptibility is somehow related to altered immunologic responsiveness in many cases. It is also probable that the diseases in question have multifactorial ideologies involving multiple gene interactions and environmental factors. When all these factors are identified, the prospects for practicing preventive medicine will be enormous!

REFERENCES

1. DAUSSET, J: *Leukoagglutinins. IV. Leukoagglutinins and blood transfusion.* Vox Sang 4:190, 1954.
2. DAUSSET, J: *Iso-leuco-anticorps.* Acta Haematol 20:156, 1958.
3. PAYNE, R: *The association of febrile transfusion reaction with leukoagglutinins.* Vox Sang 2:233, 1957.
4. VAN ROOD, JJ and VAN LEEUWEN, A: *Leukocyte grouping: A method and its application.* J Clin Invest 42:1382, 1963.
5. TERASAKI, PI and McCLELLAND, JP: *Microdroplet assay of human serum cytotoxins.* Nature 204:998, 1964.
6. TERASAKI, PI, et al.: *Microdroplet testing for HLA-A, -B, -C, and -D antigens.* Am J Clin Pathol 69:103, 1978.
7. World Health Organization: *Nomenclature for factors of the HL-A system.* Bull WHO 39:483, 1968.
8. CEPPELLINI, R, et al.: *Genetics of leukocyte antigens. A family study of segregation and linkage.* In Curtoni, ES (ed): *Histocompatibility Testing.* Munksgaard, Copenhagen, 1967, p 149.

9. SANDBERG, L, et al.: *Evidence for a third sub-locus within the HLA chromosomal region.* In Terasaki, PI (ed): *Histocompatibility Testing.* Munksgaard, Copenhagen, 1970, p 165.

10. BACH, RH and HIRSHHORN, K: *Lymphocyte interaction. A potential histocompatibility test in vitro.* Science 143:813, 1964.

11. BAIN, B and LOWENSTEIN, L: *Genetic studies on the mixed leukocyte reaction.* Science 145:1315, 1964.

12. BACH, FH and AMOS, DB: *Hu-1: Major histocompatibility locus in man.* Science 156:1506, 1967.

13. DUPONT, B, et al.: *Typing for MLC determinants by means of LD-homozygote and LD-heterozygote test cells.* Transplant Proc 5:1543, 1973.

14. VAN ROOD, JJ, et al.: *The serological recognition of the human MLC determinants using a modified cytotoxicity technique.* Tissue Antigens 5:73, 1975.

15. McDEVITT, HO and LANDY, M (eds): *Genetic Control of the Immune Responsiveness Relationship to Disease Susceptibility.* Academic Press, New York, 1972.

16. D'AMARO, J: *W4 (4a) and W6 (4b) in diverse human populations. Demonstrations of their genetic identity in population and segregation studies.* Tissue Antigens 5:386, 1975.

17. THORSBY, E: *Biological function of HLA.* Tissue Antigens 11:321, 1978.

18. KLEIN, J: *Biology of the Mouse Histocompatibility 2 Complex.* Springer, Berlin, 1975.

19. BERNOCO, R, et al.: *HLA molecules at the cell surface.* In Dausset, J (ed): *Histocompatibility Testing.* Munksgaard, Copenhagen, 1972, p 527.

20. FRANKLIN, EC: *Beta-2 microglobulin—small molecule—big role?* N Engl J Med 293:1254, 1975.

21. TERASAKI, PI, et al., op cit.

22. TROUP, CM and WALFORD, RL: *Cytotoxicity test for the typing of human lymphocytes.* Am J Clin Pathol 51:529, 1969.

23. VAN ROOD, JJ and LEEUWEN, AJ: *Leukocyte grouping. A method and its application.* J Clin Invest 42:1382, 1963.

24. GUDINO, M and MILLER, WV: *Application of the enzyme linked immunospecific assay (ELISA) for the detection of platelet antibodies.* Blood 57:32, 1981.

25. YANKEE, RA, GRUMET, FC and ROGENTINE, GN: *Platelet transfusion therapy: The selection of compatible platelet donors for refractory patients by lymphocyte HL-A typing.* N Engl J Med 281:1208, 1969.

26. DUQUESNOY, RJ, FILIP, DJ and ASTER, RH: *Hemostatic effectiveness of selectively mismatched platelet transfusions in refractory thrombocytopenic patients.* Blood 46:1056, 1975.

27. VERHEUGT, FWA, et al.: *A family with allo-immune neonatal neutropenia: Group specific pathogenicity of maternal antibodies.* Vox Sang 36:1, 1979.

28. CLIFT, RA, et al.: *Marrow transplantation from donors other than HLA-identical siblings.* Transplantation 28:235, 1979.

29. *Scandiatransplant report: HLA matching and kidney graft survival.* Lancet i:240, 1975.

30. TING, A, WILLIAMS KA and MORRIS, PJ: *HLA-DR matching and B-cell crossmatching in renal transplantation.* Transplant Proc 12:495, 1980.

31. OPELZ, G, et al.: *Effect of blood transfusion on subsequent kidney transplants.* Transplant Proc 5:253, 1973.

32. OPELZ, G and TERASAKI, PI: *Improvement of kidney graft survival with increased numbers of blood transfusions.* N Engl J Med 299:799, 1978.

33. BARBOSA, J and YUNIS, EJ: *HLA and disease.* In Miller, WC and Grumet, FC (eds): *HLA Typing.* American Association of Blood Banks, Washington, DC, 1976.

34. THORSBY, E, et al.: *Typing for HLA (LD-1 or MLC) determinants.* In Kissmeyer-Nielsen, F (ed): *Histocompatibility Testing.* Munksgaard, Copenhagen, 1975, p 415.

35. ALBRECHTSEN, D, SOLHEIM, BG and THORSBY, E: *Serological identification of five HLA-D associated (Ia-like) determinants.* Tissue Antigens 9:153, 1977.

36. BARNSTABLE, CJ, et al.: *The structure and evolution of the HLA-Bw4 and Bw6 antigens.* Tissue Antigens 13:334, 1979.

37. BOURGUIGNON, LY, et al.: *Participation of histocompatibility antigens in capping molecularly independent cell surface components by their specific antibodies.* Proc Natl Acad Sci 75:2406, 1978.

486

CHAPTER **23**

PATERNITY TESTING

MARGARET A. BROOKS

The question of how parentage is ascertained has been with us for centuries. One of the first recorded cases involving disputed parentage was recorded in the Bible. In the Old Testament,[1] two women claimed the same child. The alleged mothers came before King Solomon, who resolved the case by threatening to cut the child in half in order to allow each claimant to share the child equally. The "true" mother relinquished her claim in order to spare the life of the child, and Solomon, in his wisdom, had no further trouble in awarding custody of the child.

The concept of using blood tests to solve this kind of problem also goes back to ancient times. Dr. Herbert Silver[2] tells of two tests recorded in Japanese folklore of the 12th century describing tests in vogue at that time. When someone claimed to be heir to an estate, a drop of his blood was permitted to drip onto the skeleton of his alleged relative. If the blood soaked in, the claim was upheld; if it did not, the claimant was considered an imposter. A second test was used to determine if two persons were related. Drops of blood from each individual were allowed to fall into a basin of water. If the drops came together, a "blood relationship" was established; if they flowed apart, it was considered proof that no relationship existed.

The reliability of blood tests available to study a relationship has improved considerably, and tests are currently based on established genetic principles. Today, blood tests are based on detection of genetic "markers" in various blood components and can rule out familial relationships with greater certainty in the great majority of cases. These tests can also provide strong evidence in establishing that such relationships exist.

SOCIOLEGAL ASPECTS

In recent years these so-called "paternity tests" have come to the attention of the legal community and there has been a simultaneous marked increase in the number of disputed paternity cases examined by the courts. This trend can be explained by several social and legal changes.

From the social viewpoint, we know that illegitimacy is increasing at a remarkable rate. An American Medical Association-American Bar Association report[3] stated that more than 1,700,000 illegitimate children were born during the 5-year period from 1966 to 1970. This report also stated that the number of illegitimate children born throughout the United States exceeds 10 percent of all births; in many urban areas this rate stands at 40 percent, and in a few locations (e.g., Baltimore) the rate is as high as 50 percent. A more recent figure reported by the federal government estimates that at least 16 percent of all births are out of wedlock.

The mothers of these illegitimate children are often not able to provide the necessary child support and turn to society (social services) for help. The number of people receiving welfare is unprecedented and is creating a burden that many taxpayers find overwhelming. In the legal community new legislation has brought the economic and social problems of the illegitimate child to the attention of the public.

Beginning in 1968, the status of the illegitimate child was addressed by the Supreme Court. Decisions based on the Equal Protection Clause of the Federal Constitution established the principle that a nonmarital child has the same legal rights as a legitimate child. Supreme Court decisions have affected a number of areas:

1. Support
2. Inheritance
3. Custody

4. Birth records
5. Welfare laws

Once paternity has been established the following happens:

1. Child support should be determined on the same level as for legitimate children in a divorce case;
2. The illegitimate child has some intestate inheritance rights given by a 1977 Supreme Court decision.
3. The father may be awarded custody in some situations;
4. Birth records may be reissued or amended with reference to illegitimate status removed;
5. A nonmarital child may make claims and be compensated as a dependent.

The Uniform Parentage Act,[4] which has been adopted by many states, comments in a prefatory note that the concept of "substantive legal equality of children regardless of the marital status of their parents seemed revolutionary if one considered existing state law on the subject." This act addresses many of the problems associated with illegitimacy. The concept of illegitimacy is set aside and ways of being legitimate are defined.

In 1975, the federal government enacted legislation concerning child support enforcement described by Dr. H.D. Krause as follows:

The legislation is too new to allow conclusions to be reached whether it contains all the answers, but it is clear that it contains many. By 1977, more than one billion dollars has been collected [from the child's father] under the program. It is not exaggeration to say that this Act represents, to date, the most important federal legislative venture into family law generally, and it may revolutionize the area of Paternity.

Public Law 93-647–Title IV D[5] provides for the following:

1. States are to establish plans for child support enforcement including establishment of paternity when necessary;
2. An elaborate process is established for HEW to monitor State's performance and compliance;
3. Generous incentives are provided for effective performance, and conversely, penalties are exacted for decreased support;
4. Absent fathers are traced through Social Security records and other Federal bureaus (except the census);
5. Debt of an absent father is assigned to the State for collection;
6. Enforcement by Internal Revenue Services is used as a last resort;
7. States can save money collected over and above their AFDC (Aid to Families of Dependent Children) payment;
8. There is a legal requirement that mothers must cooperate in ascertaining paternity.

The use of scientific data that is objective and accurate can be an important factor in helping to solve sociolegal problems related to disputed parentage. It should be noted that although paternity testing constitutes the majority of laboratory investigations in disputed parentage, other issues may also be resolved. Some of these include claimed familial relatives among immigrants, claims of maternity of babies mixed up in nurseries, lost relatives, identification of missing persons and custody demands by persons claiming to be related to a child.

SELECTION OF TEST SYSTEMS

Genetic markers can be defined as recognizable characteristics inherited from parents and strictly controlled by genes on a pair of chromosomes. Recognizable characteristics can be gross physical qualities such as hair color, or serologically detectable properties of blood components, or biochemical and other attributes. The AMA-ABA report[3] lists over 60 markers they had found suitable thus far for use in paternity testing. This list is not complete and will no doubt continue to grow as our technology expands. It has been established that genetic markers are encoded by particular genes (or DNA segments) at specific sites on a specific chromosome. To be suitable for paternity testing, markers must follow Mendel's basic rules of inheritance.

1. Unit Inheritance: The unit of inheritance (gene) is transmitted through generations intact.
2. Allelic Segregation: A pair of genes (one obtained from each parent and found on separate chromosomes) is never found in the same gamete, but is always separate and passes to two different gametes.
3. Independent Assortment: Different pairs of genes assort independently of each other, unless the different genes are linked on the same chromosome.

According to Thompson and Thompson in their book *Genetics in Medicine*,[6] suitability for genetic study of a marker is determined by:

1. A single and unequivocal pattern of inheritance;
2. Accurate classification of different phenotypes by reliable techniques;
3. A relatively high frequency of each of the common alleles;
4. Absence of effect of environmental factors, age, interaction with other genes, or other variables in the expression of the trait.

Of the 60 useful markers, approximately 20 are in general use. If the list is examined closely, it becomes apparent that some of the systems are much more useful than others. Reagents (antisera) used in testing for some markers (antigens) are rare and available for selected studies only. Additionally, the cost of testing for all these markers would be prohibitive. It then becomes necessary to be selective in choosing test systems. The usefulness of a system is defined by how often it can be expected to exclude a wrongly accused man. This information is referred to as "prior probability of exclusion" (PPE).[7] The PPE can be calculated for each test system by:

1. Listing all possible mating trios that will result in an exclusion of the alleged father;
2. Calculating the occurrence of these random matings using genotype and phenotype frequency charts for a given racial group;
3. Combining the results for all trios in a system;
4. Combining the results for all systems to be used.

The results of these calculations may be different from published figures if genotype and phenotype frequencies vary for the group or geographic area in question. Listing all the matings in all systems that would result in exclusion (combined PPE of several test systems) is best accomplished by a computer, especially if HLA is one of the test systems. In addition to the usefulness of the system, it is advisable to choose markers for which both the technology and reagents are available at a reasonable cost. Other considerations are reliability of markers, numbers of cases that can be tested at one time, test simplicity, and independence of the marker systems (coded on different chromosomes). The authors of the AMA-ABA report[3] recommended the use of the seven test systems listed in Table 23-1.

DRAWING OF SAMPLES

Once test systems are chosen the next step to consider is the collection and processing of samples to be tested. In most laboratories, blood samples are drawn directly from the involved individuals (e.g., mother, child, alleged father). This is a very important procedure. Paternity cases are generally referred to a laboratory by the courts or by agencies acting for the courts. Very often the cases will not be resolved until a trial is held and a judge or jury renders a decision based on evidence presented by prosecutors and defense attorneys. If blood testing information is to be

TABLE 23-1. Test Systems Recommended by AMA-ABA[3]

Genetic Marker or System	Mean Probability of Exclusion of Non-Fathers		
Red Cell Antigens	Black	White	Japanese
ABO	.1774	.1342	.1917
MNSs	.3206	.3095	.2531
Rh	.1859	.2746	.2050
Duffy	.0420	.1844	.1159
Kell	.0049	.0354	0
Kidd	.1545	.1869	.1573
Cumulative PPE six systems	63.37	72.26	64.24
HLA	.92	.92	.92
Cumulative PPE seven systems	97.07%	97.78%	97.14%

submitted to the courts, it is wise to take all precautions necessary so the information will be acceptable.

This begins with the identification of the parties to be tested. Most laboratories find it desirable to use more than one method of identifying their clients. Some methods to consider are:

1. Confrontation may be used in which all parties are present at the same time to identify each other. This may cause problems if the parties are hostile.
2. Identification sheets may be used to record name, address, birthday, transfusion history, identifying number (social security or driver's license numbers), marital status, and so on.
3. Interview information may be checked with information provided from the referring agency.
4. Photographs of individuals or the group may be used.
5. Fingerprints of adults and heelprints of infants may be taken.

When drawing the samples the tubes used should be clearly labeled (Fig. 23-1) with the following information:

1. Name of laboratory
2. Date of sample
3. Sample number
4. Mother's name (or that of alleged father or child)
5. Case designation
6. Client's initials
7. Technologist's initials

Case designation is often not included but becomes important if several cases are under study at the same time. It is possible for two persons in two different cases to have the same name. Case designation, which is the last name of the mother and alleged father, should assure that the correct partners are grouped together. Labels should be correctly prepared before being placed on the tubes and should be checked and initialed by the client after blood is drawn. The technologist drawing samples should also check and initial tubes after drawing to verify that he checked labels and attached them correctly. It may be helpful if the mother's, alleged father's, and child's labels are color coded to provide for spot identification.

Once the samples are in the laboratory it should be possible to verify what happens to them as testing occurs (audit trail). It is necessary to assure the court that it is not possible for unauthorized persons to have access to the tubes or the test results. This constitutes a chain of custody.

If a laboratory accepts samples drawn at other locations, the drawing center is responsible for the identification and accurate drawing procedures outlined above. A laboratory's responsibility begins when the samples are received into custody. It is advisable to make written notations concerning the following items:

1. Delivery of samples—Was a common carrier, U.S. Post Office, or delivery service used, or was it picked up by laboratory personnel at an airport or

Sample # ____________ Date ________________

Mother's Name ________________________________

Case Desig. ______________ vs ____________

Patient's Ints. __________ Tech's Ints. __________

Sample # ____________ Date ____________

Put. Father ________________________________

Case Desig. ______________ vs __________

Patient's Ints. __________ Tech's Ints. ______

Sample # ____________ Date ____________

Child's Name ________________________________

Case Desig. ______________ vs ____________

Patient's Ints. __________ Tech's Ints. __________

FIGURE 23-1. Labels for tubes. For spot identification, it is helpful if the three labels are color coded (e.g., mother red, father blue, child black).

bus station, and so on? Record signature of persons receiving samples, shipping number, date, time, and how the shipping container was sealed.

2. Opening of shipping container—Record signature of person opening container, date, time, condition of samples, how tubes were sealed, and condition of labels.

All these notations should be made upon receipt of the samples (Fig. 23-2).

Generally, when court appearances are requested, considerable time has elapsed between receipt and testing of samples and court testimony. For this reason, it is desirable to have records documenting exactly what did occur at the time of collection and analysis. Once the blood samples are logged in, procedures that assure the integrity of samples drawn at the laboratory should also be followed.

SEND REPORT TO: DRAWING CENTER: DATE SAMPLES
                                                                                      WERE DRAWN:

It is very important that all requested information is provided. We need to know if any party
has received blood transfusions within four (4) months prior to testing. If so, give dates where
indicated. Also, we need to know the race of the involved parties for use in computation of
probabilities. Please use the following codes: W-White, B-Black, M-Mexican, O-Oriental,
AmI-American Indian.

PATIENT INFORMATION: PLEASE TYPE OR PRINT ALL INFORMATION

Lab #	Names:	Race	Birthdate	Trans.	Drawn By
	Mother:				
	Alleged Father #1:				
	Alleged Father #2:				
	Child #1:				
	Child #2:				

Drawing Witnessed By: Transported to Airport By:

FOR LABORATORY USE ONLY:

How did samples arrive at Lab: Delivered By: Picked up at:

Received by: Date: Time: ID/Air Bill #:

Opened By: Date: Time: Condition of Package:

Tubes Received:	Black	Red	Yellow	Stoppers Sat.	Labels Sat.	Cond. of Samples	Misc.
Mother:							
Alleged Father #1:							
Alleged Father #2:							
Child #1:							
Child #2:							

FIGURE 23-2. Information and custody sheets.

RED AND WHITE CELL TESTING

Laboratories in the United States have been performing blood tests for cases of disputed parentage for over 30 years. Early reports included results of ABO, MN, and Rh typings. These test systems could exclude about 50 percent of falsely accused men and were considered informative by the courts only when there was an exclusion. The MN system has been expanded to include S,s typings and the Kell, Duffy, and Kidd systems have been added as reagents became available. A few laboratories report results of red cell enzyme and serum protein markers. In the early 1970s technology developed that allowed for the classification of antigens found on human leukocytes (HLA). This test system has received considerable publicity in recent years as a powerful tool for paternity testing.

RED CELL TESTING

The ABO blood group system was discovered in 1901; the MNS in 1927. The Rh system has been in use since the 1940s, and Kell, Duffy, and Kidd were among the many systems that have been defined in the last 30 years. Our present laboratory test procedures have evolved because we know these antigens are expressed on red cells and because their presence can be demonstrated using relatively simple procedures. These procedures require the presenting of test cells (RBCs) to a specific antibody under optimal conditions for the reaction of the antigen indicated by the known antibody. The absence or presence of the antigen is decided according to the absence (negative reaction) or the presence (positive reaction) of agglutination (clumping). It is possible to determine whether a reaction has occurred by examination of the antigen-antibody mixture in the test tube over a magnifying mirror. In some instances, it is desirable to confirm a negative reaction by examining the mixture microscopically.

The antigens in these six systems and the technology required to demonstrate their presence is familiar to medical technologists—blood bankers in particular. ABO and Rh_o (D) types of patients requiring blood transfusions are always determined. If a patient presents no cross-match problems these are usually the only blood groups studied. In some cases, problems are encountered and additional testing is indicated. Sometimes, other antigens in the Rh system or in the MNS, Kell, Duffy, Kidd, and a host of other blood group systems must be evaluated. Suitable testing reagents, knowledge of appropriate test procedures, and knowledge of expected patterns of reaction for each of these systems are required to enable blood bankers to safely transfuse these problem patients. The antigen testing in parentage studies is similar to that in these blood bank procedures.

It is possible to purchase the reagents needed to test for most of the antigens in these six systems from commercial manufacturers who are regulated by the Food and Drug Administration. This agency approves a license for these companies after regular inspection of their facilities, approving their standard operating procedure, and evaluating their finished product. These companies, of their own accord, employ a variety of quality controls and claim to be even more stringent than the FDA in assuring antisera of specificity, avidity, and titer, as well as freedom from interference and contamination.

The knowledge of how to use these reagents and of how to solve these blood bank problems is required of technologists working in the "specials" level of blood banking.

HLA TESTING

The seventh recommended system, HLA or human leukocyte antigen, was discovered by Daussett and Ivanyi in 1954. While each of the red cell systems are defined by differing numbers of antigens, none demonstrates the polymorphism (great number of alleles) of this system. The technology developed rapidly once it became apparent that these antigens were to play an important role in the transplantation of solid organs and the transfusion of some blood components. These antigens are present on most body tissue (not red cells or trophoblasts), but for the serologic test procedures that have been developed, the lymphocyte is the test cell of choice. Present technology requires the harvesting of lymphocytes and the presenting of these cells to a panel of test sera containing reagent antibody specific for antigens of the HLA system. Testing is performed using a microtiter tray and microliters of test sera. Cells and sera are added to the wells of the trays in measured amounts using a microtiter syringe and capillary pipettes modified to deliver very small, uniform drops of reagents.

The antibody-antigen mixture is maintained at conditions expected to enhance the reaction. If any antibody-antigen reaction occurs, the addition of complement will result in loss of cell membrane integrity. The cytotoxic effect is detected by the use of a vital stain (e.g., trypan blue or eosin). Positive reactions are indicated by stained cells. In the absence of an antibody-antigen complex, the cell wall remains intact and the cell membrane excludes the dye. The cell remains clear and glistening. Absence of staining represents a negative reaction (see Color Plate 18).

A limited number of reagents for HLA testing are available commercially, but the PPE of the HLA system would be greatly reduced by using only these few antisera; therefore, it becomes necessary to find other sources. It is well established that multiparous females and multiply-transfused persons are a good source of antibody. A panel of cells of known antigen types is used to screen the sera of possible donors. Once antibody is detected and procured, the laboratory must be capable of testing and standardizing the reagent. It is often necessary to trade with other laboratories if a panel of test sera is to be maintained that will enable the laboratory to test for a sufficient number of specificities. HLA laboratories perform such studies to develop antisera, not just for paternity studies, but to insure the survival of transplants (allograph compatibility tests) and to study the major histocompatibility system of man in various disease states.

If red cell and HLA technology are compared, few similarities are found in equipment, procedures, or test results. However, the principles of the testing for paternity work rely on the same basic principle of using known antibody to detect the presence of an antigen (genetic marker) on the test cells.

EXCLUSIONS

Once accurate test results are compiled the next step is to determine if an exclusion of the alleged father has occurred. Exclusions are characterized as First Order (direct) or Second Order (indirect).[8]

FIRST ORDER EXCLUSION

It may be readily apparent after inspection of test results that a contradiction to the expected pattern of inheritance has occurred. If the child's blood type exhibits an antigen lacking in both parents, a first order exclusion is demonstrated. If neither parent can contribute one of the two allelic genes that appear in the child's phenotype it must be assumed that a child of the given phenotype could not result from a mating of the adults tested.

Since maternity is not in question, it must be assumed that the alleged father is wrongly accused. With proper testing procedures, it is rare that a first order exclusion can be false, so that only one test is considered sufficient for a determination of nonpaternity.

SECOND ORDER EXCLUSION

Second order exclusions can be explained in one of three ways[9]:

1. The child is negative for two different allelic antigens, both of which are present in the alleged father, for example:

   | Alleged Father | AB | Probable genotype | A/B |
   | Child | O | Probable genotype | O/O |

   A/B genotype indicates the A antigen from one parent and the B antigen from the other. One antigen or the other must be present in offspring. Group O type indicates the absence of both A and B antigen.

2. The child appears homozygous for an antigen demonstrated in the mother but not present in the alleged father, for example:

Alleged father	N	Probable genotype	N/N
Mother	M	Probable genotype	M/M
Child	M	Probable genotype	M/M

3. The alleged father appears homozygous for an antigen not present in the child:

Alleged Father	CCDee	Probable genotype	CDe/CDe
Mother	ccdee	Probable genotype	cde/cde
Child	ccdee	Probable genotype	cde/cde

Explanations 2 and 3 can be used interchangeably.[10] Choice depends on traditional use and clarity of expression. Pitfalls (e.g., low-frequency alleles, unidentified alleles, and amorphs) are to be found in most of the recommended blood group systems. In order to guard against false exclusions, additional testing may be indicated and it is desirable to demonstrate two second order exclusions before concluding nonpaternity.

Note that the weakness of second order or indirect exclusions is that one assumes that phenotype denotes genotype. This is not always a correct assumption. Examples of such fallacies are given below.

PITFALLS

Pitfalls may be encountered in the following blood groups:

ABO: Cis-AB (A and B on the same chromosome and inherited together from one parent).

Bombays (Oh—cells fail to react with anti-A, anti-B, anti-A,B, and anti-H, yet have anti-A, anti-B, and anti-H in their serum. A, B, and H genes may be present but not expressed because the necessary H substance has not been produced for conversion to A or B).

Suppressed A_1 typings.

MN: Mg, Mk (fail to react with either anti-M or anti-N).
Ss: S^u (amorph).

Rh: Null, C^w, C^u, E^u, Rh32, depressed antigens, and so on.

Kell: Ko.

Duffy: Fy, Fy^x.

Kidd: Jk.

Problems may be encountered when making the assumption that a given phenotype represents a specific genotype. Before it can be assumed that the following test results indicate a homozygous genotype, it is necessary to test for the low-frequency allele (i.e., Mg):

Test Sera	M	N	Possible Genotype
Alleged father	−	+	N/N
Child	+	−	M/M

If Mg testing is included:

Test Sera	M	N	Mg	Possible Genotype
Alleged father	−	+	+	N/Mg
Child	+	−	+	M/Mg

Not only would it be incorrect to conclude an exclusion, but if calculations for probability of paternity were made, with Mg as the paternal obligatory gene (necessary from the biologic father), the results would no doubt be in the "practically proven" category. If Mg typings are negative it is still not appropriate to base a conclusion of nonpaternity on this system alone, because of the possibility of other even less-frequent alleles or amorphs. In black patients, it is not appropriate to make assumptions that S+s− or S−s+ phenotypes represent homozygous genotypes of S/S or s/s. The amorph S^u (frequency of 0.11) must be considered (i.e., S/S^u or s/S^u).

In the Rh system the most common of the "low-frequency" alleles to consider is C^w. Any time test results of C+c− suggest the genotype C/C, C^w typings are indicated. This system has many pitfalls to consider, as indicated by the possible maternal exclusion encountered in the case study in Figure 23-3.

RED CELL TYPINGS

SYSTEM: ABO		MNSs								Rh								Kell		Duffy		Kidd			
NO.	Group	Mg	M	N	S	s	S^u		SUM.	D	D^u	C	E	c	e	C^w	SUM.	K	k	Fy^a	Fy^b	Jk^a	Jk^b		
MOTHER	B		+	+	-	+				+		+	-	-	+	-		-	+	-	-	+			
A.F.	B		+	-	-	+				+		-	-	+	+	-		-	+	-	-	-			
CHILD	B		+	+	-	+				+		-	-	+	+	-		-	+	-	-	-			

Possible Genotypes:

Mother	CDe/CDe	R1R1	A.F.	cDe/cDe	RoRo	Child	cDe/cDe	RoRo
	CDe/Cde	R1r		cDe/cde	Ror		cDe/cde	Ror
	CDe/ ?	R1?					cDe/ ?	Ro?

HLA TYPINGS

No.	A 1	A 2	A 3	A 9	A 10	A 11	A 28	A 29	AW 19	AW 23	AW 24	AW 25	AW 26	AW 30	AW 31	AW 32		B 5	B 7	B 8	B 12	B 13	B 14	B 18	B 27	BW 15	BW 16	BW 17	BW 21	BW 22	BW 35	BW 37	BW 40		CW 2	CW 3	CW 4
MOTHER	X		X																	X											X						
A.F.		X							X														X								X						
CHILD	X								X											X			X														

Possible HLA Haplotypes:

Mother A1,B18/A3, BW35 A.F. A2,BW35/AW19,B14 Child A1,B18/AW19,B14

MATERNAL FAMILY STUDIES

SYSTEM: ABO		MNSs								Rh								Kell		Duffy		Kidd			
NO.	Group	Mg	M	N	S	s	S^u		SUM.	D	D^u	C	E	c	e	C^w	IDAT on C typings	K	k	Fy^a	Fy^b	Jk^a	Jk^b		
MAT. GRANDMA			-	+	-	+				+		-	-	+	+	-	+	-	+	-	-	+			
MAT. SISTER			+	+	-	+				+		-	-	+	+	-	+	-	+	-	-	+			
MAT. BROTHER			+	+	-	+				+		-	-	+	+	-	-	-	+	-	-	+			

Possible Genotypes:

Mat.	cDe/cDe	RoRo	Mat.	cDe/cDe	RoRo	Mat.	cDe/cDe	RoRo
Grandma	cDe/cde	Ror	Sister	cDe/cde	Ror	Brother	cDe/cde	Ror
	cDe/ ?	Ro ?		cDe/ ?	Ro ?		cDe/ ?	Ro ?

ADDITIONAL TESTING

1. Adsorption and elution of Maternal Grandmother's and Maternal Sister's cells with anti-rh' (C) gave positive results.
2. Typing for rh'(C) variant RH:32 also gave positive results for Maternal Grandmother, Maternal Sister, Mother and Child.

Conclusion: Mother's Genotype = CDe/Rh:32De
Child's Genotype = cDe/Rh:32De

FIGURE 23-3. Case Study #1.

PROBLEMS WITH MULTIPLE CHILDREN

Not all cases consist of only three people. Some may involve more than one child. In multiple child cases, additional information must be utilized in interpreting results. Consider the following:

CASE #1

	Major Blood Group	Possible Genotype
Mother	O	O/O
Alleged father	A_1	A_1/O
Child	O	O/O

CASE #2

	Major Blood Group	Possible Genotype
Mother	O	O/O
Alleged father	A_1	A_1/O, A_1/A_1, A_1/A_2
Child	A_1	A_1/O

CASE #3

	Major Blood Group	Possible Genotype
Mother	O	O/O
Alleged father	A_1	A_1/A_2
Child	A_2	A_2/O

In each individual case no exclusion would be indicated; however, if all three children were tested as a family group, we would see the following:

	Major Blood Group	Possible Genotype
Mother	O	O/O
Alleged father	A_1	
Child #1	O	O/O
Child #2	A_1	A_1/O
Child #3	A_2	A_2/O

The three phenotypes of the children could not result from the union of a mother of group O and a man of group A_1. The genotype of a man who types A_1 may be A_1/O and he could be the father of child #1 and #2, but not of #3. If his genotype is A_1/A_2 he could father child #2 and #3, but not #1. Only additional test systems or family studies would help to determine paternity for the three children.

Linkage in some test systems can be useful in determining paternity. Consider the MNSs system in the case study of fraternal twins in Figure 23-4. If each twin is considered individually or only phenotypes are considered, an exclusion is not apparent. Because the genotype of Twin A is most likely Ns/Ns, it can be determined that the mother's genotype is MS/Ns. This child must receive Ns from each of his parents. Twin B's genotype is NS/Ns. The mother can contribute only Ns. The discernible Ns/Ns genotype of the alleged father could not produce an NS child. Because both children were tested at the same time and genotypes could be deter-

RED CELL TYPINGS

SYSTEM:	ABO		MNSs							Rh									Kell		Duffy		Kidd		
NO.	Group	Mg	M	N	S	s	U	S	SUM.	D	Dᵁ	C	E	c	e	Cᵂ	SUM.	K	k	Fyᵃ	Fyᵇ	Jkᵃ	Jkᵇ	
MOTHER	O		+	+	+	+				+		+	-	+	+			-	+	+	+	+		
▓	O		-	+	-	+				-	-	-	-	+	+			-	+	-	+	+		
TWIN A	O		-	+	-	+				+		+	-	+	+			-	+	+	+	-		
TWIN B	O		-	+	+	+				+		+	-	+	+			-	+	+	+	+		

Possible Genotypes:
Mother: MS/Ns
A.F.: Ns/Ns
Twin A: Ns/Ns
Twin B: NS/Ns

Neither parent had NS

HLA TYPINGS

No.	A1	A2	A3	A9	A10	A11	A28	A29	A19	AW23	AW24	A25	AW26	A30	AW31	AW32	B5	B7	B8	B12	B13	B14	B18	B27	BW15	BW16	BW17	BW21	BW22	BW35	BW37	BW40	CW2	CW3	CW4
MOTHER		X	X																X							X									
A.	X									X									X									X							
TWIN A	X	X																	X							X									
TWIN B		X	X																X												X				

Possible HLA Haplotypes:
Mother: A2,B8/A3,BW16
A.F.: A1,B8/A11,B35
Twin A: A2,B8 from mother; A1,B8 from A.F.
Twin B: Either A2, B8 or A3,BW16 from mother.
Did not inherit either A1 or A11 from A.F.

ADDITIONAL TESTING

	ENZYMES							SERUM PROTEINS			OTHER MARKERS		
	ADA	AK	AcP	PGM	6PGD	Hb	EsD	HP	Tf	Gc	Umpk	Gm	Km
MOTHER	1-1	1-1	AB	1-1	AA	A	2-1	2-1	CC	2-1	1-1	1,2	+
A.F.	1-1	1-1	AA	2-1	AA	A	1-1	2-2	CC	2-1	1-1	3,5;13	+
TWIN A	1-1	1-1	AA	1-1	AA	A	2-1	2-2	CC	2-1	1-1	5,13	-
TWIN B	1-1	1-1	BB	1-1	AA	A	2-2	2-1	CC	2-1	1-1	1	+

Additional testing can exclude the A.F. as the father of Twin B by Acp, EsD, and Gm. He cannot be excluded as the father of Twin A.

FIGURE 23-4. Case Study #2.

mined, it is possible to know how the MN and Ss antigens are linked. Therefore, it is possible to exclude the alleged father as the biologic father of Twin B. A second order exclusion in the HLA system confirms this finding (see Fig. 23-4). Additional test systems confirm nonpaternity of Twin B with no evidence of exclusion of Twin A. This case may be another example of superfecundation (i.e., twin pregnancy produced by fertilization of two ova produced by the same woman by spermatozoa of different males).

In the HLA system linkage can not be used as proof of exclusion. Haplotype analysis will not always produce four possible pairs of A and B locus antigens within one family. Crossing over occurs 0.8 percent of the time, allowing the possibility of five or more haplotypes.

	Phenotypes	*Possible Genotypes*
Mother	A1, A29, B12, B37	A1, B12/A29, B37
Alleged father	A2, A3, B18, BW22	
Child #1	A1, A2, B12, B18	A1, B12/A2, B18
Child #2	A2, A29, BW22, B37	A29, B37/A2, BW22

A phenotype of HLA A2, A3, B18, BW22 is consistent with paternity if crossing over occurred.

PROBABILITY

To calculate probability of paternity it is necessary to know the races of the persons in the nonexcluded paternity case and to have the phenotype frequencies for the racial group or groups to which they belong. If phenotype frequencies are available, it is possible to calculate gene frequencies. This is done using one of two methods. Gene frequencies may be determined by a direct count if the system has codominant alleles (i.e., no amorphs or recessive genes). Because amorphs exist in all blood group systems and are not always rare, it is usually more appropriate to use the second method. This method is based on the Hardy-Weinberg principle or the random mating law (selection of mates is independent of blood types and therefore is random). Likewise, the genetic markers passed by parents to an offspring are also random. This method assumes that in a two-allele system with gene frequencies of "p" and "q" that $(p + q)^2 = 1$. By squaring both sides of the equation, it can be expanded to $p^2 + 2pq + q^2$, where p^2 or q^2 would represent individuals homozygous for the gene represented by p or q; 2pq would stand for the heterozygotes. The same principle may be utilized to accommodate systems with more than two alleles and is one of the most useful tools in population genetics. Gene frequency charts are available and if the phenotype frequency of a given group agrees with the phenotype frequency the gene frequencies were derived from, it is appropriate to use those charts.

The attempt to diagnose paternity begins with the assumption that the mother is the biologic mother of the child. Consequently, the child's phenotype is, in part, the result of the mother's genetic make-up. Suppose, for example, the mother's phenotype is MNS and the child's type is MSs. Lists of genotypes and genes constituting the genotypes follow:

	Mother	*Child*
Phenotype	MNS	MSs
Genotypes	MS/NS	MS/Ms
	MS/N^u	
	M^u/NS	
Genes	MS, NS, M^u, N^u	MS, Ms

The biologic mother is obliged to pass one of the genes in her genotype to her child; it is referred to as the maternal obligatory gene (MOG). As a result, any maternal genotype not bearing a possible MOG can be dropped from consideration. In the above example, the only gene mother and child have in common is MS; therefore, the mother's genotype is either MS/NS or MS/N^u, not M^u/NS. The identification of possible MOGs enables the determination of possible paternal obligatory

502

genes (POGs). To this end, listings of the child's possible genotypes in MOG/POG-ordered combinations must be constructed:

Phenotype		Genotype	
		MOG	POG
Child	MSs	MS	Ms

Note that any accused man whose phenotype could not be expressed in part by one of the possible POGs can be excluded from paternity. In the example, the biologic father must be able to pass the "Ms" gene.

In the event the alleged father cannot be excluded, two probabilities are of interest: (1) the probability that the child resulted from the mating of the mother and alleged father, and (2) the probability that the child was the result of the mating of the mother and a random man.

The probability that a child was the result of the mating of the mother and alleged father is the summation, over all possible genotypes, of the probabilities that the following pairs of events occurred simultaneously: (1) the mother passed the MOG to her child, and (2) the alleged father would pass the POG to his child. Due to the independence of the two events, the probability of their simultaneous occurrence is the probability that the mother passed the MOG times the probability that the alleged father passed the POG. Furthermore, the probability that either event occurred is the relative frequency of its occurrence in the set of genotypes that express the mother's and alleged father's phenotypes, respectively. Consequently, the probability of the simultaneous occurrence of MOGs and POGs is the product of the frequencies with which the mother would pass the MOG to her child, and the frequency with which the alleged father would pass the POG to his child.

Given a set of genotypes, the frequency with which a particular gene will be passed to an offspring is dependent upon the following elements: (1) genotype frequency, (2) relative genotype frequency of all genotypes belonging to the set, and (3) the probability that the particular gene will be passed from the genotype. The first element, the genotype frequency, is the probability with which the two genes occur simultaneously times the number of ways the genotype could occur. Owing to the fact that the genes were inherited independently, this product is simply the product of the two gene frequencies times the number of ways the genotype could occur. Recall from our example that the mother's genotype is either MS/Ns or MS/N^u. Given the gene frequencies listed below, genotype frequencies are computed as follows:

Gene Frequencies		Genotypes	Genotype Frequencies	
MS	.2578	MS/NS	$2(.2578)(.0628)$	$= .0324$
NS	.0628	MS/N^u	$2(.2578)(.0004)$	$= \underline{.0002}$
N^u	.0004		TOTAL	.0326

The second element or the relative genotype frequency indicates the frequency with which the genotype occurs in the set of genotypes. It is easily computed by dividing the genotype frequency by the sum of the genotype frequencies:

Genotypes	Relative Genotype Frequencies
MS/NS	.0324/.0326 = .9939
MS/Nu	.0002/.0326 = .0061
	TOTAL 1.0000

Finally, the probability with which a particular gene is passed from a genotype is dependent upon whether the genotype is heterozygous or homozygous. In the event of homozygosity, the gene appearing in the genotype will be passed 100 percent of the time. On the other hand, in the heterozygous state, each gene of the genotype has a 50 percent chance of being transmitted. Consequently, the frequency with which a gene is passed from a set of genotypes is the sum of the products of the probability that a particular gene will be passed from the genotype and the relative genotype frequency. Continuing with the example, the frequency with which the mother will pass the MS, NS, or N^u gene to her child is computed as follows:

MOG	Frequency
MS	.5(.9939) + .5(.0061) = .5000
NS	.5(.9939) = .4970
Nu	.5(.0061) = .0030
	TOTAL 1.0000

The frequency with which the alleged father will pass the POGs is computed in a similar fashion; however, in this case the alleged father is not assumed to be the biologic father of the child. Consequently, all genotypes indicating the alleged father's phenotype must be considered. Suppose the alleged father's phenotype is MNSs and the gene frequencies are as follows: MS = .2578; NS = .0628; Ms = .2907; Ns = .3877; then

Phenotype	Genotypes	Genotype Frequencies
MNSs	MS/Ns	2(.2578)(.3877) = .1999
	Ms/NS	2(.2907)(.0628) = .0365
	TOTAL	.2364

Genotype	Relative Genotype Frequencies
MS/Ns	.1999/.2364 = .8456
Ms/NS	.0365/.2364 = .1544

Gene	Frequency
MS	.5(.8456) = .4228
NS	.5(.1544) = .0772
Ms	.5(.1544) = .0772
Ns	.5(.8456) = .4228

Recall that the probability that the child has resulted from the mating of the mother and alleged father is the sum of the products of the frequency with which the mother passes the MOG and the alleged father passes the required POG. The resulting number is referred to as "X."

MOG/POG   X

MS   Ms $(.5)(.0772) = .0386$

In a similar fashion, the probability that a child was the result of the mating of a mother and a random man can be computed. Once again it is the summation, over all possible genotypes, of the probability that the following pairs of events occurred simultaneously: (1) the mother passed the MOG to her child; and (2) a random man passed the POG to his child. The two events are independent; therefore, the probability of their simultaneous occurrence is the probability that the mother passed the MOG times the probability that a random man would pass the POG. Furthermore, the probability that the mother passed a possible MOG is its relative frequency of occurrence in her set of possible genotypes, whereas the probability that a random man passed the POG is simply the frequency with which the gene is found in the population. As a result, the probability of the simultaneous occurrence of MOG and POG is the product of the frequency with which the mother passes the MOG and the gene frequency of the corresponding POG. The resulting probability is referred to as "Y." Recall that the gene frequency of MS is .2578.

Child

MOG/POG   Y

MS   Ms $(.5)(.2578) = .1289$

The above logic is used to calculate X and Y values for each blood group system, and the final results must be combined. Recall that the systems appropriate for use in paternity testing adhere to Mendel's rules of inheritance. Therefore, the probability with which a specific constellation of phenotypes results from the mating of a mother and an alleged father or a mother and a random man is the product of the corresponding probabilities for each system. In other words, the probability with which the mother and alleged father produced the child is the product of all X values and the probability that the child was the result of the mating of the mother and random man is the product of the Y values. The final step is to calculate the two values that are of main interest: (1) X/Y representing the odds that a mating of the alleged father and mother would result in a child of the given phenotype as compared with the same event occurring if the mother mated with a random man, and (2) X/X + Y = the plausibility of paternity (Table 23-2).

INTERPRETATION OF RESULTS

In many laboratories using the seven test systems recommended by the AMA-ABA report[3] (with a PPE of 97 percent), exclusions are reported in approximately 25 percent of the cases tested. The enactment of Public Law 93-647, which asks for ascertainment of paternity, has made it necessary for laboratories to change their method of reporting results in the remaining 75 percent of cases. Prior to the enactment of this law and a change in the attitude of the courts, a conclusion of "can not be ex-

TABLE 23-2. Probability Calculations

System	Phenotypes			Obligatory Genes			X	Y
	Child	Mother	A. Father	Maternal	Paternal		A. Father	Random Man
ABO	A₁	O	A₁	O	A₁		0.5612	0.2038
MNSs	NSs	MNS	MNSs	NS	Ns		0.2114	0.1939
Rh	Cc D ee	Cc D ee	cc D ee	CDe cde cDe Cde	CDe cde cDe Cde		0.4998	0.4101
Kell	Kk	kk	KK	k	K		0.9984	0.0359
Duffy	a+b−	a+b−	a+b−	fya fy	fya fy		0.9985	0.4424
Kidd	a−	a+	a+	Jkb Jk	Jkb Jk		0.1645	0.2450
HLA	A-03, A-11 B-07, B-27	A-01, A-03 B-07, B-18	A-02, A-11 B-27, BW21	A-03 B-07	A-11 B-27		0.0735	0.0010

X = .0007147
Y = .0000001
X/Y = 7147 to 1
X/X + Y = 99.99%

cluded" was sufficient. A number of states had laws that provided for the admission into evidence of reports finding exclusion of paternity. This policy is being challenged and changed. A number of states have either changed their laws or introduced statutes allowing calculations of probability of paternity to be admitted as evidence. Even when the laws have not been changed, the agencies representing the mother are requesting that calculations of probabilities be reported. They find the information very helpful when counseling the involved parties and when negotiating out-of-court settlements.

Many hours of court time and many thousands of dollars are being saved and justice may be served better. When resolution of a case requires a trial, the child will already be 2 or 3 years of age. The legal scenario often runs as follows: The mother will testify she gave birth to a child and name the date of birth. She will try to determine the date of conception and verify that a relationship existed between herself and the alleged father at that critical time. There may be other witnesses called to confirm the existence of this relationship and to pinpoint the time. The alleged father may testify that such a relationship never existed or if it did, not at the "critical time." Events that can verify happenings during this critical period become important. Since it is not customary to keep records to document this kind of relationship, it is often difficult for the true facts to be presented. The attitude of the legal community regarding the use of blood tests in this kind of situation was expressed by Justice Brennan while he was a member of the Appellate Division of the New Jersey Superior Court. He wrote

> In the field of contested paternity . . . the truth is often obscured because social pressures create a conspiracy of silence or worse, induce deliberate falsity. The value of blood tests as a wholesome aid in quest for truth in the administration of justice in these matters cannot be gainsaid in this day. Their reliability as an indicator of the truth has been fully established. The substantial weight of medical and legal authority attests their accuracy, not to prove paternity, and not always to disprove it, but "they can disprove it conclusively in a great many cases provided they are administered by specially qualified experts. . . ."

Since paternity cases are usually civil cases, it is only necessary to convince a judge or jury that paternity is "more likely than not" (preponderance of the evidence) to justify a verdict of guilty or produce an order to pay child support. This differs from criminal cases, in which a verdict of innocent is mandated so long as there is "a reasonable doubt." If a criminal case is tried by a jury, the jurors must be unanimous in their verdict, but in civil cases agreement by a specified number is sufficient.

Directors of some laboratories are concerned that probability calculations that result in numbers such as 99 percent will be given undue weight and will result in time-consuming trips to court. These are valid reservations, but many laboratories are routinely including statistical calculations in the conclusion of their reports. There have been workshops addressing the problem of how to perform these calcu-

RED CELL TYPINGS

NO.	SYSTEM: ABO Group	MNSs Mg	M	N	S	s	Su	SUM.	Rh D	Du D	C	E	c	e	Cw	SUM.	Kell K	k	Duffy fya	fyb	Kidd Jka	Jkb		
MOTHER	A1	-	+	-	+				+		-	-	+	+			-	+	-		-	+		
A.F.	A1	-	+	-	+				+		-	+	+	-			-	+	-		-	+		
CHILD	A1	-	+	-	+				+		-	-	+	+			-	+	-		-	+		

Because the alleged father appears to be homozygous E/E and the child did not inherit an E antigen, a second order exclusion is possible.

HLA TYPINGS

No.	A1	A2	A3	A9	A10	A11	A28	A29	AW19	AW23	AW24	AW25	AW26	AW30	AW31	AW32	B5	B7	B8	B12	B13	B14	B18	B27	BW15	BW16	BW17	BW21	BW22	BW35	BW37	BW40	CW2	CW3	CW4
MOTHER	X																		X								X								
A.F.					X					X									X								X	X							X
CHILD	X									X																	X								

ADDITIONAL hr"(e) TESTING

	hr^s(2 sera)	hr^b(2 sera)	hr"(7 sera)	hr"(2 sera)
A.F.	w+	+	+	-
CHILD	w+	+		

Many examples of Anti-hr"(e) are mixtures of Anti-hr^s

Titers for Dosage

A.F.

Antibody = rh"(E)

Control I R2R2 cell = 1:32
Control II R2r cell = 1:8
A.F.   = 1:8

Child

Antibody = hr"(e)

Control I rr cell = 1:32
Control II R2r cell = 1:4
Child   = 1:4

ADDITIONAL TESTING

	ENZYMES PGM1	GLO	GPT	EsD	ADA	AK	6PGD	SERUM PROTEINS Hp	Gc	Tf	OTHER MARKERS Gm	Km	
MOTHER	1	2	1-2	1	1	1	AA	1	1	CD	azb	1+3+	
A.F.	1-2	1-2	1	1	1	1	AA	2	1	C	azb	1-3+	
CHILD	1	1-2	1-2	1	1	1	AA	1-2	1	C	azb	1-3+	

Additional testing did not provide an additional exclusion which is necessary for a determination of non-paternity. Results of additional hr"(e) testing and titration studies make it necessary to consider the possibility of a hr"(e) variant.

FIGURE 23-5. Case Study #3.

MODERN BLOOD BANKING AND TRANSFUSION PRACTICES

lations at recent meetings of both the American Association of Blood Banks and the American Association of Clinical Histocompatibility Testing.

The final step is to formulate a report that contains:

1. Reference to the individuals tested
2. Summary of phenotypes
3. Interpretation of results
   (a) Exclusion—List reasons
   (b) No exclusion—Report probability of paternity

The interpretation of test results should only be undertaken by knowledgeable and experienced workers with a clear understanding of the scientific content as well as the emotional and social consequences of their report. The care given should be the same as in a medical report. It should be recognized that these test results can be just as consequential for the involved parties.

The pitfalls and cases cited are only a few examples of the many complications and problems encountered when test results are interpreted. As our knowledge expands, it will be important to be aware of additional variants and possible exceptions to the expected pattern of inheritance. It may be necessary to employ other technology, such as adsorption and elution, in order to confirm the presence of a weakened or suppressed antigen and to do titrations for additional evidence of dosage. These techniques may resolve some situations, but another option to consider is referral of samples to laboratories with expertise in other test systems (Fig. 23-5). It may be necessary to utilize one or more of these alternatives before a conclusion can be drawn.

REFERENCES

1. The Bible:1 Kings 3:16–27.
2. SILVER, H: *An introduction to paternity testing.* In *Paternity Testing.* American Association of Blood Banks, Washington, DC, 1978.
3. *Joint AMA-ABA guidelines: Present status of serologic testing in problems of disputed parentage.* Family Law Quarterly 10:247, 1976.
4. National Conference of Commissioners on Uniform State Laws (1973): *Uniform Parentage Act.*
5. KRAUSE, HD: *Legal considerations.* In *Paternity Testing.* American Association of Blood Banks, Washington, DC, 1978.
6. THOMPSON, JS and THOMPSON, MW: *Genetics in Medicine.* WB Saunders, Philadelphia, 1973.
7. WALKER, RH: *Probability in the analysis of paternity test results.* In *Paternity Testing.* American Association of Blood Banks, Washington, DC, 1978.
8. RACE, RR and SANGER, R: *Blood Groups in Man,* ed 6. Blackwell Scientific Publications, London, 1975.
9. LEE, CL: *Current status of paternity testing.* Family Law Quarterly 9:615, 1975.
10. HOUTZ, TD, et al.: *Utility of HLA and six erythrocyte antigen systems in excluding paternity among 500 disputed cases.* Forensic Sci Int 17:211, 1981.

CHAPTER **24**

MEDICOLEGAL IMPLICATIONS OF BLOOD BANKING AND TRANSFUSION SERVICES

L. RUTH GUY, PH.D.

Continues—

The day-by-day medicolegal responsibilities of blood banks and transfusion services seldom get much attention from those who are closely involved and who might incur greatest losses in litigation. This disinterest is due in part to the vague wording of existing laws and to the legal jargon that confuses the lay person. Nevertheless, malpractice insurance has skyrocketed, and the tendency of people to sue for real or imagined damage has increased as large financial settlements have been awarded to patients or their families in cases involving transfusions or donors. Sometimes the suits are based on activities over which blood bank or transfusion service personnel have little control.

CAUSES OF LITIGATION

INJURY TO THE DONOR

Blood banks have been sued for negligence in the case of blood donation because of infections and excessive damage to tissues at the site of the venipuncture.[1,2] So far as this author can determine, most of these cases have been settled out of court and few appear in legal literature. The blood bank is responsible for the following:

1. Ordinary care of the donor including the taking of an adequate history to assure that the donation of blood will not harm the donor, prompt medical attention in case of donor reaction, and caution regarding strenuous activities following donation.

2. Getting the informed consent of the donor or, in cases of a minor, the consent of a parent or guardian. Interviewers and donor room attendants must explain the procedure to the donor so that the donor knows what to expect.[3] Persons who are mentally incompetent to give informed consent probably should not be accepted as donors.

3. Exercising proper arm preparation and sterile techniques during the drawing of blood. Most cases of this kind have been settled out of court, but a few have resulted in the award of damages to the plaintiff.[2]

4. Cautioning the donor to rest before resuming normal activities and informing the donor of the possible danger of strenuous exertion following donation.

5. Having properly trained personnel available in reasonable proximity to the donor area during blood drawing. If a physician is not on the premises during the drawing of blood, arrangements must be made for nearby medical care in case of emergency. The staff must be trained and prepared to deal with the various kinds of donor reactions or injuries that might be anticipated.

ERRORS IN ORDERS

The physician is responsible for the written order for transfusion and for choosing the particular component needed. This responsibility cannot be delegated to non-medical personnel. Failure to order blood in an emergency also may constitute malpractice. In one case, the court awarded damages to the plaintiff because incompatible blood was transfused during surgery that the surgeon knew he had not ordered.

ERRORS IN PATIENT IDENTIFICATION

The majority of transfusion accidents occur because of errors in identification of the patient at the time the blood sample for compatibility testing was drawn, failure to maintain the chain of identification of the sample during testing, failure to issue the blood that was intended for the patient, or failure to identify the patient with the information attached to the unit of blood issued.

The venipuncture team, the nursing personnel, the attending physician, the blood bank personnel, and the transfusionist share these responsibilities. If an error is made by any one of these people, the patient can suffer damage.

TRANSMISSION OF DISEASE

Several diseases may be transmitted by transfusion, including malaria, syphilis, yaws, cytomegalovirus, and viral hepatitis. Of these, hepatitis B and hepatitis "non-A, non-B" are the most frequently transmitted and the most likely to give rise to litigation. Blood banks are responsible for carrying out careful selection of donors and using sensitive testing procedures to detect carriers in the donor population.

In addition bacterial contamination of blood, which may produce endotoxic shock, can cause grave damage to the patient and can result in a law suit on the part of the patient's family. In such cases, the patient rarely survives.

BASIS OF LITIGATION

When litigation does occur, the suit is most frequently based on negligence, implied warranty, or assault and battery.[1-3] Negligence is argued on the basis that standard safety precautions and procedures were not exercised. Malpractice suits based on implied warranty are more likely to occur if the blood was purchased as a product rather than provided as a service. For this reason the Food and Drug Administration

(FDA) requires that blood be labeled as coming from a "paid donor" or a "volunteer donor."

Assault and battery can be charged if there is injury to a donor or transfusion was given without consent of the patient or his family. Charges are rarely made in the case of transfusion unless there has been an unfavorable reaction. Blood cannot be infused if the patient or the patient's family has specifically refused permission. In the case of a minor, a court order may be obtained to transfuse if the parents have refused permission, but court orders do not apply to adults.

OTHER LEGAL CONSIDERATIONS

DOCTRINE OF CHARITABLE IMMUNITY

For many years the doctrine of charitable immunity was absolute in the matter of liability for harm resulting from negligence if the hospital or blood bank existed as a non-profit institution or was engaged in providing a charitable service.[2] Most courts no longer favor granting immunity to charitable institutions. For this reason, most blood banks and transfusion services would be well advised to carry liability insurance rather than depend on the court's decision in the matter of charitable immunity.

STATUTE OF LIMITATIONS

The statute of limitations varies from one state to another. Generally law suits for damages must be brought within 5 years of the event, but in some states the time is shorter, 1 to 5 years. The problem is more complicated than first appears. The statutory period does not begin until the patient should reasonably know that his injury was due to negligence. In the case of a minor, the statutory period does not begin until the child has reached legal maturity.

RIGHT TO PRIVACY

The Right to Privacy Act is applicable to medical records.[3] Records cannot be transmitted from one medical facility to another without the written consent of the patient. Published case reports and data for clinical research papers require the written permission of the patients involved if the information can be traced to the findings on an identifiable patient. In times past it was permissible to refer to a patient by identifying initials, but that is no longer permissible unless the patient grants specific written permission to do so.

STATE AND FEDERAL REGULATIONS

STATE LICENSURE

In addition to licensing various categories of medical personnel, some states require inspection and licensing of blood banks and clinical laboratories. Blood banks and transfusion services must conform to state and local regulations regardless of whether or not they meet the requirements for federal licensure or registration. It is the responsibility of the institution to make sure that personnel have the required licenses for practice as well as the institution.

FEDERAL REGULATIONS

The FDA has the responsibility of regulating, inspecting, and licensing all blood banks that are engaged in interstate commerce, that is, the shipment of blood or blood products across state lines.[4] Much of the attention is focused on the selection of donors, drawing of blood, processing of blood and blood products, storage, and shipment. In addition it regulates and licenses the manufacture of biologic products, containers for collection, and so on.

Nonlicensed blood banks and transfusion services must register with the FDA on an annual basis and furnish information regarding their operations. Unannounced inspections are carried out by FDA personnel with varied scientific backgrounds. Inspection is based on compliance with the latest revision of the Code of Federal Regulations (CFR), 21, Food and Drugs Parts 600 to 1299, and such changes as may have been published in the *Federal Register*. Theoretically, the revision of the CFR is published each April 1, but it is usually several months after that date before the publication becomes available. No written report is sent by the FDA unless there is evidence of significant noncompliance.

MEDICARE AND MEDICAID REGULATIONS

The laws pertaining to Medicare and Medicaid impose regulations on all institutions that serve Medicare and Medicaid patients.[5] The agency will accept accreditation by the Joint Commission on Accreditation of Hospitals (JCAH) in lieu of its own inspections. The JCAH, in turn, accepts the inspection and accreditation of clinical laboratories, including transfusion services, by the College of American Pathologists (CAP). To fulfill these requirements, additional standards must be met, including those pertaining to compatibility, immunohematology testing, and quality control. In addition Medicare and Medicaid requires a review of transfusions and transfusion practice by the medical staff or by one of its committees.

VOLUNTARY ACCREDITING AGENCIES

As noted above, in addition to the professional organizations and certifying agencies for the various categories of personnel, three voluntary agencies have inspection and accreditation programs: the American Association of Blood Banks (AABB),[4] the CAP,[6] and the JCAH.[7] These programs are usually more comprehensive than those of the federal and state agencies because these agencies are interested not only in the selection of donors, collection of blood, processing and storage of whole blood and components, and transportation of blood or components from one institution to another, but also the quality of personnel, compatibility testing, and transfusion practices. The CAP inspection of transfusion services is part of the inspection and accreditation of a hospital's entire group of laboratory services. The JCAH inspects and accredits the entire hospital. Neither the CPA nor the JCAH inspects accredited community blood banks.

The AABB Inspection and Accreditation program is limited to the inspection and accreditation of hospital transfusion services, hospital blood banks, and independent community blood banks serving a number of hospitals. The inspection is based on the current edition of *Standards for Blood Banks and Transfusion Services.*[8] The accreditation period is 2 years from the date of the approved accreditation. To be inspected by one of the voluntary agencies, the institution must apply to the sponsoring organization for that service. The inspectors are medical or scientific directors of blood banks and medical technologists with Specialist in Blood Bank (SBB) certification. The inspection and accreditation are a form of peer review and have no legal status other than giving evidence of approved, standard practice.

RESPONSIBILITIES OF HEALTH CARE PERSONNEL

BLOOD SUPPLIER

Institutions that draw and process blood or blood components for transfusion, whether in a hospital or a community blood center, have assumed a number of responsibilities, which include the selection of a qualified medical director and a staff of technologists, nurses, and clerical personnel who have sufficient education and training to perform their duties in an acceptable manner. Selection of adequately trained personnel applies to those persons covering night, holiday, and weekend shifts, as well as the usual working hours. Equipment and supplies must be provided so that work can proceed in an orderly manner. The blood bank also has the obligation to recruit healthy donors so that there is an adequate supply of blood to meet the needs of the community and is responsible for safety precautions so that donors will not be harmed by the drawing of blood. The responsibility to patients includes the provision of the safest blood possible at the lowest cost possible.

The community has the right to expect the provision of sufficient blood and components to meet its needs. Although both blood and money are necessary for the operation of a blood bank, there should be no profiteering with regard to provision of either blood or services.

HOSPITAL PERSONNEL

The hospital has the responsibility of maintaining a transfusion service, monitoring transfusion practice, and selecting a source of safe blood, whether it be collected and processed by hospital personnel or obtained from an outside source.

It is the responsibility of the hospital to obtain the services of a qualified medical director under whose supervision other personnel will work. If the technical and clerical personnel are hospital employees, the hospital must assume the legal responsibility for the selection of an adequate number of qualified personnel and for their acts. If the blood bank personnel are employees of the medical director rather than of the hospital, then the medical director must assume those obligations.

Nursing personnel are usually employees of the hospital. The hospital must assume the responsibility of choosing an adequate number of nurses who have the skills required for patient care. The hospital is responsible for the acts of nursing, housekeeping, dietary service, x-ray, maintenance, and all other hospital employees.

When a patient is transferred from one hospital to another, copies of records should be sent to the receiving hospital. Generally, crossmatched blood or blood components should not be transferred with the patient unless special arrangements have been made with the receiving hospital's transfusion service. The second or receiving hospital becomes responsible for future transfusions and should make sure that transferred blood has been properly refrigerated and handled during transit. Storage of transfused blood should be handled by the receiving hospital and compatibility testing should be repeated to be sure that no mistakes in identification of either the patient or transferred blood have occurred.

In order to fulfill Medicare-Medicaid laws, the hospital medical staff must appoint a transfusion committee or refer the duties for peer review of transfusion practices to another standing committee. The committee must review ordering and transfusion practices, transfusion safety, transfusion reactions, and hepatitis transmission in order to evaluate means of improving the transfusion service.

In addition, the hospital must maintain some system of continuing education for all personnel involved in patient care.

MEDICAL DIRECTOR

The medical director of a blood bank or transfusion service is legally responsible for the following duties[1,3]:

1. Exercising medical judgment in the care and selection of donors.
2. Selection of procedures and techniques.
3. Medical supervision of personnel.
4. Investigation of transfusion complications.
5. Investigation of post-transfusion hepatitis and other diseases that might be transmitted.
6. Monitoring transfusion practice and serving as a consultant in hemotherapy.

MEDICAL TECHNOLOGIST

Frequently the medical director and not the laboratory personnel will be named in a malpractice law suit, but indications are that this may be changing. The time may come when technologists and nurses will have to carry malpractice insurance.

The technologist is responsible for meeting the educational requirements for licensure and/or certification as required by the state or institution in which he or she is employed. Duties must be carried out with both moral and scientific integrity. Here the technologist is in a subordinate relationship with the medical director and the practicing physician. Orders must be carried out as transmitted, and clarification must be sought if there is doubt. Meticulous record-keeping becomes as important as test performance and generation of results. Copies of results of testing must go to the patient's chart and to the laboratory record with accuracy. Such records must be stored in such a manner that they can be retrieved if the need arises. In addition, the technologist must engage in continuing education to be sure that skills have not become obsolete.

ATTENDING PHYSICIAN

The attending physician entrusted with the primary care of the patient is responsible for issuing legible, clearly understood orders for blood or blood components. Legally, he must exercise great care in deciding whether or not the patient needs transfusion based on the patient's condition. The responsibility should not be delegated to others. The attending physician must investigate signs of adverse transfusion reaction and report them to the blood bank laboratory for further study. If a serious transfusion reaction has occurred, it is the responsibility of the attending physician to instigate prompt treatment.

Post-transfusion hepatitis must be reported to both state and federal agencies. The physician should submit a written report as soon as post-transfusion hepatitis is suspected, so that blood bank personnel can begin their investigation of the transmission. The attending physician is also responsible for making sure that the patient receives prompt medical care if post-transfusion hepatitis occurs.[4]

AVOIDANCE OF LITIGATION

The best way to avoid litigation is prevention of incidents that might lead to legal intervention.

LICENSE AND REGISTRATION. Blood banks must maintain state and federal license or registration as required.

INSPECTION AND ACCREDITATION. Inspection and accreditation by one or more voluntary peer organizations are evidence that the standards of safe, scientific practice are observed.

QUALITY CONTROL. Records of quality control testing of reagents, equipment, and blood components offer substantial evidence that high standards are maintained routinely and may serve as an account of the conditions at the time the alleged malpractice act occurred.

CONTINUING EDUCATION OF PERSONNEL.   Participation of all medical and technical personnel in continuing education offers good evidence that the personnel have kept themselves informed of advances in standards and procedures.

MAINTENANCE OF METICULOUS RECORDS.   Maintenance of meticulous records of all procedures that pertain to donors or patients is one of the best defenses one can offer in litigation. Complete, signed records are far more convincing than verbal testimony of personnel who may not be able to recall the details of particular incidents. Records of investigation of unfavorable reactions in either donors or patients should be well documented and signed. If a physician is consulted, his notes made at the time of the incident carry considerable weight in court. Above all else there must not be alteration of records without signed notations of why corrections were made.

BLOOD BANK PROCEDURES AND FORENSIC MEDICINE

The application of blood bank procedures to solving forensic problems is more fascinating to medical technologists than the pursuit of knowledge of the day-by-day medicolegal responsibilities in the routine blood bank operation. The focus of this section will be on the use of hematologic testing in criminal investigation. The tests are used as a means of identification that would relate blood stains, body fluids, and so on to either a victim or a person accused of a crime. Many advances have been made since the first recorded use of blood tests in murder trials more than 700 years ago. Chinese coroners were instructed to mix a drop of the victim's blood with a drop of the person's blood who was accused of the murder. If there was an homogenous mixture of the two drops of blood, the accused man was set free. If clumping occurred, the verdict of guilty was proclaimed and the accused was promptly executed.[9] The use of blood grouping tests in modern court cases began in 1926 in Germany, when little was known about the individuality of blood samples except ABO grouping.[10] In the United States, Dr. Alexander S. Wiener[11,12] and Dr. Leon Sussman[10] were instrumental in getting court acceptance of blood grouping results for ABO, Rh, and MN. The greatest amount of research and the application of sophisticated techniques has occurred in England during the last 20 years with other significant contributions being made by workers in the United States, France, Germany, Japan, and Russia.

SUBPOENAS

Blood banks and transfusion services are most frequently involved in court cases when transfusion records and personnel are subject to subpoena to present evidence in court.[1] On receipt of a subpoena both records and personnel may be required to appear in court. Only the records requested are to be submitted. Physicians are more frequently called to the witness stand than technologists, although the latter may also have to testify. Simple answers and frequently "yes" or "no" answers are advisable if possible, although occasional defense or prosecuting attorneys may engage in elaborate questioning in an attempt to discredit the witness. This practice has done much to discourage medically and scientifically oriented individuals from offering assistance to the courts.

IDENTIFICATION OF BLOOD GROUP SUBSTANCES

A specimen submitted as evidence in criminal cases must be identified and labeled according to the source in such detail that there can be no mistake of its origin. Freshly shed blood or blood drawn from either the victim or the defendant does not pose any unusual problems in testing except that a repeat sample may not be obtainable.

As far as other samples and stains are concerned, the state of preservation and the amount of material available may limit the kinds of testing that can be done. Stains are frequently submitted from carpeting, towels, bedding, clothing, and weapons, in addition to human or animal tissue. The state of contamination and preservation is variable. Stains on clean, dry pieces of cloth pose few problems, but criminals are seldom so considerate. Examination of moist or decaying samples that have been subject to many kinds of contaminants and environmental hazards may sorely limit the kinds of examinations that can be performed.

In any case, the chain of evidence must be maintained from the time that the evidence was collected until the final testing is complete. Each person must sign that the material was received and state its disposition. If possible the samples should be maintained in locked storage so that no tampering can occur. All slides, photographs, records, and residual material with intact identifications must be preserved and available for presentation as evidence if required.

Freshly shed blood or a sample drawn from a vein can be examined in much the same way as any fresh sample with regard to blood grouping and red cell enzymes.

Blood stains require special handling. The first question to be asked in examining a stain is: Is it blood? If it is blood, is it human blood? The tests used to detect occult blood in clinical samples may be used for forensic purposes, keeping in mind the limitations of the procedure. Of these, the o-tolidine dip stick test is most frequently employed.[13-15] The leuko malachite green test is more adaptable for use with materials that are presented as physical evidence in criminal investigation.[15] The Metropolitan Police Laboratory in London includes o-tolidine and peroheme tests in kits issued to Scenes of Crimes Officers, but prefers the Kastle-Meyer test for red blood cell peroxidase, the Takayama test for hemoglobin, and spectrophotometric studies for more definitive study.[14]

In order to determine the species of origin of stain material, precipitin tests are employed by several methods. Antibodies directed against humans and various commonly encountered animals, such as cattle, sheep, hogs, horses, dogs, cats, and so on, are available. The antisera must be carefully absorbed to rule out as much cross-reactivity as possible. The tube technique is probably employed more frequently than the other variations of the test. Saline extract of the stain under examination is layered over the antiserum. If antibody to the particular species of the stain is used, a white precipitate will form at the interface of the reactants.[14,15] The same principle applies whether the antiserum and stain extract are placed in capillary tubes, Ouchterlony gel diffusion systems, or counterelectrophoresis. Counterelectrophoresis and gel diffusion systems may be preferable because the reaction can be better preserved and photographed.[13,14] Passive agglutination tests using latex particles coated with antihuman serum and antihuman globulin (AHG) inhibition tests have also been used.[16,17]

Selection of stains and unstained control samples from unstained areas of the garment or other material is important. Each location must be clearly marked on the entire specimen from which samples were taken. The unstained sample should give negative reactions if positive findings from the stain are to be creditable.

Tests for blood group substances in stains can be done by several methods. If the stain is fresh, intact red blood cells may be harvested from the material using a saline wash. The red cell suspensions can be tested by the techniques routinely employed in the blood bank. Positive and negative controls should be included for each antiserum. Frequently, intact red blood cells can be obtained from freshly macerated tissue specimens if no liquid blood can be obtained.

Blood group agglutinins, anti-A and anti-B, can be detected in clean, dried stains up to 6 to 18 months. Saline extracts are made of the stain and mixed with red blood cell suspensions, group A, group B, and group O, respectively.[10,13] The test is read in the same manner as the reverse or serum grouping in the blood bank.

There are three approaches to red blood cell typing of stains: absorption and inhibition,[10,12] mixed agglutination,[18-22] and absorption and elution.[13,14,23-28] In the absorption and inhibition of agglutination tests, several dilutions of the stain extract are added to a preselected dilution of antiserum or lectin that will demonstrate a 2+ agglutination. Dilutions of the material are added to anti-A, anti-B, and anti-H lectin. If the blood group substance is present, the antiserum will be neutralized by the stain extract preventing the agglutination of cells with the corresponding antigen. The method is not as sensitive as the mixed agglutination or the absorption and elution techniques, but it has enjoyed wide acceptance in the United States owing to promotion of the method by Dr. Alexander S. Wiener. It has been used successfully to identify ABH, Rh, MN, and some of the other antigens.[10,12]

The mixed agglutination technique was first described by Coombs and Bedford[19] and Coombs and Dodd.[20] Bits of stained material are treated with antiserum and incubated for lengths of time that vary according to the blood group system involved, then thoroughly washed in saline to remove uncombined antibodies. Fibers from the washed samples are placed on properly identified glass slides, and a drop of a weak suspension (0.5 percent) of red blood cells of the appropriate blood type is added to each of the slides. Each mixture is covered with a glass cover slip. The cell suspension and the samples are allowed to stand 15 to 30 minutes at a temperature appropriate for best reaction with the antiserum used. The preparation is then examined microscopically. If the red cell antigen present in the sample has reacted with the antiserum, the corresponding red blood cells will be agglutinated onto the sample fibers.

The coating may not be uniform because of loss of some antigenic material in the washing stage. Although the procedure has been used successfully, it has not gained widespread use because of the time required and the tediousness of the procedure.

Absorption and elution methods have gained greater acceptance in other countries than they have in the United States. Single threads from stained material or clean white cotton threads to which a stain has been transferred can be examined by modifications of the heat elution method so familiar to blood bank technologists. Threads used for the negative controls are taken from unstained portions of the same material. The samples should be thoroughly dry before use. Threads are cut in lengths of 1.5 to 2 cm and attached with cellulose acetate adhesive to polycarbonate sheets that have been marked in sections to identify the samples and the antisera to be used. Appropriate antiserum is added to the various bits of thread attached to the sheet and then the sheet is incubated at an appropriate temperature and time for the particular antiserum used. After incubation the polycarbonate sheet is rinsed by spraying with chilled saline from a wash bottle, and then it is blotted. The sheet is immersed in a container of chilled saline for 30 minutes and agitated occasionally. It is removed from the saline, blotted dry, and placed in humid chambers. Indicator red cell suspensions of the appropriate type (0.1 percent suspension in 0.3 percent bovine albumin in saline) are added to the respective thread samples. The chamber is covered and placed in an incubator at 50°C for 15 minutes. Antibodies bound to that sample will be eluted into the cell suspension and will agglutinate cells carrying the corresponding antigen. Modifications of the method have been used for identifying many blood group antigens.[14,26-28,42] Depending on the state of preservation, some of the antigens will remain detectable for several years. Although automated procedures have been described, they have not gained wide acceptance.[29,30]

RED CELL ENZYMES

The polymorphic red cell enzymes are also used as identification markers in criminal investigation. The enzymes remain detectable in stains for 8 to 30 days, depending on the enzyme.[31] Starch and polyacrylamide gel electrophoresis are the most generally accepted procedures.[13,14,17] The enzymes most useful for identification have been adenylate kinase (AK),[32] adenosine deaminase (ADA),[13,14] acid phosphatase (AcP),[13,14] glucose-6-phosphate dehydrogenase (G6PD),[13,14] 6-phosphoglucomutase (PGM),[13,14] glutamate-pyruvate transaminase (GPT),[34] and alkaline phosphatase.[24,33,35] Transfused cells may interfere with testing.

POLYMORPHIC PROTEINS

The variations of haptoglobin,[36] Gm and Inv[14,37,38] groups, hemoglobin,[13,14,39,40] and alpha fetoprotein[41] also have been used as identification markers.

BODY FLUIDS AND TISSUES

The ABH blood group substances are present in the body fluids of secretors and on many tissue cells.

Blood group substances may be detected in saliva by absorption and inhibition and by absorption and elution. Undiluted saliva and several dilutions including 1 to 10, 1 to 100, 1 to 1,000, 1 to 10,000, and 1 to 100,000 should be examined to rule out prozones and spurious reactions.[10,13,14]

Semen and vaginal stains and fluid may be examined for ABH antigens as well as several of the enzymes.

ABH antigens can be detected in both fresh and preserved tissues. Modifications of the mixed cell agglutination technique can be used for examining routine tissue sections prepared for pathologic examinations.

TESTIMONY IN COURT

When called upon to testify in court, all written reports, workbooks, and residual samples must be submitted. Questions from attorneys are best answered as briefly and concisely as possible. In any case, the witness must be prepared for tedious cross-examination. Witnesses must not allow themselves to show annoyance during questioning.

Medicolegal testing is not usually carried out in the clinical laboratory. There are forensic laboratories established for this purpose. However, the forensic laboratory does offer satisfying careers for medical technologists who are interested in this field and are willing to learn the required skills.

REFERENCES

1. HUESTIS, DW, BOVE, JR and BUSCH, S: *Practical Blood Transfusion*, ed 2. Little, Brown & Co, Boston, 1976.
2. RANDALL, CH, JR: *Medicolegal Problems in Blood Transfusion.* Joint Blood Council, Washington, DC, 1962. Reprinted by Committee on Blood, American Medical Association, Chicago, 1963.
3. FEEGAL, JR: *Legal aspects of laboratory medicine.* In Henry, JB (ed): *Clinical Diagnosis and Management by Laboratory Methods*, ed 16. WB Saunders, Philadelphia, 1979, pp 2033–2038.
4. *Code of Federal Regulations: Food and Drugs, Title 21, Parts 600 to 1299.* US Government Printing Office, Washington, DC, 1979.
5. *Code of Federal Regulations: Federal Health Insurance for the Aged, Title 20, Ch III, Part 405, HIR-10 (6/67).* US Department of Health, Education and Welfare, Social Security Administration, Washington, DC, 1967.
6. *Inspection and Accreditation Check List, Section V. Blood Bank.* College of American Pathologists, 1979.
7. *Accreditation Manual for Hospitals.* Joint Commission on Accreditation of Hospitals, 645 N. Michigan Avenue, Chicago, 60611, 1979.

8. *Standards for Blood Banks and Transfusion Services, ed 10.* American Association of Blood Banks, Washington, DC, 1981.

9. Lu, HY: *Instructions to Coroners, China, circa 1250 AD.*

10. Sussman, LN: *Blood Grouping Tests. Medicolegal Uses.* Charles C Thomas, Springfield, Illinois, 1968.

11. Wiener, AS: *Blood Groups and Transfusions.* Charles C Thomas, Springfield, Illinois, 1943.

12. Wiener, AS: *The value of anti-H reagents* (Ulex europaeus) *for grouping dried blood stains.* J Forensic Sci 3:493, 1958.

13. Culliford, BJ: *The Examination and Typing of Blood Stains in the Crime Laboratory.* US Government Printing Office, Washington, DC, 1971.

14. *Biology Methods Manual.* Metropolitan Police Forensic Science Laboratory, London, England, 1978.

15. Moenssens, AA and Wigmore, JH: *Scientific Evidence in Criminal Cases,* ed 3. The Foundation Press, Mineola, NY, 1978.

16. Cayzer, I and Whitehead, PH: The use of sensitized latex in the identification of human blood stains. J Forensic Sci 13:179, 1973.

17. Grobbelaar, BG, Skinner, D and van de Gertenbach, HN: *The antihuman globulin inhibition test in the identification of human blood stains.* J Forensic Sci 17:103, 1970.

18. Coombs, RRA: *The mixed agglutination and mixed antiglobulin reactions.* In Ackroyd, JH (ed): *Immunological Methods.* Blackwell Scientific Publications, Oxford, 1964.

19. Coombs, RRA and Bedford, D: *The A and B antigens on human platelets demonstrated by means of mixed erythrocyte-platelet agglutination.* Vox Sang 5:111, 1956.

20. Coombs, RRA, Bedford, D and Rouillard, LM: *Blood group antigens on human epidermal cells demonstrated by mixed agglutination.* Lancet i:461, 1956.

21. Coombs, RRA and Dodd, BE: *Possible application of the principle of mixed agglutination in the identification of blood stains.* Med Sci Law 1:359, 1961.

22. Fuchs, FE, et al.: *Determination of fetal blood group.* Lancet i:996, 1956.

23. Boorman, KE, Dodd, BE and Lincoln, PJ: *Blood Group Serology,* ed 5. Churchill Livingstone, Edinburgh, 1977.

24. Dodd, BE: *Some recent advances in forensic serology.* Med Sci Law 12:195, 1972.

25. Howard, HD and Martin, PD: *An improved method for ABO and MN grouping of dried blood stains using cellulose acetate sheets.* J Forensic Sci Soc 9:28, 1969.

26. Lincoln, PJ and Dodd, BE: *The detection of the Rh antigens C, C^w, c, D, E, e and the antigen S of the MNSs system in blood stains.* Med Sci Law 8:288, 1968.

27. Lincoln, PJ and Dodd, BE: *An evaluation of factors affecting the elution of antibody from blood stains.* J Forensic Sci Soc 13:37, 1973.

28. Pereira, M: *The identification of MN group in dried blood stains.* Med Sci Law 3:268, 1963.

29. Douglas, R and Staveley, JM: *Rh and Kell typings of dried blood stains.* J Forensic Sci 14:255, 1969.

30. Kind, SS and Clevely, RM: *The fluorescent antibody technique. Its application to the detection of blood group antigens in stains.* J Forensic Sci 19:121, 1970.

31. Rothwell, TJ: *Effect of storage upon activity of phosphoglucomutase and adenylate kinase enzymes in blood samples and blood stains.* Med Sci Law 10:230, 1970.

32. Culliford, BJ and Wraxall, BGD: *Adenylate kinase (AK) types in blood stains.* J Forensic Sci 8:79, 1968.

33. Gladkikh, AS and Gadakeyan, DG: *Alkaline phosphatase isoenzymes in blood serum: Their role in forensic serology* (English summary). Sud Med Ekspert 16:25, 1973.

34. Welch, SG: *Glutamate-pyruvate transaminase in blood stains.* J Forensic Sci Soc 12:605, 1972.

35. Oya, M, Asano, M and Fuwa, I: Quantitative estimation of heat stable alkaline phosphatase activity in dried blood stains and its application to forensic diagnosis of pregnancy. Z Rechtsmed 73:7, 1973.

36. Gonzalo, JC, Canales, EV and Calabuig, JAG: *Aplicación de los grupos plasmaticos Hp a la*

MODERN BLOOD BANKING AND TRANSFUSION PRACTICES

resolución de dos casos de indificualización médicolegal de manchos de sangre mediante electroforesis en gel de poliacrilamida "en disco." Zacienta 7:502, 1971.

37. NIELSON, JC and HENNINGSEN, K: *Experimental studies on the determination of the Gm groups in blood stains.* Med Sci Law 3:49, 1963.

38. BLANC, M, GÖRTZ, R and DUCOS, J: *The value of Gm typing for determining the racial origin of blood stains.* J Forensic Sci 16:176, 1971.

39. LaCAVERA, A: *Identification médico-légale des taches de sang méleés au moyen d'immunserums anti-hémoglobines animales.* Med Leg Domm Corpor (Paris) 5:43, 1972.

40. WRAXALL, BGD: *The identification of foetal hemoglobin in blood stains.* J Forensic Sci Soc 12:457, 1972.

41. PATZELT, D, GESERICK, G and LIGNITZ, E: *Spurenkundliche Identifizierung von Neugenborenenbzw. Fetalblut mittels alphal-Fetoprotein-Präcepitation* (English summary). Z Rechtsmed 74:81, 1974.

42. SAGISAKA, K, et al.: *Detection of the MN blood group of stains by means of the elution test in combination with antiglobulin test.* Jpn J Leg Med 25:103, 1971.

GLOSSARY

ABRUPTIO PLACENTAE. Premature detachment of normally situated placenta.

ABSORBED ANTI-A_1. Serum from a group B individual contains anti-A plus anti-A_1. If that serum is incubated with A_2 cells, the anti-A will absorb onto the cells. Removal of the cells then yields a serum containing only anti-A_1, thus absorbed anti-A_1.

ABSORPTION. Removal of an unwanted antibody from a serum. Often used interchangeably with adsorption.

ACID CITRATE DEXTROSE (ACD). An anticoagulant and preservative solution that was used routinely for blood donor collection at one time, but is now only occasionally used.

ACID PHOSPHATASE (AcP). A red cell enzyme used as an identification marker in paternity testing and criminal investigation.

ADENOSINE DEAMINASE (ADA). A red cell enzyme used as an identification marker in paternity testing and criminal investigation.

ADENOSINE TRIPHOSPHATE (ATP). A compound composed of adenosine (nucleotide containing adenine and ribose) and three phosphoric acid groups. When this substance is split by enzyme action, energy is produced that can be used to support other reactions.

ADENYLATE KINASE (AK). A red cell enzyme used as an identification marker in paternity testing and criminal investigation.

ADJUVANT. A variety of substances that when combined with an antigen enhance the antibody response to that antigen.

527

ADSORPTION. Providing an antibody with its corresponding antigen under optimal conditions so that the antibody will attach to the antigen. It is thus taken out of the serum. Often used interchangeably with absorption.

AGAMMAGLOBULINEMIA. A rare disorder in which there is a virtual absence of gamma globulins.

AGGLOMERATION. The reversible aggregation of red cells in the presence of a high sugar concentration.

AGGLUTINATION. The clumping together of red blood cells or any particulate matter resulting from interaction of antibody and its corresponding antigen.

AGGLUTININ. An antibody that agglutinates cells.

AGGLUTINOGEN. A substance that stimulates the production of an agglutinin, thereby acting as an antigen.

AGRANULOCYTOSIS. An acute disease in which the white blood cell count drops to extremely low levels and neutropenia becomes pronounced.

ALBUMIN. The protein found in the highest concentration in human plasma. It is used as a diluent for blood typing antisera and a potentiator solution in serologic testing to enhance antigen-antibody reactions.

ALKALINE PHOSPHATASE (AlkP). A red cell enzyme used as an identification marker in paternity testing and criminal investigation.

ALLELE. One of two or more different genes that may occupy a specific locus on a chromosome.

ALLO-. Prefix indicating differences within a species. For example, an alloantibody is produced in one individual against the red cell antigens of another individual.

ALLOGRAFT. A tissue transplant between individuals of the same species.

ALLOSTERIC CHANGE. A change in conformation that exposes a new reactive site on a molecule.

ALPHA ADRENERGIC RECEPTOR. A site in autonomic nerve pathways wherein excitatory responses occur when adrenergic agents, such as norepinephrine and epinephrine, are released.

ALPHA METHYLDOPA (ALDOMET). A common drug used to treat hypertension; frequently the cause of a positive direct Coombs' test.

ALUM PRECIPITATION. A method for obtaining an enhanced response when producing antibody. See Adjuvant.

AMNIOCENTESIS. Transabdominal puncture of the amniotic sac, using a needle and syringe, in order to remove amniotic fluid. The material may be then studied to detect genetic disorders or maternal-fetal blood incompatibility.

AMNIOTIC FLUID. Liquid or albuminous fluid contained in the amnion.

AMORPH. A gene that does not appear to produce a detectable antigen; a silent gene, such as Jk, Lu, O.

ANAMNESTIC RESPONSE. An accentuated antibody response following a secondary exposure to an antigen. Antibody levels from the initial exposure are not detectable in the patient's serum until the secondary exposure, when a rapid rise in antibody titer is observed.

ANAPHYLAXIS. An allergic hypersensitivity reaction of the body to a foreign protein or drug.

ANASTOMOSIS. A connection between two blood vessels, either direct or through connecting channels.

ANEMIA. A condition in which there is reduced O_2 delivery to the tissues. It may result from increased destruction of red cells, excessive blood loss, or decreased production of red cells. APLASTIC A. Caused by aplasia of bone marrow or its destruction by chemical agents or physical factors. AUTOIMMUNE HEMOLYTIC A. Acquired disorder characterized by premature erythrocyte destruction owing to abnormalities in the individual's own immune system. HEMOLYTIC A. Caused by hemolysis of red blood cells resulting in reduction of normal red cell life span. IRON DEFICIENCY A. Resulting from a greater demand on stored iron than can be met. MEGALOBLASTIC A. Anemia in which megaloblasts are found in the blood. SICKLE CELL A. Hereditary, chronic hemolytic anemia characterized by large numbers of sickle-shaped red blood cells occurring almost exclusively in blacks.

ANGINA PECTORIS. Severe pain and constriction about the heart caused by an insufficient supply of blood to the heart.

ANION. An ion carrying a negative charge.

ANTECUBITAL. In front of the elbow; at the bend of the elbow. Usual site for blood collection.

ANTENATAL. Occurring before birth.

ANTI-A$_1$ LECTIN. A reagent anti-A$_1$ serum produced from the seeds of the plant *Dolichos biflorus*. It reacts with all A$_1$ cells but not with A subgroup cells, such as A$_2$, A$_3$, and so on. It does react weakly with A$_{int}$ cells.

ANTI-B LECTIN. A reagent anti-B serum produced from the seeds of the plant *Bandeiraea simplicifolia*.

ANTIBODY. A protein substance developed in response to, and interacting specifically with, an antigen. In blood banking, it is found in serum, from either a commercial manufacturer or a patient. It is secreted by plasma cells. CROSS-REACTING A. An antibody that reacts with antigens functionally similar to its specific antigen. FLUORESCENT A. An antibody reaction made visible by incorporating a fluorescent dye into the antigen-antibody reaction and examining the specimen with a fluorescent microscope. MATERNAL A. An antibody produced in the mother and transferred to the fetus in utero. NATURALLY-OCCURRING A. An antibody present in a patient without known prior exposure to the corresponding red cell antigen.

ANTIBODY SCREEN. Testing the patient's serum with group O reagent red cells in an effort to detect atypical antibodies.

ANTICOAGULANT. An agent that prevents or delays blood coagulation.

ANTICODON. A sequence of three bases that is found on tRNA which also carries an amino acid residue. The anticodon recognizes its complementary codon on mRNA at the ribosome and deposits the amino acid on the ribosome, generating the amino acid sequence of the protein.

ANTI-DL. An antibody implicated in warm autoimmune hemolytic anemia (WAIHA), which reacts with all Rh cells including Rh_{null} and Rh deleted cells.

ANTIGEN. A substance that is recognized by the body as being foreign, thus it can elicit an immune response. In blood banking, antigens are usually, but not exclusively, found on the blood cell membrane.

ANTIGLOBULIN SERUM. *See* Antihuman serum.

ANTIGLOBULIN TEST (AGT). Test to ascertain the presence or absence of red cell coating by immunoglobulin (IgG) and/or complement. This test utilizes a xenoantibody (rabbit antihuman serum) to act as a bridge between sensitized cells, thus yielding agglutination as a positive result. **DIRECT AGT (DAT).** Used to detect in-vivo cell sensitization. **INDIRECT AGT (IAT).** Used to detect antigen-antibody reactions that occur in vitro.

ANTI-H LECTIN. A reagent anti-H produced from the seeds of the plant *Ulex europaeus.*

ANTIHEMOPHILIC FACTOR. *See* Hemophilia A.

ANTIHEMOPHILIC GLOBULIN. *See* Hemophilia A.

ANTIHISTAMINE. Drug that opposes the action of histamine.

ANTIHUMAN GLOBULIN. *See* Antihuman serum.

ANTIHUMAN SERUM. An antibody prepared in rabbits or other suitable animals that is directed against human immunoglobulin and/or complement. It is used to perform the antiglobulin or Coombs' test. The serum may be either polyspecific (anti-IgG plus anticomplement) or monospecific (anti-IgG or anticomplement).

ANTI-M LECTIN. A reagent anti-M serum produced from the plant *Iberis amara.*

ANTI-N LECTIN. A reagent anti-N serum produced from the plant *Vicia graminea.*

ANTI-NL. An antibody implicated in WAIHA, which reacts with all normal Rh cells except Rh_{null} cells and deleted Rh cells.

ANTI-PDL. An antibody implicated in WAIHA, which reacts with all normal Rh cells and deleted Rh cells but not with Rh_{null} cells.

ANTIPYRETIC. An agent that reduces fever.

ANTISERUM. A reagent source of antibody, as in a commercial antiserum.

ANTITHETICAL. Refers to antigens that are the product of allelic genes, for example, Kell (K) and Cellano (k).

APHERESIS. A method of blood collection in which whole blood is withdrawn, a desired component separated and retained, and the remainder of the blood returned to the donor. *See also* Plateletpheresis and Plasmapheresis.

APLASIA. Failure of an organ or tissue to develop normally.

ARACHIS HYPOGAEA. A peanut lectin used to differentiate T polyagglutination from Tn polyagglutination.

ASPHYXIA. Condition caused by insufficient intake of oxygen.

ASTHMA. Paroxysmal dyspnea accompanied by wheezing caused by a spasm of the bronchial tubes or by swelling of their mucous membrane.

ATYPICAL ANTIBODIES. Any antibody other than anti-A, anti-B, or anti-A,B.

AUSTRALIA ANTIGEN. Old terminology referring to the hepatitis B associated antigen.

AUTO-. Prefix indicating self. For example, an autoantibody is reactive against one's own red cell antigens. This is usually associated with a disease state.

AUTOABSORPTION. A procedure for the removal of a patient's antibody using the patient's own cells.

AUTOLOGOUS CONTROL. Testing the patient's serum with his own cells in an effort to detect autoantibody activity.

AUTOSOME. Any of the chromosomes other than the sex (X and Y) chromosomes.

BACTERICIDAL. Destructive to or destroying bacteria.

BANDEIRAEA SIMPLICIFOLIA. *See* Anti-B lectin.

BFU-E (BURST FORMING UNIT COMMITTED TO ERYTHROPOIESIS). A primitive stem cell committed to erythropoiesis and thought to be a precursor to the GFU-E.

BILIRUBIN. The orange-yellow pigment in bile carried to the liver by the blood. It is produced from hemoglobin of red blood cells by reticuloendothelial cells in bone marrow, in the spleen, and elsewhere. DIRECT B. The conjugated water soluble form of bilirubin. INDIRECT B. The unconjugated water insoluble form of bilirubin.

BILIRUBINEMIA. Pathologic condition in which excessive destruction of red blood cells occurs, increasing the amount of bilirubin found in the blood.

BINDING CONSTANT. The "goodness of fit" in an antigen-antibody complex.

BIPHASIC. Reactivity occurring in two phases.

BLOOD GASES. Determination of pH, pCO_2, PO_2, and HCO_3^- performed on a blood gas analyzer.

BLOOD GROUP SPECIFIC SUBSTANCES (BGSS). Term used for soluble antigens present in fluids that can be used to neutralize their corresponding antibodies. Some systems that demonstrate BGSS are ABO, Lewis, and P.

BOMBAY. Individuals who possess normal A or B genes but are unable to express them because they lack the gene necessary for production of H antigen, the required precursor for A and B. They often have a potent anti-H in their serum, which reacts with all cells except other Bombays.

BOVINE. Pertaining to cattle.

BRADYKININ. A plasma kinin.

BROMELIN. A proteolytic enzyme obtained from the pineapple.

BUFFY COAT. Light stratum of a blood clot seen when the blood is centrifuged or allowed to stand in a test tube. The red blood cells settle to the bottom and, between the plasma and the red blood cells, there is a light colored layer that contains mostly white blood cells.

C3a. A biologically active fragment of the C3 molecule, which demonstrates anaphylactic capabilities upon liberation.

C3b. A biologically active fragment of the complement C3 molecule, which is an opsonin and promotes immune adherence.

C3d. A biologically inactive fragment of the C3b complement component formed by inactivation by the C3b inactivator substance present in serum.

C4. A complement component present in serum, which participates in the classic pathway of complement activation.

C5a. A biologically active fragment of the C5 molecule, which demonstrates anaphylactic capabilities as well as chemotactic properties upon liberation. This fragment has also been reported to be a potent aggregator of platelets.

CARDIAC OUTPUT. The amount of blood discharged from the left or right ventricle per minute.

CATECHOLAMINES. Biologically active amines, epinephrine and norepinephrine, derived from the amino acid tyrosine. They have a marked effect on nervous and cardiovascular systems, metabolic rate, temperature, and smooth muscle.

CATION. An ion carrying a positive charge.

CENTRAL VENOUS PRESSURE. The pressure within the superior vena cava reflecting the pressure under which the blood is returned to the right atrium.

CFU-C (COLONY FORMING UNIT—CULTURE). Generation of stem cells using tissue culture methods. Current synonym is CFU-GM, which is a colony forming unit committed to the production of myeloid cells (granulocytes and monocytes).

CFU-E (COLONY FORMING UNIT COMMITTED TO ERYTHROPOIESIS). A stem cell that is committed to forming cells of the red blood cell series.

CHEMICALLY MODIFIED ANTI-D. IgG anti-D reagent antisera in which the immunoglobulin has been chemically modified to react in the saline phase of testing by breaking disulfide bonds at the hinge region of the molecule, converting the Y-shaped antibody structure to a T-shaped form through the use of sulfhydryl reducing reagents.

CHEMOTAXIS. Describes movement toward a stimulus, particularly the movement displayed by phagocytic cells toward bacteria and sites of cell injury.

CHIMERA. An individual who possesses a mixed cell population.

CHLOROQUINE. White crystalline powder used for its antimicrobial action, especially in the treatment of malaria and used in treating lupus erythematosus.

CHROMOGEN. Any principle that may be changed into coloring matter.

CHROMOSOME. The structures within a nucleus that contain a linear thread of DNA, which transmits genetic information. Genes are arranged along the strand of DNA and constitute portions of the DNA.

CIS POSITION. The location of two or more genes on the same chromosome of a homologous pair.

CITRATE. Compound of citric acid and a base; used in anticoagulant solutions.

CITRATE PHOSPHATE DEXTROSE (CPD). The anticoagulant preservative solution that replaced ACD in routine donor collection. It has been replaced by CPD-A1 in routine use.

CITRATE PHOSPHATE DEXTROSE ADENINE (CPD-A1). The anticoagulant preservative solution in current use. It has extended the shelf-life of blood from 21 days (in ACD and CPD) to 35 days.

CODOMINANT. A pair of genes in which neither is dominant over the other, that is, they are both expressed.

CODON. A sequence of three bases in a strand of DNA that provides the genetic code for a specific amino acid. The complementary triplets are found on mRNA, which is synthesized from the DNA and then proceeds to the ribosomes for protein synthesis.

COLLOID. A gluelike substance, such as protein or starch, whose particles when dispersed in a solvent to the greatest possible degree remain uniformly distributed and fail to form a true solution.

COLOSTRUM. Breast fluid secreted 2 to 3 days after birth but before the onset of true lactation. A thin yellowish fluid that contains a great quantity of proteins and calories as well as antibodies and lymphocytes.

COMPATIBILITY TESTING. All pretransfusion testing performed on a potential transfusion recipient and the appropriate donor blood. This testing is an attempt to ensure that the product will survive in the recipient and induce improvement in the patient's clinical condition. The crossmatch between recipient's serum and donor's cells.

COMPLEMENT. A series of proteins in the circulation that, when sequentially activated, causes disruption of bacterial and other cell membranes. Activation occurs via one of two pathways, and once activated, the components are involved in a great number of immune defense mechanisms including anaphylaxis, chemotaxis, and phagocytosis. Red cell antibodies that activate complement may be capable of causing hemolysis.

COMPLEMENT FIXATION (CF). An immunologic test.

COMPONENT THERAPY. Transfusion of specific components for treating a patient rather than whole blood. These components, such as red blood cells, platelets, and plasma, are separable by physical means, such as centrifugation.

COMPOUND ANTIBODY. An antibody whose corresponding antigen is an interaction product of two or more antigens.

COMPOUND ANTIGEN. Two or more antigens that interact and are recognized as a single antigen by an antibody.

CONGLUTININ. A substance present in bovine serum that will agglutinate sensitized cells in the presence of complement.

CONSTANT REGION. That portion of the immunoglobulin chain that shows a relatively constant amino acid sequence within each class of immunoglobulin. Both light and heavy chains have such constant portions and they originate at the carboxyl region of the molecule.

CONVULSION. Involuntary muscle contraction and relaxation.

COOMBS' SERUM. *See* Antihuman serum.

COOMBS' TEST. *See* Antiglobulin test.

CORD CELLS. Fetal cells obtained from the umbilical cord at birth. They may be contaminated with Wharton's jelly.

COUMARIN (COUMADIN). A commonly employed anticoagulant that acts as a vitamin K antagonist that prolongs the PTT.

COUNTERELECTROPHORESIS (CEP). An immunologic procedure.

CROSSMATCH. Testing a patient and prospective donor for compatibility. MAJOR C. Recipient serum tested with donor cells. MINOR C. Recipient cells tested with donor serum or plasma.

CRYOPRECIPITATE. A concentrated source of coagulation factor VIII prepared from a single unit of donor blood. The product also contains fibrinogen, factor XIII, and von Willebrand's factor.

CRYOPROTECTANT. A substance that protects blood cells from damage caused by freezing and thawing. Glycerol and dimethyl sulfoxide (DMSO) are examples.

CRYSTALLOID. A substance capable of crystallization; opposite of colloid.

CYANOSIS. Slightly bluish or grayish discoloration of the skin resulting from accumulations of reduced hemoglobin or deoxyhemoglobin in the blood caused by oxygen deficiency or carbon dioxide buildup.

CYTOMEGALOVIRUS (CMV). One of a group of species-specific herpesviruses.

CYTOPHERESIS. A procedure utilizing a machine by which one can selectively remove a particular cell type normally found in peripheral blood of a patient or donor.

CYTOTOXICITY. Ability to destroy cells.

CYTOTOXICITY TESTING. Procedure commonly used in HLA typing and crossmatching.

DANE PARTICLE. Term referring to hepatitis B virion.

DEGLYCEROLIZATION. Removal of glycerol from a unit of red cells after thawing has been performed. Required to return the cells to a normal osmolality.

DELETION. The loss of a portion of a chromosome.

DEOXYRIBONUCLEIC ACID (DNA). The chemical basis of heredity and the carrier of genetic information for all organisms except RNA viruses.

DEXAMETHASONE. A topical steroid with anti-inflammatory, antipruritic, and vaso-constrictive actions.

DEXTRAN. A plasma expander that may be used as a substitute for plasma. It can be used to treat shock by increasing blood volume. Rouleaux may be observed in the recipient's serum or plasma.

DIAPHORESIS. Profuse sweating.

DIASTOLIC PRESSURE. The point of least pressure in the arterial vascular system; the lower or bottom value of a blood pressure reading.

DIELECTRIC CONSTANT. A measure of the electrical conductivity of a suspending medium.

DIFFERENTIAL COUNT. Counting 100 leukocytes to ascertain the relative percentages of each.

2,3-DIPHOSPHOGLYCERATE (2,3-DPG). An organic phosphate in red blood cells that alters the affinity of hemoglobin for oxygen. Blood cells stored in a blood bank lose 2,3-DPG, but once infused the substance is resynthesized or reactivated.

DIPLOID. Having two sets of chromosomes for a total of 46.

DISSEMINATED INTRAVASCULAR COAGULATION. Clinical condition of altered blood coagulation secondary to a variety of diseases.

DITHIOTHREITOL (DTT). A sulfhydryl compound used to disrupt the disulfide bonds of IgM, yielding monomeric units rather than the typical pentameric molecule.

DIURESIS. Secretion and passage of large amounts of urine.

DIURETIC. Increasing or an agent that increases the secretion of urine. Action is in two ways: by increasing glomerular filtration or by decreasing reabsorption from the tubules.

DIZYGOTIC TWINS. Twins who are the product of two fertilized ova (also fraternal twins).

DNA POLYMERASE. Also known as the HBeAg (antigen) of the hepatitis B virion.

DOLICHOS BIFLORUS. See Anti-A₁ lectin.

DOMAIN. Portions along the immunoglobulin chain that show specific biologic function.

DOMINANT. A trait or characteristic that will be expressed in the offspring even though it is only carried on one of the homologous chromosomes.

DONATH-LANDSTEINER TEST. A test usually performed in the blood bank to detect the presence of the Donath-Landsteiner antibody, which is a biphasic IgG antibody with anti-P specificity found in patients suffering from paroxysmal cold hemoglobinuria.

DONOR. An individual who donates a pint of blood.

DOPAMINE. A catecholamine synthesized by the adrenal gland used especially in the treatment of shock.

DOSAGE. A phenomenon whereby an antibody reacts more strongly with a red cell carrying a double dose (homozygous inheritance of the appropriate gene) rather than a single dose (heterozygous inheritance) of an antigen.

DYSCRASIA. An old term now used as a synonym for disease.

ECCHYMOSIS. A form of macula appearing in large irregularly formed hemorrhagic areas of the skin; originally a blue black color changing to greenish brown or yellow.

EDEMA. A local or generalized condition in which the body tissues contain an excessive amount of tissue fluid.

EDTA (ETHYLENEDIAMINOTETRAACETIC ACID). An anticoagulant useful in hematologic testing and preferable when direct antiglobulin testing is indicated.

ELECTROLYTE. A substance that in solution conducts an electric current. Acids, bases, and salts are common electrolytes.

ELECTROPHORESIS. The movement of charged particles through a medium (paper, agar gel) in the presence of an electrical field. Useful in the separation and analysis of proteins.

ELISA (ENZYME-LINKED IMMUNOSORBENT ASSAY). An immunologic test.

ELUATE. *See* Elution.

ELUTION. A process whereby cells that are coated with antibody are treated in such a manner as to disrupt the bonds between the antigen and antibody. The freed antibody is collected in an inert diluent such as saline or 6 percent albumin. This antibody serum then can be tested to identify its specificity using routine methods. The mechanism to free the antibody may be physical (heat, shaking) or chemical (ether, acid) and the harvested antibody-containing fluid is called an eluate.

EMBOLISM. Obstruction of a blood vessel by foreign substances or a blood clot.

EMBOLUS. A mass of undissolved matter present in a blood or lymphatic vessel brought there by the blood or lymph circulation.

ENDEMIC. A disease that occurs continuously in a particular population but has a low mortality; used in contrast to epidemic.

ENDOGENOUS. Produced or arising from within a cell or organism.

ENDOTHELIUM. A form of squamous epithelium consisting of flat cells that line the blood and lymphatic vessels, the heart, and various other body cavities; derived from mesoderm.

ENDOTOXEMIA. The presence of endotoxin in the blood; endotoxin is present in the cell of certain bacteria, for example, gram-negative organisms.

ENZYME. A substance capable of catalyzing a reaction. Enzymes are proteins that induce chemical changes in other substances without being changed themselves.

ENZYME TREATMENT. A procedure in which red blood cells are incubated with an enzyme solution that cleaves some of the membrane's glycoproteins. The cells are then washed free of the enzyme and used in serologic testing. Enzyme treatment cleaves some antigens and exposes others.

EPISTAXIS. Hemorrhage from the nose; nosebleed.

EPITOPE. The portion of the antigen molecule that is directly involved in the interaction with the antibody; the antigenic determinant.

EQUIVALENCE ZONE. The zone in which antigen and antibody concentrations are optimal and lattice formation is most stable.

ERYTHROBLAST. Any form of nucleated red corpuscles. Nucleated red cells are not normally seen in the circulating blood. Erythroblasts contain hemoglobin.

ERYTHROBLASTOSIS FETALIS. *See* Hemolytic disease of the newborn.

ERYTHROCYTE. The blood cell that transports oxygen and carbon dioxide. A mature red blood cell.

EUGLOBULIN LYSIS. Coagulation procedure testing for fibrinolysins.

EXOGENOUS. Originating outside an organ or part.

EXTRACORPOREAL. Outside of the body.

EXTRAVASCULAR. Pertaining to outside the blood vessel.

FACTOR ASSAY. Coagulation procedure to assay the concentration of specific plasma coagulation factors.

FACTOR VIII CONCENTRATE. A commercially prepared source of coagulation factor VIII.

FEBRILE REACTION. A transfusion reaction caused by leukoagglutinins that is characterized by fever. Usually observed in multiply transfused or multiparous patients.

FIBRIN. A whitish filamentous protein or clot formed by the action of thrombin on fibrinogen, converting it to fibrin.

FIBRINOGEN. A protein produced in the liver that circulates in plasma. In the presence of thrombin, an enzyme produced by the activation of the clotting mechanism, fibrinogen is cleaved into fibrin, which is an insoluble protein that is responsible for clot formation.

FIBRINOLYSIN. The substance, also called plasmin, that has the ability to dissolve fibrin.

FIBRINOLYSIS. Dissolution of fibrin by fibrinolysin caused by the action of a proteolytic enzyme system that is continually active in the body but that is increased greatly by various stress stimuli.

FIBROBLAST. Cells found throughout the body that synthesize connective tissue.

FICIN. A proteolytic enzyme derived from the fig.

FICOLL. A macromolecular additive that enhances the agglutination of red cells.

FICOLL-HYPAQUE. A density gradient media utilized for the separation and harvesting of specific white blood cells, most commonly lymphocytes.

FORMALDEHYDE. A disinfectant solution.

FORWARD GROUPING. Testing unknown red cells with known reagent antisera to determine which ABO antigens are present (cell type).

FRESH FROZEN PLASMA (FFP). A frozen plasma product (from a single donor) that contains all clotting factors, especially the labile factors V and VIII. Useful for clotting factor deficiencies other than hemophilia A, von Willebrand's disease, and hypofibrinogenemia.

FREUND'S ADJUVANT. Mixture of killed microorganisms, usually mycobacteria, in an oil and water emulsion. The material is administered to induce antibody formation and yields a much greater antibody response.

FUROSEMIDE (LASIX). An oral diuretic.

G6PD (GLUCOSE-6-PHOSPHATE DEHYDROGENASE). A liver enzyme used to monitor liver function.

GAMETE. A mature male or female reproductive cell.

GAMMA GLOBULIN. A protein found in plasma and known to be involved in immunity.

GAMMA MARKER. Allotypic marker on the gamma heavy chain of the IgG immunoglobulin.

GENE. A unit of inheritance within a chromosome.

GENOTYPE. An individual's actual genetic makeup.

GESTATION. In mammals, the length of time from conception to birth.

GLOBIN. A protein constituent of hemoglobin. There are four globin chains in the hemoglobin molecule.

GLOMERULONEPHRITIS. A form of nephritis in which the lesions involve primarily the glomeruli.

GLUTEN ENTEROPATHY. A condition associated with malabsorption of food from the intestinal tract.

GLYCEROL. A cryoprotective agent.

GLYCEROLIZATION. Adding glycerol to a unit of red cells for the purpose of freezing.

GLYCINE SOJA. Soy bean extract or lectin used to differentiate different forms of polyagglutination.

GLYCOPHORIN A. A major glycoprotein of the red cell membrane. MN antigen activity is found on it.

GLYCOPHORIN B. An important red cell glycoprotein. SsU antigen activity is found here.

GLYCOSYL TRANSFERASE. A protein enzyme that promotes the attachment of a specific sugar molecule to a predetermined acceptor molecule. Many blood group genes code for transferases, which reproduce their respective antigens by attaching sugars to designated precursor substances.

GOODPASTURE SYNDROME. A disease entity that represents a rapidly progressive glomerulonephritis associated with pulmonary lesions. Usually the patients possess an antibody to the basement membrane of the renal glomeruli.

GPT (SGPT, SERUM GLUTAMIC PYRUVATE TRANSAMINASE). A liver enzyme used to monitor liver function.

GRANULOCYTOPENIA. Abnormal reduction of granulocytes in the blood.

GVH DISEASE (GRAFT VS HOST DISEASE). A disorder in which the grafted tissue attacks the host tissue.

HAGEMAN FACTOR. Synonym for the XII coagulation factor.

HALF-LIFE. The time that is required for the concentration of a substance to be reduced by one half.

HAPLOID. Possessing half the normal number of chromosomes found in somatic or body cells. Seen in germ cells (sperm and ova).

HAPLOTYPE. A term used in HLA testing to denote the five genes (HLA-A,B,C,D,DR) on the same chromosome.

HAPTENE. The portion of an antigen containing the grouping on which the specificity depends.

HAPTOGLOBIN. A mucoprotein to which hemoglobin released into plasma is bound; it is increased in certain inflammatory conditions and decreased in hemolytic disorders.

HBcAg. Hepatitis core antigen referring to the nucleocapsid of the virion.

HBeAg. Hepatitis DNA polymerase of the nucleus of the virion.

HBsAg. Hepatitis B surface antigen.

HEMANGIOMA. A benign tumor of dilated blood vessels.

HEMARTHROSIS. Bloody effusion into cavity of a joint.

HEMATINIC. Pertaining to blood; an agent which increases the amount of hemoglobin in the blood.

HEMATOCRIT. The proportion of red blood cells in whole blood expressed as a percentage.

HEMATOMA. A swelling or mass of blood confined to an organ, tissue, or space and caused by a break in a blood vessel.

HEMATURIA. Blood in the urine.

HEME. The iron-containing protoporphyrin portion of the hemoglobin wherein the iron is in the ferrous (Fe^{++}) state.

HEMODIALYSIS. Removal of chemical substances from the blood by passing it through tubes made of semipermeable membranes. The tubes are continually bathed by solutions that selectively remove unwanted material. Used to cleanse the blood of patients in whom one or both kidneys are defective or absent; and to remove excess accumulation of drugs or toxic chemicals in the blood.

HEMODILUTION. An increase in the volume of blood plasma resulting in reduced relative concentration of red blood cells.

HEMOGLOBIN. The iron-containing pigment of the red blood cells. Its function is to carry oxygen from the lungs to the tissues.

HEMOGLOBINEMIA. Presence of hemoglobin in the blood plasma.

HEMOGLOBIN-OXYGEN DISSOCIATION CURVE. The relationship between the percent saturation of the hemoglobin molecule with oxygen and the environmental oxygen tension.

HEMOGLOBINURIA. The presence of hemoglobin in the urine freed from lysed red blood cells. Occurs when hemoglobin from disintegrating red blood cells or from rapid hemolysis of red cells exceeds the ability of the blood proteins to combine with the hemoglobin.

HEMOLYSIN. An antibody that activates complement leading to cell lysis.

HEMOLYSIS. Disruption of the red cell membrane and the subsequent release of hemoglobin into the suspending medium or plasma.

HEMOLYTIC DISEASE OF THE NEWBORN (HDN). A disease characterized by anemia, jaundice, enlargement of the liver and spleen, and generalized edema (hydrops fetalis). Due to maternal IgG antibodies that cross the placenta and attack fetal red cells when there is a feto-maternal blood group incompatibility. Usually caused by ABO or Rh antibodies. Synonym is erythroblastosis fetalis.

HEMOPHILIA A. An hereditary disorder characterized by greatly prolonged coagulation time. The blood fails to clot and bleeding occurs, especially in males because of the inheritance of a deficiency of factor VIII.

HEMOPHILIA B. "Christmas disease," which is a hemophilia-like disease caused by a lack of factor IX.

HEMOPOIESIS. Formation of blood cells. Synonym is hematopoiesis.

HEMORRHAGE. Abnormal internal or external bleeding. May be venous, arterial, or capillary from blood vessels into the tissues, into or from the body.

HEMORRHAGIC DIATHESIS. Uncontrolled spontaneous bleeding.

HEMOSIDERIN. An iron-containing pigment derived from hemoglobin from disintegration of red blood cells. It is one method whereby iron is stored until it is needed for making hemoglobin.

HEMOSTASIS. Arrest of bleeding; maintaining blood flow within vessels by repairing rapidly any vascular break without compromising the fluidity of the blood.

HEMOTHERAPY. Blood transfusion as a therapeutic measure.

HEPARIN. An anticoagulant used for collecting whole blood that is to be filtered for the removal of leukocytes.

HEPATITIS. Inflammation of the liver.

HEPATITIS ASSOCIATED ANTIGEN (HAA). Older terminology currently replaced by the designation HBsAg.

HEPATITIS B IMMUNE GLOBULIN (HBIG). An immune serum given to individuals exposed to the hepatitis B virus.

HETEROZYGOTE. An individual with different alleles for a given characteristic.

HETEROZYGOUS. Possessing different alleles at a given locus.

HIGH-FREQUENCY ANTIGEN. Also known as high-incidence antigen, which is one whose frequency in the population is 98 to 99 percent.

HISTOCOMPATIBILITY. The ability of cells to survive without immunologic interference; especially important in blood transfusion and transplantation.

HLA. Human leukocyte antigen.

HOMEOSTASIS. State of equilibrium of the internal environment of the body that is maintained by dynamic processes of feedback and regulation.

HOMOZYGOTE. An individual developing from gametes with similar alleles and thus possessing like pairs of genes for a given hereditary characteristic.

HOMOZYGOUS. Possessing a pair of identical alleles.

HORMONE. A substance originating in an organ or gland that is conveyed through the blood to another part of the body, stimulating it by chemical action to increased functional activity and increased secretion.

HTR. Hemolytic transfusion reaction.

HYALURONIDASE. An enzyme found in the testes; present in semen.

HYBRIDOMA. A hybrid (cross) between a plasmacytoma cell and a spleen (or Ab producing) cell that produces a monoclonal antibody. This results in a malignant cell line that can grow indefinitely in culture and can produce high quantities of Ab. This antibody is monoclonal because only one Ab producing cell combined with the plasmacytoma cell is present.

HYDATID CYST FLUID. Source of P_1 substance.

HYDROCORTISONE. A corticosteroid that possesses anti-inflammatory properties.

Hydrops fetalis. *See* Hemolytic disease of the newborn.

Hydroxyethyl starch (HES). A red cell sedimenting agent used to facilitate leukocyte withdrawal during leukapheresis.

Hypertension. Increase in blood pressure.

Hyperventilation. Rapid breathing that results in CO_2 depletion and accompanying hypotension, vasoconstriction, and fainting.

Hypogammaglobulinemia. Decreased levels of gamma globulins seen in some disease states.

Hypotension. Decrease in blood pressure.

Hypothermia. Having a body temperature below normal.

Hypovolemia. Diminished blood volume.

Hypoxia. Deficiency of oxygen.

Iberis amara. *See* Anti-M lectin.

Icterus. A condition characterized by yellowish skin, eyes, mucous membranes, and body fluids caused by deposition of excess bilirubin.

Idiopathic. Pertaining to conditions without clear pathogenesis, or disease without recognizable cause, as of spontaneous origin.

Idiopathic thrombocytopenic purpura (ITP). Bleeding owing to a decreased number of platelets; the etiology is unknown, with most evidence pointing to platelet autoantibodies.

Idiothrombocythemia. An increase in blood platelets with unknown etiology.

Idiotype. That portion of the immunoglobulin variable region that is the antigen-combining site, which interacts with the antigenic epitope.

Immune response. The reaction of the body to substances that are foreign or are interpreted as being foreign. Cell-mediated or cellular immunity pertains to tissue destruction mediated by T cells, such as graft rejection and hypersensitivity reactions. Humoral immunity pertains to cell destruction response during the early period of the reaction.

Immune serum globulin. Gamma globulin protein fraction of serum containing antibodies.

Immunoblast. A mitotically active T or B cell.

Immunodeficiency. A decrease from the normal concentration of immunoglobulins in serum.

Immunodominant sugar. In reference to glycoprotein or glycolipid antigens, that sugar molecule that gives the antigen its specificity. An example is D-galactose, which confers B antigen specificity.

Immunogen. Any substance capable of stimulating an immune response.

IMMUNOGENICITY. A descriptive term indicating the ability of an antigen to stimulate an antibody response.

IMMUNOGLOBULIN. One of a family of closely related though not identical proteins that are capable of acting as antibodies. They are IgA, IgD, IgE, IgG, and IgM. IgA is the principal immunoglobulin in exocrine secretions such as saliva and tears. IgD may play a role in antigen recognition and the initiation of antibody synthesis. IgE is produced by the cells lining the intestinal and respiratory tracts and is important in forming reagin. IgG is the main immunoglobulin in human serum. IgM is a globulin formed in almost every immune response during the early period of the reaction.

IMMUNOLOGIC MEMORY. The development of T and B memory cells that have been sensitized by exposure to an antigen and respond rapidly under subsequent encounters with the antigen.

IMMUNOLOGIC UNRESPONSIVENESS. Development of a "tolerance" to certain antigens that would otherwise evoke an immune response.

IMMUNOPRECIPITIN. An antigen-antibody reaction that results in precipitation.

INCUBATION. In-vitro combination of antigen and antibody under certain conditions of time and temperature to allow antigen-antibody complexes to occur.

INITIATION. The deposition of N-formyl methionine on the ribosome, which begins the synthesis of all proteins.

IN LU. A rare, dominant gene that inhibits the production of all Lutheran antigens as well as i, P_1, and Au^a (Auberger). The quantity of antigen on the red cell is markedly reduced in the presence of In Lu; it may be virtually undetectable.

INTRAOPERATIVE SALVAGE. A procedure to reclaim a patient's blood loss during an operation by reinfusion.

INTRAVASCULAR. Within the blood vessel.

IN UTERO. Within the uterus.

INV. Light chain marker on the lambda light chains of the IgG immunoglobulins.

INVERSION. The breaking of a chromosome during division with subsequent reattachment occurring in an inverted or "upside-down" position.

IN VITRO. Outside the living body, as in a laboratory setting.

IN VIVO. Inside the living body.

ION EXCHANGE RESIN. Synthetic organic substances of high molecular weight. They replace certain positive or negative ions, which they encounter in solutions.

IONIC STRENGTH. Refers to the number of charged particles present in a solution.

IR GENES. Immune response genes found within the region of the major histocompatibility complex. Ir genes in humans are likely to exist; preliminary evidence shows genes at the DR locus may be analogous to the Ir genes of mice.

ISCHEMIA. Local and temporary deficiency of blood supply caused by obstruction of the circulation to a part.

ISOAGGLUTININS. A term used to denote the ABO antibodies, anti-A, anti-B, and anti-A,B.

ISOIMMUNE. An antibody produced against a foreign antigen in the same species.

ISOTYPE. Refers to the subclasses of an immunoglobulin molecule.

JAUNDICE. A condition characterized by yellowing of the skin and the whites of the eyes. One cause is excess hemolysis, which results in increased circulating bilirubin. Another cause is liver damage caused by hepatitis.

KARYOTYPE. A photomicrograph of a single cell in the metaphase stage of mitosis that is arranged to show the chromosomes in descending order of size.

KERNICTERUS. A form of icterus neonatorum occurring in infants. Develops at 2 to 8 days of life. Prognosis is poor if untreated.

KININ. A general term for a group of polypeptides that have considerable biologic activity, for example, vasoactivity.

KLEIHAUER-BETKE TECHNIQUE. Quantitative procedure used to determine the amount of fetal cells present in the maternal circulation.

KM. Light chain marker on the kappa light chains of the IgG immunoglobulins.

LABILE. Describes a substance that deteriorates rapidly on storage.

LD. Lymphocyte defined antigens.

LECTIN. An extract prepared from seeds, which with the appropriate manipulation can demonstrate antibody specificity.

LEUKEMIA. Malignant proliferation of leukocytes, which spill into the blood yielding an elevated leukocyte count.

LEUKOAGGLUTININS. Antibodies to white blood cells.

LIGATURE. Process of binding or tying. A band or bandage. A thread or wire for tying a blood vessel or other structure in order to constrict it.

LINKAGE. The association between distinct genes that occupy closely situated loci on the same chromosome. This results in an association in the inheritance of these genes.

LINKAGE DISEQUILIBRIUM. Genes associated in a haplotype more often than would be expected on the basis of chance alone.

LOCUS. The site of a gene on a chromosome.

LOW-FREQUENCY ANTIGEN. Also known as low-incidence antigen. One whose frequency in a random population is very low, less than 10 percent.

LOW IONIC POLYCATION TEST. A compatibility test that incorporates both glycine (low ionic) and protamine (polycation) in an effort to obtain maximal sensitivity and minimize the need for antibody screening.

LOW IONIC STRENGTH SOLUTIONS (**LISS**). A type of potentiating medium in use for serologic testing. Reducing the ionic strength of the red cell suspending medium increases the affinity of the antigen for its corresponding antibody such that sensitivity can be increased and incubation time can be decreased. The solutions contain glycine or glucose in addition to saline.

LYMPHOCYTE. A type of white blood cell involved in the immune response. Lymphocytes normally total 20 to 45 percent of total white cells. T-lymphocytes mature during passage through the thymus or after interaction with thymic hormones. These cells function both in cellular and humoral immunity. There are several subsets: helper T cells (T_h), which enhance B cell antibody production, and suppressor T cells (T_s), which inhibit B cell antibody production. B-lymphocyte cells are not processed by the thymus. Through morphologic and functional differentiation, they mature into plasma cells that secrete immunoglobulin.

LYMPHOMA. A solid tumor of lymphocytic cells.

LYSOSOMES. Part of an intracellular digestive system that exists as separate particles in the cell. Even though their importance in health and disease is certain, all the precise ways lysosomes effect changes are not understood.

MACROGLOBULINEMIA. Abnormal presence of high molecular weight globulins (IgM) in the blood.

MACROPHAGE. End stage development for the blood monocyte. Macrophages have the ability to ingest (phagocytose) a variety of substances for subsequent digestion or storage. The cells are located in a number of sites in the body (e.g., spleen, liver, lung) and may exist as free, mobile cells or as fixed cells. Functions include elimination of senescent blood cells and participation in the immune response.

MAJOR HISTOCOMPATIBILITY COMPLEX (**MHC**). Present in all mammalian and ovarian species. Analogous to human HLA complex. HLA antigens are within the MHC at a locus on chromosome 6.

MAJOR XM. Major crossmatch. Compatibility testing procedure using recipient's serum and donor red cells.

MALARIA. An acute and sometimes chronic infectious disease caused by the presence of parasites within red blood cells. The parasite is *Plasmodium* (*P. vivax, P. falciparum, P. malariae, P. ovale*), which is introduced through bites of infected female *Anopheles* mosquitoes or through blood transfusion.

MEIOSIS. Type of cell division of germ cells in which two successive divisions of the nucleus produce cells that contain half the number of chromosomes present in somatic cells.

MENORRHAGIA. Excessive bleeding at the time of a menstrual period, either in number of days or amount of blood or both.

2-Mercaptoethanol (2-ME). A sulfhydryl compound used to disrupt the disulfide bonds of IgM, yielding monomeric units rather than the typical pentameric units.

Metastasis. Movement of bacteria or body cells, especially cancer cells, from one part of the body to another. Change in location of a disease or of its manifestations or transfer from one organ or part to another not directly connected. Spread is by the lymphatics or blood stream.

Methemoglobin. An abnormal form of hemoglobin wherein the ferrous (Fe^{++}) iron has been oxidized to ferric (Fe^{+++}) iron.

Microaggregates. Aggregates of platelets and leukocytes that accumulate in stored blood.

Microglobulin (β-2). A protein of unknown function; thought to be the light chain of the HLA molecule with structural similarities to the light chain in immunoglobulins.

Microspherocytes. Red blood cells, small and shaped like spheres seen in certain kinds of anemia.

Minor XM. Minor crossmatch. Compatibility testing procedure using recipient's red cells and donor's serum.

Mitosis. Type of cell division in which each daughter cell contains the same number of chromosomes as the parent cell. All cells except sex cells undergo mitosis.

Mixed field. A type of agglutination pattern in which there are numerous small clumps of cells amid a sea of free cells.

MLC. Mixed lymphocyte culture.

MLR. Mixed lymphocyte reaction.

Monoclonal. Antibody derived from a single ancestral antibody-producing parent cell.

Monocytes. *See* Macrophage.

Monozygotic twins. Two offspring that develop from a single fertilized ovum.

Mosaic. An antigen that is composed of several subunits, such as the Rh_0 (D) antigen. A mixture of characteristics that may result from a genetic crossing over or mutation.

Multiparous. Having borne more than one child.

Multiple myeloma. A neoplastic proliferation of plasma cells, which is characterized by very high immunoglobulin levels of monoclonal origin.

Mutation. A change in a gene potentially capable of being transmitted to offspring. Point m. A change in a base in DNA that can lead to a change in the amino acid incorporated into the polypeptide. The change is identifiable by analyzing the amino acid sequences of the original protein and its mutant offspring. Frameshift m. A change in which a message is read incorrectly either because a base is missing or an extra base is added. This results in an entirely new polypeptide since the triplet sequence has been shifted one base.

MYELOFIBROSIS. Replacement of bone marrow by fibrous tissue.

MYELOPROLIFERATIVE. An autonomous, purposeless increase in the production of the myeloid cell elements of the bone marrow, which includes granulocytic, erythrocytic, and megakaryocytic cell lines as well as the stromal connective tissue.

N-ACETYL NEURAMINIC ACID (**NANA**). *See* Sialic acid.

NEONATE. A newborn infant up to 6 weeks of age.

NEURAMINIDASE. An enzyme that cleaves sialic acid from the red cell membrane.

NEUTRALIZATION. Inactivating an antibody by reacting it with an antigen against which it is directed.

NEUTROPHIL. A leukocyte that ingests bacteria and small particles and plays a role in combating infection.

NONDISJUNCTION. Failure of a pair of chromosomes to separate during meiosis.

NONRESPONDER. An individual whose immune system does not respond well in antibody formation to antigenic stimulation.

NORMAL SERUM ALBUMIN. *See* Albumin.

O$_h$. *See* Bombay.

OLIGURIA. Diminished amount of urine formation.

OPSONIN. A substance in serum that promotes immune adherence and facilitates phagocytosis by the reticuloendothelial system (RES).

ORTHOSTATIC. Concerning an erect position.

OSMOLALITY. The osmotic concentration of a solution determined by the ionic concentration of dissolved substances per unit of solvent.

OUCHTERLONY DIFFUSION. An immunologic procedure in which antibody and antigen are placed in wells of a gel media plate and allowed to diffuse in order to visualize the reaction by a precipitin line.

OXYHEMOGLOBIN. The combined form of hemoglobin and oxygen.

P50. The partial pressure of oxygen or oxygen tension at which the hemoglobin molecule is 50 percent saturated with oxygen.

PALLOR. Paleness, lack of color.

PANAGGLUTININ. An antibody capable of agglutinating all red blood cells tested, including the patient's own cells.

PANCYTOPENIA. A reduction in all cellular elements of the blood, including red cells, white cells, and platelets.

PANEL. A large number of group O reagent red cells that are of known antigenic characterization and are used for antibody identification.

PAPAIN. A proteolytic enzyme derived from papaya.

PARAGLOBOSIDE. The immediate precursor for the H and P_1 antigens of the red cell.

PAROXYSMAL. A sudden, periodic attack or recurrence of symptoms of a disease.

PAROXYSMAL COLD HEMOGLOBINURIA (PCH). A type of cold autoimmune hemolytic anemia usually found in children suffering from viral infections in which a biphasic IgG antibody can be demonstrated with anti-P specificity. *See* Donath-Landsteiner test.

PAROXYSMAL NOCTURNAL HEMOGLOBINURIA (PNH). Caused by an intrinsic defect in the red blood cell membrane rendering it more susceptible to hemolysins in an acid environment and characterized by hemoglobins in the urine following periods of sleep.

PERFUSION. Supplying an organ or tissue with nutrients and oxygen by passing blood or a suitable fluid through it.

PERIORAL PARESTHESIA. Tingling around the mouth occasionally experienced by apheresis donors resulting from the rapid return of citrated plasma, which contains citrate bound calcium and free citrate.

PEROXIDASE. An enzyme that hastens the transfer of oxygen from peroxide to a tissue that requires oxygen; this process is essential to intracellular respiration.

PHAGOCYTOSIS. Ingestion of microorganisms, other cells, and foreign particles by a phagocyte.

PHENOTYPE. The outward expression of genes (e.g., a blood type). On blood cells, serologically demonstrable antigens constitute the phenotype except those sugar sites that are determined by transferases.

PHENYLTHIOCARBAMIDE (PTC). A chemical used in studying medical genetics to detect the presence of a marker gene. About 70 percent of the population inherit the ability to taste PTC, which tastes bitter. The remaining 30 percent find PTC tasteless. The inheritance of this trait is due to a single dominant gene of a pair.

PHLEBOTOMY. To take blood from a person.

PHOSPHOGLYCEROMUTASE (PGM). A red cell enzyme.

PHOTOTHERAPY. Exposure to sunlight or artificial light for therapeutic purposes.

PLASMA. The liquid portion of whole blood containing water, electrolytes, glucose, fats, proteins, and gases. Plasma contains all the clotting factors necessary for coagulation, but in an inactive form. Once coagulation occurs, the fluid is converted to serum.

PLASMA CELL. A B-lymphocyte derived cell that secretes immunoglobulins or antibodies.

PLASMAPHERESIS. A procedure utilizing a machine by which one can remove only plasma from a donor or patient.

PLASMA PROTEIN FRACTION (PPF). Also known as plasmanate. Sterile pooled plasma stored as a fluid or freeze-dried. Used for volume replacement.

PLASMINOGEN. A protein found in many tissues and body fluids important in preventing fibrin clot formation.

PLASMODIUM. *See* Malaria.

PLASMODIUM KNOWLESI. A parasite that causes malaria in monkeys.

PLATELET. A round or oval disc, 2 to 4 microns in diameter, that is derived from the cytoplasma of the megakaryocyte, a large cell in the bone marrow. Platelets play an important role in blood coagulation, hemostasis, and blood thrombus formation. When a small vessel is injured, platelets adhere to each other and the edges of the injury and form a plug that covers the area and stops the loss of blood.

PLATELET CONCENTRATE. Platelets prepared from a single unit of whole blood or plasma and suspended in a specific volume of the original plasma. Also known as random donor platelets.

PLATELETPHERESIS. A procedure utilizing a machine by which one can selectively remove platelets from a donor or patient.

POLYACRYLAMIDE GEL. A type of matrix used in electrophoresis upon which substances are separated.

POLYAGGLUTINATION. A state in which an individual's red cells are agglutinated by all sera regardless of blood type.

POLYBRENE. A polycation used to enhance antigen-antibody reactions because it promotes red cell aggregation, thus enhancing agglutination. Used to detect polyagglutination.

POLYCLONAL. Antibodies derived from more than one antibody-producing parent cell.

POLYCYTHEMIA VERA. A chronic life-shortening myeloproliferative disorder involving all bone marrow elements, characterized by an increase in red blood cell mass and hemoglobin concentration.

POLYMER. Combination of two or more molecules of the same substance.

POLYMORPHISM. A genetic system that possesses numerous allelic forms, such as a blood group system.

POLYSPECIFIC COOMBS' SERA. A reagent that contains antihuman globulin sera against IgG immunoglobulin and C3d.

POLYVINYLPYRROLIDONE (PVP). A neutral polymeric substance used to increase blood volume in patients with extensive blood loss. It is also used to enhance antigen-antibody reactions in vitro.

PORTAL HYPERTENSION. Increased pressure in the portal vein as a result of obstruction of the flow of blood through the liver.

POSTPARTUM. Occurring after childbirth.

POTENTIATOR. A substance that, when added to a serum and cell mixture, will enhance antigen-antibody interactions.

PRECIPITATION. The formation of a visible complex (precipitate) in a medium containing soluble antigen (precipitinogen) and the corresponding antibody (precipitin).

PRECIPITIN. An antibody formed in the blood serum of an animal by the presence of a soluble antigen, usually a protein. When added to a solution of the antigen, it brings about precipitation. The injected protein is called the antigen and the antibody produced is the precipitin.

PRECURSOR SUBSTANCE. A substance that is converted to another substance by the addition of a specific constituent (e.g., a sugar residue).

PRIVATE ANTIGEN. An antigenic characteristic of the red blood cell membrane that is unique to an individual or a related family of individuals and, therefore, not commonly found on all cells (usually less then 1 percent of the population).

PRODROME. A symptom indicative of an approaching disease.

PROPOSITUS. The initial individual whose condition led to investigation of a hereditary disorder or to a serologic evaluation of family members. Feminine form is proposita. Synonyms are proband and index case.

PROSTHESIS. An artificial substitute for a missing part, such as an artificial extremity.

PROTAMINE. A polycation with applications similar to Polybrene.

PROTAMINE SULFATE. A substance used to neutralize the effects of heparin.

PROTHROMBIN COMPLEX. A concentrate of coagulation factors II, VII, IX, and X in lyophilized form.

PROZONE. Incomplete lattice formation resulting from an excess of antibody molecules relative to the number of antigen sites. This results in false-negative reactions.

PRP. Platelet rich plasma.

PUBLIC ANTIGEN. An antigenic characteristic of the red blood cell membrane found commonly among individuals, usually greater than 98 percent of the population.

PULMONARY ARTERY WEDGE PRESSURE. Pressure measured in the pulmonary artery at its capillary end.

PULSE PRESSURE. The difference between the systolic and the diastolic pressures.

RADIOIMMUNOASSAY (RIA). A very sensitive method for determination of substances present in low concentrations in serum or plasma by using specific antibodies and radioactively labeled or tagged substances.

RAPID PASSIVE HEMAGGLUTINATION ASSAY (RPHA). A third generation procedure used in hepatitis testing.

RAPID PASSIVE LATEX ASSAY (**RPLA**). A second generation procedure used in hepatitis testing.

RAYNAUD'S DISEASE. A peripheral vascular disorder characterized by abnormal vasoconstriction of the extremities upon exposure to cold or emotional stress. A history of symptoms for at least 2 years is necessary for diagnosis.

RECESSIVE. A gene that, in the presence of its dominant allele, does not express itself. Expression of recessive genes occurs when they are inherited in the homozygous state.

RECIPIENT. Refers to a patient who is receiving a transfusion of blood or a blood product.

REFRACTORY. Obstinate, stubborn, resistant to ordinary treatment. Resistant to stimulation—said of a muscle or nerve.

RESPIRATORY DISTRESS SYNDROME (**RDS**). A condition, formerly known as hyaline membrane disease, accounting for more than 25,000 infant deaths per year in the United States. Clinical signs, including delayed onset of respiration and low Apgar score, are usually present at birth.

RETICULOCYTE. The last stage of development prior to a mature erythrocyte. The reticulocyte has lost its nucleus but retains some residual RNA in its cytoplasm, which is stainable by special techniques. It may be slightly larger than the mature red cell. Sometimes referred to as a neocyte.

RETICULOENDOTHELIAL SYSTEM (**RES**). A term applied to the fixed phagocytic cells of the body, such as the macrophage, having the ability to ingest particulate matter.

REVERSE GROUPING. Testing a patient's serum with commercial or reagent A and B red blood cells to determine which ABO antibodies are present.

Rh IMMUNE GLOBULIN (**RhIG**) (**RHOGAM**). A concentrated, purified anti-RH_0(D) prepared from human serum (of immunized donors), which is given to Rh_0(D) negative mothers after they have given birth to an Rh_0(D) positive baby or after abortion or miscarriage. It acts to prevent the mother from becoming immunized to any Rh_0(D) positive fetal cells that may have entered her circulation and thereby prevents formation of anti-Rh_0(D) by the mother.

RIBONUCLEIC ACID (**RNA**). A nucleic acid that controls protein synthesis in all living cells. There are three different types and all are derived from the information encoded in the DNA of the cell. Messenger RNA (mRNA) carries the code for specific amino acid sequences from the DNA to the cytoplasm for protein synthesis. Transfer RNA (tRNA) carries the amino acid groups to the ribosome for protein synthesis. Ribosomal RNA (rRNA) exists within the ribosomes and is thought to assist in protein synthesis.

RIBOSOME. A cellular organelle that contains ribonucleoprotein and functions to synthesize protein. Ribosomes may be single units or clusters called polyribosomes or polysomes.

Rickettsia. Term applied to any of the microorganisms belonging to the genus *Rickettsia*.

Ringer's lactated injection. An aqueous solution suitable for intravenous use.

Rouleaux. Coin-like stacking of red blood cells in the presence of plasma expanders or abnormal plasma proteins.

Saline anti-D. A low protein (6 to 8 percent albumin) IgM anti-D reagent.

Salvia horminum. Plant lectin used in the differentiation of various forms of polyagglutination.

Salvia sclarea. Plant lectin with anti-Tn activity, which is used in the differentiation of different forms of polyagglutination.

Screening cells. Group O reagent red cells that are used in antibody detection or screening tests.

SD. Serologically defined antigens.

Secretor. An individual who is capable of secreting soluble, glycoprotein ABH soluble substances into saliva and other body fluids.

Sensitization. A condition of being made sensitive to a specific substance (e.g., an antigen) after the initial exposure to that substance. This results in the development of immunologic memory that evokes an accentuated immune response with subsequent exposure to the substance.

Sepsis. Pathologic state, usually febrile, resulting from the presence of microorganisms or their poisonous products in the blood stream.

Septicemia. Presence of pathogenic bacteria in the blood.

Serologic test for syphilis (STS). First developed in 1906 by Wasserman, present tests are of three main types based on complement fixation, flocculation, and detection of specific antitreponemal antibodies.

Serotonin. A chemical present in platelets that is a potent vasoconstrictor.

Serum. The fluid that remains after plasma has clotted.

Sex chromosome. Chromosomes associated with determination of sex.

Sex linkage. A genetic characteristic located on the X or Y chromosome.

Shelf-life. The amount of time blood or blood products may be stored upon collection.

Shock. A clinical syndrome in which the peripheral blood flow is inadequate to return sufficient blood to the heart for normal function, particularly transport of oxygen to all organs and tissues. Shock may be caused by a variety of conditions including hemorrhage, infection, drug reaction, trauma, poisoning, myocardial infarction, or dehydration. Symptoms include paleness of skin (pallor), a bluish-gray discoloration (cyanosis), a weak and rapid pulse, rapid and shallow breathing, or blood pressure that is decreased and perhaps unobtainable.

SIALIC ACID. A group of sugars found on the red cell membrane attached to a protein backbone. They are the major source of the membrane net negative charge.

SICKLE TRAIT. Blood that is heterozygous for the gene coding for the abnormal hemoglobin of sickle cell anemia.

SIDEROSIS. A form of pneumoconiosis resulting from inhalation of dust or fumes containing iron particles.

SINGLE DONOR PLATELETS. Platelets collected from a single donor by apheresis.

SODIUM DODECYL SULFATE (SDS). An anionic detergent that renders a net negative charge to substances it solubilizes.

SPECIFICITY. Refers to the affinity of an antibody and the antigen against which it is directed.

SPLENOMEGALY. Enlargement of the spleen.

STEATORRHEA. Increased secretion of the sebaceous glands.

STEROID HORMONES. Hormones of the adrenal cortex and the sex hormones.

STERTOROUS. Pertaining to laborious breathing.

STORAGE LESION. A loss of viability and function associated with certain biochemical changes that are initiated when blood is stored in vitro.

STROMA. The red cell membrane that is left after hemolysis has occurred.

SUBGROUP. Antigens within the ABO group that react less strongly with their corresponding antisera than do A and B antigens.

SURVIVAL STUDIES. A measure of the in-vivo survival of transfused blood cells. Usually performed with radioactive isotopes. Normal red cells survive approximately 100 to 120 days in circulation.

SYNGENEIC. Possessing identical genotypes as monozygotic twins.

SYNTENY. Genes that are closely situated on a chromosome but cannot be shown to be linked.

SYSTEMIC LUPUS ERYTHEMATOSUS (SLE). A disseminated autoimmune disease characterized by anemia, thrombocytopenia, increased IgG levels, and the presence of four IgG antibodies: antinuclear antibody, antinucleoprotein antibody, anti-DNA antibody, and antihistone antibody. Believed to be caused by "suppressor" T cell dysfunction.

SYSTOLIC PRESSURE. Maximum blood pressure that occurs at ventricular contraction. The upper value of a blood pressure reading.

TACHYCARDIA. Abnormal rapidity of heart action, usually defined as a heart rate over 100 beats per minute.

TACHYPNEA. Abnormal rapidity of respiration.

TEMPLATE BLEEDING TIME. The elapsed time a uniform incision made by a template and blade stops bleeding is a test of platelet function assuming a normal platelet count.

TETANY. A nervous affection characterized by intermittent spasms of the muscles of the extremities.

THALASSEMIA MAJOR. The homozygous form of deficient beta chain synthesis, which is very severe and presents itself during childhood. Prognosis varies; however, the younger the child when the disease appears, the more unfavorable the outcome.

THERMAL AMPLITUDE. The range of temperature over which an antibody demonstrates serologic and/or in-vitro activity.

THROMBIN. An enzyme that converts fibrinogen to fibrin so that a soluble clot can be formed.

THROMBOCYTOPENIA. A reduction in the platelet count below the normal level. Decreased platelet counts are associated with spontaneous hemorrhage.

THROMBOTIC THROMBOCYTOPENIC PURPURA (TTP). A coagulation disorder characterized by (1) increased bleeding owing to a decreased number of platelets, (2) hemolytic anemia, (3) renal failure, and (4) changing neurologic signs. The characteristic morphologic lesion is thrombotic occlusion of small arteries or capillaries in various organs.

THYMIDINE. An essential ingredient used in DNA synthesis and incorporated by T-lymphocytes undergoing blast transformation in response to foreign HLA-D antigens in the mixed lymphocyte culture test.

TITER. A measure of the strength of an antibody by testing its reactivity at increasing dilutions against the appropriate antigen.

TITER SCORE. A method used to evaluate more precisely than simple dilution by comparing the titers of an antibody. Agglutination at each higher dilution is graded on a continuous scale; the total is the titer score.

TRAIT. A characteristic that is inherited.

TRANSCRIPTION. The process of RNA production from DNA, which requires the enzyme RNA polymerase.

TRANSFERASE. An enzyme that catalyzes the transfer of atoms or groups of atoms from one chemical compound to another.

TRANSFUSE. The act of performing a transfusion.

TRANSFUSION. The injection of blood, a blood component, saline, or other fluids into the bloodstream. CADAVER BLOOD T. Using blood obtained from a cadaver within a short time after death. DIRECT T. Transfer of blood directly from one person to another. EXCHANGE T. Transfusion and withdrawal of small amounts of blood repeated until blood volume is almost entirely exchanged; used in infants born with hemolytic disease. INDIRECT T. Transfusion of blood from a donor to a suitable storage container and then to a patient. INTRAUTERINE T. Transfusion of blood into a fetus in utero.

TRANSFUSION REACTION. An adverse response to a transfusion.

TRANSLATION. The production of protein from the interactions of the RNAs.

TRANSLOCATION. Transfer of a portion of one chromosome to its allele.

TRANSPOSITION. The location of two genes on opposite chromosomes of a homologous pair.

TRYPSIN. A proteolytic enzyme formed in the intestine.

TYPE AND SCREEN. Testing a patient's blood for ABO group, Rh type, and atypical antibodies. The sample is then retained in the event that subsequent crossmatching is necessary.

ULEX EUROPAEUS. See Anti-H lectin.

ULTRACENTRIFUGATION. Rapid and prolonged centrifugation used to separate by density gradients substances of various specific gravities.

URTICARIA. A vascular reaction of the skin similar to hives.

VACCINE. A suspension of infectious organisms or components of them that is given as a form of passive immunization to establish resistance to the infectious disease caused by that organism.

VALVULAR. Relating to or having a valve.

VARIABLE REGION. That portion of the immunoglobulin light and heavy chains where amino acid sequences vary tremendously. These amino acid variations permit the different immunoglobulin molecules to recognize different antigenic determinants. In other words, the variable region determines the antigen against which the antibody will react, thus providing each antibody molecule with its unique specificity. The variable region is located at the amino terminal region of the molecule.

VASCULITIS. Inflammation of a blood or lymph vessel.

VASOCONSTRICTION. Constriction of the blood vessels.

VASODILATATION. Dilatation of blood vessels, especially small arteries and arterioles.

VASOVAGAL SYNCOPE. Syncope resulting from hypotension caused by emotional stress, pain, acute blood loss, fear, or rapid rising from a recumbent position.

VENESECTION. See Phlebotomy.

VENIPUNCTURE. Puncture of a vein for any purpose.

VENULE. A tiny vein continuous with a capillary.

VIABILITY. Ability of a cell to live or survive for a reasonably normal life span.

VICIA GRAMINEA. See Anti-N lectin.

VIRION. A complete virus particle; a unit of genetic material surrounded by a protective coat that serves as a vehicle for its transmission from one cell to another.

VON WILLEBRAND'S DISEASE. A congenital bleeding disorder.

VON WILLEBRAND'S FACTOR. Factor VIII.

WAIHA. Warm autoimmune hemolytic anemia.

WHARTON'S JELLY. A gelatinous intercellular substance consisting of primitive connective tissue of the umbilical cord.

X CHROMOSOME. The chromosome that determines female sex characteristics. The normal female has two X chromosomes and the normal male has an X and Y chromosome.

XENO-. Prefix indicating differing species. For example, a xenoantibody is an antibody produced in one species against an antigen present in another species. Synonym is hetero-.

YAWS. An infectious nonvenereal disease caused by a spirochete, *Treponema pertenue*, found mainly in humid, equatorial regions.

ZETA POTENTIAL. The difference in charge density between the inner and outer layers of the ionic cloud that surrounds red cells in an electrolyte solution.

INDEX

Italics indicate a figure.
A *t* indicates a table.

complex problems in, 276–280, *277,*
278, 279
enzyme pretreatment and, 281
high-frequency antibodies in, 276, *279*
inconclusive, resolution of, 280–282
increased serum: cell ratio in, 281
incubation in, 281
multiple antibodies in, 276, *278*
neutralization in, 281–282
one-stage enzyme technique in, 281
panel in, 273–276, *274, 275, 277, 278,*
279
phenotyping and, 280
profile of screening cells in, *273*
rare cells in, 281
reference laboratories and, 282
serum acidification in, 281
two-stage enzyme technique in, 281
maternal, fetal red blood cells and, 78–79
testing for. *See* Alloantibody, identification of.
Alloantigens, 59
Allotypes, immunoglobulin, 67
Alpha-methyldopa, red cell sensitization reactions and, 82
A$_m$ allotypes, 67
Amberlite IR-45 anion-exchange resin, 17
Amniocentesis, hemolytic disease of the
newborn and, 406, *407, 408*
Anaerobic glycolytic pathway, 3–4
Anaphylactic reactions
causes of, 370
investigation of, 370–371
treatment of, 370
Anemia
autoimmune hemolytic. *See* Autoimmune hemolytic anemia.
chronic compensated, McLeod phenotype and, 190
hemolytic disease of the newborn and,
405
hydrops fetalis in, 405
late, 405
sickle cell. *See* Sickle cell anemia.
transfusion in
assessment of need for, 330–331
effect of, 331
monitoring, 331
product selection and, 331
Anti-A$_1$, sources of, 97
Anti-A,B
ABO antigens and, 93
activity of, 92–93
Antibodies. *See also specific antibodies;* Al-

loantibodies; Autoantibodies; Immunoglobulins.
allotypes and, 67
antigen-combining sites and, excess, 72–
73
clinical significance of, 77–79
cold reacting, 92
compatibility testing and, 249, 251–253.
See also Compatibility testing.
complete, definition of, 69–70
detection of. *See* Antiglobulin test.
donor blood screening for, 228–229
high-frequency, identification of, 276, *279*
high-titered low-avidity, HLA related
systems and, 209t
idiotype of, 63–64
incomplete, definition of, 69–70
laboratory detection of, 78–79
monoclonal, definition of, 62–63
mononuclear phagocyte assay and, 79
multiple, identification of, 276, *278*
naturally occurring, 91, 92
Anticoagulants. *See also specific anticoagu-*
lants.
apheresis and, 357–358
exchange transfusion and, 413
oral, bleeding disorders and, 342
whole blood collection and, 223
Anticomplement
hybridoma technology and, 296
immune hemolytic anemia and, 84
uses of, 84
Antigenic determinant, definition of, 61
Antigens. *See also specific antigens and*
blood group systems.
characteristics of, 60–61
classification of, 59
high-incidence, miscellaneous, 210t
red blood cell structure and, 61
structure of, 60–61
T, 110–111
tissue distribution of, 61
Antiglobulin serum
broad-spectrum, 83, 85
fluorescein dye and, 85
monospecific, 83–84
production of, 83
Antiglobulin test
anticomplement and, 84
applications of, 82
control for, 86–87
direct
applications of, 82, 85
autoimmune hemolytic anemia and, 424

MODERN BLOOD BANKING AND TRANSFUSION PRACTICES

MODERN BLOOD BANKING AND TRANSFUSION PRACTICES

MODERN BLOOD BANKING AND TRANSFUSION PRACTICES

Phlebotomy
  donor care after, 225. *See also* Donor re-
    actions.
  donor care before, 222–223, 223t
  hematomas and, 227–228
  procedure for, 224–225
Phototherapy, hemolytic disease of the
  newborn and, 409
PIPA solution, 13
Plant lectin, polyagglutination and, 463,
  464–465, 467–468
Plasma
  anaphylactic reactions and, 371
  apheresis and. *See* Plasma exchange.
  bacteria and, 368
  compatibility test and, 258
  exchange of. *See* Plasma exchange.
  federal regulations and, 303–305, 304t,
    309
  fresh-frozen
    coumadin overdosage and, 342
    disseminated intravascular coagulation
      and, 343
    hemophilia and, 335
    liver disease and, 344
    plasma exchange with, 357
    single donor, 238–239
    von Willebrand's disease and, 338
  reagent production and, 357
  single donor, 238–240
Plasma exchange
  autoimmune condition and, 356
  fresh-frozen plasma in, 357
  indications for, 356–357
  solution selection in, 356–357
  therapeutic application of, 357
Plasma expanders, rouleaux and, 110
Plasma protein fraction, fluid replacement
  with, 325–326
Platelet. *See also* Platelet concentrates.
  federal regulations and, 301–302, 309
  hemostatic functions of, 331
  liver disease and, 344
  metabolism of, 10–12
  preservation of
    agitation in, 12
    concentration in, 12
    container material in, 11–12
    factors in, 11
    history of, 10–11
    oxygen in, 11–12
    pH in, 11
    temperature in, 11

  time limits on, 11
  random donor. *See* Platelet concentrates.
  transfusion with
    assessment of, 334
    HLA system and, 482
    indications for, 331–332
    platelet increment and, 334
    prophylactic, 332
    thrombocytopenia and, 333–334
Platelet concentrates. *See also* Platelets.
  anaphylactic reactions and, 371
  bacteria and, 368
  disseminated intravascular coagulation
    and, 343
  plasma volume of, 12
  preparation of, 11, 237–238
  quality control and, 238
  uses of, 237
Platelet increment, 334
Plateletpheresis
  indications for, 354
  procedure in, 354
  side effects in, 354
  stem cells and, 353
  therapeutic application of, 355
Pneumonia, atypical, anti-I and, 183
Polyagglutination
  ABO discrepancy in, 461, 461t
  categories of, 460
  causes of, 460
  disease states and, 462
  history of, 459–460
  infection and, 110–111
  laboratory recognition of, 462–465, 463t,
    464t, 467–468
    ABO testing in, 461t, 462
    autologous control in, 463
    enzyme treatment in, 463–464
    Glycine soja in, 463, 467, 468
    papain in, 463–464
    plant lectins in, 463, 464–465, 467–468
    Polybrene in, 463, 467, 468
    sialic acid levels in, 463, 467, 468
  Rh typing in, 461–462
  T antigen and, 110–111
  transfusion and, 462
Polybrene
  agglutination and, 71
  polyagglutination and, 463, 467, 468
Polycythemia, therapeutic phlebotomy
  and, 355–356
Polyvinylpyrrolidone (PVP)
  agglutination and, 71

Red blood cells—*continued.*
   rouleaux and, 69
   stages of, 68
   antibody-mediated destruction of, 76, 76, 78–79
   buffy-poor, 233–235
   concentrated, 232–233
   drug-induced sensitization of. *See also specific drugs.*
      autoantibody formation in, 455
      drug adsorption mechanism in, 450–454, *452,* 453t
      immune complex mechanism in, 448–450, *448,* 449t, 451t, 457
      membrane modification in, 454, *454*
      penicillin in, 450–454, 457–458
      suspicion of, 447–448
   federal regulations and, 301, 307–308, 309
   freezing of, 14–15, 235–236, 413
   lesion of storage and, 3
   leukocyte-poor, 233–235
   metabolism of
      chemical modifiers of, 12–13
      pathways of, 3–6, *5*
   packed
      transfusion with, 326–327
      viscosity of, 327
   phagocytes and, 77
   polyagglutination of. *See* Polyagglutination.
   preservative and, 9–10
   reagent, quality control and, 294–295
   sialic acid-deficient, 137
   structure of, antigens in, 61
   substitute for
      perfluorochemicals as, 16
      stroma-free hemoglobin solution as, 15–16
   survival time of, 3, *4*
   transfusion with
      anaphylactic reactions and, 371
      anemia and, 331
      neocytapheresis and, 355
      product choice and, 326–327
   viability of
      adenosine triphosphate in, 3, 4, *4*
      container material in, 10
      freezing in, 14–15
      glucose utilization in, 10
      lesion of storage in, 3
      metabolism and, 3–6
      rejuvenation solutions in, 13

   resin system in, 16–17
   SAG system in, 13
   solid buffers in, 16–17
   young, transfusion of, 355
Red blood cell autoantibodies
   anti-I, 429–431, 432
   anti-i, 429–431
   anti-IH, 431
   anti-H, 431
   autoimmune hemolytic anemia and, 424, 425
   cold reactive
      autoabsorption technique and, 443
      benign, 425–431. *See also* Autoagglutinins, cold, benign.
      pathologic, 432–434. *See also* Autoagglutinins, cold, pathologic.
   drug-induced, 455
   mechanism of, 423–424
   unaffected individuals with, 424–425
   warm reactive
      autoabsorption technique and, 444–445
      laboratory testing and
         ABO grouping, 435
         alloantibody detection in, 438–439, 439t, 440t, 444–445
         blood selection and, 439–440
         direct antiglobulin, 436
         Rh grouping, 435–436
         specificity in, 436–438, 437t, 438t, 444
   serology of, 434, 434t
Regulations. *See also* Quality control.
   agencies and, 284–287
   federal
      antihemophilic factor and, 302–303
      blood bank checklist and, 312–322
      cryoprecipitate and, 302–303
      distribution and, 305
      equipment and, 298, 299t
      inspection of blood and, 305–306
      instruction circular and, general information in, 308–309
      labeling and
         antibodies in, 307
         anticoagulants in, 307
         autologous infusion in, 308
         general information in, 306–307
         incomplete tests in, 308
         nontransfusion, 308
         recovered plasma in, 308
         red blood cells and, 307–308

Wharton's jelly, rouleaux and, 110
White blood cells, transfusion of. *See* Leukapheresis.
Whole blood
  collection of. *See* Collection, whole blood.
  donor selection for. *See* Donor selection, whole blood.
  federal regulations and, 298–300, 307–308, 309
  transfusion with
    product choice and, 326–327
    thrombocytopenia and, 333

Wr^a and Wr^b antigens, 206
Wright system, 206

XENOANTIBODIES, 59
Xenoantigens, 59
Xg^a antigen, 206

Yk^a ANTIGENS, 209t
York blood group system, 209t
Yt^a and Yt^b antigens, 206–207

ZETA POTENTIAL, 70–71

MODERN BLOOD BANKING AND TRANSFUSION PRACTICES